Pediatric Nursing
An Introductory Text

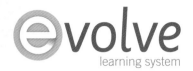
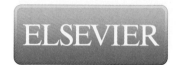
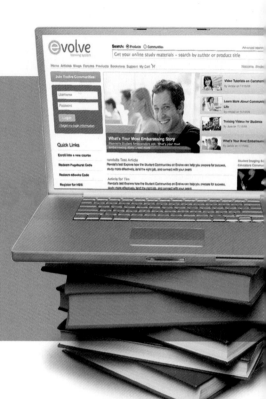

Pediatric Nursing

An Introductory Text

Debra L. Price, MSN, RN, CPNP
Assistant Professor of Nursing
Tarrant County College
Fort Worth, Texas

Julie F. Gwin, MN, RN
Associate Professor of Nursing
Tarrant County College
Fort Worth, Texas

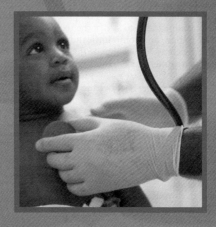

11th Edition

ELSEVIER

3251 Riverport Lane
St. Louis, Missouri 63043

PEDIATRIC NURSING: AN INTRODUCTORY TEXT   ISBN: 978-1-4377-1709-9

Copyright © 2012, 2008, 2005, 2001, 1997, 1992, 1987, 1981, 1976, 1970, 1965 by Saunders, an imprint of Elsevier Inc.

Notices

Knowledge and best practice in this field are constantly changing. As new research and experience broaden our understanding, changes in research methods, professional practices, or medical treatment may become necessary.

Practitioners and researchers must always rely on their own experience and knowledge in evaluating and using any information, methods, compounds, or experiments described herein. In using such information or methods they should be mindful of their own safety and the safety of others, including parties for whom they have a professional responsibility.

With respect to any drug or pharmaceutical products identified, readers are advised to check the most current information provided (i) on procedures featured or (ii) by the manufacturer of each product to be administered, to verify the recommended dose or formula, the method and duration of administration, and contraindications. It is the responsibility of practitioners, relying on their own experience and knowledge of their patients, to make diagnoses, to determine dosages and the best treatment for each individual patient, and to take all appropriate safety precautions.

To the fullest extent of the law, neither the Publisher nor the authors, contributors, or editors, assume any liability for any injury and/or damage to persons or property as a matter of products liability, negligence or otherwise, or from any use or operation of any methods, products, instructions, or ideas contained in the material herein.

Library of Congress Cataloging-in-Publication Data

Price, Debra L.
  Pediatric nursing : an introductory text / Debra L. Price, Julie F. Gwin.—11th ed.
    p. ; cm.
  Includes bibliographical references and index.
  ISBN 978-1-4377-1709-9 (pbk. : alk. paper)   1. Pediatric nursing.   I. Gwin, Julie F.   II. Title.
  [DNLM: 1. Pediatric Nursing—methods. WY 159]
  RJ245.T475 2012
  618.92′00231—dc23

                                      2011024880

Acquisitions Editor: Teri Hines Burnham
Associate Developmental Editor: Heather Rippetoe
Publishing Services Manager: Jeff Patterson
Senior Project Manager: Clay S. Broeker
Design Direction: Karen Pauls

Printed in China

Last digit is the print number: 9 8 7 6 5 4 3

For my three beautiful granddaughters

Natalie, you are your great-grandmother Price's angel and our first;
Addison, you are our second little angel whose smile lights up the room; and
Lauren, you are your mother's daughter and our third little angel.

You are all the light of my life and I love you!

And of course to my husband Jeff
whose dedication as a spouse is unsurpassed.

Debra L. Price

For my three boys and their new families

Aaron and Erin, and our first wonderful grandson Austin;
Adam and April, and our second sweet grandson Carter; and
Alex and the girl in his life—Lily, the pound puppy.

I am so proud of the young men and fathers you have become.
And I am so thankful for the honor of being a grandmother to your children.

And to my husband John
who has accompanied me on this journey with his support.

Julie F. Gwin

Reviewers

Janice Ankenmann-Hill, RN, MSN, CCRN, FNP-C
Professor
Napa Valley College
Napa, California

Maryanne Barra, DNP, FNP-L, RN
Faculty
Union County College
Plainfield, New Jersey

Emily Cannon, RN, MSN
Associate Professor
Ivy Tech Community College
Infection Control Practitioner
Union Hospital
Terre Haute, Indiana

Michele Cislo, RN, MA
Associate Professor
Practical Nursing Department
Union County College
Plainfield, New Jersey

Pamela Cleveland, RN, MSN, FNP
ADN Faculty
Program Chair
South Texas College
McAllen, Texas

Belinda Douglas, MSN, PMHNP-BC, GNP-BC
Four Rivers Nursing Director
Tennessee Technology Center
Ripley, Tennessee

Marian Theresa Doyle, MSN, MS
Associate Professor of Nursing
Northampton Community College
Bethlehem, Pennsylvania

Pat Floro, RN
Faculty
Nancy J Knight School of Nursing
Bellefontaine, Ohio

Kristine M. Gill, RN, PhD
Associate Professor Emeritus, College of Nursing
The University of Akron
Member, Summit County Board of Health
Consultant, Akron Children's Hospital
Consultant, Cleveland Clinic
Faculty, Northcoast Medical Training Academy
Akron, Ohio

Jeanne Hately, MSN, RN, PLNC
Regional Nursing Director
Nursing Program Research and Development
Corinthian Colleges, Inc.
Aurora, Colorado

Nancy Humphries, RN, BSN
Faculty
Georgia Northwestern Technical College
Rome, Georgia

T. Camille Lindsey Killough, RN, BSN
Instructor Nursing Department
Pearl River Community College
Hattiesburg, Mississippi

Teresa McNabb, RN
Faculty
South Plains College
Levelland, Texas

Laurie Peyronel, MA, MSN, RN
Instructor of Practical Nursing
Mercyhurst Northeast
Northeast, Pennsylvania

Trena Rich, RN, MSN, APRN, CIC
Director Quality Assurance, Patient Care Center
Western University of Health Sciences
Pomona, California

Allison St. Clair, RN, MSN
Coordinator
Summers County School of Pediatric Nursing
Hinton, West Virginia

Elise J. Webb, RN, MSN
CE Health Program Coordinator
Wilson Community College
Wilson, North Carolina

To the Instructor

Pediatric Nursing: An Introductory Text, **11th edition**, has been updated and revised to provide the novice pediatric nursing student with the fundamental knowledge needed to practice in a pediatric setting. We have retained many of the book's strengths, including its easy-to-read, clear writing style and the nursing interventions focus.

ORGANIZATION

Newly organized by systems, the book covers pediatric nursing from infant to adolescent (in individual chapters) and also contains a separate chapter on end-of-life care for children and their families. Each chapter begins with **Objectives** and then lists **Key Terms** (with phonetic pronunciations for many terms) and their page reference numbers. Key Terms are in color at first mention and are defined in the **Glossary**. At the end of every chapter, **Key Points** of the chapter are briefly summarized and students will have the opportunity to test what they've learned with additional **NCLEX® Examination Review Questions**.

A perforated **Study Guide** at the end of this book may be used for review or as an assignment to be turned in by students. Included are matching exercises, multiple-choice questions, more Study Questions, new Community Search activities, Case Studies with Critical Thinking Questions, and Internet Activities for each chapter. Guidelines to the Case Studies are provided in the TEACH Instructor Resources.

CRITICAL CONTENT

Community-based care and care of the family are given special emphasis throughout. *Healthy People 2010* **Objectives** form the basis for health promotion and are integrated into the text to provide a basis for student study.

End-of-life care is addressed in a separate chapter that includes recommendations by Last Acts, the National Task Force on Palliative Care. Topics include both psychosocial and physiologic issues in providing nursing care for the terminally ill child. **Pain content** reflects current views on pediatric pain assessment and therapy. **Complementary and alternative therapies** are located throughout the text. **Cultural content** is found in Chapter 2, and more coverage on cultural influences and diversity in pediatric care has been added to this edition.

NEW TO THIS EDITION

The new 11th edition has an abundance of expanded content, including **evidence-based nursing**, cultural influences, and more nutrition information, as well as the following new features:

- **Content Reorganization.** A systems approach along with developmental chapters from newborn to adolescence help students understand basic growth and development in a logical sequence as the foundation for information about specific disorders commonly seen in children. Several new topics have been included, such as Kawasaki disease, near-drowning, and colic.
- **Critical Thinking Snapshots**. Several Critical Thinking Snapshots have been added to enhance students' clinical reasoning.
- **Safety Alerts** highlight 2010/2011 Joint Commission National Patient Safety Goals, with special consideration for serious and potentially fatal medication errors.
- **Global Perspectives** enlighten the reader on health issues impacting various part of the world.
- **Icons** in the **Nursing Skills** features reinforce common practices for all nurses before performing skills. The **margin icons** will direct students to animations and videos on Evolve that reinforce the content of the text. Rationales have been provided for the steps of the procedures.

LEARNING AIDS

The following learning aids are designed to guide and instruct:

- **Nursing Care Plans** with **Critical Thinking Questions** reinforce the nursing process as applied to pediatric disorders. Answers to the **Critical Thinking Questions** are provided in the Instructor Resources. Several Nursing Care Plans include **Critical Thinking Snapshots**, which give brief scenarios for students to evaluate.
- **Skills** teach basic techniques used in pediatric nursing settings.
- **Nursing Briefs** stress important content-related points.
- **Communication** boxes identify key tips to establish successful nurse-patient-family communication.
- **Community Considerations** address home care and community-based care issues.

- **Did You Know?** boxes list assessment data to cue the nurse to recognize possible pediatric disorders.
- **Health Promotion** boxes are found throughout the book, accentuating wellness and disease prevention in light of *Healthy People 2010* objectives
- **Home Care Considerations** are located throughout the book. Strategies are provided to help families and caregivers understand how to minister to their child's ongoing needs.
- **The Joint Commission Lists of Dangerous Abbreviations, Acronyms, and Symbols** provide guidelines for the prevention of medication administration errors, especially serious in pediatric dosages.
- **Internet Activities**, found in the **Study Guide,** provide students with the opportunity to practice online research on content-related topics.
- **Online Resources** included in the Bibliography section direct students to current websites related to chapter content.

ANCILLARIES

FOR THE INSTRUCTOR

Supplemental teaching aids include the Evolve Learning Resources website.

EVOLVE LEARNING RESOURCES WEBSITE

- Open-Book Quizzes, Answers to the Study Guide with Guidelines for Internet Activities and Case Studies, guidelines for the Critical Thinking Questions and Snapshots in the Nursing Care Plans, and Suggestions for Working with English as a Second Language Students.
- A **PowerPoint presentation** of text and image slides has been expanded substantially from the previous edition with new Audience Response Questions incorporated.
- An **Image Collection** includes all the illustrations and photographs from the textbook.

- A **Test Bank** of approximately 700 NCLEX® Examination multiple-choice and alternate-item format questions includes the following categories: Correct Answer, Rationale, Topic, Nursing Process Step, Objective, Cognitive Level, NCLEX® Category of Client Needs, and Text Page Reference.
- Fully revised for the 11th edition, the **TEACH Lesson Plans** are based on the learning objectives for each chapter in the book, providing a roadmap to link and integrate all parts of the educational package.
- An Online Course Management System is also provided.

FOR THE STUDENT

EVOLVE LEARNING RESOURCES WEBSITE

- Over 90 **Video Assessments** of newborns, infants, toddlers, and children offer a unique opportunity for students to combine visual and textbook information as they apply what they have learned.
- **3-D Animations** of neonatal procedures and physiology allow students to see procedures and difficult anatomy and physiology clearly, colorfully, and accurately portrayed for better comprehension.
- A **Glossary of Audio Pronunciations** of commonly used terms includes all Key Terms and more to help students learn and apply difficult terminology.
- **Answers with rationales** for the NCLEX® Examination Review Questions are provided.

Our knowledge and extensive experience in pediatrics have guided us in the development of this new edition. It is our hope that students will find the information clearly presented and easily understood. As reflected in our writing, we aspire to show our love of pediatrics, the children involved, their families, and the nurses who choose to pursue pediatric nursing.

DEBRA L. PRICE
JULIE F. GWIN

Advisory Board

To the Student

READING AND REVIEW TOOLS

Objectives introduce the chapter topics.

Key Terms are listed with page number references, and difficult medical, nursing, or scientific terms are accompanied by simple phonetic pronunciations. Key terms are considered essential to understanding chapter content and are defined within the chapter. Key terms are in color the first time they appear in the narrative and are briefly defined in the text, with complete definitions in the Glossary.

Each chapter ends with a *Get Ready for the NCLEX® Examination!* **section** that includes (1) **Key Points** that reiterate the chapter objectives and serve as a useful review of concepts, (2) a list of **Additional Resources**, and (3) an extensive set of **Review Questions for the NCLEX® Examination,** with answers located in Appendix H.

A complete **Bibliography** in the back of the text cites evidence-based information and provides resources for enhancing knowledge.

CHAPTER FEATURES

Skills are presented in a logical format with defined *purpose,* relevant *illustrations,* and clearly defined and numbered nursing *steps.* Each Skill includes icons that serve as reminders to perform the basic steps applicable to *all* nursing interventions:

 Check orders.

 Gather necessary equipment and supplies.

 Introduce yourself.

 Check patient's identification.

 Provide privacy.

 Explain the procedure/intervention.

 Perform hand hygiene.

 Don gloves (if applicable).

Not listing the exact supplies or equipment needed encourages you to think critically about what you might need to do or gather according to hospital protocol prior to performing the specific Skill.

 Nursing Care Plans, developed around specific case studies, include nursing diagnoses with an emphasis on patient goals and outcomes and questions to promote **critical thinking.** Four types of sample care plans are presented as valuable tools that can be used as a guideline in the clinical setting. The critical thinking aspect empowers you to develop sound clinical decision-making skills.

 Nursing Brief boxes highlight pertinent information applicable in the clinical setting.

 Did You Know? boxes list assessment data to prompt the nurse to recognize possible pediatric disorders.

 Safety Alert boxes emphasize the importance of maintaining safety in patient care to protect patients, family, health care providers, and the public from accidents and the spread of disease.

 Health Promotion boxes emphasize a healthy lifestyle, preventive behaviors, and screening tests to assist in the prevention of accidents and illness.

 Cultural Considerations boxes explore select specific cultural preferences and how to address the needs of a culturally diverse patient and family when planning nursing care and teaching.

 Global Perspectives boxes discuss the issues facing patients and caregivers on a global scale.

 Communication boxes focus on communication strategies with real-life examples of nurse-patient dialogue.

 Home Care Considerations boxes discuss the issues facing patients and caregivers in the home setting.

 Community Considerations boxes address home care and community-based care issues.

Acknowledgments

To Johanna Rosser, whose expertise in neonatal intensive care was invaluable in providing updated information. To the Child Life Organization who assisted with new approaches in pediatric care. To Cook Childrens Medical Center for sharing clinical pathway information.

And finally, to Julie Gwin, my dear friend and teaching partner, with whom I so often collaborate and also share a love of pediatrics.

DEBRA L. PRICE

I would especially like to express my appreciation to all the nurses at Cook Children's Medical Center, who assist me in providing a positive learning environment for my students. Also to my family and friends who helped by providing encouragement during the writing of this book.

And lastly, to Debbie Price, my friend and co-editor, who provides me with the support needed in my teaching position and in the writing of this book.

JULIE F. GWIN

Contents

Child Health Evolution

Objectives

1. Define the vocabulary terms listed
2. List government programs that have affected the care of children
3. Contrast present-day causes of morbidity and mortality with those of the past
4. Discuss current health care trends in pediatrics and the effect they have on nursing care
5. Identify the role of the pediatric nurse
6. Discuss critical thinking as it relates to the nursing process
7. Describe the philosophy of evidence-based practice
8. Discuss legal implications for the pediatric nurse

Key Terms

anticipatory guidance (ăn-TĬS-ĭ-pa-TŌR-ē; p. 5)
critical thinking (p. 5)
emancipated minor (e-MĂN-sĭ-pāt-ed; p. 6)
evidence-based practice (p. 5)
Healthy People 2010 (p. 2)
HIPAA (Health Insurance Portability and Accountability Act (p. 6)
holistic (p. 1)

infant mortality rate (mŏr-TĂL-ĭ-tē; p. 2)
informed consent (p. 6)
mature minor doctrine (p. 6)
morbidity (mŏr-BĬD-ĭ-tē; p. 4)
Nursing Interventions Classification (NIC) (p. 5)
Nursing Outcomes Classification (NOC) (p. 5)
pediatrics (pē-dē-ĂT-rĭks; p. 1)

EVOLUTION OF CHILD HEALTH

Pediatrics is the branch of medicine that deals specifically with children, their development, childhood diseases, and the treatment of such diseases. The word *pediatrics* is derived from the Greek *pais/paisos*, meaning "child," and *iatreia*, meaning "cure." The study of pediatrics began under the influence of Abraham Jacobi (1830-1919), a Prussian-born physician. Known today as the Father of Pediatrics, Jacobi paved the way for the promotion of children's health through the establishment of "milk stations," where mothers could bring sick children for treatment and learn the importance of pure milk and its proper preparation. The emergence of pediatric nursing as a specialty paralleled the establishment of pediatric departments in medical schools, the founding of children's hospitals, and the development of separate units for children in general hospitals.

The nursing care of children has evolved dramatically over the past 100 years. From its initial connection with the specialty of pediatric medicine, it has evolved into a holistic approach for providing health care to children and families. Pediatric nursing views children as having a physical, intellectual, emotional, and spiritual nature and as having needs that differ according to developmental level. In the early part of the twentieth century, the nursing of children was primarily focused on illness. Children frequently became ill and died during epidemics of communicable diseases such as measles and polio. With improved sanitation, the advent of antimicrobials, and the institution of preventive measures such as immunizations and improved prenatal care, children no longer encounter the obstacles that prevented them from reaching adulthood. As the organic causes of death and disability have declined, pediatric nursing has become focused on improving the quality of care by providing an environment for optimal growth and development, as well as health promotion, health maintenance, and health restoration. Over the years, many advances have been made in medical and surgical techniques, giving rise to medical and nursing subspecialties within the area of pediatrics. For example, children with heart problems are treated by a pediatric cardiologist and cared for by pediatric cardiology nurse specialists. The complex surgery necessary for the newborn infant with a congenital defect is provided by the pediatric surgeon. Equipment to diagnose and treat illness in infants and children has become more sophisticated

1

and specialized. Chromosomal studies and biochemical screening have made identification and family counseling more significant than ever. Acutely ill children are being cared for in special diagnostic and treatment facilities, where they receive expert attention. Many conditions that were once treated in inpatient settings are now treated in clinics, same-day surgery units, and other ambulatory settings.

GOVERNMENT PROGRAMS

In the past 40 or more years, several federal programs have positively affected child health care. In 1965, Medicaid and the Children and Youth Project were formed to provide care for children in low-income and inaccessible areas. The Child Nutrition Act (1966) provides meals, either free or at a reduced rate, for low-income children. The Special Supplemental Food Program for Women, Infants, and Children (WIC) was established in 1972. This program serves to safeguard the health of low-income women, infants, and children up to age 5 who are at nutritional risk by providing nutritious foods to supplement diets, information on healthy eating, and referral to health care. In 1982, the Missing Children's Act was passed, which established a clearinghouse for missing children.

There are more than 8 million uninsured children in the United States, and millions more are underinsured. Uninsured children are more likely than insured children to have unmet medical needs. Regular health screenings are crucial to a child's healthy development. Uninsured children are also more likely to perform poorly in school. The Children's Defense Fund advocates for children's health care reform. In addition, the Balanced Budget Act of 1997 established the State Children's Health Insurance Program (SCHIP) as Title XXI of the Social Security Act to expand insurance coverage to a large portion of uninsured children who are ineligible for Medicaid. Many children are eligible for SCHIP and Medicaid. The Patient Protection and Affordable Care Act and the Health Care and Education Reconciliation Act of 2010 are new government programs designed to address the issue of inadequate health care coverage for children and will also make immunizations for children easier to access. Education is also needed to break down barriers. The nurse is often in a position to provide this education.

Health promotion and disease prevention have become priorities. In 1990, the United States Department of Health and Human Services released a document entitled *Healthy People 2000: National Health Promotion and Disease Prevention Objectives*. This document builds on previously developed objectives to present an opportunity for Americans to take responsibility for their own health. It emphasizes equal access to health care for all segments of the population, particularly the most vulnerable. Many of these objectives apply to infants and children and are being researched and updated on an ongoing basis.

Healthy People 2010 is a follow-up to *Healthy People 2000*. Its objectives are promotion of healthy behaviors, promotion of healthy and safe communities, improvement of systems for personal and public health, and prevention and reduction of diseases and disorders. *Healthy People 2020* will continue work on many of the same issues as it strives to build a healthier nation.

Table 1-1 summarizes federal programs that affect maternal-child health, and Table 1-2 compares the leading health indicators for *Healthy People 2010* with selected proposed objectives of *Healthy People 2020*.

◉ Global Perspective

Two international organizations concerned with children are the United Nations Children's Fund (*www.unicef.org*) and the World Health Organization (*www.who.int/en*); *www.unicef.org/rightsite/sowc/* includes a video link regarding the rights of children around the globe. In addition, the American Academy of Pediatrics is an organization of pediatricians that is committed to the promotion of health for all pediatric patients (*www.aap.org*).

MORTALITY AND MORBIDITY

The infant mortality rate (number of infant deaths per 1000 live births) has declined from approximately 200 deaths in 1900 to 20 in 1970 to 6.77 in 2007. Infant mortality among infants of non-Hispanic black mothers, however, is still much higher than non-Hispanic whites and Hispanic mothers (Heron et al., 2010).

Despite declines in infant mortality, the United States continues to rank poorly in international comparisons. Although the exact reason is unclear, countries that rank higher have national health programs. Low birth weight (LBW) has been well documented as a primary contributor to infant mortality in developed countries. Other contributing factors include African-American race, male gender, socioeconomic status, lower level of maternal education, and gestational age (longer or shorter). According to the 2010 statistics, the leading causes of infant mortality are congenital malformations, deformations, and chromosomal abnormalities; disorders relating to short gestation and unspecified LBW; sudden infant death syndrome (SIDS); maternal complications; and accidents or unintentional injuries (Heron et al., 2010).

Positive steps are being taken to help with the continual decline of infant mortality. Education on cigarette smoking during pregnancy and early prenatal care are stressed. The Healthy Start program (*www.hrsa.gov*), which works to expand the availability and accessibility of prenatal health care in more than

Table 1-1   Summary of Federal Programs That Affect Maternal-Child Health

NAME	YEAR	COMMENT
White House Conference on Children and Youth	1909	Issued 15 recommendations, one of which was for the formation of a Children's Bureau for child welfare
Social Security	1935	Provides matching state/federal funds for maternal/child care and for children with disabilities, supports preventive health programs (immunizations, screenings)
Fair Labor Standards Act	1938	Establishes minimum working age of 16 years
Maternal-Child Health Infant Care Project	1963	Effort to decrease infant and child mortality
Children and Youth Project	1965	Targets low-income children and children in less accessible areas who need health care
Medicaid EPSDT	1965	Early and periodic screening, diagnosis, and treatment (EPSDT) for low-income children
Crippled Children's Service	1965	Services disabled children under 21 years
Head Start	1965	Assists disadvantaged preschool children, increases educational skills
National School Lunch Act and Child Nutrition Act	1966	Provides reduced or free meals to low-income families
WIC	1972	Supplemental food program for low-income women, infants, and children (WIC)
Education for All Handicapped Children	1975	P.L. 94-142, free public education for all disabled children ages 3-21 years; provides necessary supportive services
CMHCs (Community Mental Health Centers)	1982	Effort to increase availability of mental health centers to low-income families
Missing Children's Act	1982	Nationwide clearinghouse for missing children (National Crime Information Computer)
Comprehensive Child Immunization Act	1993	Ensures that all children in the United States are protected against vaccine-preventable infectious diseases at the earliest appropriate age
Family and Medical Leave Act (FMLA)	1993	Enables eligible employees to take up to 12 weeks of unpaid leave from their jobs every year to care for newborn or newly adopted children; to care for children, parents, or spouses who have serious health conditions; or to recover from their own serious health conditions; after the leave, the law entitles employees to return to their previous jobs or the equivalent jobs with the same pay, benefits, and other conditions
Health Insurance Portability and Accountability Act (HIPAA)	1996	Developed by the Department of Health and Human Services to protect patient's medical records and other health information provided to health plans, doctors, hospitals, and other health care providers
State Children's Health Insurance Program (SCHIP)	1997	Provides health care coverage for children in families that earn too much money to qualify for Medicaid but cannot afford private health insurance
Children's Online Privacy Protection Act	2000	Regulates the collection of personally identifiable information online from children under 13 years

100 communities nationwide with higher-than-average infant mortality rates, has received increased funding to help with the problem of infant mortality.

Childhood mortality rates have also declined. The overall leading cause of death in children 1 year to 19 years of age is injury from unintentional injuries; the majority of these are motor vehicle–related. Homicide is the second leading cause of death for this broad age group. Malignant neoplasms and intentional self-harm (suicide) rank third and fourth, respectively. This

Table 1-2	Comparison of *Healthy People 2010* and *Healthy People 2020*
LEADING HEALTH INDICATORS *HEALTHY PEOPLE 2010*	**SELECTED PROPOSED *HEALTHY PEOPLE 2020* OBJECTIVES**
Physical Activity	Physical Activity and Fitness
Overweight and Obesity	Nutrition and Weight Status
Tobacco Use	Tobacco Use
Substance Abuse	Substance Abuse
Responsible Sexual Behavior	Sexually Transmitted Diseases
Mental Health	Mental Health and Mental Disorders
Injury and Violence	Injury and Violence Prevention
Environmental Quality	Environmental Health
Immunization	Immunization and Infectious Diseases
Access to Health Care	Access to Health Services

From U.S. Department of Health and Human Services: Healthy People 2010: understanding and improving health (2nd ed.). Washington, DC, 2000, US Government Printing Office and Healthy People 2020: The Road Ahead. Retrieved May 18, 2010, from *http://www.healthypeople.gov/hp2020*.

Box 1-1	Leading Causes of Childhood Death in Specified Age Groups: United States

1 TO 4 YEARS
Accidents (unintentional injuries)
Congenital malformations, deformations and chromosomal abnormalities
Malignant neoplasms
Assault (homicide)
Diseases of heart

5 TO 9 YEARS
Accidents (unintentional injuries)
Malignant neoplasms
Congenital malformations, deformations and chromosomal abnormalities
Assault (homicide)
Diseases of heart

10 TO 14 YEARS
Accidents (unintentional injuries)
Malignant neoplasms
Intentional self harm (suicide)
Assault (homicide)
Congenital malformations, deformations, and chromosomal abnormalities

15 TO 19 YEARS
Accidents (unintentional injuries)
Assault (homicide)
Intentional self-harm (suicide)
Malignant neoplasms
Diseases of heart

Data from Centers for Disease Control and Prevention/NCHS, National Vital Statistics System: Mortality, 2007 and 2006. Retrieved from *www.cdc.gov/nchs/nvss/mortality_tables.htm*.

reflects a continued shift in societal values and greatly affects the approach to health care for children in this age group. Box 1-1 illustrates a breakdown of causes of death in specified age groups.

Childhood morbidity (i.e., illness, chronic disease, disability) is affected by general health, socioeconomic status, access to health care, and psychosocial factors. Acute illnesses, such as respiratory and gastrointestinal disorders, are common in children. At-risk children, such as those who are homeless, live in poverty, attend daycare regularly, or have decreased access to the health care system, often have more frequent illnesses.

Because of technological advances, many premature and low–birth weight infants who formerly would have died are surviving. Although this improvement in survival rates is encouraging, many of these infants develop chronic health problems such as bronchopulmonary dysplasia (BPD). See Chapter 11 for further discussion on BPD.

Children with formerly fatal conditions, such as severe congenital heart disease and cystic fibrosis, are also surviving into adulthood. The AIDS epidemic has presented a spectrum of new challenges for nurses who care for infected infants and children. As incidents of childhood injury increase, the incidence rate of associated disabilities rises as well. A final important concern is the number of children and adolescents with severe emotional and behavioral problems that are caused by, or result in, school failures, violence, substance use, and risky sexual behavior.

CURRENT PRACTICE

EDUCATION REQUIREMENTS

Because of the rapid changes taking place in health care today, it is the nurse's responsibility to update his or her knowledge continually. As the role of the pediatric nurse expands, the issue of accountability becomes more important. Nurses have a responsibility to the community and to their profession. Today, involvement in community and professional organizations is not simply encouraged; it is absolutely essential for continued growth in an ever-changing society.

Nursing Brief

The Society of Pediatric Nursing is a professional organization for pediatric nurses; its mission is to "promote excellence in nursing care of children and their families through support of our members' clinical practice, education, research, and advocacy" (*www.pedsnurses.org*).

RESEARCH AND ROLES

Nurses are also expected to provide the best practice, and thereby the best outcomes, for their patients. Simply saying, "Because we have always done it this way" is no longer acceptable. Health care professionals need to question current practices and find better alternatives. Through examination of research literature, nurses can analyze important evidence and improve the quality of care for their patients. This philosophy is known as evidence-based practice. In the future, nurses will make more nursing care decisions based on evidence, rather than opinion. This will improve the quality of nursing care, improve nursing practice, and promote nursing professionalism.

The pediatric nurse may serve in a variety of roles, ranging from teaching in various settings to providing hands-on care in the hospital or clinic. Disease prevention is a focus for current health care. Health promotion and anticipatory guidance continue to play important roles in pediatric nursing. Caring for children in today's society requires careful assessment and early identification of children and families at risk. Working with families in a variety of settings helps to ensure the safety and needs of all children. Advocating for children and families involves helping families to be fully informed regarding their child's care. The pediatric nurse works with other members of the health care team and with the family in providing care. Coordination and collaboration with other professionals becomes the norm. The nurse must be able to give competent, skillful care to children while maintaining a caring, holistic attitude. Ethical decision making is an issue that nurses must deal with. Nurses must determine the most beneficial or least harmful action within the scope of the practice guidelines, standards, laws, and society.

CRITICAL THINKING AND THE NURSING PROCESS

Nurses today are charged with making decisions in the clinical setting that affect their patient's lives. In order to make the correct decision, the nurse utilizes critical thinking skills. Critical thinking is an expanded, systematic way of thinking. It emphasizes process, inquiry, and reasoning, as well as creativity and ingenuity, so that the nurse can draw the best conclusion regarding a situation. Critical thinking requires insight into one's ability to think and find solutions that provide the most effective nursing care. It also involves understanding why things are done in a certain manner. The nurse should never be satisfied with the "status quo" and needs to always seek to understand the rationale for why things are done; for example, physicians' orders. Several critical thinking exercises are used throughout this text.

Both critical thinking and the nursing process involve problem solving. The nursing process incorporates five steps: assessment, diagnosis, planning, implementation (intervention), and evaluation. In pediatrics, *both* the child and the family are the focus of the nursing process. The *care plan* is the result. See Chapter 2 for further discussion.

Assessment involves the collection of data and the analysis of the data, and it is the basis for decision making. During the assessment, the data-gathering phase of the process, the nurse obtains essential information about the child's physical, social, and emotional health and about the family's adaptation to health alterations. Problems that emerge from the assessment are stated in diagnostic format. Those diagnoses approved by the North American Nursing Diagnosis Association (NANDA) are listed on the inside back cover of this text. The nurse next plans care for problems that were identified during assessment and are stated as nursing diagnoses. Priorities are set, and goals or outcomes are developed. Nursing *outcomes* and *goals* are sometimes used interchangeably; however, outcome statements are more measurable and state specific outcome criteria. In general, goal setting and outcome criteria constitute the planning phase and are the organizing structure for nursing interventions. The NANDA, Nursing Outcomes Classification (NOC), and Nursing Interventions Classification (NIC) are three standardized nursing languages that were developed to facilitate communication, improve data collection and prioritizing, and assist in nursing research. Linkages between the three classifications show the connections between the patient's problem, the patient outcomes, and the nursing actions that resolve or decrease the problem. For example, if the NANDA diagnosis is *anxiety*, the NOC label might be *anxiety control*, and the NIC label might be *active listening*. The focus is on the actions necessary to reduce or eliminate a specific problem or to promote health. The evaluation phase appraises the changes experienced by the child or family in relation to achieving goals or outcomes.

DOCUMENTATION

The nurse must document assessment findings throughout the child's stay; this is important regardless of the setting. Data collection and assessment findings would be documented in a physician office just as they would in a hospital or clinic setting. Note any changes in the child's condition as well as the follow-up, for example, if the physician is notified because of a drop in blood pressure. Document patient care needs and interventions done to meet those needs as well as the patient's response to the nursing care provided. Always document according to a specific time, as this is important legally. Documentation of discharge needs, and the ability of the patient and/or parents to manage the care after discharge is important as well. Always chart with legal requirements in mind because each patient's chart is a legal document. In lawsuits, juries often assume that *if something was not charted, it was not done.*

CONFIDENTIALITY AND INFORMED CONSENT

The enactment of the HIPAA (Health Insurance Portability and Accountability Act) regulations in 1996 required strict observance of confidentiality within the hospital setting. This requirement is for the protection of the patient and is extremely important when caring for children. Adults and older children could easily overhear and misinterpret information discussed about a child.

In addition, respecting an older school-age child or teenager's right to confidentiality is essential to establishing trust (Figure 1-1). In general, the nurse does not divulge or share information without the patient's consent. Many problems can be avoided if the confidentiality of the relationship is clearly defined during initial meetings. At this time, nurses explain to older children and teenagers that certain situations must be reported, such as plans to harm themselves or harm others or any abuse that may have occurred. Patient records must be carefully monitored to avoid loss or access by unauthorized personnel. The nurse should not give any private information about any patient to telephone callers or visitors.

For children younger than 18 years of age, informed consent is generally obtained from the parent or legal guardian. Informed consent is obtained when written approval is needed in order for surgery or a procedure to be performed. This occurs after the physician explains the reason for the procedure as well as potential adverse effects. It is the responsibility of the nurse to witness the signing of the informed consent. The procedure is explained to the child in age-appropriate terminology and level of understanding. The child is prepared for the procedure in order to minimize anxiety and stress. See Chapter 2 for further discussion.

The term emancipated minor generally refers to adolescents younger than 18 years of age who are no longer under their parents' authority. Married minors or minors in the military are automatically considered

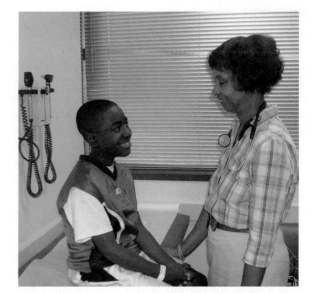

FIGURE 1-1 Nurses need to be respectful and nonjudgmental when discussing issues with adolescents.

emancipated and may give consent for medical treatment for themselves and their children. The mature minor doctrine recognizes that individuals mature at different rates. In most parts of the United States, the young adolescent may receive medical assistance for certain conditions such as sexually transmitted diseases, contraception, pregnancy, and drug abuse without parental awareness. These laws are designed to afford the young person immediate medical help without fear of reprisal. However, they are subject to controversy. In addition, many states now require at least one parent be notified if a minor requests an abortion. Some states require parental consent. All states allow minors to obtain treatment in life-threatening situations when legal guardians are not available. Because laws vary from state to state, nurses must be continually informed about the policies and the legislation within their practice state. This information is usually available from the local medical or nursing association office.

Get Ready for the NCLEX® Examination!

Key Points

- Child health care has grown over the past several years as a result of federal programs and federal funding.
- The infant mortality rate continues to decline, although LBW is still the major contributor to infant death. An alarming increase in childhood mortality rates can be attributed to increases in homicide and suicide.

- *Healthy People 2000, Healthy People 2010,* and *Healthy People 2020* have documented the need for Americans to take responsibility for their own health and have outlined government goals regarding health promotion and disease prevention.
- Through evidence-based practice, nurses can analyze important evidence and improve the quality of care for their patients.

- Critical thinking and the nursing process are methods of problem solving that guide the care of the hospitalized child.
- An awareness of the legalities involved in documentation and informed consent with pediatric patients is important for sound nursing care.

Additional Learning Resources

evolve Go to your Evolve website (*http://evolve.elsevier.com/Price/pediatric/*) for the following FREE learning resources:
- 3-D Animations
- Answer Keys
- Appendixes
- Audio Glossary
- Spanish/English Glossary
- Video Clips

Review Questions for the NCLEX® Examination

1. A government program designed in 2010 to address the issue of inadequate health care coverage for children is the:
   1. Children and Youth Project
   2. Children's Defense Fund
   3. State Children's Health Insurance Program (SCHIP)
   4. Health Care and Education Reconciliation Act

2. Infant mortality is highest among infants born to:
   1. Non-Hispanic white mothers
   2. Hispanic mothers
   3. Non-Hispanic black mothers
   4. European mothers

3. The majority of deaths in children ages 1 year to 19 years of age are due to:
   1. Homicide
   2. Motor vehicle accidents
   3. Malignant neoplasms
   4. Suicide

4. The focus for current health care is:
   1. Symptom management
   2. Identification of disease processes
   3. Disease prevention
   4. Increased provision of nursing services

5. The step in the nursing process that is considered the data-gathering phase is:
   1. Diagnosis
   2. Evaluation
   3. Planning
   4. Assessment

Care of the Child with Medical/Surgical Needs

Objectives

1. Define the vocabulary terms listed
2. Discuss the variety of settings in which the pediatric nurse may work
3. Describe the physical facilities of a children's hospital unit, and explain their significance to the child's adjustment to hospitalization
4. Discuss five measures the nurse can take to make hospitalization less threatening for the child
5. Describe how illness affects the child and family
6. Discuss the nurse's role in a hospital admission
7. Discuss nursing implications when caring for children of different cultures and religions
8. Discuss how to perform a systems review
9. Discuss five guidelines or suggestions that may be useful to parents at discharge
10. List five safety measures applicable to the care of the child
11. Plan care for a child who is in isolation
12. Discuss care of the child before and after surgery
13. Discuss both pharmacologic and nonpharmacologic pediatric pain management

Key Terms

adventitious (ad-ven-TĬ-shes; p. 18)
case manager (p. 9)
contaminated (kĕn-TA-mĕ-nāt-ed; p. 24)
critical pathways (p. 20)
disinfected (dĭ-sĕn-FEKT-ed; p. 24)
dramatic play (dre-MA-tik; p. 13)
hospice (hŏs-pĭs; p. 9)

hypnosis (hĭp-NŌ-sĭs; p. 31)
pediatric nurse practitioner (PNP) (prak-TI-sh[e]ner; p. 8)
reconciled (RE-ken-sīled; p. 16)
standard precautions (pre-KŌ-shens; p. 25)
therapeutic holding (thĕr-ă-PŪ-tĭk; p. 23)
triage (trē-AZH; p. 8)

HEALTH CARE DELIVERY SETTINGS

Although children are hospitalized when illnesses or injuries warrant, in general, they are most often cared for in a variety of other settings. These include, but are not limited to, community and school clinics, pediatrician and family practice offices, home care, children's camps, and pediatric long-term care facilities.

CLINICS AND OFFICES

Most large hospitals today have well-organized outpatient facilities and satellite or community clinics for preventive medicine and care of the child who is ill. Although substantial socioeconomic disparities are still involved in the procurement of routine preventive services, Medicaid and other similar programs have made these services available to more low-income families. In many institutions, information is distributed and education is offered on childhood immunizations, injury prevention, and parenting skills. Specialty clinics such as cardiac, orthopedic, respiratory, and so forth exist to facilitate ongoing care on an outpatient basis.

In many cities, groups of pediatricians practice in office settings or clinic settings removed from the hospital. Such services aid in the distribution of health services and often provide evening and weekend health coverage. In most offices or clinics, nurses constantly triage (prioritize) and respond to telephone inquiries.

The pediatric nurse practitioner (PNP) may care for children in the pediatric or family practice office, give routine physical examinations at the clinic, and otherwise collaborate with the physician so that a higher quality of individual care may be attained. This nurse frequently is the primary contact person for children in the health care system. The PNP may also work in school-based clinics or health centers along with school nurses and other health care providers. School-based health centers are often an ideal location to provide primary health care for children and adolescents.

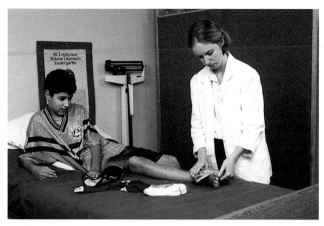

FIGURE 2-1 School-based clinics provide accessible and affordable health care services to students.

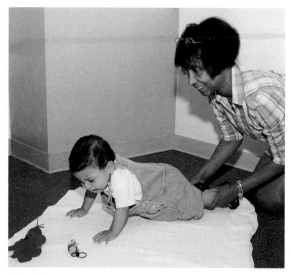

FIGURE 2-2 A home care nurse helps the child attain an optimal level of functioning within the home setting.

(Access to quality health care for all is the number-one focus area for *Healthy People 2010*.) The role of the school nurse has expanded at the same time that school-based health centers have increased in number (Figure 2-1). Most school-based health centers provide the basics of primary health care. Health assessments, anticipatory guidance, screenings, immunizations, acute illness care, lab services, dental care, sexually transmitted disease precautions, pregnancy testing, and family planning may be incorporated into these centers. School nurses provide health counseling and education and act as advocates for students with disabilities. School nurses and nurse practitioners also partner with community physicians and community organizations and may collaborate with state programs, such as SCHIP (State Children's Health Insurance Program).

Nursing Brief

Another area of outpatient care is the pediatric research center, such as the one at St. Jude's Hospital in Memphis, Tennessee. St. Jude's is one of the world's premiere centers for research and treatment of catastrophic diseases in children, particularly pediatric cancers, often at little or no expense to the patient. Research is also done at Shriners Hospitals, a network of pediatric specialty hospitals where children younger than 18 years of age receive medical care absolutely free of charge. Shriners Hospitals mainly treat children with orthopedic conditions and burn injuries.

Elective surgery for children with uncomplicated conditions, such as tonsillectomy or hernia repair, is also routinely done in outpatient settings. Advantages of same-day surgery include a reduction in cross-infection and hospital costs. Outpatient clinics also eliminate the need to separate the child from the family, making it less stressful for the child. In this type of

setting, careful preparation and teaching must be done, and the child's home environment must be adequate to meet the child's recovery needs.

As more and more medical care occurs in outpatient settings, there is an even greater reduction in the number of children who need hospitalization. It is expected that, for many children, the only exposure to medical personnel will be through brief clinic appointments. The nurse's responsibility is to make these encounters positive for children and their families.

HOME CARE

Because hospitalizations are now briefer for most children, home care may be an acceptable alternative to a prolonged hospital stay (Figure 2-2). Technical improvements and research in specific disease entities have helped to advance the movement in home care. The result is often lower cost, increased patient satisfaction, and overall general well-being. Ongoing intravenous therapy is often maintained through home care, as is phototherapy for the newborn with jaundice. Home care, however, is not merely a matter of supplying equipment, appliances, and nursing care; it requires assessment of the total needs of children and their families. Families need to be linked to a wide variety of network services. These services are often established by a case manager, who plays a vital role in home care arrangements. Case managers oversee a continuum of care for the child by managing medical care.

For families who are facing the loss of a child, hospice is a service that offers unique help. Hospice is a program offered to children who are terminally ill, usually those with only 4 to 6 months left to live. Parents, with the help of hospice nurses and caregivers, often provide the care for their dying child at home. See Chapter 22 for further discussion on hospice.

OTHER SETTINGS

Local and national support groups for specific problems afford opportunities for families to share and support one another and to learn from others' successes and failures. Special groups and camps for children with chronic illnesses are also available. Many different types of organized camps exist in the United States. Examples include camps for children with asthma or children with cancer. Many of these camps are held in the summer months. Camp nurses perform assessments, dispense medications, provide first aid, triage health problems, and may also provide training to other staff.

Parish nurses provide specialized practice of professional nursing that focuses on the promotion of health within the context of the values, beliefs, and practices of a faith community. Parish nursing focuses on the health care needs of all ages and provides health promotion, health maintenance, and illness prevention programs, as well as community resources and support groups. Children and adults can benefit from the services provided.

Group therapy for children who have undergone stressful situations is important in prevention of mental health problems. Children coping with depression or suicidal tendencies often need the support of group therapy. Many children also need group support if their parents are divorced, abusive, or abusing substances. Group support programs not only have the potential for improving life for the child and family but may also help reduce the high cost of medical care.

Long-term care facilities may be necessary for children with severe or profound mental retardation or for those with multiple disabilities. Placing a child in a long-term care facility is a difficult decision for any family to make. A thorough assessment of the facility, with the needs of the child kept in mind, is essential not only for the child's well-being but for the family's peace of mind as well.

THE HOSPITAL SETTING

Children are usually hospitalized in a pediatric hospital. They may also be hospitalized in a community hospital. Regardless of where the child is hospitalized, the pediatric setting differs in many respects from an adult setting. The pediatric unit or hospital is designed to meet the needs of children and their parents. A cheerful, casual atmosphere helps bridge the gap between home and hospital and is in keeping with the child's emotional and physical needs. Children may wear their own clothing while they are hospitalized, and nurses wear colorful scrubs or pastel uniforms.

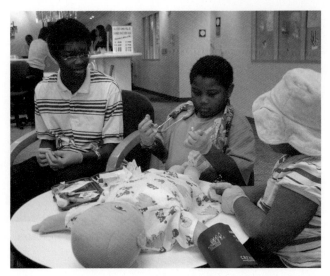

FIGURE 2-3 A child-friendly atmosphere on the pediatric unit may help children feel less anxious when hospitalized.

The physical structure of a pediatric unit includes furniture of the proper height for the child, colorful furnishings, and child-friendly décor (Figure 2-3). Even transportation is suited to the child; wagons are often used to take younger children to and from procedures in the hospital setting.

 Communication

Always meet and speak with children at their eye level. Figures that tower over them can be frightening.

Most pediatric departments include a playroom in the structural plan. This room is generally equipped with toys for various age groups. Some playrooms are equipped with a fish aquarium or blossoming plants because most children love living things. Computers are also often available for use by the child. The playroom may be under the supervision of a play therapist or a child life specialist. Parents usually enjoy taking their children to the playroom and observing the various activities. The nurse should allow each child freedom to develop independently and should make observations about the child's play. See Chapter 8 for further discussion on the value of play to the child.

Community Considerations

Child life specialists apply knowledge of child development, therapeutic play, treatment of stress, and other psychosocial principles in working with children and their families to help them cope effectively with potential stressful situations, primarily in hospitals, but also in a variety of other settings (www. childlife.org).

Some children are not able to be taken to the playroom because of their physical condition. In such cases, the nurse should provide age-appropriate toys for the child in his or her room. If the child is in isolation, the toys generally stay in the room until the child goes home. The nurse ensures that cleaning procedures are followed once the child is discharged.

The daily routine in the pediatric setting also differs widely for obvious reasons. Although rigid schedules are not encouraged, children do benefit from a certain amount of routine. Meals, rest, and play are carried out at approximately the same time each day. Such questions about the child's routine are asked on admission. Children should have choices in food selection, and the same protocols are followed for children at mealtimes as for adults: No urinals should be in view, the tray table should be clean, and so on. For the school-age child, time needs to be included in the daily routine for school work. Observe the time the child is with a teacher, and keep interaction to a *minimum*. It is important for children to carry on school work while in the hospital.

Nursing care is often delivered by consistent caregivers, which provides comfort to the child in the hospital. Oftentimes nurses and children form bonds, especially if the child returns frequently to the same unit in the hospital. Visiting hours on the pediatric unit are usually liberal and depend on the child's condition. Parents are encouraged to stay with their child whenever possible, and most hospitals provide beds for parents.

THE CHILD'S REACTION TO HOSPITALIZATION

How a child reacts to hospitalization depends on the child's age, preparation, previous illness-related experiences, support of family and health professionals, and the child's emotional status. The major stressors of hospitalization include separation, loss of control, and bodily injury and pain (Hockenberry and Wilson, 2009).

Infants and Toddlers

For infants and toddlers, separation anxiety is the major stressor during hospitalization. Unless toddlers are extremely ill, their grief and sense of abandonment are obvious. They protest loudly, watch and listen for their mother, and cry continuously until they fall asleep from sheer exhaustion. The second stage occurs as anger turns to despair. The children look sad and lonely and may refuse to eat. They may become depressed and move about less than usual. In the third stage—denial—children may try to deny the need for their mother or father by appearing detached and uninterested during visits. On the surface, children may seem to have settled in, but this is only a disguise to prevent further emotional pain. The nurse who comprehends the various separation stages sees parental

visits as essential, even though the process of separation and reunion is painful. Education of the parents helps promote their continued visits and decreases feelings of inadequacy.

Toddlers also react to the loss of control they experience while hospitalized. According to Erikson, these children are involved in the task of autonomy. (See Chapter 4 for further discussion.) Activity limits, decreased opportunities for choices, and interrupted rituals contribute to a feeling of powerlessness. It is not unusual for toddlers to respond to this feeling with regression. They abandon recently acquired skills and may demand assistance with tasks that they have previously mastered. Without preparation for this, parents often do not understand the child's behavior. They need to be reminded that in this situation, this is normal behavior. Parents, however, do need to reinforce appropriate behavior, and the nurse needs to maintain a sense of sameness whenever possible.

Toddlers also are often affected by fear of injury and remember previous painful experiences. A brief explanation of the procedure followed by comfort after the procedure is often the best way to deal with this stressor.

Box 2-1 lists interventions for dealing with the stressors of hospitalization. In addition, toddlers need to be allowed choices, within reason, which helps them to achieve control. However, questions such as, "Do you want to take your nap now?" could lead to answers such as, "I don't want to take a nap." Thus, questions such as, "Do you want to take your nap now or after a story?" are better. Sometimes limits on behavior are necessary, especially if the behavior is intolerable. Parents are encouraged to support the child and use sensible limit setting if necessary.

Children should be forewarned, in keeping with their level of understanding, about any unpleasant or

Box 2-1 Nursing Interventions for Stressors of Hospitalization

Explain all procedures with honesty.
Include parents in the care of the child.
Encourage parents to stay with the child.
Maintain the routines and rituals of home.
Encourage parents to bring familiar objects from home (e.g., stuffed animal, blanket, doll).
If the parents cannot stay with the child, encourage them to call, leave photographs, and visit when possible.
Perform all invasive procedures in the treatment room to keep the child's room a safe place for the child.
Provide for a consistent caretaker when possible.
Comfort the child after traumatic procedures if the parent is not present to care for the child.
Provide age-related diversionary activities.

new experience that they may have to undergo while in the hospital. Be truthful about procedures that may hurt; this prevents a child from feeling betrayed and losing trust. Preparation and explanation should be done immediately before a procedure so that the child does not worry needlessly for an extended period of time. During the procedure, explain what is happening step by step. Children should be allowed to discuss how they feel after the procedure. It is better not to put preconceived ideas in the child's mind, such as suggesting how something might feel. The child should be allowed to describe the experience after the procedure is over. Reassure the child that it is all right to cry or say "ouch." Allow toddlers to master the threatening experience through the use of play and fantasy.

 Communication

Using a stuffed animal, doll, or puppet decreases fear and helps the toddler to communicate. The nurse can use the inanimate object to assist in gaining the child's cooperation. For instance, pretending to "count the heart rate" on a stuffed animal prior to the child will often elicit cooperation.

Toddlers are encouraged to play with safe equipment used in their care, for example, tongue blades and stethoscopes. Provide other toys that are appropriate to the developmental level, such as blocks, stacking toys, balls, and wooden puzzles. Whenever possible, toddlers should also be allowed out of the crib because being confined is frustrating for little ones who have just begun to enjoy walking (Figure 2-4). Supervised playroom activity contributes to intellectual, social, and motor development. Whenever possible, treatments should be done in the treatment room. The child's room should remain a "safe place,"

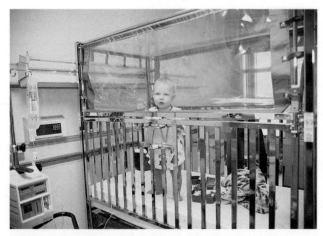

FIGURE 2-4 To facilitate autonomy, young toddlers should be allowed outside of their cribs whenever possible.

and the playroom should *never* be used for anything but play.

Preschoolers

Preschoolers exhibit separation anxiety, although not as obviously as the toddler. Preschoolers may act uncooperatively and ask frequently for their parents. Preschoolers are, however, significantly affected by loss of control. Not only have their schedules changed, but they are physically restricted. Children at this age are pre-logical in their thinking and have a difficult time distinguishing between fantasy and reality. They believe they are all-powerful and control the world around them and, in fact, may believe that their illness was caused by something they did or thought. They may feel guilty, particularly if an accident happened because of some mischief on their part, as in the case of a burn or a fall. It is important to help hospitalized preschoolers realize that hospitalization is not a punishment for something they have done wrong. Preschoolers also need choices so that they can regain some sense of control.

One of the major ways preschoolers cope with their environment is by fantasizing. Unfortunately, when in an unfamiliar environment, preschoolers' use of fantasy also contributes to their fears. Hospitalized preschoolers often have nightmares and are afraid of the dark or of unfamiliar sights and sounds. Preschoolers may also worry that inanimate objects are alive; for this reason, they may fear hospital machinery and equipment. This causes them to feel powerless. See Chapter 8 for further discussion on the preschooler.

Preschoolers fear mutilation during hospitalization and do not understand body integrity. They are afraid of bodily harm, particularly by invasive procedures and procedures that involve the genital area. Because they still have limited understanding of the inside of the body, preschool children often imagine that bodies are filled with air and will collapse when punctured or that bodies are filled with blood, which could all leak out through any artificial opening. This is why bandages (Band-Aids, for example) are so important to cover any injury, real or imagined.

Preschoolers tend to attach literal meanings to words such as *dye, draw blood, take,* or *test.* These words can have more than one meaning for the child and can be confusing. Avoid these words when describing procedures to children, and try to rephrase information in terms that are clear and understandable.

In addition to the interventions listed in Box 2-1, nurses should use their communication skills to assist the child in dealing with feelings of separation or fear. For example, the nurse might say, "Some boys and girls feel afraid in the hospital. Do you feel that way?" This assists the child in expressing fears. Nurses and parents should not tell a child that they will return unless they definitely intend to do so.

Communication

Preschool children do not have a concept of time as it relates to the clock. If the child asks a question regarding time, the nurse might reply, "We will do that after cartoons" or "Mommy will come back after you eat your lunch."

The nurse must be aware of verbal and nonverbal cues from children this age. The child may withdraw or act in an aggressive manner. Parents may tell their children to "be brave" or to "act like a grown-up." This can prevent the child from verbalizing fears and discomfort.

 Communication

Use of the first person can help a child express feelings. The nurse might say, "Sometimes when *I* am in a new place, *I* feel afraid." The child can either agree, disagree, or remain silent. Silence might indicate that the child agrees but is still unable to express feelings.

The preschool child relieves tension through magical thinking, fantasy, and role playing. Nurses should participate readily in the child's fantasy if the fantasy is positive and appears to be helping the child achieve control. For example, if the child views the cardiac monitor as threatening because it is so loud, help the child write or draw a sign telling it to "talk softly" or "be quiet." Many children this age have imaginary friends with whom they converse and behave as though the friends were really present in the room. Participation in this form of imagination is acceptable because displacing fears and feelings onto an imaginary friend helps a child feel more powerful.

Play is important to help the child adjust to hospitalization (Figure 2-5). Through dramatic play, children can act out situations that are part of their hospital experience. Dramatic play through the use of hospital equipment enables children to "work through" emotions they may be dealing with. Giving a "shot" to a doll is an example of dramatic play. Puppets also help young children work through feelings. Nurses can encourage children to communicate through puppets; dolls and puppets may also be an avenue to play out situations with children.

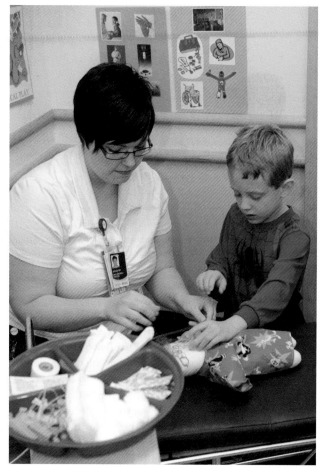

FIGURE 2-5 A child life specialist engaged in play therapy.

should be assured that these behavior changes are temporary and the child will soon return to his or her "old self."

School-Age Children

School-age children may show some signs of parental separation anxiety, especially when they are ill. Even more so, these children miss their friends. They may fear that their peers will forget them while they are away from school. On the other hand, their more sophisticated concept of time generally allows them to be patient and wait for a parent's return or a peer's visit.

School-age children are in the process of developing confidence in their abilities to control their feelings and actions. Hospitalization places them in the position of feeling out of control because it interrupts their routine and limits their independence. They may demonstrate resistive behaviors and have changes in vital signs in response to stress. Anger, boredom, frustration, and disinterest are other common manifestations of loss of control in the school-age child. These children appreciate the familiarity of objects from home and should be encouraged to bring such items to the hospital (Figure 2-6).

Nursing Brief

In addition to toys appropriate for the child's age group, everyday hospital supplies such as tongue depressors and bandages may become works of art.

Preschool children may regress in their behavior when they are ill. An example of this regression would be bedwetting after the child has not had an "accident" for some time. Children may also be irritable and demanding when they are hospitalized. The parent

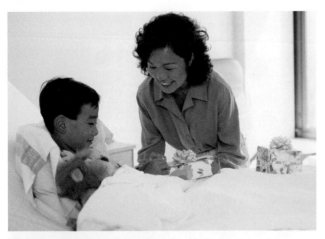

FIGURE 2-6 While gifts can brighten a child's hospital experience, objects from home provide comfort and familiarity.

The school-age child fears pain and bodily harm. These children are more concerned with permanent disability or body disfigurement than are younger children. The older school-age child may also fear death.

In addition to the interventions listed in Box 2-1, school-age children can benefit from drawing and talking about drawings. This activity allows them to get in touch with their feelings because they may not have the ability or vocabulary to express their fears, worries, and concerns verbally. The use of drawings allows a child to express his or her feelings in an abstract manner, and the nurse can then discuss these drawings with the child.

 Communication

Playing a board game often facilitates communication with a school-age child, who may feel uncomfortable talking to an adult. As the two participants become involved in the game, therapeutic conversation can be directed and begin to flow.

Encourage the hospitalized school-age child to be as independent as possible. Most school-age children are capable of complete self-care and can perform most daily activities independently within the limitations of their illness. Maintaining a school-age child's privacy is extremely important.

The education of the school-age child must continue throughout any illness. This gives the child a sense of continuity with the outside world, provides periods of socialization, and may reinforce weak academic areas. Some pediatric hospitals have areas designated for school-learning activities. The local school district may provide teachers to do on-site teaching. If this service is not available, family or friends may bring in school work from the child's regular teacher. This will ensure that the child does not fall behind in his or her studies.

Education involves the parents, who may act as liaisons between the school and hospital. The teacher needs to be informed of the child's physical and emotional health to deal effectively with him or her. The nurse provides the children with opportunities to study undisturbed so that they are prepared for their classes. Whenever possible, diagnostic tests and treatments should be scheduled around established school routines.

Teachers should be notified if a child will be out of school for any length of time, and classmates should be encouraged to send cards, draw pictures, call, and visit if appropriate. The nurse should assist the child in displaying the cards and pictures. If possible, care should be planned around the visit of classmates and friends. Children need to maintain as much control as possible while in the hospital.

Adolescents

Adolescents may still want their parents present when they are hospitalized. They too miss their friends. However, some are hesitant to have friends visit because they are not sure how their friends will handle their illness or injury. They do not want to appear different or act differently, so compliance may be a problem if the child lives with a chronic disease. Even though adolescents may give the impression that they are not afraid, they actually may be terrified of being in the hospital. The whole process of why they are there and having to undergo different procedures may be very frightening to them. They may feel that they will no longer "fit in" with their friends. Encouraging adolescents to express their fears helps alleviate these stressors and allows them to work toward maintaining or reestablishing their identity. Offer choices; this helps them maintain control and independence.

In general, fear of the unknown affects all hospitalized children. The nurse must explain in an age-appropriate manner what the child can expect, whether it pertains to unit routines or to procedures that need to be performed.

Unclear limits and expectations can best be minimized by explaining the rules and the expectations to the child. Once children understand what is expected of them, they feel less threatened and confused.

THE FAMILY'S REACTION TO HOSPITALIZATION

When a child is hospitalized, the whole family is affected. If the caregiver stays with the child in the hospital, then normal duties at home are neglected. Parents may be concerned about small children who are being cared for by relatives or friends. If the parents are unable to stay at the hospital, they may feel guilty about leaving the child. They may also attempt to rearrange their schedules to spend as much time as possible with the hospitalized child. Whatever the situation, the parents' needs should be identified by the nurse, and efforts should be made to decrease the anxiety the parents experience.

Parents may initially feel guilty, helpless, and anxious. They often blame themselves for the child's illness because they did not recognize early symptoms of a disease, may have delayed treatment, or were behind in preventive care. However, parents seldom are the direct cause of a child's hospital admission. Even in cases of child abuse, nothing is gained by blaming the parents. The nurse must realize that developing a trusting relationship with parents is often at the center of helping the child. This can be done only if the nurse remains objective and empathetic. The nurse should listen, acknowledge feelings, and support the family.

Parents may also fear the unknown. They may be unfamiliar with the hospital setting, procedures, treatments, and the disease itself. Explaining the rules and protocol of the hospital unit will reduce anxiety. Discussing procedures ahead of time and educating the parents on the disease process will also help to allay anxious feelings. Many children's hospitals now have educational areas designed for parents. Hospital librarians or other resource persons help parents to be *empowered* in the care of their child.

Hospitalization may cause financial problems for the family. This is especially true in the case of long-term illnesses and treatment. In addition to the obvious expense of the hospital and physician, families often have the added costs of travel, lodging, food, and missed work. The nurse must be aware of these needs and make the appropriate referrals to social services as necessary.

As with the child, the nurse assesses the family's needs and develops interventions to meet these needs. Some of these interventions include the following:

- Assist parents in obtaining written and verbal information concerning the condition of the child and the treatment plan (Figure 2-7).
- Orient the family to the hospital.
- Explain all procedures.
- Refer parents as needed to social services to assist in areas of medical expenses, food, and lodging.
- Listen to parents' concerns, and clarify information.
- Involve parents in the care of the child.
- Provide for rooming-in.
- Reinforce positive parenting.
- Provide educational resources as necessary.

Siblings are also affected when a family member is hospitalized. They may experience anger, resentment, jealousy, and guilt. Suddenly attention is focused on the sick family member, and siblings may feel neglected. When routines are changed and members are separated, the needs of the siblings may not receive attention. Siblings may feel resentment. This can lead them to feel guilty about their ill family member. The nurse can assist the parents in identifying and meeting the needs of siblings in the following ways:

- Keep siblings informed of the child's illness and progress.
- Allow siblings to visit the hospitalized child.
- Encourage siblings to provide pictures, make cards, and call.
- Allow siblings to assist with the care of the ill child if they seem comfortable doing so and if the child's condition permits (Figure 2-8).

THE NURSE'S ROLE

ADMISSION PROCESS

A child must be prepared for outpatient procedures or hospitalization. If a planned, nonemergency hospitalization is required, the nurse should provide a tour of the pediatric unit to the parents and the child before admission. This is advisable and enables the parents to meet the people who will be caring for their child. Children and their families are often overwhelmed by the size of an institution and fear becoming lost.

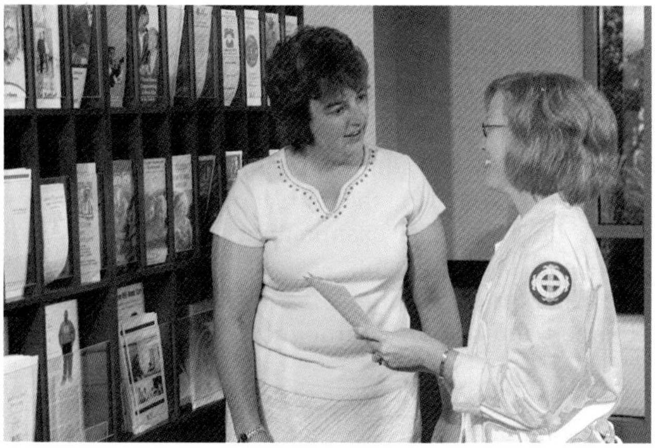

FIGURE 2-7 A variety of educational tools should be used to instruct the family.

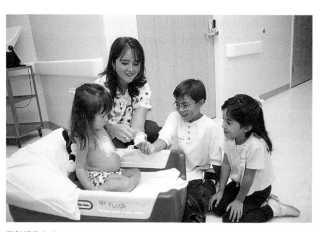

FIGURE 2-8 Siblings need to be fully informed about their sibling's care needs and condition and should be allowed to participate in care activities as much as they wish.

Beginning as early as age 6 months, the child is worried about being separated from the parents. Increased stress can lead to increased separation anxiety. After age 3 years, children may become more fearful about what is going to happen to them. Parents should try to be as matter-of-fact about this new experience as possible. Unless they have been hospitalized before, children can only try to imagine what will happen to them. Much detail is not provided because giving information beyond a child's understanding may create unnecessary fears. It is better to focus on the more pleasant and positive aspects—but not to the point where hospitalization seems to involve no discomforts. For example, one might mention that meals are served on a tray, that baths are taken from a basin at the bedside, and that the child will be with other children. The fact that there is a buzzer to call the nurse if necessary may add to the child's sense of security. The parents may also plan with the child what favorite toy or book to bring to the hospital. Security objects from home will help reduce anxiety in an unfamiliar setting.

In addition to explaining certain procedures, it is important to listen to children and encourage questions. Parents should prepare children a few days, not weeks, in advance of a hospital admission. They should never lure children to the hospital under the pretense that they are actually going someplace else. In emergency situations, however, there may be little time for any preparation. In such cases, the entire medical team must try to give added emotional support to the child.

The nurse prepares the child's room for the admission (including equipment needed for determining weight, length, vital signs, and so forth) well in advance. This saves time and frustration. Once the technical details are attended to, the nurse should concentrate on the approach to the child and the family. The initial greeting should show warmth and friendliness. Smile and introduce yourself to the family and the child. When addressing the child, position yourself at eye level. If the child is shy, talk to the parents first. Children may need time to feel comfortable. Speak in a quiet and unhurried manner. When the child and parents are taken to the child's room, parents should be seated comfortably. Explain the admission procedure carefully. Avoid discussing information in front of the child that he or she will not understand. The parents are encouraged to do as much for their child as possible, such as removing the child's clothes. This is also true throughout the hospital stay. Be prepared to meet the family's emotional needs because many parents are stressed when their child is hospitalized.

The admission form asks about the child's statistical information, health history, family history, lifestyle, and home routine. This includes questions about nutrition, elimination, sleep, activity, previous hospitalization, terminology used by the child, and so on. The

| Box 2-2 | Complementary and Alternative Medicine |

- Complementary therapy refers to nontraditional therapy that is used with traditional or conventional therapy.
- Alternative therapy replaces traditional or conventional therapy.
- In 2005, the American Academy of Pediatrics reaffirmed its position statement on CAM for children with chronic illnesses or disabilities. The AAP recommends that physicians provide balanced advice about therapeutic options, guard against bias, and establish a trusting relationship with families. Physicians need to be informed and be willing to actively listen to the family and child with a chronic illness, realizing that many families may want to provide CAM as a treatment option.
- Often, a perception exists that CAM is more "natural" and "does no harm." Some parents do not realize that herbal remedies can actually cause health problems for their children. The concept of "natural" may also disillusion parents.
- Consumers have no guarantee of quality because the Food and Drug Administration (FDA) does not require testing of herbal remedies for therapeutic or adverse effects.

questions are generally directed to the parent; the child can help answer if old enough. The nurse also inquires about the use of medications at home, including complementary medicine. Complementary and Alternative Medicine (CAM) is often used by parents with conventional treatments; the nurse needs to document the use of any alternative medicine products including herbs because of potential drug interactions or surgical complications (Box 2-2 and Table 2-1).

Safety Alert

All medications the child takes at home are recorded at the time of admission. Medications are reconciled not only on admission, but if the child is transferred, and also at discharge.

2010 National Patient Safety Goals, The Joint Commission. Retrieved from *www.jointcommission.org/PatientSafety/NationalPatientSafetyGoals*.

After essential admission information is documented (Figure 2-9), the nurse performs a systems review and physical examination of the child. Vital signs and measurements are obtained and recorded (see Chapter 3). Continued assessment findings are obtained and recorded throughout the stay.

SYSTEMS REVIEW

When examining the child, proceed in a general head-to-toe manner while collecting vital signs. In very young children, it is often helpful to examine heart,

Table 2-1	Selected Common Herbs and Uses
HERB	**TYPICAL USES/CONCERNS**
Echinacea *(Echinacea purpurea)*	Has traditionally been used to treat or prevent colds, flu, and other infections. Believed to stimulate the immune system to fight infections. May cause allergic reactions including rashes, increased asthma, and anaphylaxis. Gastrointestinal side effects have also been reported. NCCAM is studying the effects on the immune system and upper respiratory infections.
Ginkgo *(Gingko biloba)*	Used to treat asthma, bronchitis, fatigue, and tinnitus (ringing in the ears). Hope is to improve memory and improve dementia, decrease intermittent claudication, and treat sexual dysfunction, multiple sclerosis, and other health conditions. May cause headache, nausea, gastrointestinal upset, diarrhea, dizziness, or allergic skin reactions. May increase bleeding risk, so use caution with anticoagulant drugs, bleeding disorders, or scheduled surgery or dental procedures.
Kava *(Piper methysticum)*	Used to help people fall asleep and fight fatigue, as well as to treat asthma and urinary tract infections. Topically has been used as a numbing agent. Today is used primarily for anxiety, insomnia, and menopausal symptoms. May cause liver damage, hepatitis, or liver failure. The U.S. Food and Drug Administration has issued a warning that the use of kava supplements has been linked to a risk of severe liver damage, and NCCAM-funded studies on kava were suspended after the FDA warning.
St. John's wort *(Hypericum perforatum)*	Used for centuries to treat mental disorders and nerve pain. Also used as a sedative; treatment for malaria; and as a balm for wounds, burns, and insect bites. Used by some for depression, anxiety, and/or sleep disorders. Possible side effects include increased sensitivity to sunlight, anxiety, dry mouth, dizziness, gastrointestinal symptoms, fatigue, headache, or sexual dysfunction. May interact with indinavir, digoxin, warfarin, birth control pills, antidepressants, cyclosporine, and irinotecan. NCCAM is studying the use of St. John's wort in a wider spectrum of mood disorders, including minor depression.

Data from the National Center for Complementary and Alternative Medicine (NCCAM) Fact Sheets. (2005-2006). National Institutes of Health. Updated 2008. Retrieved from *http://nccam.nih.gov/health/herbsataglance.htm*.

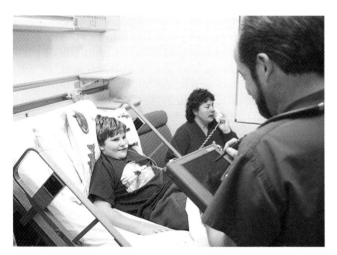

FIGURE 2-9 Documenting admission assessment findings in a computerized database organizes the information and makes it accessible to all health care providers.

lungs, and bowel sounds first, especially if the child is quiet. Children can sit up if they prefer during the examination, or the parent can hold the child during the exam. Keep the child warm during the examination. Perform the least distressing aspects of the examination before those that are more upsetting to the child. Use puppets or dolls to ease the anxiety of younger children. A simple magic trick can allay

anxiety. Explain procedures using simple language. Allow children to handle the equipment (e.g., the blood pressure cuff or stethoscope) before the examination, but keep potentially frightening equipment out of sight. Provide privacy, especially for older children and adolescents. Perform the most invasive procedures (such as rectal temperatures) last. In addition, always examine painful areas last. Discuss findings with the child (as age permits) and parents. Parents are often very interested in learning and appreciate the candor of the nurse. When finished with any procedure, praise the child and provide stickers or small toys as age permits.

Note the facial expression and general appearance of the child. Observe posture, positioning, and body movement. Note the hygiene, any odor, drainage, discharge, or unusual skin conditions. Determine the child's nutritional status and any growth or developmental alterations. Observe the child's behavior. If the child is not alert and responsive, the child may be seriously ill. Inform the nurse in charge immediately if the child is lethargic or unresponsive. Always talk to the parents about how *they* think their child is doing because they know their child best. Be sure to perform a systems review on all hospitalized children at least once a shift or as directed by hospital policy. All hospitals have a method of recording the systems review. Be sure to document and report any unusual or

Table 2-2   Review of Body Systems

Integument	Observe for odor, color, moisture, texture, scars, bruising, and lesions of the skin. Check for edema and turgor. Look at the hair for texture, quality, and distribution. Inspect the nails for color, shape, and condition.
Head and neck	Observe the shape and symmetry of the head; observe and palpate the fontanel. Inspect the neck for any masses or swollen lymph nodes. Observe range of motion of the neck.
Eyes and ears	Look for symmetry. Check for any drainage. Does the child have trouble seeing or hearing?
Nose and mouth	Check for any drainage, observe the oral mucosa for color and moisture; check condition of the teeth.
Chest and lungs	Evaluate respiratory rate, rhythm, and depth. Note any retractions. Check symmetry. Listen to breath sounds with a stethoscope utilizing a side-to-side sequence. Always compare both sides when auscultating lung sounds. Look at the color and consistency of sputum; note any cough. Note any breast development in females.
Heart	Note rate and rhythm of heartbeat with stethoscope. Listen for murmurs (blowing, swooshing sound).
Abdomen	Listen for bowel sounds in all quadrants. Note peristalsis, hernias. Check the umbilicus in the newborn for drainage, odor, and redness.
Genitalia and rectum	Observe for lesions, discharge, and descended testes. Note if the penis is circumcised or not. Observe for patency of the rectum.
Back and extremities	Look for curvature of the spine. Note gait, posture, and movement. Evaluate range of motion of extremities. Look for asymmetry of gluteal folds in an infant.

abnormal findings. Table 2-2 provides a review of the body systems.

All areas of the systems review are important. It is especially important, however, to note that when auscultating the heart and lungs, the heart should have a regular rhythm. If extra sounds are detected or if the rhythm is irregular, notify the nurse in charge. The lungs should be clear to auscultation with no **adventitious** or abnormal breath sounds. If wheezing, crackles, diminished lung sounds, or other unusual sounds are heard, report this to the nurse in charge also. Additional assessment information is located within each systems chapter.

CULTURAL AND RELIGIOUS PREFERENCES

The nurse must also be aware of cultural and religious preferences. Today, as in the past, cultural beliefs affect how a family perceives health and illness. Incorporation of cultural and religious awareness and understanding of the family structure are essential in providing competent nursing care. (See Chapter 4 for discussion on the family unit.) Each culture has its own beliefs and values. These values and beliefs are generally passed on from generation to generation. The more nurses know and understand different cultural beliefs, the easier it is to gain cooperation and trust from families. Holistic nursing includes awareness of cultural diversity and integration of this information with nursing care. It is important that one remain respectful and open-minded in discussions of cultural beliefs with the child and family. Beliefs generally cannot be changed, but the nurse should try to

negotiate with the family to achieve desired goals when caring for the child. The nurse needs to have an understanding of, and respect for, the beliefs of various cultures. When interviewing the family, it is crucial that one discuss cultural and religious preferences and determine the language that the family speaks most frequently. The nurse should discuss methods or preferences of treatment, any use of cultural and/or religious healers, and any home remedies that may have been used recently (Table 2-3).

Active listening is a key component of effective communication. Major blocks to listening are environmental distraction and premature judgment. Observe interactions with others to determine which body gestures (e.g., shaking hands or direct eye contact) are appropriate; ask when in doubt. Speak slowly and clearly to families with limited language comprehension. If possible, learn basic words and sentences of a family's language. Offer the services of an interpreter when necessary. When an interpreter is needed, be sure the interpreter knows the reason for the interview and the type of questions that will be asked. Try to use the same interpreter each time, to provide consistency. To avoid confusion, pose questions to elicit only one answer at a time. Refrain from interrupting the family member and interpreter while they are conversing. Avoid medical jargon whenever possible. These reminders help to bring down the communication barriers that exist when two people speak different languages.

The nurse also needs to determine whether practices and beliefs are beneficial to the child. Some

Table 2-3   Worldview: Examples of Cultural Influences on Health Care Beliefs and Practices

CULTURAL GROUP	HEALTH CARE BELIEFS AND PRACTICES
Mexican American	An individual who is believed to possess a special power admires or covets the child of another and looks at but does not touch the child can bring about *mal ojo* (evil eye). The remedy is for that individual to touch the child, or to mix a hen's egg with water and place this under the head of the child's bed (drives out the bad influence). Cold remedies are used to treat hot diseases, and hot remedies are used to treat cold diseases. Often seek *curandero,* or a folk healer, for treatment remedies and spiritual healing ceremonies. May be very modest when it comes to physical examination. Father has the dominant role; mother may influence decision making. Family values and roles need to be considered in the child's treatment and recovery.
African American	Believe illness can be from natural causes (exposure to wind, rain) or unnatural causes (witchcraft, voodoo, punishment for sin). "Granny" or "old lady" is woman in community with knowledge of herbs to treat common illnesses; many rely on folk remedies passed on from one generation to the next before seeking care from physician. "Spiritualist" will combine rituals, spiritual beliefs, and herbal medicines to cure ailments or illnesses. Some believe in the voodoo priest or priestess. Family structure is matrifocal or oriented around women.
Vietnamese American	Direct eye contact should be avoided when talking with someone who does not have equal standing in education, social standing, age, or gender. Beckoning with one's hand or finger with an upturned palm is the gesture used to beckon dogs and is considered insulting when used with people. Forces of yang (light, heat, or dryness), and yin (darkness, cold, or wetness) influence the balance and harmony of a person's state of health; an imbalance causes disease. Natural elements can cause illness, such as bad food or contaminated water. Medicinal herbs and therapeutic diets can counteract the effects of natural causes. Supernatural causes of disease may be from gods, demons, or spirits. The *shaman* can restore the individual's spirit. Copper or silver bracelets, necklaces, or anklets prevent the spirit from leaving. Germs may also cause illness. Antimicrobials have healing powers.
Chinese American	Forces of yang and yin influence the balance and harmony of a person's state of health. Excessive eye contact may be considered impolite. May not ask questions when they do not understand. Normally, do not touch another person during conversation. "Yes" may mean "I heard you" and not indicate agreement. Family is based on a hierarchical structure; boys may be valued more than girls. Colors and numbers may take on significance. The number 8 is lucky, as is the color red. The number 4 and the color white are considered unlucky. Traditional Chinese medicine is sought first before Western medicine. Acupuncture, herbal medicines, massage, and so on, are used as therapies to restore yin and yang. Cultural healing practices can cause visible bruising or injury to child's skin.
Navajo	Eye contact is considered a sign of disrespect. Pointing is considered insulting. Children are taught to respect tradition and are viewed as assets. It is taboo to touch a dead or dying person and items associated with death. Many members of the extended family will stay in or close to the hospital until the child is discharged. Must live in harmony with nature and supernatural forces. Medicine men and medicine women use sacred items for healing and blessing. Mother is responsible for domestic duties; father maintains the family and home.

Adapted from Giger, J., and Davidhizar, R. (2008). *Transcultural nursing* (5th ed.). St. Louis: Mosby.

practices raise concerns of abuse. An example of a cultural practice possibly considered abusive is *coining,* a Vietnamese practice that may produce weltlike lesions on the child's back when a coin, held on edge, is repeatedly rubbed lengthwise on the oiled skin to rid the body of disease (Figure 2-10). Families need to know that some strict disciplinary practices can place them in jeopardy with Child Protective Services.

Anticipatory guidance is an important intervention in exploring alternative means of discipline. However, any time beliefs and practices are detrimental to the health and welfare of the child, legal intervention may become necessary.

Religious beliefs also must be respected when caring for the child. Discussion with the family about religious beliefs and wishes is important. Many religions

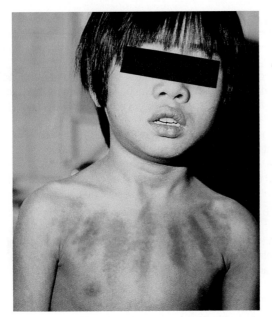

FIGURE 2-10 Oil is applied using vigorous stroking of the skin of a child with a fever. This produces a bruising pattern called *coining* and may be incorrectly interpreted as abuse.

Table 2-4	Global Perspective: Religious Dietary Practices
RELIGIOUS GROUP	**DIETARY PRACTICES**
Hinduism	Some sects are vegetarians. The belief is not to kill *any* living creature.
Buddhism	Some are vegetarians; many will fast on holy days.
Judaism	Some observe the kosher dietary restrictions (e.g., avoid pork and shellfish, do not prepare and eat milk and meat at the same time).
Jehovah's Witnesses	Members avoid food prepared with or containing blood.
Native Americans	Individual tribal beliefs influence food practices.
Islam	Prohibits consumption of pork; fasts during the month of Ramadan.

Modified from Potter, A., and Perry, A. (2009). *Fundamentals of nursing* (7th ed.). St Louis: Mosby Elsevier.

have special rites or practices that need to be respected. Religion is an important aspect of health care. Many religions have health care beliefs that could affect the health of the child. Roman Catholics have the priest perform "last rites" for those who are seriously ill. Jehovah's Witnesses may not allow blood transfusions. The court sometimes must take action on the child's behalf. In the Jewish religion, circumcision is performed on the eighth day of life by a trained *mohel* in the baby's home (Giger and Davidhizar, 2008). In the Muslim faith, cremation is not permitted. Religions may also have dietary restrictions the nurse needs to be alert to. These are discussed in Table 2-4.

CARE PLANS AND CRITICAL PATHWAYS

Most hospitals and institutions use nursing care plans—individualized guidelines for care of the child and family. Some hospitals use preprinted, standardized care plans that are broad in nature and can be individualized to a particular child. Care plans serve as communication tools among members of the health care team. They are a written expression of the nursing process. They state specifically what is to be done for each child and keep the focus on the child, not on the condition or the therapy. Care plans should be reviewed and updated daily. Nursing care plans appear throughout this book to illustrate the treatment of selected illnesses.

Because hospital stays, even for acutely ill children or those who have had major surgery, are becoming shorter (sometimes only 24 to 48 hours), many hospitals use written care plans and critical pathways.

Critical pathways (also referred to as *clinical pathways*) convert expected medical, nursing, social, and emotional outcomes for a particular problem into actions necessary to achieve the outcomes within a specified time frame. Additional information regarding the care of the child is discussed in a report. Box 2-3 and Figure

---

Box 2-3	Asthma Decision Points

ON ADMISSION
1. Initiate age appropriate asthma education on Get Well Network.
2. Initiate intervention regarding activity tolerance, rounds, education, etc.

BY HOUR 6
1. Is child on room air? If not, do we have them up moving around?
2. If not tolerating ambulation, may suggest incentive spirometry or bubbles for younger children.
3. Encourage PO intake. Offer choices.
4. Find out if child has a home nebulizer.
5. Does child need asthma education?

BY HOUR 12
1. Continue to encourage ambulation.
2. Does child have a primary care physician? If not, may need social work consult to assist with needs for management of asthma.
3. Does the family have any other need for resources?

Decision Points are clinical pathways developed for a variety of diagnoses on a short stay unit. They use a plain language checklist and clinical expectation timeline to guide nurses in planning care.
Information courtesy of Cook Children's Medical Center, Ft. Worth, TX. Used with permission.

ASTHMA

5 Pavilion Report

Patient Name_____ Age_____

Diagnosis_____Allergies_____

Time of arrival to 5P_____

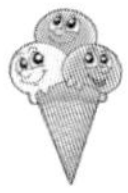

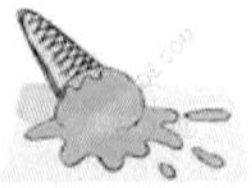

Specific symptoms that caused patient to be admitted_____

_____

Duration of symptoms_____

Significant medical history_____

Has the patient ever been admitted to the hospital with asthma?_____

Ever been admitted to the ICU?_____

IV location_____D51/2+20KCI@_____Other_____

What medications are ordered?_____

Where is pt with neb treatments?_____

Are there any social issues that need to be addressed (e.g., insurance, transportation, car seat)?

_____

_____

Have vital signs been within acceptable range?_____

O_2 settings_____Sats_____ Lung sounds?_____

What interventions have been done to improve lung volume, and how is patient tolerating?

_____

Does patient have a home neb?_____MDI?_____Spacer?_____PCP?_____

Did they get asthma education consult?_____ Did they collect a mycoplasma? ___

What specific Decision Points have not been accomplished, preventing discharge?

_____

FIGURE 2-11 Report form to accompany Asthma Decision Points.

2-11 depict a clinical pathway and report information that would be obtained for a child with asthma. Nurses need to be especially vigilant with critical pathways to ensure that teaching and preparation for discharge are adequately provided for the child and family and that the appropriate referrals are made for follow-up care and health promotion.

DISCHARGE PLANNING

Ideally, preparation for the child's discharge begins on admission, because the goal of hospitalization is to return a more healthy and happy child to the parents. Good physical management of the child's disease is necessary, but this is not enough. The nurse must also consider the emotional growth of the child and the education of the child and family. This should provide a positive learning experience for all involved.

If a child needs specific home treatment, such as hyperalimentation, colostomy care, crutches, a special diet, or insulin therapy, instructions should be given to the parents gradually throughout their child's hospitalization. These instructions should be provided in writing so that parents can refer to them as needed. If older children are to administer any treatments to themselves, they need careful explanations and supervision until both they and the parents are confident that the procedure will be carried out correctly at home. This may require home health care services.

Parents must also be prepared for behavioral problems that may arise after hospitalization. Severe stress is obvious during the child's stay and requires in-service care and professional follow-up. In guiding the parents, the following suggestions may prove helpful:

- Recognize that after hospitalization the child may display such behaviors as clinging, regression in bowel and bladder control, aggression, fears, nightmares, and negativism.
- Allow the child to become a participating family member as soon as possible. Return former family responsibilities within the limits of the child's present abilities.
- Try not to make the child the center of attention simply because of the illness. Praise accomplishments unrelated to it.
- Be kind, firm, and consistent if the child misbehaves.
- Be truthful so that the child continues to trust you.
- Provide suitable play materials such as clay, paints, and doctor and nurse kits. Allow free play.
- Listen to the child, and clear up any misconceptions about the illness.
- Do not leave the child alone for a long period or overnight until a sense of security is regained.
- Allow the child to visit hospital staff when returning for routine clinic visits.

Whenever possible, parents should be given as much notice of their child's discharge from the hospital as possible so that they can make necessary arrangements. This is particularly important if both parents work or if transportation is a problem. First, the physician writes the discharge order. Next, the approximate hour of dismissal is relayed to the parents. The intravenous (IV) or heparin lock is removed (as ordered by the physician), the child is dressed, and all personal belongings are collected. Parents are given any prescriptions written by the doctor, and discharge paperwork is completed. Most hospitals have a special discharge sheet that provides the family with written instructions regarding medications, diet, activity, and any other special precautions or procedures the child may need. The nurse prepares the discharge sheet, reviews it with the parent to determine understanding, and then has the parent sign the sheet. A copy is given to the parent, and a copy is retained on the child's chart. Parents visit the hospital business office according to hospital procedure. According to condition, the child usually is placed in a hospital wagon, wheelchair, or stretcher and accompanies the family to the exit. The nurse assists the child into the car as needed. State law requires that parents have car seats for infants and small children. Families without car seats may be provided with them on either a permanent or a loan basis. Charting includes time of departure and person with whom the child departs, the child's behavior (smiling, alert, crying), method of transportation from the unit, any instructions or medications given to the child or parents, and possibly the child's weight and vital signs. Always check the institution's policy on dismissal.

 Nursing Brief

Discharge planning includes the identification and follow-up of children who may be at risk for child abuse, neglect, poverty, or a number of other conditions associated with their health problem or family lifestyle.

SAFETY

The nurse must be especially conscious of safety measures in any area where children are cared for. This includes physician offices, outpatient surgery centers, clinics, and inpatient hospital units. By showing concern about safety regulations, nurses not only reduce unnecessary accidents but also set a good example for the parents of children who are placed in their care.

DO

- Wash your hands before and after caring for each child.
- Check wheelchairs and stretchers before placing children in them.
- Use safety straps with children when they are in a highchair, swing, infant seat, stroller, and so on.
- Always look for small objects that can become choking hazards.
- Inspect toys for sharp edges and removable parts.
- Apply restraints correctly to prevent constriction of a part. Check institutional policy on frequency of releasing restraints and providing range of motion.
- Identify the child properly before giving medications.
- Keep medications and solutions out of reach of the child.
- Keep the medication room locked when not in use.
- Keep lotions, tissues, disposable pads and diapers, and safety pins out of the infant's reach.
- Handle infants and small children carefully. Use elevators rather than stairs. Walk at the child's pace.
- Locate fire exits and extinguishers on the unit, and learn how to use them properly. Become familiar with the facility's fire manual.
- Protect children from entering the treatment room, elevator, utility rooms, and stairwells.
- Keep crib sides up at all times when the child is unattended in bed. Use enclosed (bubble top) cribs for older infants and toddlers to keep them from falling or climbing out of the crib.
- Turn an infant *perpendicular* to the side of the bed when rails are down. This helps ensure that the infant will not roll off when side rails are down.
- Place a hand on the infant's or child's back or abdomen when you turn your back to the child (Figure 2-12).
- Place cribs so that children cannot reach electrical outlets and appliances.

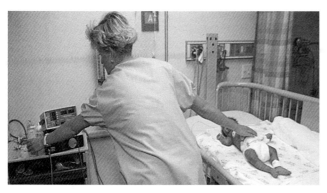

FIGURE 2-12 Safety is always a priority. The nurse maintains hand contact when her back is turned.

- Supervise playroom activity.
- Prevent cross-infection. Diapers, toys, and materials that belong in one child's unit should not be borrowed for another child's use. Properly disinfect any item brought out of an isolation room.
- Take proper precautions when oxygen is in use.
- Use electrical outlet safety plugs on the unit.
- Check hospital policy for children who are alone (for instance, policy may recommend that the door be kept open).

 Safety Alert

Identify child by Identiband and at least one other identifier, such as date of birth or medical record number. *Never* use the room number as an identifier.

DO NOT

- Do not prop nursing bottles or force-feed small children. There is a danger of choking, which may cause lung disease or sudden death.
- Do not allow ambulatory children to use wheelchairs or stretchers as toys.
- Do not leave a child unattended in a highchair, infant seat, or swing.
- Do not leave a child unattended on an examination table. *Always* keep your hand on the child.
- Do not leave medications at the bedside.
- Do not leave any medication administration materials in the child's bed or infant's crib.
- Do not leave a child unattended in an infant seat if it is placed on any area above the floor.
- Do not leave small children unattended out of their cribs in their rooms.
- Do not leave a child unattended in the bathtub.

Many other safety measures must be carried out as each nurse becomes more familiar with the hazards of individual units. The nurse needs to continually assess the setting for safety issues.

 Nursing Brief

QSEN (Quality & Safety Education for Nurses) is a comprehensive resource for quality and safety education for nurses. Nurses are able to gain the knowledge, skills, and attitudes to continuously improve health care for promoting quality and safety competency in nursing (*www.qsen.org*).

TRANSPORTING, POSITIONING, AND RESTRAINING THE CHILD

The means by which the child is transported within the unit and to other parts of the hospital depends on age, level of consciousness, and how far the child has to travel. Older children are transported in the same way as adults. Younger children are often transported in their cribs, in a wagon or wheelchair, or on a stretcher. The side rails on a stretcher are raised during transport. Ensure that the child's identification band is secured before leaving the unit. A notation is made about where the child is being taken and for what purpose.

Figure 2-13 shows three safe methods for holding a baby. Head and back support is necessary for young infants. The movements of small children are often random and uncoordinated; therefore they must be held securely. The football hold is useful when one hand needs to be free, such as for bathing the baby's head.

Restraints should rarely be used in the care of children because they restrict movement, limit autonomy, and create distress. Today's health care facilities and regulating agencies clearly specify policies regarding application of restraints. When necessary, they are used to immobilize a child for diagnostic and therapeutic procedures and for safety. Documentation is required that identifies why restraints are necessary and what type of restraint is used. Restraint may be accomplished by simply holding the child or using the *least* restrictive type of physical device. Many procedures can be performed when a child is held in a secure, comfortable manner that provides close physical contact with the parent or caregiver (therapeutic holding). An example of therapeutic holding is when a parent securely holds the child for an injection. Restraint should be used only when other measures have failed and *never* as punishment. When restraint is necessary, it must be accompanied by increased emotional support such as rooming-in, additional attention from nurses, and suitable diversions. Always keep the child's safety in mind when choosing the appropriate restraint. Restraints must be checked every 1 to 2 hours or more frequently as necessary, depending on the circumstances. To ensure that they are applied correctly, they also need to be *removed at least* every 1-2 hours so that they do not impair circulation or sensation, or compromise skin integrity. *Always*

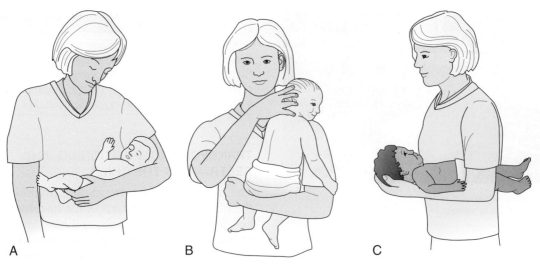

A   B   C

FIGURE 2-13 Three safe ways to hold a baby. **A,** The cradle position. **B,** The upright position. **C,** The football position.

Table 2-5	Restraints for Children
RESTRAINT*	**DESCRIPTION**
Mummy	Immobilizes infant or small child for short time while procedure is performed or child is examined. Arms and legs are secured so that child cannot wiggle free. Useful for starting scalp IVs or performing nasogastric insertion.
Elbow (sometimes referred to as "no-no's")	Keeps child from reaching face or head. Covers most of arm. Must be correct size and positioned so that it does not rub against axilla or wrist. Useful for preventing touching of face, IV line, and so on.
Jacket	Keeps child in bed, chair, or wheelchair. Tied in back of child and to frame of bed. Never tied to side rails.

*Check all restraints at least every 1 to 2 hours.

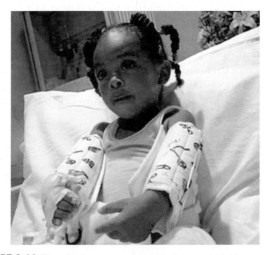

FIGURE 2-14 The most common form of elbow restraint is a padded, firm material that reaches from just below the axilla to the wrist.

check the institution policy on restraint use. Table 2-5 describes some restraints for children. Figure 2-14 depicts a child in elbow restraints.

MEDICAL ASEPSIS

The purpose of the medical aseptic technique is to prevent the spread of infection from one child to another or from the child to the nurse. A person (or object) is considered contaminated if that person has touched an infected child or any equipment that has come in contact with the child. People or articles that have not had any contact with the child are considered clean.

Articles that have come in direct contact with the child must be disinfected before they can be used by others. When something is disinfected, microorganisms in or on it are killed physically or chemically. The autoclave, which uses steam under pressure, is considered effective in killing most germs when the article is adequately exposed and sterilized for the proper length of time. The autoclave is used for certain nondisposable reusable items only. Items such as highchairs, IV line poles, cribs, and so forth must be properly disinfected (by chemical means) before the next child can use them. Disinfection is done according to hospital policy, usually by the housekeeping department. Disposable items, such as needles, syringes, suction catheters, lumbar puncture trays, suture sets, nursing bottles, and oxygen tubing, are supplied to hospitals for medical asepsis purposes.

Nursing Brief

Used needles are not recapped and should be disposed of in a properly labeled, puncture-proof container. These special containers should be available in each patient room and in other areas where disposal is likely.

PREVENTING THE TRANSMISSION OF INFECTION

Children in the hospital need to be protected from nosocomial (hospital-acquired) infections. Likewise, health care workers need to be protected from infectious agents transmitted by children. Any child who is suspected of having a contagious disease must be isolated until a definite diagnosis has been established. The Centers for Disease Control and Prevention (CDC) publish guidelines for isolation precautions that are readily available in health care institutions. These guidelines are usually located in an infection control manual. Many hospitals also have an infection control department with personnel who are specially trained to be resources in the hospital.

Pediatric hospitals and smaller children's units in general hospitals have isolation rooms or isolation setups. The nurse admitting the child must follow isolation protocol. The purpose of the medical aseptic technique is to prevent the spread of the disease to the nurse and others. Proper hand hygiene cannot be overemphasized.

The child is admitted to a private room. Equipment for daily care is placed in the room. This equipment includes a thermometer, stethoscope, bath equipment, and so on. Such equipment remains there until the child is discharged, and then it is disinfected. Disposable equipment is discarded in the proper receptacle. Linen is usually changed daily. Having on hand an ample supply of gowns, masks, and gloves also saves time and energy. A clean area is prepared according to hospital procedure. Remember that the floor is always considered contaminated. Anything that touches the floor must be properly cleaned or discarded (in or out of isolation). Toys must be washable. They may be borrowed from the playroom but must be disinfected before they can be returned. Because there is no satisfactory method of disinfecting books, reading should be limited to magazines or materials that are not highly prized by the owner. In the case of highly communicable diseases, reading material is discarded when the child is discharged.

When blood pressure is taken, a disposable blood pressure cuff is used. Built-in wall units reduce the danger of contamination. If electronic blood pressure equipment is used, it must be disinfected after use and before taking it into another patient room. When a flashlight, otoscope, or ophthalmoscope is used, it is protected by a technique paper. Any equipment that comes in direct contact with the child must be disinfected. All the specimens that leave the room are placed in a clean outer container according to hospital procedure. The hot water and detergents used in hospital dishwashers are sufficient to decontaminate dishes, glasses, cups, and eating utensils, so no special precautions are needed.

Throughout this book, emphasis is placed on the role of the nurse in preparing a safe environment for the child and parents. Of all the dangers in surroundings, none is more serious than disease-bearing organisms. Nurses must understand the importance of protecting themselves and others. This is accomplished with standard precautions. Standard precautions are followed because a history and physical examination cannot identify all patients infected with HIV or other blood-borne pathogens. Therefore body fluid precautions are taken with *all* patients. In addition to standard precautions, transmission-based precautions are designed to prevent/interrupt transmission of pathogens in the hospital. The three types of transmission-based precautions include *airborne, droplet,* and *contact* precautions (see Appendix B). Although it is vital to remember and use precautionary measures, the nurse must not forget that the patient is the primary concern. As the student's confidence increases with repetition of the details of isolation, the approach to the patient and the patient's problems is also more effective.

The following are specific techniques to be used with standard and transmission-based precautions.

Hand Hygiene

Hand hygiene is the most important barrier against transmission of disease. Hands should be washed before and after contact with every patient, regardless of whether or not the nurse wore gloves during the contact. Gloves may be torn during use, and hands can become contaminated if the gloves are not properly removed. Many hospitals use gels or foams that do not require water. Dispensers are affixed either just outside or just inside the patient's door. Using these on entry and exit is now a requirement of most facilities. Soap and water are still required for visible soiling and for *Clostridium difficile (C. diff)* organisms.

Gloves

Gloves are worn to protect the health care worker from contact with pathogens. They must be worn when health care workers are likely to have contact with mucous membranes, nonintact skin, blood, body fluids, secretions, excretions, and contaminated items. Gloves must be changed between patient contacts.

Masks

Masks are worn to protect the health care worker from pathogens that are shed through respiratory droplets. A mask is also worn if there is a risk of blood or body fluid being splashed or splattered. A supply of disposable masks is kept outside the child's room or in a designated location on the nursing unit. A fresh one should be donned each time the health care worker enters the room. A mask is used once and discarded. It should *never* be allowed to hang around the neck and then be placed back over the face. It should cover the nose and mouth and should be changed at least once every hour. Do not touch a mask once it is in place. Remove it after removing the gown when leaving the unit, and do not touch the part that comes in contact with the face. Discard the mask in the room.

Gowns

When giving direct care to the child in isolation, the health care worker wears a gown to protect clothing from contamination. A gown is also worn to protect skin when procedures and patient care activities are likely to generate splashes or sprays of blood or body fluids. Without a gown, bacteria and other disease-causing organisms could be carried on the uniform, endangering the health of other patients. Sweaters should not be worn in isolation units. On the children's unit, the nurse must be particularly conscientious because small children need to be held for feedings and comforting. The nurse's relationship with the child is very direct. Caregivers wear disposable paper gowns that are used only once and then discarded. When the gown is put on, it is tied in the back. To remove, first untie the waist strings and the neckband, remove gloves if worn, and then discard. Remember to wash your hands. Use technique papers to open the door. Be sure to discard these papers in the patient's room and to close the door. The health care worker's shoes are always a source of contamination, so hands need to be thoroughly washed if they come into contact with shoes. Contaminated linen and trash are disposed of according to hospital procedure.

Protective Eyewear

Goggles or face shields are worn if there is a risk of blood or body fluid being splashed or splattered. They are for one-time use and are disposed of with the trash.

EDUCATION OF THE FAMILY

Visitors are usually restricted to members of the immediate family. Check the hospital policy on sibling visits. Isolation information is posted near the patient's door. Box 2-4 lists patient and family teaching tips when the child is in isolation.

Education of family members is an ongoing process. Points that need to be emphasized include the importance of immunizing children, the proper care of food (particularly perishables), the proper cooking of meats, the need for cleanliness in food preparation, and the importance of hand hygiene. Review with the family the primary ways in which infectious diseases are spread. Other modes of transmission, such as crowded

Box 2-4	Patient/Family Teaching Tips for the Child in Isolation

Wash hands on entering and exiting.
Gowns, masks, and even gloves may be required while in the child's room.
Articles brought to the child must be washable or disposable.
Always remove gowns, masks, and gloves before leaving the child's room.
Do not take articles from the room.

living conditions, insects and rodents, and sandbox hazards, may also be topics to explore.

IMPLICATIONS OF PEDIATRIC SURGERY

The pediatric surgical patient needs to be shown the part of the body that requires surgery. The nurse can sketch a body outline and draw a circle around the operative site. The nurse should give simple information about the system that will be affected and stress that this is the only area of the body that will be involved. It may also be helpful to use anatomically correct dolls. The nurse must be careful if any procedure involves the genital area, especially if the child is a preschool boy. Preschool boys are very afraid of castration. Therefore, when possible, the male child should be allowed to look at his penis after the procedure to reassure himself that it has been fixed and not cut off.

Safety Alert

The procedure site is to be marked, and a "time-out" is conducted immediately before starting an invasive procedure or making the incision

National Patient Safety Goals, The Joint Commission, 2010.

Children need to know what to expect on the day of surgery. Whenever possible, the child should attend a preoperative class. Children are particularly fearful of surgery and need both physical and psychological preparation. The child should be able to easily understand explanations and information. In addition, listening to the child is especially valuable for clarifying misunderstandings. Ask the child to point to the operative site on a body outline and then ask, "Can you show me what they are going to fix?" After explaining anesthesia, allow the child to play with the mask (Figure 2-15). Both children and adults need reassurance that they will not awaken during surgery. Be careful of expressions such as being "put to sleep" because a child may associate this phrase with the death of a pet. It is important to always be truthful

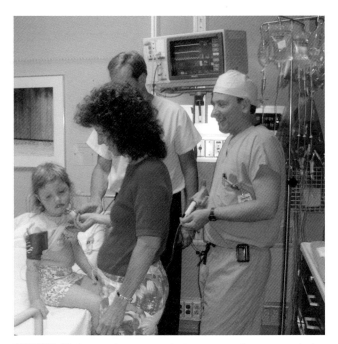

FIGURE 2-15 A parent's presence in the preoperative area can help reduce the child's separation anxiety.

because this establishes trust. A short waiting time reduces anxiety. Finally, nursing interventions after surgery are aimed at helping the child master a threatening situation and at minimizing physical and psychological complications. (See the Index for specific surgical procedures.)

Tables 2-6 and 2-7 summarize preparation for surgery and postoperative care.

THE CHILD IN PAIN

DEFINITION AND CHALLENGES

Pain in children has long been researched. Historically, children have not always been medicated properly for pain control. There is still a concern that pain in children is not controlled appropriately. It is now known that children of all ages experience pain and are entitled to appropriate pain management. Pain is an individual, subjective experience, and health care providers need to identify and treat pain adequately. Pain is considered the fifth vital sign and is to be

Table 2-6 Preparation of the Child for Surgery

PROCEDURE	MODIFICATION
Consent	Parent or legal guardian
Lab work	Age-appropriate restraint
Urinalysis	Age-appropriate collection (U-bag) Assist school child Age-appropriate instructions
Evaluation for illness	Use more objective observations in infants and toddlers because of limited verbal skills
Allergies	Indicate clearly on chart and patient wrist band
NPO	May increase fluids before NPO; IV generally started Length of time may vary with age and type of surgery (6 to 12 hours) Remove goodies from bedside stand No gum Supervise hungry ambulatory patients carefully
Vital signs	Approach child carefully, explain, demonstrate
Void before surgery	Not always possible in infants and toddlers
Gown	Hospital gown; may wear underwear or pajama bottoms depending on age, type of surgery
Identification	Identification bracelet
Teeth	Check for loose teeth, orthodontic appliance
Skin preparation	May be done in operating room
Nails	Remove nail polish
Glasses or contact lenses	Have children and adolescents remove glasses and contact lenses
Enemas	Not routine
Transportation	Crib or stretcher Parents may accompany to OR door
Emotional preparation	Preoperative tour Group and individual puppet play Body drawings of parts involved Support parents during surgery
Sedation	In pre-op holding area
Record all pertinent data	On patient chart

NPO, Nothing by mouth.

Table 2-7	Summary of Postoperative Care of the Child
PROCEDURE	**MODIFICATION**
Return from recovery room	Notify parents (parents may be allowed in recovery room) Smaller patients generally in crib Age-appropriate safety precautions
Note general condition, alertness	Evaluate per pain scale as appropriate
Vital signs	Every 15 to 30 minutes until stable
Assessment of operative site for bleeding, dressing intactness	Monitor as ordered Elevate casted extremities Circle drainage
Restraints	May be necessary to protect IV line and other tubes (e.g., NG, catheter) Remove periodically for range of motion per hospital policy
Connect dependent drainage (urinary catheter), Levin tubes, oxygen	Prepare child for sight and noises of equipment, teach purpose of tubes, and so on.
Position patient	As ordered
IVs	Infusion pump with ordered rate Measure and record I&O (intake and output)
Assess elimination	Record I&O
Relief of pain	Hold, comfort small children unless contraindicated Evaluate pain according to pain scale suitable for developmental level of child Administer pain relievers as ordered Involve parents in care Provide transitional object such as blanket, favorite toy, pacifier Be aware of transcultural considerations that provide familiarity and comfort
NPO	Until fully awake Babies are started on clear fluids by bottle unless contraindicated Monitor bowel sounds
Consider diet	Advance from clear to full liquids to soft to regular diet
Observe for complications	Turn, cough, deep-breathe, dangle feet, ambulate early; less of a problem in children; splint operative site (with small pillow) when child coughs

NPO, Nothing by mouth.

documented as such. In 2001, the American Pain Society wrote a policy statement in collaboration with the American Academy of Pediatrics (AAP) to ensure that all children receive adequate treatment of pain *(http://aappolicy.aappublications.org/).*

EVALUATION

When evaluating pain in children, always ask them about past pain experiences and known coping mechanisms. Also ask the parents about the child's past pain experiences. Be sure to identify words the child uses for pain, reaction to pain, and management of pain.

In addition, when evaluating the child, include precipitating factors, location, onset, duration, quality, intensity, and characteristics of the pain. Assess the physiologic characteristics of pain. Observe behavioral and nonverbal cues as well. For accurate assessment of pain, several pain scales have been developed. Depending on the developmental stage, children use different strategies to deal with pain. Pain is assessed

using self-report if the child is old enough. Similar to adults, most older school-age children and adolescents are able to report pain on a scale of 1 to 10. A pictorial tool often used for preschool and young school-age children is the Wong-Baker FACES Pain Rating Scale (Figure 2-16). With this tool, the child looks at several pictures of faces ranging from happy to sad and then chooses whichever face reflects his or her pain. A second pictorial pain assessment tool is the Oucher Scale for 3-year-old to 7-year-old children. It consists of six photographs of a Caucasian child's face representing levels ranging from "no hurt" to "biggest hurt you could ever have" and includes a vertical scale with numbers from 0 to 100. There are scales for African-American and Hispanic children also.

For infants and very young children, behavior is observed to assess pain. The FLACC (Face, Legs, Activity, Cry, and Consolability) scale is one tool that can be used for this young age group (Table 2-8). The FLACC scale measures each of the five identified categories on

FACES PAIN RATING SCALE* (WONG AND BAKER, 1988)

Consists of 6 cartoon faces ranging from smiling face for "no pain" to tearful face for "worst pain"

Original instructions:
Explain to child that each face is for a person who feels happy because there is no pain (hurt) or sad because there is some or a lot of pain. FACE 0 is very happy because there is no hurt. FACE 1 hurts just a little bit. FACE 2 hurts a little more. FACE 3 hurts even more. FACE 4 hurts a whole lot, but FACE 5 hurts as much as you can imagine, although you don't have to be crying to feel this bad. Ask child to choose face that best describes own pain. Record number under chosen face on pain assessment record.

Brief word instructions:
Point to each face using the words to describe the pain intensity. Ask child to choose face that best describes own pain, and record appropriate number.

For children as young as 3 years. Using original instructions without affect words, such as happy or sad, or brief words resulted in same range of pain rating, probably reflecting child's rating of pain intensity. For coding purposes, numbers 0, 2, 4, 6, 8, 10 can be substituted for 0-5 system to accommodate 0-10 system.

FACES provides three scales in one: facial expressions, numbers, and words.

Research supports cultural sensitivity of FACES for Caucasian, African-American, Hispanic, Thai, Chinese, and Japanese children.

| 0 No hurt | 1 or 2 Hurts little bit | 2 or 4 Hurts little more | 3 or 6 Hurts even more | 4 or 8 Hurts whole lot | 5 or 10 Hurts worst |

FIGURE 2-16 Wong's Faces of Pain Rating Scale.

Table 2-8 FLACC Scale

CATEGORY	SCORE 0	1	2
Face	No particular expression or smile	Occasional grimace or frown, withdrawn, disinterested	Frequent to constant frown, clenched jaw, quivering chin
Legs	Normal position or relaxed	Uneasy, restless, tense	Kicking or legs drawn up
Activity	Lying quietly, normal position, moves easily	Squirming, shifting back and forth, tense	Arched, rigid, or jerking
Cry	No cry (awake or asleep)	Moans or whimpers, occasional complaint	Crying steadily, screams or sobs, frequent complaints
Consolability	Content, relaxed	Reassured by occasional touching, hugging, or talking to; distractible	Difficult to console or comfort

From Merkel, S.I., Voepel-Lewis, T., Shayevitz, J.R., et al. (1997). The FLACC: a behavioral scale for scoring postoperative pain in young children. *Pediatr Nurs,* 23(3), 293-297. Used with permission. © The Regents of the University of Michigan and the University of Michigan Health System. Can be reproduced for clinical and research use.

a scale of 0 to 2, resulting in a total score between 0 and 10. According to the tool, the higher the total score, the more pain the child is experiencing.

INTERVENTION

Nursing Care Plan 2-1 provides examples of nursing diagnoses related to pain in children. Management of pain in children includes pharmacologic interventions. Physicians will order pain medications for children depending on the intensity of the pain. Oral administration is generally used for mild to moderate pain. When the child needs immediate pain relief for more intense pain, intravenous administration is indicated. For moderate to severe pain expected to persist, continuous dosing or around-the-clock dosing at fixed intervals is recommended. Dosage is always adjusted, depending on patient response. When giving opioids or nonopioids, be sure the dosages are appropriate for the child's weight and age. (See Chapter 3 for dosage calculations.) Pediatric drug reference books are readily

⭐ Nursing Care Plan 2-1   **The Child in Pain**

NURSING DIAGNOSIS *Pain, acute, related to surgery, injury, etc.*

Goals/Outcome Criteria	Interventions	Rationale

Patient demonstrates decrease in pain, as evidenced by:
  Vocalizing decreased pain
  Nonverbal signs (relaxed body position, decreased crying)
  Vital signs within normal limits
	Assess and record subjective and objective signs of pain
	Use an assessment tool to measure pain
	Use nonpharmacologic techniques of pain control as needed
	Use pharmacologic methods to control pain as needed
	
	Include the parents in the care
	
	Medicate before painful procedures
	Monitor vital signs at least every 4 hours
	
	Evaluate follow-up to pain medication (generally within 15 to 30 minutes)
		Documentation serves as a baseline and ongoing evaluation
		Provides for consistency in assessment
		May be less painful; child has control
		
		Keeping pain under control helps child move more easily, preventing complications of immobilization
		Parents' presence may reduce fear and anxiety, therefore reducing the amount of pain experienced
		Helps child cope with painful procedures
		Changes can indicate a change in level of pain
		To ensure that the pain medication was effective

NURSING DIAGNOSIS *Anxiety related to anticipation of pain*

Goals/Outcome Criteria	Interventions	Rationale

Child shows a decrease in anxiety by:
  Verbalizing decreased anxiety
  Decreased crying
  Interacting with staff
  Participating in activities
	Assign a consistent caregiver
	Involve parents in care of child
	Explain all procedures to child
	
	Follow home rituals when possible
	Allow the older child some control
	Reassure preschool children that they are not to blame for illness and are not being punished
		Can make child more at ease
		Reduces anxiety
		Knowing what to expect helps reduce anxiety
		Routines make child less anxious
		Control helps child cope with situation
		Are "magical thinkers" and believe they can cause illness

Critical Thinking Question

1. How does the nurse identify and treat pain in an infant versus pain in a school-age child?

---

available in hospitals that care for children. Safe dosage guidelines should *always* be followed.

Nonopioid analgesics are often used to control children's pain. They are most effective for mild to moderate pain and have antipyretic effects as well. They do not produce dependence or tolerance, but recommended/prescribed dosages must be carefully followed. Examples of nonopioid analgesics are acetaminophen and ibuprofen.

Opioids are used to manage most forms of moderate to severe acute and chronic pain. They can be administered by most routes; generally, they are given orally or intravenously. Although opioid analgesics can cause psychological and physical dependence, it is important not to withhold pain medication when this type of pain control is necessary. Tolerance or physical dependence may develop if opioids are used over a long period of time. Reducing doses over several days will help prevent withdrawal symptoms. Side effects of opioids may include respiratory depression, sedation, mental confusion, constipation, pruritus, nausea, and/or vomiting. Children often sleep after receiving

an analgesic, but this does not mean they are pain free. Always evaluate the opioid's effect on pain, and monitor vital signs after administering any analgesic. Examples of opioids commonly given orally in pediatrics are codeine and oxycodone; morphine is often given by the IV route. In pediatrics, the use of meperidine (Demerol) is controversial and therefore uncommon.

Pain medication may also be administered rectally, by intramuscular (IM) injection, transdermally, or topically. The subcutaneous and intranasal routes are also mentioned in the literature but are seldom used. The rectal route is occasionally used. Acetaminophen suppositories, for example, may be ordered rectally if the child has been vomiting or has difficulty swallowing. Children generally fear needles; therefore the IM route is rarely used. The transdermal route (patch) is generally reserved for chronic pain control. Topical application is often aimed at eliminating or reducing pain from most procedures involving skin puncture (intramuscular injection or intravenous insertion). EMLA (eutectic mixture of local anesthetics) cream is one example. It must be applied as a "dollop" over the site and covered by an occlusive dressing 1 hour or more before the procedure to be effective. The anesthetic cream LMX can also be used; it only requires 30 minutes prior to the skin puncture in order to be effective. Vapocoolant sprays also may be used immediately before injections. In addition, the intradermal route is often used for local (skin) anesthesia such as lidocaine (Xylocaine). Finally, nonnutritive sucking is effective as is concentrated sucrose with or without nonnutritive sucking when an infant is undergoing a painful procedure (Hockenberry and Wilson, 2009).

Patient-controlled analgesia (PCA) has also been used successfully with children. Typically, children are old enough to understand PCA when they are school age and older. This programmable infusion pump is used to self-administer medication boluses at preset dose and time intervals, generally via the IV route. There is a lockout interval between doses so that the patient cannot inadvertently self-deliver too much medication. Morphine is often the drug of choice to use with the PCA pump. The epidural/intrathecal route has been used successfully when short-term or long-term analgesia is needed. The direct effect of the analgesia (in the epidural space of the spinal column) produces few and rare side effects.

Pain management may also include nonpharmacologic interventions, which may be used in conjunction with pharmacologic interventions or by themselves. Such interventions are often referred to as *complementary or alternative medicine (CAM)*, and it is important to evaluate the success of these methods as well. For instance, music therapy (Figure 2-17) may be used to promote guided imagery or relaxation. (See Chapter 22 for a discussion of guided imagery, relaxation, biofeedback, and distraction.) Hypnosis is another complementary form of pain management. In this altered state of consciousness, suggestions can lead to changes in behavior or, in the case of pain, altered physical sensations (The National Pain Foundation, 2006). The

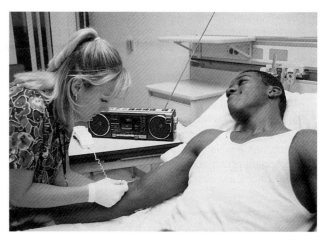

FIGURE 2-17 The adolescent listens to soothing music to promote relaxation and coping during stressful procedures.

TENS (transcutaneous electric nerve stimulation) *unit* has also proven helpful in pain management and uses electric stimulation to relieve pain. *Acupuncture* is based on a theory that energy, or *chi*, flows through the body along channels (meridians) that are connected by acupuncture points. Pain occurs when the flow of energy is obstructed. With insertion of fine needles at specific (acupuncture) points along the meridians involved, health can be restored because the flow of energy is no longer obstructed and balance is achieved.

Chiropractors see pediatric patients as well as adult patients. Chiropractors use a holistic approach to treating all patients. They treat patients whose health problems are associated with the body's muscular, nervous, and skeletal systems, specifically the spine. Two other forms of manual healing include massage therapy and healing touch (practitioners place their hands on or near the patient's body to direct energy). Many hospitals now include a massage therapist on site; however, insurance companies generally do not pay for massage.

Get Ready for the NCLEX® Examination!

Key Points

- There are a variety of settings in which health care for children is available.
- The pediatric hospital unit is designed to create a cheerful, casual atmosphere to help meet the needs of children.
- All children react differently to hospitalization. Parents and health care providers need to minimize the stressors of hospitalization as much as possible.
- Actively involve both parents and child in the admission process to allay anxiety.

- Carefully observe the child's behavior when performing a systems review. Discuss the child's normal behavior with the parent. Changes in behavior can be indicative of abnormal assessment findings and need to be closely monitored.
- Respect cultural and religious differences when caring for children.
- The plan of care serves as a communication tool among the health care team.
- Discharge planning begins on admission, and teaching is done throughout the child's hospitalization, not just when the child is about to leave the hospital.

- Following safety measures is of the utmost importance when caring for children in any health care setting.
- Restraints are only used when absolutely necessary and according to institution policy.
- Medical asepsis guidelines must be strictly followed to prevent the spread of infection.
- Fears of a child who is about to undergo surgery need to be alleviated before surgery.
- A thorough evaluation of a child with pain and appropriate pharmacologic or nonpharmacologic interventions are essential for the child's well-being.

Additional Learning Resources

evolve Go to your Evolve website (*http://evolve.elsevier.com/Price/pediatric/*) for the following FREE learning resources:

- 3-D Animations
- Answer Keys
- Appendixes
- Audio Glossary
- Spanish/English Glossary
- Video Clips

Review Questions for the NCLEX® Examination

1. Which of the following inpatient pediatric patients would not be able to be taken to the playroom because of their physical condition?

   1. A 7-year-old with new onset diabetes mellitus
   2. A 12-year-old with a fractured femur
   3. A 4-year-old with respiratory syncytial virus
   4. A 10-year-old postoperative appendectomy

2. A 2-year-old is hospitalized for dehydration secondary to gastroenteritis. The nurse is aware that the **major** stressor during hospitalization for a toddler is:

   1. Loss of control
   2. Separation anxiety
   3. Bodily injury
   4. Pain

3. A 5-year-old has a bedwetting episode while hospitalized. The most likely explanation is:

   1. An allergic reaction to medication
   2. A probable urinary tract infection
   3. Regression due to illness
   4. Excessive fluid intake

4. The nurse can assist parents in identifying and meeting the needs of the siblings of the hospitalized child in the following ways: (**Select all that apply.**)

   1. Inform siblings of the child's illness and progress.
   2. Allow siblings to visit.
   3. Encourage phone calls from siblings.
   4. Require siblings to assist in care of the hospitalized child.

5. When performing an assessment on a hospitalized child, the nurse observes weltlike lesions present on the child's back. The parents report that these welts are secondary to a cultural practice called coining. Coining is a cultural health care practice that may be implemented by:

   1. Mexican Americans
   2. Vietnamese Americans
   3. African Americans
   4. Chinese Americans

Pediatric Procedures

Objectives

1. Define the vocabulary terms listed
2. Discuss preparation techniques for the different developmental stages
3. Explain the necessary safety precautions when bathing an infant
4. Describe the collection of urine and stool specimens with infants and children
5. Discuss how to collect blood, throat, and nasopharyngeal specimens with infants and children
6. Describe the pediatric implications of assisting with a lumbar puncture
7. Contrast the administration of medicines to children and adults

8. Describe the preferred sites for intramuscular injections in infants and small children
9. Discuss precautions necessary when a child is receiving parenteral fluids and the rationale for each precaution
10. Compare and contrast gastrostomy button and gavage feedings with infants and children
11. Discuss care of the child with a tracheostomy
12. Describe oxygen therapy related to children
13. Explain how to measure an infant's or child's height, weight, and head circumference
14. Discuss how to obtain pediatric vital signs

Key Terms

alimentation (ĂL-ĕ-mĕn-TĀ-shŭn; p. 50)
azotemia (p. 50) (ă-zō-TĒ-mē-ă; p. 50)
enteral (ĔN-tĕ-ral; p. 51)
extravasation (ik-stră-vĕ-SĀ-shŭn; p. 50)
hyperalimentation (hī-per-a-le-men-TĀ-shŭn; p. 50)
hyperthermia (hī-per-THER-mē-ă; p. 35)
lumbar puncture (p. 41)
midstream specimen (p. 38)

nomogram (NŎM-ŏ-grăm; p. 43)
ostomy (ĂS-tĕ-mē; p. 53)
palpation (păl-PĀ-shŭn; p. 60)
pulse oximeter (ŏk-SĬM-ĕ-tĕr; p. 56)
surface area (p. 43)
thrombosis (thräm-BŌ-ses; p. 50)
tracheostomy (trā-kē-OS-to-mē; p. 53)

PREPARATION FOR PROCEDURES

Preparation of the child for a procedure is one of the most important tasks of the nurse. Children fear pain and bodily injury, so it is important for nurses to prepare the child with honest, age-appropriate explanations and carry out the procedure in the least stressful manner to the child. Hockenberry and Wilson (2009) refer to this as atraumatic care or care without trauma. Once nurses understand the stressors that affect hospitalized children, the effect of these stressors can be minimized with providing atraumatic care.

With infants, the parents are given the explanation and will want to comfort the infant after the procedure. Toddlers can be given brief, simple explanations just before the procedure and may need to be restrained while the procedure is performed. Be sure the toddler does not view this as punishment. Parents may want to be there during the procedure to provide comfort

but should not be viewed as the restrainer. An exception would be therapeutic holding done by the parent. The nurse always provides comfort after the procedure. Preschoolers need simple explanations and should be allowed to touch and handle equipment if possible. Preschoolers engage in "magical thinking" and believe they have all-powerful thoughts. They may feel responsible for bad thoughts that coincide with events and need to be reassured that their thoughts did not cause the event and that a procedure is not a punishment. They may need to be restrained as well. Always provide comfort (adhesive bandages, stickers) after a procedure. The school-age child needs explanations through the use of drawings, pictures, and contact with equipment. Restrain only if needed. Praise cooperation, and explain steps as you proceed. School-age children may be able to perform stress-reducing techniques such as visualization during the procedure. The adolescent generally needs no restraint, only clear explanations and praise for cooperation. Remember that child life specialists not only provide education before procedures, but often help children through procedures as well by providing distraction and other assistance. These specialists are helpful in the hospital and clinic setting.

 Nursing Brief

Always perform procedures in the treatment room.

BASIC HYGIENE AND CARE

BATHING

Bathing not only promotes cleanliness and stimulates circulation to the skin, but also provides exercise and may help the child relax and feel more comfortable (Skill 3-1). Explain the procedure in appropriate terms. **Always remain with the child when bathing occurs.**

Be sure to check any allergies the child may have. Always assess conditions that influence the type of bath given, such as a recent surgical incision, EEG monitor, a cast, an intravenous (IV) line or Foley catheter in place, and so on. Examine the infant or child for skin abnormalities such as rashes, birthmarks, bruises, breaks in the skin, and so on. *Never* use baby powder after the bath because the powder can be inhaled and cause breathing problems. Skill 3-1 can be taught to parents for home use.

 Nursing Brief

Always wash hands before and after *any* procedure performed.

BULB SUCTIONING

A bulb syringe is used when it is necessary to provide an open airway by removing secretions from an infant's

Skill 3-1   Bathing an Infant or Small Child

Equipment

✓ Wash basin or tub
✓ Washcloth
✓ Towels
✓ Shampoo (as appropriate)
✓ Mild soap
✓ Cotton balls
✓ Clean clothing
✓ Diapers
✓ Lotion (as appropriate)

Safety Issues *(Rationale)*

- Never leave a child unattended around water *(children can drown in as little as 1 inch of water)*.
- Place a towel or rubber mat on the bottom of the tub or basin *(prevents the child from slipping)*.
- Verify that the room temperature is warm enough and draft-free *(prevents chilling)*.
- Only sponge bathe the baby until the cord has fallen off *(the cord should be kept dry to promote healing)*.
- Only sponge bathe the baby until the circumcision has healed *(the circumcision should not get wet in order to promote healing)*.
- Always run cold water first *(prevents burns)*.
- Hold on to infant securely, supporting the head while bathing *(babies are slippery when wet)*.

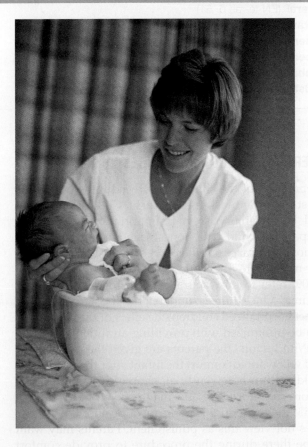

Method (Rationale)

1. Explain procedure (allays anxiety).
2. Assemble equipment.
3. Wash hands. Use gloves if body fluid precautions are warranted (ensures that standard precautions are followed).
4. Run water. Temperature should be 100° F (38° C). Check the temperature by submerging your wrist in the water or placing drops on the inside surface of your forearm. It should feel comfortably warm. (May use bath thermometer if available.) (Helps prevent burns as skin is actually thinner than an adult's).
5. Begin by removing secretions from the child's eyes with cotton ball immersed in plain water. Use a separate cotton ball for each eye (ensures cleanliness and prevents any cross-contamination).
6. Shampoo hair (if necessary); wash the scalp of an infant younger than 1 year of age as necessary. Pour water over head. Apply shampoo, and rinse. Avoid eyes. Dry head with towel when finished (helps prevent chilling).
7. Bathe remainder of body. End with the perineal area. Remember to wash from front to back (always wash from clean to dirty) Wrap in towel when finished (prevents chilling).
8. Apply lotion as needed (provides moisturizing and hydration)
9. Dress in clean clothing. Keep top edge of diaper below umbilicus site if cord has not fallen off (promotes healing and reduces irritation).
10. Teach hygiene practices to the parents as needed: frequency of bathing, shampooing hair, cleaning genitals, avoiding bubble bath (can cause vaginal irritation), and so on.

Skills Checklist

✓ Prepare the child and family.
✓ Assemble equipment.
✓ Wash hands.
✓ Prepare basin, check temperature.
✓ Clean infant's eyes, wash hair and scalp.
✓ Bathe the rest of the child; prevent chilling.
✓ Dry. Apply lotion as needed.
✓ Wash hands.
✓ Teach as appropriate.
✓ Document procedure. Be sure to note any abnormal skin conditions. (e.g., bath performed per hospital policy. Cried briefly but consoled easily by parents. No abnormal skin conditions noted~signature).

mouth and nose (Skill 3-2). Secretions may be the result of mucus or regurgitation of a feeding. Always assess the condition of the child after suctioning. There should be no sign of respiratory distress. Be sure parents know how to suction their baby's mouth and nose prior to discharge from the hospital.

FEVER, HYPERTHERMIA, AND SPONGE BATHING

Fever is defined as body temperature above 38° C (100.4° F) rectally. The child's metabolic rate will increase 10% for every 1° C increase. The physician may only recommend monitoring the fever, since it is the body's way of defending itself against illness and is part of the immune process. Fever with temperatures less than 39° C (102.2° F) does not require treatment if the child is generally healthy (Kliegman et al., 2007). Antipyretic agents such as acetaminophen (10 to 15 mg/kg orally every 4 to 6 hours) and ibuprofen (5 to 10 mg/kg orally every 6 to 8 hours) may be ordered because they are considered safe and effective in proper doses for treatment of fever for children. (Always refer to a drug reference manual for specific information.) Ibuprofen should only be used for children older than 6 months of age. Aspirin is not recommended because of the risk for Reye syndrome. Cooling the child by reducing the room temperature and removing blankets and clothing may be beneficial if an antipyretic has been given approximately 1 hour beforehand. The antipyretic works to lower the "set point" associated with the fever, much like regulating a thermostat (body temperature is regulated by the hypothalamus).

Hyperthermia is defined as the body temperature exceeding the set point, such as from heat stroke or seizures. Tepid sponge bathing in warm water may be ordered to reduce hyperthermia (Hockenberry and Wilson, 2009). Tepid sponge bathing, however, is not effective in treating fever. When performed, the sponge bath may be given in a tub or in the child's bed (Skill 3-3). The child should not be permitted to shiver because shivering causes vasoconstriction and increased metabolism and can lead to a rise in temperature. The bath is given for approximately 20 minutes. **Alcohol should never be added to the water because it reduces the heat too rapidly and can be absorbed (leading to brain damage or even death in infants).** A table of Celsius (centigrade) and Fahrenheit temperature equivalents is provided in Appendix E.

Skill 3-2   Suctioning with a Bulb Syringe

Equipment
✓ Bulb syringe
✓ Tissues
✓ Washcloth

Safety Issues (Rationale)
- Be sure infant shows no signs of respiratory distress after the procedure.
- Do not insert bulb straight to the back of the throat (could result in a vagal response or gagging).
- Suction nares carefully (avoids traumatizing tissue).

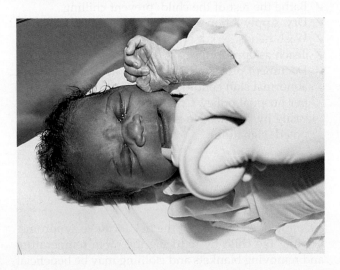

Method (Rationale)
1. Explain the procedure to the parent (allays anxiety).

2. Gather equipment.
3. Wash hands; wear gloves (ensures that standard precautions are followed).
4. Hold infant's head (stabilizes head).
5. Compress bulb and insert into mouth (along side of mouth), and release bulb slowly (releasing the bulb will pull secretions into the bulb tip).
6. Remove bulb syringe, and empty by compressing several times as needed onto tissues or washcloth (removes secretions).
7. Suction nares carefully if necessary in same manner (suctioning the mouth first ensures that nasal secretions are not placed in the mouth).
8. Discard tissues, or place washcloth with soiled linen.
9. Rinse bulb syringe with water, or take it apart and clean if applicable.
10. Remove gloves, and wash hands (ensures that standard precautions are followed).

Skills Checklist
✓ Assess need for suctioning.
✓ Explain procedure.
✓ Wash hands; glove.
✓ Position infant.
✓ Compress bulb.
✓ Insert into mouth, release bulb.
✓ Suction nose if needed
✓ Remove gloves, and wash hands.
✓ Document procedure (e.g., mouth and nares suctioned; minimal white secretions removed. No distress noted during procedure~signature).

COLLECTION OF SPECIMENS

COLLECTION OF URINE SPECIMENS

Urine specimens are often collected in doctors' offices and clinics, as well as in the hospital (Skill 3-4). All urine specimens need to be labeled and sent to the lab immediately because bacteria accumulate at room temperature. If there is a delay, the urine specimen is to be kept refrigerated or on ice. An example would be if the patient were taking a urine specimen that was obtained at home, to a laboratory. Documentation of the procedure, including child's reactions, is also done. The physician may request that the specimen be

collected with the clean-catch method, catheterization, or 24-hour collection.

The physician may also order a specimen so that the nurse can check certain lab results immediately, either in the clinic or the hospital. Examples of this may include specimens such as protein, albumin, glucose, ketones, or blood. These are checked with a urine dipstick without being sent to the lab. Results are recorded on the patient's chart.

Obtaining a Clean-Catch Specimen
Children who can voluntarily void can assist in obtaining a clean-catch specimen. Be sure to use familiar

Skill 3-3   Sponge Bath to Reduce Hyperthermia

Equipment
✓ Basin of tepid water (see Method)
✓ Three washcloths, towel(s)
✓ Two bath blankets
✓ Waterproof sheet

Safety Issues
• *Never* leave a child unattended around water.
• Sponge bath should take approximately 20 minutes.
• If the child shivers, stop the procedure.
• Assess color and pulse frequently.
• Record temperature before and 30 minutes after the procedure.
• *Never* add alcohol to water.

Method *(Rationale)*
1. Explain the procedure to the patient and family *(allays anxiety)*.
2. Assemble the equipment at the bedside.
3. Water temperature should be 37° C (98.6° F); needs only be 1° C or 2° F less than the child's temperature to be effective (Hockenberry and Wilson, 2009).
4. Wash hands. Apply gloves if applicable *(ensures that standard precautions are followed)*.
5. Record temperature, pulse, and respirations *(establishes a baseline)*.
6. The child is placed in the tub, and water is put over the back and chest *or (if done in the bed)*
7. Cover the patient with a bath blanket or sheet. Fanfold linens to the foot of the bed. Place a waterproof sheet and bath blanket beneath the patient. Remove patient's gown.
8. Wash the patient's face and neck with tepid water.
9. Lift the corner of the bath blanket, and bathe the child's body, one area at a time.
10. Place moist, folded cloths over blood vessels that lie close to the skin (underarms and groin).
11. Turn the patient and repeat the procedure, beginning with the neck, and then going to the shoulders, the back, and so forth.

12. Check color and pulse to be sure that the child is tolerating the procedure without adverse effects *(report changes to charge nurse as patient's condition may be changing)*.
13. If the child begins to shiver, the procedure should be immediately stopped *(shivering causes vasoconstriction, increases temperature)*.
14. When the bath is completed, remove the waterproof sheet and blanket. Rub the skin dry *(stimulates circulation)*, and replace the hospital gown and cover with sheet.
15. Arrange pillows and bedding for the patient's comfort.
16. Take the patient's temperature within 30 minutes of the time the procedure ended, and record it. If the temperature has not started to go down, check to see whether the procedure should be repeated. Note: The temperature is not expected to drop to normal but merely to a more reasonable level. Also record pulse and respirations *(report changes to charge nurse as patient's condition may be changing)*.
17. *Document:* Time procedure began, length of time administered, untoward reactions, patient's vital signs before and after procedure.

Skills Checklist
✓ Prepare the child and family.
✓ Assemble equipment.
✓ Wash hands.
✓ Record temperature, pulse, respirations.
✓ Drape patient (if done in the bed)
✓ Remove gown.
✓ Wash face, neck, other body parts, one at a time.
✓ Place cloths; proceed to back of patient.
✓ Check color, pulse.
✓ Pat dry; regown.
✓ Assess comfort.
✓ Record temperature, pulse, respirations.
✓ Wash hands.
✓ Document procedure.

terms that the young child understands, such as "pee-pee" or "tinkle" when describing what the child is to do. Many children will be reluctant to void into a specimen container; have the parents assist as much as possible. Always wear protective equipment for

standard precautions such as gloves when handling *any* specimen.

Special sterile containers are available for clean-catch specimens; follow the directions of the manufacturer. All require cleansing of the perineum or tip of

Skill 3-4   Obtaining a Specimen for Urinalysis

Equipment
✓ Sterile container
✓ Urine collection bag (infant)

Safety Issues (Rationale)
- Wear gloves because of contact with body fluids.
- Check urine collection bag frequently.
- Label specimen clearly.
- Deliver specimen immediately to the laboratory (*bacteria may grow at room temperature*).

Method (Rationale)
1. Explain the procedure (*allays anxiety*).
2. Wash hands; wear gloves (*ensures that standard precautions are followed*).
3. Use a sterile container, or apply a urine collection device.
4. If a bag is used, secure the diaper over the bag or cut a slit so that the bag is outside the diaper (*prevents leakage*).
5. Check bag every 20 to 30 minutes (*prevents leakage*).
6. Label all specimens clearly, and attach the proper laboratory slip. Collected specimens should be transported in a plastic bag (check institution policy).
7. Record in nurse's notes. Document time; also color, amount, and any odor (*e.g., 30 ml clear yellow odorless urine collected in urine bag and sent to lab~signature*).

Skills Checklist
✓ Explain procedure.
✓ Obtain container/urine collection device (infant).
✓ Wash hands; glove.
✓ Apply urine collection device (infant) or have child void.
✓ Recover specimen.
✓ Remove gloves and wash hands.
✓ Label, send to laboratory.
✓ Document procedure.

When applying newborn and pediatric urine collectors, the skin must be clean and perfectly dry. (Avoid oils, baby powders, and lotion soaps that may leave a residue on the skin and interfere with the ability of the adhesive to stick.) Apply the collection bag first to the area between the anus and genitals for boys and start at the narrow bridge of skin separating the vagina from the anus for girls. Press adhesive firmly against the skin and avoid wrinkles. Remove paper from the adhesive patch, working upward to finish applying the collection bag. Monitor closely for urine output.

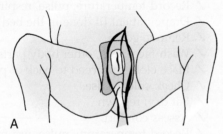 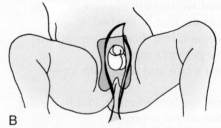

A   B

the penis. When cleaning girls, cleanse the perineum with a soap or antiseptic agent, wiping from front to back. Repeat twice and follow with sterile water to prevent contamination of the specimen. After the urine stream has started, and the first few milliliters of urine are voided, the midstream specimen should be caught in the sterile container, with care taken not to contaminate the container.

Infants and young children may have a sterile urine bag applied (see Skill 3-4). Check frequently under the diaper as leakage from the bag may occur. A slit may also be cut in the diaper to allow the bag to remain on the *outside* of the diaper where it is more visible.

Obtaining a Specimen with Catheterization
Obtaining a specimen with a catheter is the same as for adults, except that the size of the catheter is usually an 8 or 10 Foley catheter (check institution policy). When necessary for surgical patients, the catheter may

be inserted once the child has undergone anesthesia. This is less traumatic for children, who are usually frightened by this procedure. It is also difficult to keep the awake child still for catheter insertion, which increases the risk of contamination.

Home Care Guidelines for Intermittent Catheterization Using a "Clean" Technique

Some children require frequent catheterization such as those with spina bifida. Parents can be taught how to catheterize their child at home. When children are old enough, they too can learn this procedure. A mirror is helpful for girls. Remember, repeated exposure to latex can cause latex allergies; therefore non-latex catheters are recommended. A clean technique is generally used. Always be sure the bladder is completely emptied to reduce the risk for urinary tract infections (UTIs). Steps include the following:

- Thoroughly cleaning the perineum or tip of penis with mild soap and water or povidone-iodine (*be sure there are no allergies to iodine*).
- Using the appropriate size lubricated catheter, inserting until urine is obtained.
- Urine can flow freely into a clean container, urinal, bedpan, or toilet (if the child is old enough)
- Cleansing the area when finished.

It is preferred practice to use a sterile catheter each time to avoid potential UTIs. However, if sterile catheters are not always available, additional guidelines may be recommended by the physician.

Obtaining a 24-Hour Urine Specimen

At times, a 24-hour urine specimen may be requested to determine the rate of urine production and to measure the excretion of specific chemicals from the body. This requires close supervision by the nurses on each shift to maintain accuracy of the test because lost specimens necessitate restarting the test. Older children can help with collection of their own specimens; collection bags are required for infants and small children. A sign may be posted to alert personnel of a 24-hour urine collection.

 Nursing Brief

The rule of thumb for urine output is 0.5 to 2 mL/kg/hr.

COLLECTION OF STOOL SPECIMENS

Stool specimens from older children are obtained as for an adult (Skill 3-5). This is embarrassing for most children, who are turned off by the suggestion. The ambulatory child can use a collection device (potty hat) placed beneath a toilet seat. It is difficult for a child to tell the nurse that the sample has been collected. The nurse can acknowledge these feelings by giving the

---

Skill 3-5 Obtaining a Stool Specimen

Equipment
✓ Clean container
✓ Tongue blade

Safety Issues
- Wash hands. Wear gloves to obtain specimen.
- Label specimen appropriately.

Method *(Rationale)*
1. Explain procedure to child or parent (*allays anxiety*).
2. Wash hands; wear gloves (*ensures that standard precautions are followed*).
3. Obtain stool specimen directly from the diaper (if it has not been contaminated by urine) with the tongue blade, or use the tongue blade to retrieve the specimen from the collection device.
4. The specimen is labeled properly, and the laboratory slip is attached.
5. Some specimens must be sent to the laboratory while they are warm.
6. The nurse documents the time; also the color, amount, consistency of the stool and the purpose for which it was collected (e.g., blood, ova, parasites, bacteria); and any related information (e.g., 20 ml. loose, brown stool specimen obtained for culture and sent to lab~signature).

Skills Checklist
✓ Explain procedure.
✓ Wash hands; glove.
✓ Obtain specimen.
✓ Remove gloves, wash hands.
✓ Label, send to laboratory.
✓ Document procedure.

child permission to express them without being critical. The nurse might say, "I know this must be embarrassing for you. It is for grown-ups, too, but we need this because …"

COLLECTION OF BLOOD SPECIMENS

Blood specimens are generally collected by the laboratory technician or a specially trained nurse. Children generally fear this procedure. EMLA (eutectic mixture of lidocaine and prilocaine) cream can be used to lessen the pain. Remember, however, that the cream needs to be in place approximately 60 minutes before the blood sample is taken (if LMX or lidocaine cream is used, allow 30 minutes). If time permits, have the blood specimen obtained in the treatment room, keeping the child's bed a safe place. The antecubital fossa is a common site for venipuncture in children older than 2 years of age. The dorsum of the hand or foot can also be used (Figure 3-1). The heel is often used in infants (Figure 3-2). If blood is to be collected from the heel, it needs to be warmed with a warmed washcloth or commercial warmer to increase the blood flow. The external jugular vein can be used in infants when other sites have not worked. The femoral vein may be used when other sites have been exhausted. Jugular and femoral venipuncture are only performed by the physician. Both the jugular and the femoral veins are large; therefore, after venipuncture, the child is checked frequently to ensure that there is no bleeding. The child is soothed accordingly if either of these sites is used, because crying and thrashing may precipitate oozing or hemorrhage. If a child has a central venous catheter or port, specially trained nurses can obtain the blood specimen by following hospital procedure. Always use standard precautions when obtaining or assisting with blood specimens. Regardless of the location used to obtain the blood specimen, the nurse charts the site used, the name of the blood test, and any untoward developments.

Communication

Many children fear losing blood, and reminding children who are old enough to understand that they are continuously producing blood helps to reassure them. Application of an adhesive bandage reassures them that their body fluids will not leak out. This is particularly helpful for preschoolers.

COLLECTION OF THROAT CULTURES

A throat culture is frequently ordered by the physician when a child has a "sore throat" or a strep infection is suspected (Skill 3-6). The child may need to be temporarily restrained when a throat specimen is obtained. The child needs to stick out the tongue and say "ah" while the nurse swabs the pharyngeal area and tonsils. If the child is unable to cooperate, a tongue depressor should be used to hold down the tongue while obtaining the swabbed specimen. **If the child has a diagnosis**

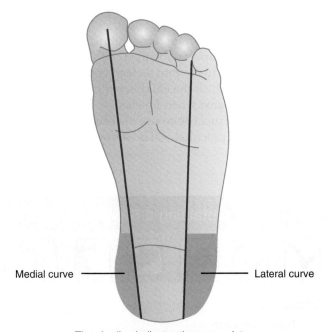

Medial curve — Lateral curve

The shading indicates the appropriate area for making the puncture.

A

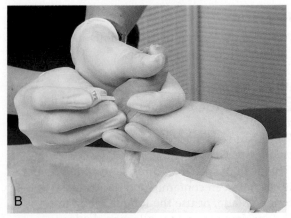

B

Figure 3-2 Sites for heel punctures on an infant.

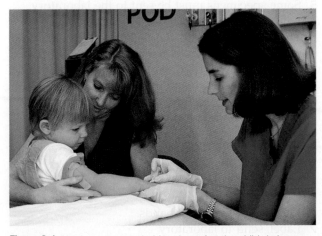

Figure 3-1 Using a parent to hold and comfort the child during a blood specimen procedure.

Skill 3-6   Obtaining a Throat Culture

Equipment

✓ Throat swab(s)
✓ Tongue depressor
✓ Media culture
✓ Pen light if necessary

Safety Issues

• Nurse may need to wear mask/eye goggles for protection.
• Label specimen appropriately.

Method *(Rationale)*

1. Explain procedure to child/parents *(allays anxiety)*.
2. Gather equipment.
3. Wash hands; wear gloves; apply mask and eye goggles if necessary *(ensures that standard precautions are followed)*.
4. Have child stick out tongue and say "ah" *(helps visualize throat area for swabbing)*.
5. Depress anterior half of tongue with tongue depressor if necessary *(use caution as this may elicit the gag reflex)*.

6. Swab area with exudate or redness, one time only per swab (avoid teeth, tongue, cheeks, lips, and palate).
7. Place swab(s) into media culture without touching sides of tube *(ensures that bacteria will be placed directly into the medium)*.
8. Be sure parents or nurse comfort child *(provides reassurance once procedure is over)*.
9. Label, obtain requisition.
10. Transport to laboratory.
11. Document the time of the procedure, including description of pharyngeal area if you can see it.

Skills Checklist

✓ Explain procedure.
✓ Wash hands; glove; apply mask and goggles (if necessary).
✓ Obtain specimen.
✓ Place in media culture.
✓ Provide comfort.
✓ Remove mask, goggles, and gloves, and wash hands.
✓ Label, obtain requisition.
✓ Take to laboratory.
✓ Document procedure.

suspicious of epiglottitis, the throat culture should not be done because the airway may become edematous (swollen) and occlude (block air movement) from the trauma of specimen collection.

COLLECTION OF NASOPHARYNGEAL CULTURES

A nasopharyngeal culture may be ordered to rule out certain respiratory infections such as pertussis in children. Have the child look up, dip the swab tip into saline, and with the wire bent, insert the swab to the back of the nares and into the nasopharyngeal area. Remove after several seconds, place the swab into the culture media, label, and transport to the lab with the specimen requisition form. Comfort the child after the procedure. Record the specimen collection and the child's response.

Other respiratory secretion specimens may be ordered to rule out such conditions as respiratory syncytial virus (RSV) or tuberculosis. An adequate specimen may be obtained using a suction device such as a mucus trap with a catheter inserted into the trachea. A nasal washing may also be attempted to obtain an RSV

culture. This involves instillation of sterile saline, followed by aspiration of the contents (Hockenberry and Wilson, 2009).

COLLECTION OF SPINAL FLUID FOR CULTURE

The nurse assists the physician with a lumbar puncture, which is done to obtain cerebrospinal fluid (CSF) for diagnosis and treatment. Disposable lumbar puncture sets are available. EMLA cream should be applied to the site at least 1 hour previous to the lumbar puncture. Children may require additional analgesia or anesthesia, depending on the physician's orders.

Normal spinal fluid is clear. The pressure ranges from 60 to 180 mm Hg. It is somewhat lower in infants. The procedure for children is essentially the same as for adults. The main difference lies in the child's ability to cooperate with positioning. The nurse explains that the child must lie quietly and that there will be help in doing this. Sensations during a lumbar puncture include a cool feeling when the skin is cleansed and a feeling of pressure when the needle is inserted.

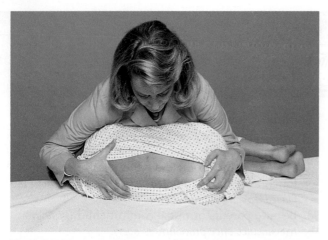

Figure 3-3 The nurse holds the child in a side-lying position with the head flexed and the knees drawn upward toward the chest during a lumbar puncture. This position enlarges the spaces between the vertebral spines, thereby improving access to the spinal fluid spaces.

The child lies on the side with the back parallel to the side of the treatment table. The knees are flexed, and the head is brought down close to the flexed knees. The nurse can keep the child in this position by placing the child's head in the crook of one arm and the knees in the crook of the other arm. The nurse then clasps hands together at the front of the child and leans forward, gently placing his or her chest against him or her (Figure 3-3). Infants may be supported in the sitting position with their backs curved and head flexed forward. The way in which the child is held can directly affect the success of the procedure and prevent serious complications. **Always monitor the child's respiratory status during a lumbar puncture. There is a potential for airway obstruction related to neck flexion.**

Once the child is positioned, the physician cleans the skin and numbs the area for needle insertion. A long, hollow spinal tap needle is inserted into the child's lower back, and the spinal fluid is collected into different culture tubes. These are labeled for different studies. Once the procedure is complete, a sterile adhesive bandage is applied over the injection site and the child is comforted. The site should be checked for any drainage or redness. The charge nurse is notified if drainage or redness is present. Vital signs are monitored according to hospital policy. Specimens are then labeled and taken to the laboratory with the appropriate requisition form.

Children need to be monitored for headaches after a lumbar puncture. Headaches can occur because cerebral spinal fluid was removed. Post–lumbar puncture headaches may be avoided by having the child lie flat for a period of time after the procedure.

The nurse charts the date and time of the lumbar puncture and the name of the attending physician. Also charted are the amount of fluid obtained, its character (cloudy, bloody), whether or not specimens were sent to the laboratory, and the reaction of the child to the procedure. The nurse then cleans and restocks the treatment room.

ADMINISTERING MEDICATIONS

VARIATIONS IN CHILDREN

The responsibility for giving medications to children is a serious one. Although a full technical description of drug administration is beyond the scope of this book, the following considerations and hazards are applicable to children.

Many drugs currently on the market are unsuitable for children because of their toxicity or because of lack of information about their effect on children. Children have a smaller body mass than adults, and their medications have to be adapted to their size and age. Neonates and preterm infants are in particular jeopardy because of the immaturity of their body systems. In these children, simply adjusting the dosage is insufficient. Drugs must be individualized and tailored to a multitude of factors (Figure 3-4).

The nurse should always ask whether the calculated dose makes sense. It is also helpful to remember that children usually receive small doses and amounts, and if either of these is in larger amounts, the nurse should recheck the orders. Most pediatric medications are prescribed in milligrams per kilogram of body weight per 24 hours (Box 3-1). A specific dose per kilogram of

Box 3-1	Doses for Children Based on Weight in Kilograms

STEPS

1. Weigh and record child's weight in kilograms (convert from pounds by dividing by 2.2).
2. Determine recommended safe range in milligrams/kilogram (mg/kg) by checking (pediatric) medication reference.
3. Multiply child's weight by the lower and upper limits of the dose range.
4. Compare child's ordered dose with dose range to determine whether medication dose falls within the "safe range."
5. Any dose that does not fall within the "safe range" needs to be verified by the physician.

EXAMPLE

Child weighs 44 lb

Conversion: 1 kg = 2.2 lb

44 lb ÷ 2.2 = 20 kg

If reference text states that the recommended dose range is 50 to 100 mg/kg of body weight/24 hr in four divided doses:

1. 50 mg × 20 kg = 1000 mg/24 hr
2. 100 mg × 20 kg = 2000 mg/24 hr
3. Safe Range = 1000 to 2000 mg/24 hr
   Child's ordered dose is 400 mg every 6 hr
4. 400 mg given every 6 hr = 400 × 4 = 1600 mg/24 hr
   Conclusion: Dose falls in safe range

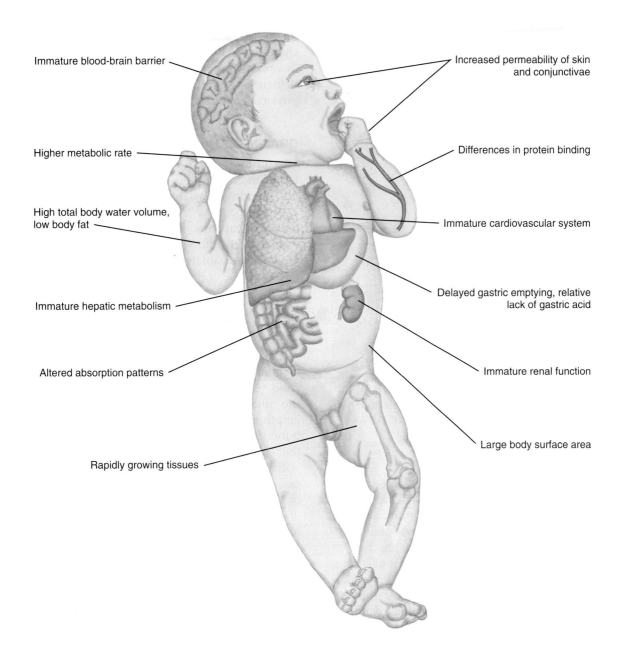

Immature blood-brain barrier

Higher metabolic rate

High total body water volume, low body fat

Immature hepatic metabolism

Altered absorption patterns

Rapidly growing tissues

Increased permeability of skin and conjunctivae

Differences in protein binding

Immature cardiovascular system

Delayed gastric emptying, relative lack of gastric acid

Immature renal function

Large body surface area

Figure 3-4 Some of the multiple factors that modify drug interaction in children. Physiologic differences in the body systems make the effects of drug interactions more dramatic in the newborn.

body weight may also be prescribed, such as 10 mg/ kg. A hospital drug formulary is usually available on the unit to enable the nurse to determine the safety of a particular dose. If there is any question with dosages or other drug information, the nurse should also consult another nurse, the physician who wrote the order, the hospital pharmacist, or the charge nurse.

Depending on the child's diagnosis and condition, the physician may need to calculate a specific dosage of a medication. One method, calculation by *body surface area* (BSA), is considered to be a very accurate method. In this method, a nomogram is used (Figure

3-5). The child's height is located on the left scale, and weight is located on the right scale. A line is drawn between the two points. The point at which the line transects the surface area (SA) gives the BSA. If the child is roughly of average size, the SA also can be estimated from the weight alone with the enclosed (shaded) area. The results are inserted into a formula. The average adult BSA is approximately 1.7 square meters.

BSA (child)/BSA (adult) × Average adult dose

= Child's dose

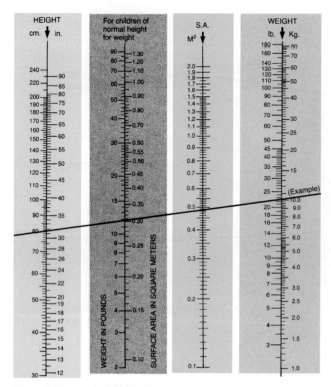

Figure 3-5 Nomogram for estimating BSA. The SA is indicated where a straight line that connects the height and weight levels intersects the SA column. If the patient is of average size, the SA can be deduced on the basis of weight alone *(see shaded area)*.

In addition to knowing the correct amount and route of a drug, the nurse must also be aware of the side effects that might occur. The absorption, distribution, metabolism, and excretion of drugs differ substantially in children. Drug reactions are not as predictable as in adult patients. The impact of a drug on normal growth and development must be considered. Drug information must be read carefully to determine suitability of a particular drug for children. **Drugs should be given only by the route indicated.** Double-check with another nurse if using calculated dosages or for any drug or dosage that may give reason for concern.

⚠ Safety Alert

Most hospitals require that two nurses verify dosages of digoxin, insulin, heparin, narcotics, and so on. Students may not be authorized to administer these medications. Always check institution policy.

The child should be correctly identified with the hospital identification band and a second identifier, such as the child's birthday. *Never* call out a child's name for identification. The nurse must always know what medications the child is receiving, whether or not the nurse administers them personally. The nurse should review the medications with the parent prior to administering them to the child, to ensure accuracy. If there is any discrepancy, always double-check the physician's orders.

ORAL MEDICATIONS

The administration of medication by mouth is preferred in children but is not always possible because of vomiting, malabsorption, or refusal. Children younger than 5 years of age find it difficult to swallow tablets or capsules, so many pediatric medications are available in liquid, suspension, or chewable tablets. Only scored tablets should be divided. Scored tablets have a crease or line on them allowing them to be split in half easily. Suspensions must be fully shaken before use. Always measure liquid medications with an oral syringe or medicine measuring cup as measuring spoons are inaccurate.

Capsules may have to be emptied and the powder disguised in a pleasant-tasting medium to get the child to take the medication. Be sure to check with the pharmacist to ascertain that capsules can be emptied. Also check with the pharmacist to determine if pills can be crushed. This is also necessary if the child cannot swallow the capsule or pill. Mix with a sweet-tasting substance such as cherry syrup or jelly for example, when the medication is bitter or otherwise unpalatable. Use of important sources of nutrients such as orange juice, formula, or milk for this purpose is discouraged because the child may develop distaste for them. *Never* refer to the medication as candy. **Elevate the child's head and shoulders (as long as their condition allows),** and administer medication slowly (especially if the child is crying) to avoid aspiration and/or choking. The child may attempt to push the medicine away. In anticipation of this, the child is held in the nurse's lap in a semisitting position with the hands restrained (Figure 3-6). "Chasers" of water, fruit juice, or a carbonated beverage are helpful. In choosing a chaser, the child's age, diet, and preference are considered.

If a nasogastric tube is in place, test for proper placement (see institution policy) of the tube before pouring medication into the syringe barrel (see Procedures to Assist Nutrition, Digestion, and Elimination later in this chapter). Administer a small amount of water afterward to cleanse the tube and to ensure delivery of all the medication. If the child has a gastrostomy button (G-button) in place, administer the medication into the G-button with an oral syringe. This may be followed by a small amount of water. Record the intake.

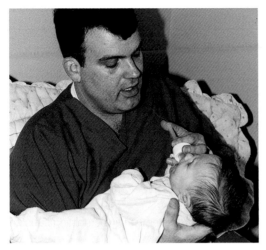

Figure 3-6 Administering oral liquid medication to an infant.

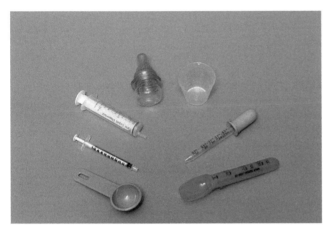

Figure 3-7 Medications can be administered to children with an oral syringe, calibrated nipple, medicine cup, calibrated dropper, or hollow-handled medicine spoon. Note: Measuring spoons (lower left) should not be used for administering medications to children because they can be inaccurate.

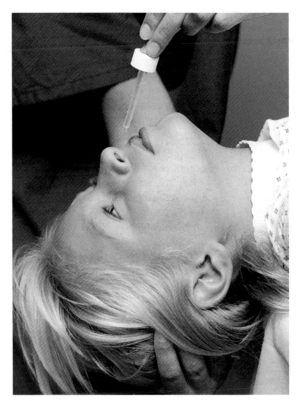

Figure 3-8 Technique of instilling nosedrops requires proper positioning for instillation.

For infants, an oral syringe is an excellent device for measuring and administering small quantities of liquid medication. Apply a bib to an infant. Place the syringe midway back at the side of the mouth. An empty nipple may also be used to take the liquid medication through. Do not place medication in a bottle of juice, milk, or water; if some of the contents is refused, there is no way to determine how much of the drug was consumed. A plastic medicine dropper is useful and may be provided with the medication by the drug manufacturer (Figure 3-7). Use only for the medication specified because these droppers are not intended for measuring other liquids. A drug ordered in teaspoons should be measured in milliliters to ensure accuracy (5 mL = 1 teaspoon). When administering medications in pediatric units, it is particularly important to keep all medications in sight at all times, so that a child does not take or play with any medicine. **Medication should**

never be left at the bedside. See Table 3-1 for further considerations about administering oral pediatric medications.

NOSEDROPS, EARDROPS, AND EYEDROPS

Except for a few differences, the principles of administering nosedrops, eardrops, and eyedrops to children are essentially the same as for adults. Infants and small children may need to be restrained. If restraint is necessary, a second person can help or a mummy restraint can be used. Warm all medications to room temperature. Explain the procedure to the child in age-appropriate detail.

Nosedrops

To administer nosedrops, first wipe mucus from the nose with a tissue. Position the infant or child lying flat with the head over the edge of a pillow. Encircle the child's cheeks and chin with your nondominant arm to hold the head steady. Instill the drops with the dominant hand. Keep the child in this position with head back for 1 minute to allow the drops to reach the proper area (Figure 3-8).

After instilling the drops, chart the time, name of medication, strength, number of drops instilled, how child tolerated the procedure, and untoward reactions.

Table 3-1   Selected Considerations in Giving Oral Medications to Children

AGE	CONSIDERATIONS
Infant	Apply bib, or use towel under chin. Support and elevate head and shoulders. Use calibrated oral syringe for measuring liquid medications. Depress chin with thumb to open mouth. Slowly insert medication along side of infant's mouth; this helps prevent gagging. Allow time for swallowing; monitor infants closely for respiratory distress.
Toddler	May require help of another person and therapeutic holding. Do not give choices regarding taking or not taking medication; give choices such as type of juice to take with medication. Explain reasons for medication. Review medication with parent(s). Crush tablets (only if pharmacy indicates) if not chewable variety; administer with sweet-tasting substance if diet allows. If cooperative, child may hold medicine cup or oral syringe. Allow child to drink at own pace; praise upon completion.
Preschool	Chewable tablets and liquids are preferred. May or may not be able to swallow pills. Watch for loose teeth that could be swallowed. Avoid prolonged reasoning; only give choices when there is one. Involve parents if appropriate. Praise child.
School-Age	Determine if child can take pills and capsules; instruct child to place pill near back of tongue and immediately swallow water or fluid of choice. Some children continue to have a difficult time swallowing pills, and other forms of the medication should be explored (many come in suspensions); never ridicule child. Children can be unpredictable from day to day in their cooperation; allow more time for the giving of pediatric medications. Always ascertain that child is fully awake (particularly after naptime and during night shift). Always inform child of what you are about to do. Remain with fearful child after procedure until composure is regained.
Adolescent	Prepare patient with explanations suitable to understanding. Always ensure privacy. Teach adolescent what side effects to report. Remain with patient until medicine is consumed (particularly if patient has a behavioral disorder). Anticipate mood swings in compliance.

🏠 Home Care Considerations

Parents and Caregivers Need to Know the Following When Medicating Children:
- Name and purpose of the medication
- Route used to deliver the medication. Many medications are given orally, but parents may be taught other routes such as IM, subcutaneous (subQ), or rectal.
- How much is to be given (always measure *accurately*)
- Time(s) of day medication is to be given
- Whether or not the medication is to be taken with food
- Possible side effects of the medication
- Possible drug or food interactions (including herbal medications)
- Follow medication schedule as prescribed (such as completing *all* of an antimicrobial)

Parents need to let their doctor know if the medication does not appear to be working or if there are any adverse effects or side effects.

Eardrops

The doctor may prescribe a drug to be instilled into the ear. Eardrops should be warmed to room temperature before instilling (cold drops would be painful). The infant and young child may need to be restrained during this procedure. Cooperation may be gained through the use of games and the involvement of parents. In the child under 3 years of age, the infected ear is drawn down and back to straighten the ear canal and the correct number of drops is instilled. In the older child, the earlobe is pulled up and back to obtain a straight canal. Children remain supine or on their side for a few minutes to permit the fluid to be absorbed. The nurse charts the time, name of drug, number of drops administered, the area (right or left ear), untoward reactions, and whether or not the child obtained relief.

The area in front of the ear may be gently massaged to aid in the entry of the drops into the ear canal. A sterile cotton pledget may be placed in the canal to prevent leakage of medication; however, this should be loose enough to allow for drainage.

Eyedrops

Ophthalmic medication is administered to a child in the same manner as for an adult. Ascertain which eye requires treatment. Gloves should be worn with eyedrop administration. Hands should be washed well before and after application of eyedrops. The child should be either supine or in the sitting position. The infant and small child may need to be restrained.

With the thumb and index finger, use gentle pressure in opposite directions to open the eye. Instruct the child to "look up." Supporting the hand on the child's forehead, instill the medication into the center of the lower lid (conjunctival sac). Instruct the child to close the eye but not to squeeze it because this could expel some of the solution. Infants may clench their eyes shut. When this happens, the drops can be placed in the nasal corner of the eye where the lids meet. When the child opens the lids, the medication flows onto the conjunctiva. Wipe excess medication with a separate tissue for each eye from the inner to the outer canthus.

Ointment is applied into the same conjunctival sac as the eyedrops (Figure 3-9). Excess ointment may be wiped outward with a tissue. If both drops and ointment are ordered, apply drops first, wait 3 minutes, then apply ointment (Hockenberry and Wilson, 2009).

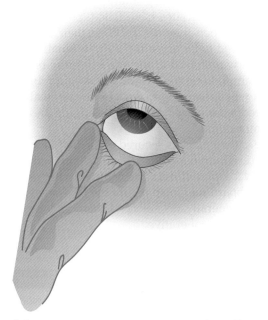

Figure 3-9 Administration of eye ointment or eyedrops. The eye ointment/eyedrops should fall in the center of the lower conjunctival sac, never directly on the eyeball.

RECTAL MEDICATIONS

Some drugs (Tylenol, glycerin) come in the form of suppositories. Children's suppositories are long and thin in comparison with the cone-shaped types administered to adults. The nurse, wearing gloves, inserts the unwrapped, lubricated suppository well beyond both of the rectal sphincters; about half as far as the forefinger reaches. The nurse applies pressure to the anus by gently holding the buttocks together until the child's desire to expel the suppository subsides.

INTRAMUSCULAR INJECTIONS

Intramuscular (IM) injections are rarely administered to children, especially if an intravenous (IV) line is present. However, physicians do order certain medications by the IM route, and most immunizations are still being given by this route.

The ventrogluteal site is free of major blood vessels and nerves and is not associated with complications. According to Cook and Murtagh (2006), this site is suitable for infants and toddlers, as well as older children. The vastus lateralis is also recommended for infants and young children. This site is well developed at birth, is the largest muscle mass in infants and small children, and has few major nerves and blood vessels. The dorsogluteal site is not recommended in infants and young children because it is insufficiently developed to be a safe site. The deltoid is also avoided in young children because the small muscle mass cannot hold large volumes of medication, nor should it be used if medications need to be injected into deep muscle mass. It should be used only for very small amounts of medication. According to Hockenberry and Wilson (2009), the deltoid muscle can only accomodate 0.5 to 1 mL.

Figure 3-10 shows the location of preferred injection sites.

The size of the syringe and needle to be used depends on several factors: the size of the child, the amount of medication to be given, the amount of muscle tissue available, and the viscosity of the medication. A 22-gauge to 25-gauge needle 0.5 to 1 inch long is usually used. Generally, 1 mL is the maximum volume to be administered at one site in older infants and small children (Hockenberry and Wilson, 2009). Figure 3-10 provides guidelines for IM injections.

The nurse should anticipate some protest from children in regard to injections. EMLA cream should be applied at least 1 hour prior to the injection. LMX cream can also be used and does not require as much time to numb the area. Whenever possible, a second nurse should be available to distract and restrain the child when necessary. If discomfort is minimized, the child is less likely to fear a return visit. If a parent chooses to be present, he or she should not be asked to restrain the child but rather should be there for distraction before and comforting after the procedure.

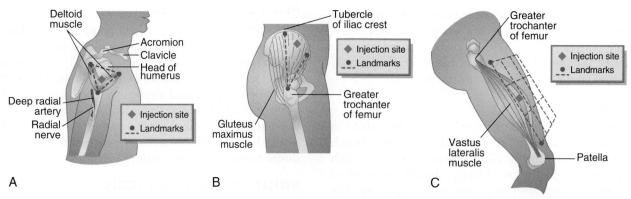

Figure 3-10 Intramuscular injection sites. **A,** Deltoid. Identify lower edge of acromion process and the point on the arm that is in line with the axilla. Site is one to three fingerbreadths (depending on the size of the child) below the acromion process and just above the axilla. Inject into mid-deltoid region. Guidelines: insert needle (½ to 1 inch size) into muscle at 90 degrees, pointed slightly toward acromion process. Use small volumes (0.5 to 1 mL) due to limited muscle mass. Radial nerve lies under the deltoid muscle. **B,** Ventrogluteal. Use the hand opposite the side for injection to locate landmarks (e.g., to give in child's left hip, use your right hand to locate the landmarks). Place your palm on the greater trochanter, index finger on the anterior superior iliac spine, and middle finger on the posterior edge of the iliac spine (or tubercle of the iliac crest). Inject into center of the V formed by the index and middle fingers. Guidelines: insert needle (⅝ to 1 inch size) into muscle at 90 degrees, pointed slightly up toward iliac crest. Use 0.5 mL in infant, up to 2 mL in child (Hockenberry and Wilson, 2009). Site is free from major nerves and blood vessels. **C,** Vastus lateralis. Palpate greater trochanter and knee (patella). Divide into thirds; site is in middle third and midlateral anterior thigh. Guidelines: insert needle (⅝ to 1 inch size) at 90 degrees. This is the largest muscle available in infants and young children. Use 0.5 mL in infants and up to 2 mL in child (Hockenberry and Wilson, 2009). Site is relatively free from major nerves and blood vessels. It can be used in older children but is more painful than other sites.

The nurse should remain with the child until the child is calm and can focus attention on more pleasant things. Child life specialists are excellent resources to utilize to help calm a child's fears.

 Communication

When children ask whether a procedure will hurt, the nurse should be truthful. The nurse might say, "Some children say it feels a little like a mosquito bite. I want you to tell me what you think after we are finished."

SUBCUTANEOUS AND INTRADERMAL MEDICATIONS

Subcutaneous and intradermal medications may also be ordered for children. Subcutaneous injections are given in the abdomen, the center third of the lateral aspect of the upper arm, and the center third of the anterior thigh for infants and toddlers. Insulin, hormone replacement, and allergy desensitization are ordered subcutaneously. Some vaccines are also ordered by this route. Small needles (25- to 27-gauge) and small amounts (up to 0.5 mL) with short needles (½- to ⅝-inch) are generally used. Always check institution policy for procedural guidelines

The intradermal route is ordered for medications such as tuberculin testing. Generally a 25-gauge, ½-inch needle is used. The amount is small (0.1 mL). Administered at a 10- to 15-degree angle, the needle will barely penetrate the skin on the inner aspect of the forearm. A bleb should be observed if technique is correct. Record the forearm used and patient tolerance.

INTRAVENOUS MEDICATIONS

Medications are routinely administered by the IV route in children. When IVs are started, patient education is provided and consideration is given to making the procedure as *atraumatic* as possible. IV infusion sites are illustrated in Figure 3-11. The scalp may be used for IV infusion in young infants. This IV site is only used when other sites have failed. Some parents are distressed when they see an IV in their baby's head. Parents need to be reassured that the small amount of hair that was shaved at the site will grow back. Some may want to keep the lock of hair. Avoid foot veins in a child who is learning to walk or already walking. All IVs need to be protected from dislodging and be carefully monitored.

The catheter hub is secured at the insertion site and covered with transparent dressing. A protective covering may be placed over the catheter insertion site. A padded board may help secure the IV; however, older children generally do not need them as long as they are alert and cooperative.

 Safety Alert

The IV and identification band should not be located on the same extremity. If the IV infiltrated, the band would act much like a tourniquet, obstructing adequate venous return and causing circulatory impairment.

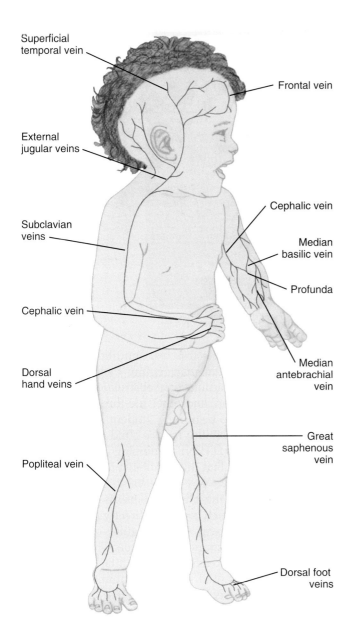

Figure 3-11 Sites for IV infusion in children.

- Superficial temporal vein
- Frontal vein
- External jugular veins
- Cephalic vein
- Subclavian veins
- Median basilic vein
- Profunda
- Cephalic vein
- Median antebrachial vein
- Dorsal hand veins
- Great saphenous vein
- Popliteal vein
- Dorsal foot veins

 Nursing Brief

Many institutions require hourly notations when an IV is infusing. The nurse charts such information as time, name, and amount of the solution; amount infused; rate of infusion; location of infusion site; condition of the site; and so on.

Compatibility is always checked between the fluid that is infusing and the medication to be given. The IV line must be flushed before and after the medication if it is not compatible with the IV solution. If two drugs are ordered to be given at the same time, compatibility must be checked again. Only one antimicrobial should be administered at a time. Medication is *never* administered with blood products.

When fluids are given IV, regardless of the site, the infant must be **closely observed.** Fluids given by vein are passing into a closed space that can be distended only to a certain point without serious problems. If the circulation becomes overloaded with fluid that is infused too rapidly, cardiac failure can result. IV medications should *always* be administered to a child via an infusion pump. For purposes of calculating fluid volume and IV rate in children, the child receives 60 mini- or micro-drops per cubic centimeter rather than the usual 10 or 15 drops from the standard adult setup.

The nurse should observe the child for these changes:
- Swelling or redness at the insertion site
- Moisture at the site or on the dressing covering the site
- Complaint of pain or inconsolable crying when fluids or medications are infusing.

IV pumps are now designed specifically for medication administration with children (Figure 3-12). Depending on the manufacturer, the precision-controlled syringe pump, or *autosyringe*, may still be used in some hospitals. Occasionally, medications are added to the Soluset (calibrated burette), but this practice is seldom used anymore. Although the use of this equipment provides a safety factor, the nurse must remember that it is a machine and is subject to failing. For this reason, children receiving IV fluids must be observed closely. The *piggyback* method may be used in older children. In general, antimicrobials should infuse within 30 minutes to 1 hour. Always check the IV medication book or pharmacy for time frames.

Some drugs are more effective and are absorbed more rapidly if given by the IV route. IV medications usually require a specified dilution and rate of administration. **Always refer to an IV medication book for specific information on pediatric dosages and administration information.** It is also less traumatic for the child to receive some medications, such as pain medications and antimicrobials, by the IV route rather than by the IM route. The nurse assesses the IV site carefully for infiltration, inflammation, and patency, particularly before administration of the medication. **Always check institution policy to determine who can administer IV medications.**

 Nursing Brief

Children fear having their IV removed. Once the physician order is verified, explain the procedure to the child, remove the tape from around the IV site with adhesive remover, and then quickly remove the IV cannula. Apply an adhesive bandage, and then praise the child. Document the time, procedure, if the cannula was intact, site appearance, and how child tolerated the procedure.

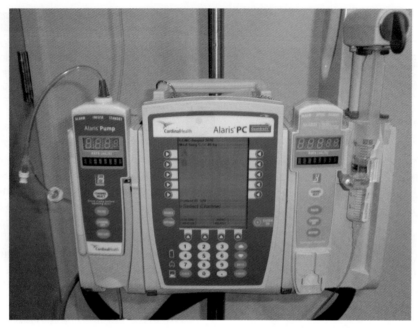

Figure 3-12 Intravenous medication delivered via syringe pump (right side of pump).

Long-Term Venous Access Devices

The heparin or saline lock is usually used as an alternative for a keep-open infusion when long-term access is needed for administration of medication. The cannula remains in place and is flushed with heparin or saline solution, according to the protocol of the hospital. The child is not continuously connected to IV tubing, which allows the child more freedom.

Peripherally inserted central catheters (PICCs) can be used for short- to moderate-term therapy. They are inserted by specially trained nurses or physicians, most commonly above the antecubital area. The catheter is threaded into the superior vena cava and can be used for total parenteral nutrition (TPN), IV fluids, and IV medications.

Tunneled catheters (Broviac® or Hickman® catheters), Groshong® catheters, and implanted ports (mediport, Port-A-Cath®) are other methods of obtaining long-term venous access. Medications, TPN, chemotherapy, IV fluids, and blood products can be given through the catheters. IV tubing is changed daily on a child with a central venous access device, to reduce the risk for infection. The child and the parents are taught how to care for the catheter at home. They are also taught how the catheters are flushed with saline and heparin (Groshong catheters are not flushed with heparin) to maintain patency and prevent clotting. The approach to care of these catheters varies, and each institution provides this information. Older children and parents need to be taught signs of infection, regardless of which IV device is used.

Total Parenteral Nutrition

Intravenous alimentation solutions are complex combinations of crystalline amino acids, glucose, vitamins, trace minerals, and electrolytes. Conditions other than low birth weight that may require their use include severe burns, chronic intestinal obstruction, intractable diarrhea, irradiation, and other life-threatening maladies. Although the beginning student would not be given total responsibility for the child receiving total parenteral nutrition (TPN), all nursing personnel must be alert to the fact that this is not just the usual superficial vein infusion.

To infuse TPN, the physician inserts a central line silastic catheter, which is passed directly into the superior vena cava by way of the jugular or subclavian vein, with careful surgical technique. The catheter is secured in place, and a filter may be attached. An infusion pump is essential for hourly monitoring of the flow. The child receiving TPN must be carefully supervised and evaluated. If an infusion gets behind, it must be reported to the charge nurse; it is *never* adjusted to "catch up." Increasing or decreasing the rate of TPN can cause hyperglycemia or hypoglycemia. Complications of TPN can be serious and are related to both the catheter and the metabolism of the infusate. The bag, IV tubing, and filter (if used) must be changed every 24 hours to prevent infections. All connections should be taped to prevent accidental separation. Contamination via catheter or solution is particularly dangerous because infectious organisms have direct access to body circulation. Thrombosis (development of a blood clot), dislodgment of the catheter, or extravasation (the escape of fluid into surrounding tissue) can occur. Metabolic complications include hyperglycemia because of the high glucose content of the solution, osmotic diuresis, dehydration, and azotemia (the presence of nitrogenous bodies in the blood). Home hyperalimentation is being successfully used for selected children. This requires specific instruction and demonstration by specialty teams. Continuous support and supervision are vital to success. The parents' insurance coverage should be reviewed because home hyperalimentation is costly.

Peripheral vein hyperalimentation may be used for short-term therapy or as a supplement to IV alimentation, but this practice is rare in children. A more dilute concentration is generally used. Infiltration must be avoided because severe tissue sloughing from dextrose irritation may occur. Because hyperalimentation provides no fatty acids, fat or lipid emulsions are usually ordered with TPN. Lipids must be added aseptically below the filter because the fat particles are too large to pass through it.

PROCEDURES TO ASSIST NUTRITION, DIGESTION, AND ELIMINATION

GASTROSTOMY

A gastrostomy (*gastro*, stomach; *stoma*, opening) is made for the purpose of introducing feedings directly into the stomach through the abdominal wall. The physician surgically places a gastrostomy tube or button and secures it in place (Figure 3-13). It is used in children who cannot take food by mouth because of anomalies or corrosive strictures of the esophagus or who are severely debilitated or in a coma. Skin care is a concern with gastrostomy buttons. Drainage may be present. Special attention should be paid to the area under the wings of the button. The wings are periodically rotated. If breakdown does occur, the button is changed to one that has a longer shaft. The area around the stoma should be cleansed frequently with mild soap and water. If a small gauze dressing is used, it should be kept dry.

GASTROSTOMY BUTTON (G-BUTTON) FEEDING

The gastrostomy feeding button may be used with children requiring long-term enteral feeding. Buttons

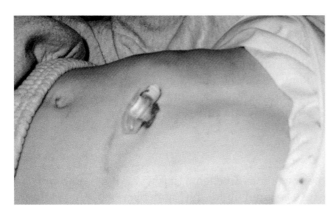

Figure 3-13 Child with skin-level gastrostomy device (MIC-KEY), which provides for secure attachment of extension tubing to gastrostomy opening.

are small, flexible silicone devices. The stomach end has a mushroom-like dome. The skin end has a flat surface that allows the child a more normal lifestyle (see Figure 3-13). There is a one-way valve to prevent reflux of stomach contents. Feedings are done either by gravity bolus (Skill 3-7) or by pump. A disposable bag is used for the feeding, and the rate is set on the pump. It is connected to the child in the same manner as the gravity bolus. The feeding pump is almost always used for feeds that last an hour or more. It is always used if a continuous feed is ordered and is available for home use.

GAVAGE FEEDING

If gavage (orogastric or nasogastric) feedings are ordered, placement is verified prior to the start of the feeding. Determine and document the pH and color of the aspirate before each feeding to confirm tube placement. The pH results need to match the stomach pH results according to the test strip manufacturer. These feedings may be done by gravity bolus feed or via pump, as with G-button feedings. The head of the bed (HOB) should be elevated unless contraindicated. Position the child onto the right side following the feeding as with G-button feeds. Intake is recorded upon completion of the feeding as well as the time of the feeding, type of formula, any residual, and how the feeding was tolerated.

🏠 Nursing Brief

Insertion of a nasogastric tube on an infant or child is similar to an adult. Measure from the nose to the bottom of the earlobe to the end of the xiphoid process. Mark the tube with tape. Verify institution policy for tube size and procedure. Be alert for signs of respiratory distress, and withdraw the tube immediately if noted. Once in place, the tube is secured according to institution policy.

ENEMA

Administering an enema to a child is essentially the same procedure as enema administration for an adult; however, the amount, type, and insertion depth require modification (Table 3-2). Mineral oil enemas are considered safe for children, as are saline enemas (Schmitt,

Table **3-2**   Enema Administration Guidelines

AGE	VOLUME AMOUNT (ML)	INSERTION DEPTH (IN)
Infant	120-240	1
2 to 4 years	240-360	2
4 to 10 years	360-480	3
11 years and older	480-720	4

Skill 3-7   Gastrostomy Button Feeding

Equipment

✓ Room-temperature formula
✓ Funnel or syringe barrel
✓ Tubing
✓ Syringe for aspiration, to flush G-button as ordered (may be up to 15 to 30 mL)

NOTE: Equipment should be sterile for premature and newborn infants.

Safety Issues *(Rationale)*

- Always use formula at room temperature *(cold formula can cause abdominal discomfort).*
- Position child with head elevated unless contraindicated *(helps prevent aspiration).*
- Check for residual volume *(may need to hold feed if too much residual).*
- Do not allow air to get into feeding tube *(causes air to enter stomach).*
- Never force a feeding.
- Stop feeding if signs of respiratory distress, vomiting, cyanosis, or abdominal distention occur.
- Leave patient with head of bed elevated and positioned on right side unless contraindicated *(aids in digestion).*

Method *(Rationale)*

1. Explain procedure *(allays anxiety).*
2. Gather equipment.
3. Wash hands; apply gloves *(ensures that standard precautions are followed).*
4. Position child comfortably, with head slightly elevated if not contraindicated. Provide pacifier to relax a baby *(promotes sucking reflex).* An infant can be held and cuddled during the feeding; an older child can sit in a highchair.
5. Check residual stomach contents by attaching syringe to gastrostomy button and aspirating. (Authors vary on their approach to checking and replacing residual. Always check the policy on this.) Residual is always checked because overloading the stomach can cause reflux and increase the danger of aspiration. If the residual

amount continues or increases, report this to the physician.
6. Attach syringe barrel to tubing, then to gastrostomy button. Fill with formula. Remove clamp *(prevents air from entering the stomach and causing distention).*
7. Elevate receptacle. Allow formula to flow slowly by gravity—*never* use force.
8. Continue to add formula to the syringe before it empties completely. The feeding should take 20 to 25 minutes to complete to prevent regurgitation, vomiting, or aspiration. Always observe for signs of respiratory distress, vomiting, cyanosis, or abdominal distention. Stop feeding if any of these occur, and notify the charge nurse.
9. Clamp the tube as the final formula or water (prescribed flush amount) is passing through the lower part of the syringe; close button.
10. Whenever possible, hold the patient quietly after feeding. Reposition in Fowler's position or on the right side if awake *(promotes gastric emptying).*
11. Record the type (gastrostomy feeding), the amount given, the amount and characteristics of the residual, and how the patient tolerated the procedure. If the patient is on measured fluids, record on intake and output section.

Skills Checklist

✓ Explain procedure.
✓ Assemble equipment.
✓ Wash hands; apply gloves.
✓ Check residual.
✓ Attach syringe barrel and extension set; add formula.
✓ Elevate receptacle.
✓ Continue to add formula.
✓ Clamp tube at end of procedure.
✓ Remove gloves, and wash hands.
✓ Position or hold patient.
✓ Document procedure.

2009). Mineral oil enemas can be purchased at a drug store or pharmacy without a prescription. Saline enemas can be made at home by mixing 2 level teaspoons of table salt to a quart of lukewarm distilled water. Do not use soapsuds, hydrogen peroxide, or plain water as an enema (tap water is isotonic and can cause a rapid fluid shift and overload). In addition, Fleet's phosphate enemas (labeled as saline enemas) can cause serious side effects and are not recommended for children.

Always be certain to know what type of enema solution is intended. This is an invasive procedure for the child; therefore careful age-appropriate explanations are necessary. Other invasive procedures related to the gastrointestinal tract include barium enema, intestinal biopsy, endoscopy, and colonoscopy. These are usually performed by the gastroenterologist.

To administer the enema, place a towel under the child, lubricate the enema tube or nozzle with a lubricant such as KY jelly, and insert 1½ to 2 inches into the rectum. Instill the solution slowly without pressure for approximately 10 to 15 minutes; the tubing should be clamped at intervals, especially if the child has cramping. Encourage the older child to "hold" the solution for 3 to 5 minutes if possible. Record the time of procedure; name, amount, and temperature of solution used; amount and character of results; untoward reactions; and child's response.

OSTOMY

An *ostomy* is a general term referring to any operation in which an artificial opening is formed between two hollow organs or between one or more such viscera and the abdominal wall for discharge of intestinal contents or of urine. Conditions requiring a child to have an **ostomy** (**colostomy,** involving the large intestine, or **ileostomy,** involving the small intestine) include necrotizing enterocolitis, Hirschsprung's disease, imperforate anus, inflammatory bowel syndrome, spina bifida, tumor, or trauma. A **urostomy,** or urinary diversion, is performed if the bladder or urinary tract is involved.

Parents of a child with an ostomy need to understand many things before discharge. They need to know the reason for the surgery, any special nutritional needs, dietary modifications, signs and symptoms of complications, supplies needed for care, and resources in the community. They also need to know how to provide the care. The procedure is similar to the adult procedure with size modification, except that with the infant, the stoma is covered with a dressing. Dressings are changed after each bowel movement. Once the stoma has healed and the infant is large enough to wear a pouch, care is similar to that for an adult. Skin management can be a challenge with infants and children because of the fragility of the skin. Always provide good skin care to prevent breakdown at the stoma site.

CARE OF THE CHILD WITH A TRACHEOSTOMY

A **tracheostomy** is a surgical procedure in which an opening is made in the trachea to enable the child to breathe. This artificial airway may be used in emergency situations, may be an elective procedure, or may be combined with mechanical ventilation. Some of the childhood conditions that may require tracheostomy are acute laryngotracheobronchitis, epiglottitis, head injury, burns, or any condition in which the child is unconscious or debilitated for an extended period. Nursing care is indispensable to the survival of the child because blockage of the tube by mucus or other secretions can lead to suffocation. In many hospitals, the child is placed in the intensive care unit immediately after surgery because this is a critical period requiring frequent suctioning and very close observation. When the condition stabilizes, the child is transferred to a regular unit.

The child with a tracheostomy is placed in an area of high visibility. Infants and small children normally communicate their needs by crying, but the tracheostomy prohibits vocalization. Whenever possible, one nurse is assigned to the child and to work with the parents and to reinforce preoperative teaching. Explain what has happened in an age-appropriate manner. For example, "You were having a lot of trouble breathing. This operation called a tracheostomy helps you breathe easier. A small opening has been made in your neck. A hollow tube was inserted to keep the area open. It is frightening not to be able to speak. When you are better, the hole will close by itself and your voice will return." An explanation of suction might be, "We have to keep the area in your neck open. This tube goes into the airway and clears it." Demonstrate use of suction in a glass of water. Prepare the child for the unfamiliar sound. "You might feel like gagging, but afterward you will feel better. I know this is difficult for you, and I'm sorry there is no easier way." Another approach is to make up a story involving the child's favorite toy, which goes to the repair shop because the toy is having trouble breathing.

The nursing care of the child with a tracheostomy is a significant responsibility. The anatomical differences between children and adults and the small child's inability to communicate through writing increase the need for close observation. Added moisture and humidity are provided by the use of a special tracheostomy collar, or direct attachment to a mechanical ventilator. This is necessary because the nose and mouth no longer warm and moisten the inspired air. Toddlers and infants often have short, stubby necks that become easily irritated with tracheostomy ties.

Maintaining patency of the tracheostomy tube is of utmost importance. Plastic or Silastic tubes are generally used because they are flexible and reduce crust formation. They are lightweight and disposable, and most do not have inner cannulas. Cuffed tubes are not usually necessary in infants and small children because their air passages are smaller and the tracheostomy tube provides a sufficient seal. The surgeon chooses a tracheostomy tube that is appropriate for the size of the child's neck and condition.

Skill 3-8 Suctioning the Tracheostomy

Equipment

✓ Sterile suctioning catheters
✓ Sterile gloves
✓ Bag-valve mask for hyperventilating
✓ Sterile saline solution

Safety Issues

- Maintain sterile technique during procedure.
- Monitor the amount of time suction is applied.
- Provide reoxygenation between suctioning attempts.
- Monitor for signs of respiratory distress during procedure.

Method *(Rationale)*

1. Explain procedure *(allays anxiety)*.
2. Gather equipment.
3. Wash hands; put on sterile gloves *(ensures that standard precautions are followed and prevents infection in the trachea)*.
4. If necessary, hyperventilate the child with 100% oxygen *(prevents hypoxia)*.
5. Lubricate the tube with sterile saline solution, and insert the catheter without applying suction.
6. Withdraw the catheter while applying suction (**5 seconds only**) *(prevents the airway from being obstructed for too long)*.

7. Allow the child to rest. Some children may need a few breaths via a resuscitation bag.
8. Clear the catheter with sterile saline solution between insertions; child may need to be suctioned more than once. Saline solution should also be discarded to prevent growth of *Pseudomonas* in the standing solution.
9. Document: Time and frequency of suctioning, the character of the secretions, the relief afforded the patient, the patient's behavior, the appearance of the stoma, and any other pertinent data.

Skills Checklist

✓ Explain procedure.
✓ Gather equipment.
✓ Wash hands; put on sterile gloves.
✓ Instill normal saline solution per institutional policy.
✓ Insert catheter.
✓ Apply suction while withdrawing the catheter.
✓ Allow/provide ventilation.
✓ Rinse catheter tubing.
✓ Repeat as necessary.
✓ Discard equipment and saline solution.
✓ Remove gloves, and wash hands.
✓ Document procedure.

SUCTIONING

Selection of an appropriately sized suction catheter by the nurse is important so that the tracheostomy tube isn't blocked or dislodged during suctioning. The diameter should be approximately one half that of the tracheostomy tube. Measure the length of the tracheostomy tube (use an extra one), and pass the suction catheter only the measured length to prevent trauma to the mucosa. Instilling a small amount of sterile isotonic saline solution into the tube before suctioning is no longer recommended.

Suctioning is performed when there are signs of secretions in the airway (Skill 3-8). Signs of secretions in the airway may include coughing, noisy breathing, or a bubbling sound. When suctioning the tracheostomy tube, do not apply suction as the catheter is introduced. Withdraw the catheter while applying suction by covering the port on the catheter with the thumb. Hold suction no more than **5 seconds** (Hockenberry and Wilson, 2009). The child should be allowed to rest

for about a minute (and take two or three breaths) between suctioning. Most institutions advise the use of hyperventilating with 100% oxygen between suctioning to prevent hypoxia. The use of pulse oximetry can provide a measure of the child's oxygenation during and after the procedure. Nurses should be aware of any variations in this procedure that might be unique to the agency in which they are working.

 Nursing Brief

Many institutions teach tracheostomy suctioning for home care as a clean rather than sterile technique.

CARE OF THE TRACHEAL STOMA

The tracheal stoma is treated as a surgical wound. The area should be kept free of secretions and exudate to minimize the risk for infection. Nonsterile gloves and eye protection should be used when caring for a tracheostomy. Cotton-tipped applicators dipped in half-strength hydrogen peroxide can be used to remove crusted mucus. Rinse by dipping an additional applicator in sterile water. Change the gauze square or Telfa pad under the tracheostomy site as needed. Some companies manufacture split gauze or dressings for use around the stoma. If this dressing remains wet, it causes skin irritation. Always check the stoma site for signs of infection and breakdown of the skin.

Ties around the child's neck should be snug but loose enough that one finger can be inserted easily. Place the knot to the side of the neck. Assess the condition of the skin beneath the ties. Document the skin condition. Change the ties daily and as necessary. Two people should be used for this procedure, one to hold the cannula and the other to change the ties. It works best if the new ties are looped through the flanges and tied snugly in a triple knot at the side of the neck *before* the soiled ties are cut and removed. Velcro straps are also now used and are much more convenient for home use.

The nurse observes the child for such symptoms of complications such as restlessness, rising pulse rate, fatigue, apathy, dyspnea, sternal retractions, pallor, cyanosis, and inflammation or drainage around the incision. Possible complications include tracheoesophageal fistula, stenosis, tracheal ischemia, infection, atelectasis, cannula occlusion, and accidental extubation. Baseline assessment of the child is done on each shift and before suctioning. The child's mental status, respirations, pulse rate and rhythm, and chest sounds are of particular importance. Accurate recording of observations is essential to evaluation.

A sterile hemostat or clamp is kept at the bedside for emergency use. Accidental **extubation** or expulsion of the tube, although uncommon, can occur from severe coughing if the ties are too loose. Patency of the airway is maintained by spreading the edges of the wound with the sterile hemostat or clamp until another tube is inserted. Extra tracheostomy tubes, **one the same size and one smaller (in case the same size tube can't be reinserted),** and the equipment needed for its replacement are always kept in a visible, easily reached area at the bedside for use in such emergencies. As the child's condition improves, he or she is weaned from the tube. The opening gradually closes with granulation. Children whose tubes must remain in place longer require periodic tube change. This is generally done on a weekly basis once healing has occurred.

Additional nursing measures include frequent change of position, the use of arm restraints ("no no's"), oral feedings unless contraindicated, and careful bathing to prevent water from entering the tube. Range-of-motion exercises are a must for long-term patients, and in acute cases, arm restraints are removed one at a time to allow for passive exercises.

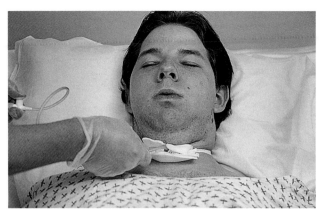

Figure 3-14 Caretakers should be given ample opportunity to take care of the child's tracheostomy before the child is discharged.

The diet is ordered by the physician. Although children initially may have nothing by mouth (NPO), as their condition improves, they progress to a soft or normal diet. Fowler's position is preferred during feedings. Older children can cooperate by holding their head flexed with the chin down. This decreases swallowing difficulties because the esophagus opens and the airway narrows. Monitor feeding of an infant closely so that no food particles are aspirated through the tracheostomy.

Some children are discharged with a tracheostomy. This should be anticipated, and instruction and demonstration for the parents should begin early (Figure 3-14). Parents who are comfortable with the procedure during hospitalization feel more secure when the child returns home. It is advisable for the parents to be "checked off" on tracheostomy procedures before discharge, and most hospitals now require this. Parents should also learn CPR if their child has a tracheostomy. Information about parent groups and the visiting nurse and other referrals are made before discharge.

OXYGEN THERAPY FOR CHILDREN

GENERAL SAFETY CONSIDERATIONS

It is important that all equipment used for oxygen therapy be inspected periodically to determine that materials are intact and that no pieces are missing. Keep combustible materials and potential sources of fire away from oxygen equipment. These materials are essentially the same as for adults; however, for the child, friction toys should also be avoided. Know where the nearest fire extinguisher is located.

Infection control is extremely important. It is imperative that cross-infection via unclean equipment be prevented. Humidifiers and nebulizers, which are warm and moist, provide an excellent medium for the growth of disease-producing organisms. Although most masks, tents, and cannulas that come into direct contact with the child are disposable, other pieces of

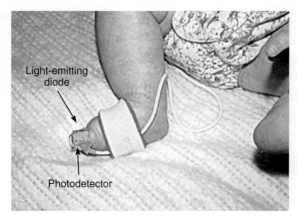

Figure 3-15 Pulse oximeter sensor. Note that the sensor is positioned with light-emitting diode (LED) opposite photodetector.

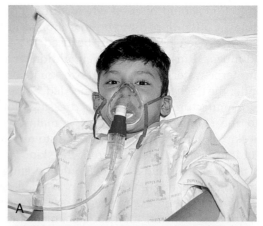

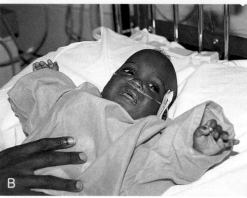

Figure 3-16 Oxygen delivery. **A,** Child receiving oxygen via a face mask. **B,** Infant with a nasal cannula.

mechanical equipment cannot be discarded. **They require periodic cleaning if therapy is extended and terminal cleaning according to product directions.**

Prolonged exposure to high oxygen concentrations can be toxic to some body tissues (e.g., the retina and lungs in premature infants). In addition, *oxygen-induced carbon dioxide narcosis* can occur in persons with chronic pulmonary disease, such as cystic fibrosis or asthma. These patients have higher $PaCO_2$ levels, and hypoxia is the drive for respiratory efforts. If oxygen is administered at too high of a level, the drive for respiratory effort is reduced, causing hypoventilation and increased $PaCO_2$ levels. It is therefore necessary to measure oxygen content at regular intervals. The amount of oxygen administered depends on the child's arterial oxygen concentration. Frequent blood gas determinations (PO_2 and PCO_2) ensure safe and accurate therapy. Noninvasive techniques that measure blood oxygen tension via the skin are available. One example is the pulse oximeter (Figure 3-15).

Oxygen is a dry gas and requires the addition of moisture to prevent irritation of the respiratory tree. **Oxygen therapy should be terminated gradually.** This allows the child to adjust to *ambient* (environmental) oxygen. Slowly reduce the liter flow, open the air vents in incubators, or open zippers in the oxygen tent. Constantly monitor the child's response. An increase in restlessness, a decrease in pulse oximeter readings, and an increase in pulse and respirations generally indicate that the child is not tolerating withdrawal from the oxygen-enriched environment.

METHODS OF ADMINISTRATION

Oxygen is administered to children as age-appropriate via Isolette, nasal cannula, mask, hood, or tent (Table 3-3). The method of delivery is often determined by what method the child tolerates (Figure 3-16). If uncooperative in a tent or with a mask, the child may receive oxygen with the oxygen tubing held near the mouth and nose of the child. Regardless of the method used, the child is observed frequently to determine the effectiveness of the oxygen. **The desired goals include decreased restlessness and improved breathing, vital signs, and color.** The highest concentrations of oxygen are delivered with a plastic hood. Warmed, humidified oxygen is delivered directly over the child's head. It may be used in an incubator or warming unit.

Oxygen tents are available from various manufacturers to deliver humidified oxygen to the child. Often the respiratory therapist sets these up. Nurses need to be aware of certain precautions in case they are required to set up the oxygen tent. The directions for the specific apparatus should be closely followed. Before assembling the tent, carefully examine the plastic for tears. Oxygen tents consist of a plastic canopy suspended from an overhead rod that is attached to a cabinet containing a machine. When adjusted, the machine regulates the ventilation and temperature of the tent and may also provide increased humidity in connection with the oxygen flow. General recommendations include the following:

- Prepare the bed; place a bath blanket and an absorbent pad over the mattress.
- Select the tent according to the age and size of the child. This information should be ascertained

Table 3-3 **Selected Considerations for the Child Receiving Oxygen**

AGE	COMMENTS
General Considerations	• Signs of respiratory distress include an increase in pulse and respiration, restlessness, flaring nares, intercostal and substernal retractions, and cyanosis; in addition, children with dyspnea frequently vomit, which increases the danger of aspiration. • Maintain a clear airway with suctioning if needed. • Organize nursing care so that interruptions are kept to a minimum. • Observe children carefully because your vision may be obstructed by mist and young children are unable to verbalize their needs.
Neonate	Oxygen may be provided via hood, which may be used in the incubator or warming unit. May be provided via Isolette; keep sleeves closed to decrease oxygen loss. Oxygen needs to be warmed to prevent neonatal stress from cold. Analyze concentration carefully to avoid pulmonary disease. Parents are primary focus of preparations; help develop good parenting skills and self-confidence in their ability to care for the child who is ill.
Infant	Nose may need to be suctioned with bulb syringe to remove mucus. A device such as a Danny Sling may be used to keep the infant from slipping down in the bed when the HOB is elevated; blankets or towels can also be rolled and placed under the infant's buttocks. Make sure crib sides are up; a canopy often gives the illusion of safety. Avoid the use of baby oil, A and D ointment, Vaseline, or other oil-based or alcohol-based substances. Anticipate stranger anxiety at around 8 months of age; baby clings to parents, turns away from nurse. An extremely irritable baby may benefit from comforting in parent's lap, followed by sleeping in tent; clarify at report time. Frequently children can be removed from oxygen tent for bathing and eating; determine before proceeding.
Toddler	Anticipate that a toddler will be distressed by a tent. Anticipate regression. A restless and fussy child may pull tent and covers apart. Toddler cannot tell nurse if tent is "too hot" or "too cold." Change clothing and bed linen when damp. Toddler may be comforted by transitional object such as a blanket. Parents may have suggestions as to how to keep child happy in the tent.
Preschool	Tent plastic distorts view. Because thought processes are immature in preschool children, reality and fantasy are inseparable. Prepare child for all procedures to decrease fear. Anticipate that child will feel lonely and isolated. Child will enjoy stories, puppets, and dramatic play. An extremely restless and anxious child may benefit from holding parent's hand through small opening in zippers. Helpful if child can be out of tent for meals and can eat with peers.
School-age	Schoolchildren usually are less frightened by tent; fears center around body mutilation and loss of control. Preparation information continues to focus on what the child will see, hear, feel, and be expected to do. Child may benefit from writing a story about the experience; nurse reviews story with child and clarifies misconceptions; posting story on unit affirms child's self-esteem and mastery (always ask permission to post). Allow child to make realistic choices before, during, and after procedures. Draw "what it feels like to be in a tent," and discuss it.
Adolescent	Needs more time to process information; needs to know the results of blood studies and other tests. Nurse remains available to the patient to answer questions as they arise. Trust is extremely important as adolescent attempts to move beyond the nuclear family. Anticipate problems of being restricted by apparatus. May feel "weird" when visited by peers; wavers between feeling self-confident and feeling ineffective. Reiterate no smoking and other safety precautions with patient and peers. Include patient in therapy; may be able to manage own oxygen needs. Review safe use of oxygen in the home if required for comfort and survival.

before admission for children in acute respiratory distress.

- Bring the canopy and control unit to the bedside; extend the overhead bar, and fold the tent out along the bar.
- Follow manufacturer directions for setup and maintenance.
- Select toys that retard absorption and do not produce static electricity.

RECORDING MEASUREMENTS

WEIGHT

Weight must be recorded accurately on admission. Pounds are generally converted to kilograms for the child in the hospital (see Appendix C). The weight of a child provides a means of determining progress and also is necessary to determine the dosage of most medications. The child who has been undressed for weighing is observed for such objective symptoms as skin coloring, abrasions, bruises, rashes, swelling, or other unusual skin conditions or markings. The way in which the nurse weighs the child depends on the age.

The infant is weighed on a scale completely naked in a warm room. A fresh diaper or scale paper is placed on the scale. This prevents cross-contamination—the spread of germs from one infant to another. The scale is balanced to compensate for the weight of the diaper. There are various ways of balancing scales; the nurse should request specific instruction for the particular scale used. The infant is placed gently on the scale. Most scales are automatic; however, if the scale has weights that must be regulated, the nurse's nondominant hand is held slightly above the infant to ensure that the infant does not fall. The nurse regulates the weights with the dominant hand. The scale should be read when the infant is lying still. If the parent is present, he or she may distract the child by waving or speaking softly. Once the exact weight is determined, the infant is removed from the scale, wrapped in a blanket, and given to the parent to soothe. Record the weight immediately. The scale paper is disposed of in the proper receptacle. An unsoiled diaper is returned with the infant. Digital pediatric scales that provide readouts in pounds and kilograms are used in many institutions. They do not require the regulation of weights. It is best to use the same scale for each measurement.

Older infants and young toddlers can be weighed in the same manner as infants but may prefer to sit up on the scale. Always protect the child from falls.

The older child is weighed in the same manner as an adult. The child is generally weighed in underwear or a hospital gown. The shoes are removed. If the child is unable to stand on the scale, the nurse may need to hold the child and read the combined weights. The nurse then is weighed and subtracts the weight from the combined weights to obtain the child's weight. Occasionally, a child who is wearing a cast is weighed. The nurse records this as, for example, "weight 34 pounds (15.45 kg) with cast on right arm." Weight is recorded on the growth chart (see Appendix C).

Community Considerations

Children's temperature and weight are recorded on nearly all sick and well visits to the physician's office or clinic.

HEIGHT

The older child's height is measured at the time of weighing. Have the child stand straight (barefoot or in stocking feet), and measure with the attached marker, to the nearest 0.1 cm (0.03 inches). The infant must be measured while lying on a flat surface beside a tape measure or on a measuring board. The infant's knees should be pressed flat on the table. Place the head in the midline position; measure from the top of the head to the heel and record. Height is recorded on the growth chart (see Appendix C).

HEAD CIRCUMFERENCE

Head circumference should be measured on all children less than 36 months of age and on children with neurological defects. Place a paper measuring tape around the head from slightly above the eyebrows and pinnae of the ears to the occipital prominence of the skull. Head circumference is recorded on the growth chart (see Appendix C). Check institutional policy to determine whether chest or abdominal circumferences need to be measured (Figure 3-17).

MEASUREMENT OF VITAL SIGNS

PULSE

When the nurse counts the pulse, the wave of blood is felt as it is forced through the artery. The pulse rate

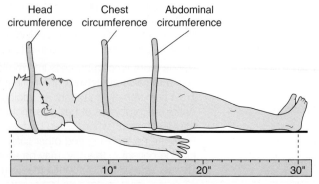

Figure 3-17 Crown-to-heel recumbent measurements.

Table 3-4	Vital Signs at Various Ages		
AGE	**HEART RATE (BEATS/ MIN)**	**BLOOD PRESSURE (MM HG)**	**RESPIRATORY RATE (BREATHS/ MIN)**
Premature	120-170*	55-75/35-45†	40-70‡
0-3 mo	100-150*	65-85/45-55	35-55
3-6 mo	90-120	70-90/50-65	30-45
6-12 mo	80-120	80-100/55-65	25-40
1-3 yr	70-110	90-105/55-70	20-30
3-6 yr	65-110	95-110/60-75	20-25
6-12 yr	60-95	100-120/60-75	14-22
12 yr	55-85	110-135/65-85	12-18

From Kliegman, R., Behrman, R., Jenson, H., et al. (2007). *Nelson textbook of pediatrics* (18th ed.). Philadelphia: Saunders.
*In sleep, infant heart rates may drop significantly lower, but if perfusion is maintained, no intervention is required.
†A blood pressure cuff should cover approximately two thirds of the arm; too small a cuff yields spuriously high pressure readings, and too large a cuff yields spuriously low pressure readings.
‡Many premature infants require mechanical ventilatory support, making their spontaneous respiratory rate less relevant.

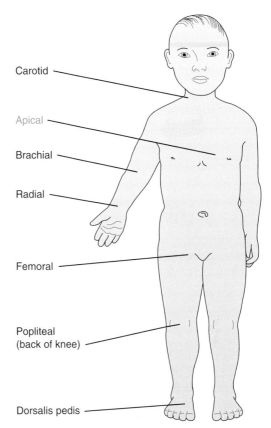

Figure 3-18 Location of pulses. The apical pulse, heard through the stethoscope, needs to be counted for 1 full minute.

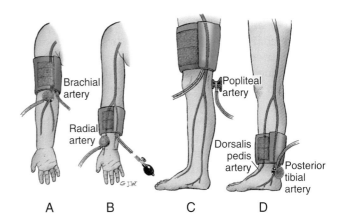

Figure 3-19 Common sites for measuring blood pressure in children. **A,** Upper arm. **B,** Lower arm or forearm. **C,** Thigh. **D,** Calf or ankle.

varies considerably in different children of the same age and size (Table 3-4). The normal pulse rate and respiratory rate of the newborn infant are high. Both pulse and respiratory rates gradually decrease with age until adult values are reached.

The pulse may be counted at any of the peripheral pulse points. However, an apical pulse is recommended for infants and small children. The apical pulse is heard through a stethoscope at the apex of the heart. The nurse counts the rate for 1 full minute. As previously mentioned, listen for any irregularities in rhythm. Report any irregularities to the charge nurse. Figure 3-18 shows the location of the pulses.

RESPIRATIONS

The respirations of the infant and small child are counted by observing the movement of the abdominal wall because respirations are primarily abdominal at this time. The rate is counted for 1 full minute because respirations tend to be irregular during infancy. After about 7 years of age, the child's respirations are measured in the same way as in the adult. Table 3-4 shows normal respiratory rates for children.

BLOOD PRESSURE

Blood pressure is defined as the pressure of the blood on the walls of the arteries. It is an index to the elasticity of the arterial walls, peripheral vascular resistance, efficiency of the heart as a pump, and blood volume. Blood pressure is lower in children than in adults. Common sites for measuring blood pressure in children are the brachial artery, radial artery, popliteal artery, and posterior tibial artery (Figure 3-19).

In the hospital setting, blood pressure is obtained on admission and at regular intervals throughout the hospital stay. In the community setting, children older than 3 years of age should have their blood pressure measured at the time of their physical examination. Children younger than 3 years of age need blood pressure evaluation if they have certain medical conditions such as congenital heart defects or renal disease (see Table 3-4 for normal blood pressure readings). It is important to remember that the child's blood pressure

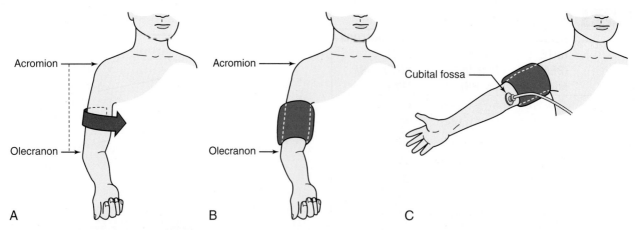

Figure 3-20 Determination of proper blood pressure cuff size. **A,** The cuff bladder width should be approximately 40% of the circumference of the arm measured at a point midway between the olecranon and acromion. **B,** Cuff bladder length should cover 80% to 100% of the circumference of the arm. **C,** Blood pressure should be measured with the cubital fossa at heart level. The arm should be supported. The stethoscope bell is placed over the brachial artery pulse, proximal and medial to the cubital fossa, and below the bottom edge of the cuff.

may be affected by time of day, age, gender, exercise, pain, medication, and emotion.

When obtaining blood pressure readings, the nurse needs to explain to the child what is about to happen. For example, the nurse might say, "This will hug your arm and feel tight for a few seconds." The child also needs to be allowed to examine the sphygmomanometer and cuff. This is followed by giving the child an age-appropriate explanation of the procedure. Afterward, the reading should be rechecked if a significant change or abnormal numbers are obtained. All readings are charted, and abnormal readings are reported to the appropriate charge nurse.

The general rule of thumb has been that the width of the cuff should cover approximately two-thirds of the upper arm, and the cuff (the inner inflatable bladder) should be long enough to encircle the extremity. See Figure 3-20 for a description of proper blood pressure cuff size. In general, systolic pressure in the lower extremities (thigh or calf) is greater than pressure in the upper extremities. In addition, a cuff that is too small causes a falsely elevated blood pressure; a cuff that is too large causes a falsely lowered blood pressure. The most common ways to measure blood pressure are through auscultation and automated devices.

Auscultation

This is the preferred method for measuring blood pressure. Measure blood pressure as for an adult, with the pediatric stethoscope and cuff. Use the correct size. Record the systolic blood pressure at the onset of the "tapping" Korotkoff (K1) sounds. The fifth Korotkoff sound (K5), or the disappearance of Korotkoff sounds, has been established as the diastolic blood pressure (National High Blood Pressure Education Program, 2004).

Automated Devices

Devices such as the Dinamap® are commonly used in pediatric settings. These can be set to measure blood pressure repeatedly and at short intervals. Remember to measure cuff size appropriately. Both systolic and diastolic pressures are recorded. An accurate reading can be obtained only if the child's arm (or leg) is held still. If the reading shows a major change from the child's baseline blood pressure, the measurement should be repeated because the machines are sensitive to movement. It is recommended that blood pressures exceeding the 90th percentile be repeated by auscultation. (Percentiles are listed in Appendix G.)

Palpation

The nurse may occasionally obtain blood pressure readings through palpation. Palpation is one of the oldest methods of blood pressure measurement and is useful in obtaining neonatal blood pressure. Apply the cuff, and inflate above the expected pressure. Place the fingers over the brachial or radial artery. Record the systolic pressure as the point where the pulse reappears. Diastolic pressure is unobtainable using this method.

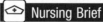
Nursing Brief

Electronic blood pressure measurements are frequently used, but hypertension or hypotension that has been assessed electronically should always be verified with a manual cuff.

TEMPERATURE

Temperature measurement can be oral, axillary, rectal, or tympanic (taken from the tympanic membrane, or eardrum). Several types of thermometers are used, including electronic (digital), plastic strip, and tympanic. According to the U.S. Environmental Protection Agency (EPA), glass thermometers made of mercury are no longer used because of the risk for breakage and leakage of mercury that could create an exposure risk. Electronic thermometers can be used to obtain oral, axillary, or rectal temperatures and are supplied with different probes and probe covers, which are always used. Plastic strips are not routinely used in hospitals. The tympanic thermometer is considered a rapid, efficient, and noninvasive device for measurement of temperature. Temperatures are generally recorded in Celsius (centigrade). See Appendix E for conversions to Fahrenheit.

Rectal Temperature

A rectal temperature measurement may be preferred for the infant and for the small child who cannot hold a thermometer in the mouth without danger of biting it. Because a rectal temperature measurement may be traumatic to children, some institutions use only axillary temperatures for children who are not seriously ill. Research is ongoing in this area as measurement accuracy and temperature differences are examined. If the temperature is to be taken rectally, it should be the last vital sign obtained because it may make the child cry, which influences the pulse, respirations, and blood pressure. Table 3-5 shows normal temperature ranges.

When obtaining the rectal temperature, place the child in a comfortable position, either on the side with the knees slightly flexed or on the stomach. Infants may be in the supine position with their legs held around the ankles and then raised up. Insert the lubricated (electronic) thermometer a maximum of 1 inch into the rectum. Rectal temperatures are contraindicated in newborns because of the danger of rectal perforation and in children who have had rectal surgery or who are immunosuppressed or receiving chemotherapy.

Table **3-5**	Normal Temperature Ranges for Children	
METHOD	**RANGE**
Oral	97.6° to 99.3° F (36.4° to 37.4° C)
Rectal	98.6° to 100.0° F (37.0° to 37.8° C)
Axillary	96.6° to 98.0° F (35.8° to 36.6° C)
Tympanic	98.4° to 99.5° F (36.9° to 37.5° C)

Nursing Care Plan 3-1   The Child with a Fever

NURSING DIAGNOSIS *Knowledge deficit, related to fever*

Goals/Outcome Criteria	Nursing Interventions	Rationale
Parent understands and verbalizes the cause and treatment of fever	Determine parent's knowledge of fever	Determines how much the parent already knows, and serves as an introduction to teaching
	Explain nature of fever (normal body reaction to infection); too vigorous control may mask signs of illness	Fever may actually enhance body's defense mechanisms and increase antibody activity
	Emphasize administration of acetaminophen or ibuprofen, explain appropriate dosage based on child's weight; explain that they may remove excess clothing when child has a fever	Antipyretics lower set point of body's "thermostat" in hypothalamus
	Call physician if child looks sick and acts in a way other than normal	Parent knows child better than anyone else; degree of fever does not always reflect severity of illness
	Have parent return-demonstrate how to read a thermometer and identify normal temperature parameters	Gives parent sense of control and knowledge for home care and guidelines for calling the physician

NURSING DIAGNOSIS *Knowledge deficit, related to possible seizure activity*

Goals/Outcome Criteria	Interventions	Rationales
Parent understands potential for and knows how to give appropriate treatment during a convulsion	Discuss with parent potential for convulsion	Only a small number of children ever convulse with fever; however, discussion is advisable to allay anxiety
	Review management of a convulsion	Knowledge allays anxiety

Continued

✴ Nursing Care Plan 3-1   The Child with a Fever—cont'd

NURSING DIAGNOSIS *Fluid volume, risk for deficient, related to dehydration, from increased metabolic rate*

Goals/Outcome Criteria	Interventions	Rationales
Child is hydrated, as evidenced by: • Good skin turgor • Moist mucous membranes • No weight loss	Increase fluid intake, offer "oral rehydration solutions," water, juice, popsicles, as age-appropriate	Body's metabolic rate increases with fever; children have a higher proportion of body water; therefore more water can be lost rapidly with fever
	Monitor for dehydration at least every shift	By monitoring for evidence of dehydration, the nurse can alert the physician if changes occur
	Monitor intake and output at least once each shift	By monitoring for intake and output, the nurse can alert the physician of deviations from norm
	Weigh daily and record	Weight is a good indicator of the overall hydration status

NURSING DIAGNOSIS *Injury, risk for, related to possible seizure activity*

Goals/Outcome Criteria	Nursing Interventions	Rationale
Child remains free of injury, as evidenced by the absence of: • Bruising • Aspiration • Breaks in the skin	Keep side rails and/or pad up, according to hospital policy	Prevents injury from falls; prevents injury from hitting side rails
	Observe child frequently	Promotes safety by detecting subtle changes and possibly reducing complications
	Maintain suction at bedside	Keeps airway clear and prevents aspiration
	Remain with child if tub bath is given	Prevents head injury or drowning should seizure occur

Critical Thinking Questions
1. How would parents care for a child experiencing a febrile seizure at home?
2. How would parents care for a child experiencing heat stroke at home?

Oral Temperature

The procedure is the same as for adults. Remember, *never* measure the temperature orally in a child who has had oral surgery or is at risk for seizures.

Axillary Temperature

The thermometer is held in the axilla with the child's arm pressed close to the body until the temperature is measured. This is a particularly good method for preschoolers who may fear invasive procedures.

Tympanic Temperature

Many hospitals, doctors' offices, and clinics use the infrared tympanic thermometer (ITT), or ear thermometer. Advantages include safety, noninvasiveness, convenience, and rapid results. Ear thermometers, however, are not as accurate, especially in younger children, specifically those younger than 3 months of age. In children 3 years of age and younger, pull the ear down and back during this temperature measurement.

Body temperature does not remain at 98.6° F (37° C), and slight variations are considered normal. Rectal temperatures are slightly higher and axillary temperatures slightly lower than oral, but not the full degree Fahrenheit that was once thought. When temperature findings are recorded, the nurse notes the route used. If the reading is abnormal, the appropriate charge nurse should be notified. Managing fever in children is depicted in Nursing Care Plan 3-1; home care guidelines are included for parents.

Get Ready for the NCLEX® Examination!

Key Points

- The medical care providers should provide atraumatic care by fostering child-parent relationships, providing information to the child regarding treatments or procedures, controlling pain, providing privacy, providing play therapy, and giving choices.
- Have someone with the child at all times when bathing.
- Sponge bathing is recommended for hyperthermia conditions such as heat stroke; use acetaminophen or ibuprofen to reduce fever
- Sterile techniques are necessary when obtaining a clean-catch urine specimen or a specimen with catheterization.
- Have an assistant help in the procedure when obtaining specimens from small children who cannot hold still.

- During lumbar puncture, always monitor the child's respiratory status.
- Dosages for children's medications are usually smaller and in lesser amounts. The nurse should determine safe dose ranges of medication before administering.
- Children should be given age-appropriate explanations for impending procedures. If a procedure is painful, the child should be told.
- EMLA or LMX cream can be applied to decrease painful insertions of needles.
- When giving medications by the IV route, always check for compatibility of the IV fluid and the medication.
- Monitoring patency of a tracheostomy tube is a priority. Children should be watched for early signs of respiratory distress. A pulse oximeter can assist in monitoring respiratory distress by providing measurements of blood oxygen.
- Oxygen-induced carbon dioxide narcosis can occur in persons with chronic pulmonary disease; oxygen should be administered only at low levels to prevent this.
- Accurate measurement of vital signs is crucial to perform a thorough and accurate evaluation of the child.
- Know the hospital policy before performing any procedures.

Additional Learning Resources

Ⓔvolve Go to your Evolve website (*http://evolve.elsevier.com/Price/pediatric/*) for the following FREE learning resources:
- 3-D Animations
- Answer Keys
- Appendixes
- Audio Glossary
- Spanish/English Glossary
- Video Clips

Review Questions for the NCLEX® Examination

1. Interventions that may be used with fever in a 5-year-old pediatric patient include: (**Select all that apply.**)
   1. Aspirin administration
   2. Reduction of room temperature
   3. Removal of blankets and clothing
   4. Acetaminophen administration
   5. Monitoring the fever

2. Which of the following statements is true regarding obtaining a 24-hour urine specimen on a pediatric patient?
   1. An 8 or 10 Foley catheter is used to obtain the urine specimen.
   2. The perineum or tip of the penis is cleansed with an antiseptic agent prior to obtaining the specimen.
   3. A urine dipstick is used to identify results.
   4. Lost specimens necessitate restarting the test.

3. EMLA cream has been applied to the antecubital fossa of a child to lessen the pain of venipuncture. The nurse is aware that in order for this cream to produce the desired effect it needs to be in place for approximately:
   1. 10 minutes
   2. 30 minutes
   3. 45 minutes
   4. 60 minutes

4. Which of the following is a contraindication to obtaining a throat culture on a child with a "sore throat"?
   1. Diagnosis of tonsillitis
   2. Strep infection
   3. Potential nasopharyngitis
   4. Suspected epiglottitis

5. Head circumference should be measured on all children: (**Select all that apply.**)
   1. Older than 12 months of age
   2. Younger than 36 months of age
   3. With neurological defects
   4. Who are hospitalized
   5. Postoperatively

Growing Children and Their Families

Objectives

1. Define the vocabulary terms listed
2. List the stages of development from the newborn period to adolescence
3. Describe characteristics of growth and development
4. Read a growth chart
5. List six factors that influence growth and development

6. Show an understanding of the influence of the family on the developing child
7. Identify four growth and development theorists
8. Describe the predictable physical changes that take place in normal growth and development
9. Explain why nurses must have an understanding of growth and development

Key Terms

autosome (AW-tō-sōm; p. 64)
body mass index (BMI) (p. 69)
cephalocaudal development (sĕf-ă-lō-KAW-dăl; p. 67)
chromosome (KRŌ-mō-sōm; p. 64)
cognition (kŏg-NǏ-shŭn; p. 71)
development (p. 67)
Erikson (p. 71)
growth (p. 67)

karyotype (KĂR-ē-ō-tīp; p. 64)
Kohlberg (p. 73)
maturation (MĂCH-u-RĂ-shŭn; p. 67)
metabolic rate (MĔT-ah-BŎL-ĭk; p. 68)
ossification (ŏs-ĭ-fĭ-KĀ-shŭn; p. 68)
Piaget (pē-ă-ZHĀ; p. 72)
proximodistal development (PRŎK-sĭ-MŌ-DǏS-tal; p. 67)

HEREDITY AND THE DEVELOPING CHILD

Most of us understand that something inherited is received from one's ancestors. The inheritance may be money or a desired heirloom. It is also possible to inherit physical traits and sometimes even a disorder, such as hemophilia. A person's gender and all inherited characteristics are determined at the moment of conception, when the male sperm cell unites with the female ovum. There are 23 pairs of chromosomes: 22 pairs of autosomes (chromosomes common to both genders) and one pair of sex chromosomes (XX in females and XY in males). Modern cytogenetics (*cyto,* cell; *genetic,* origin) has led to the identification of chromosomes as bearers of **genes** and of **DNA** as the key molecule of the gene. Like chromosomes, genes are paired. Although matching genes in a pair of chromosomes have the same basic function, they do not act with equal power. Some are **dominant,** and others are **recessive.** If a gene is dominant, its instructions are expressed. If a gene is recessive, its instructions are overpowered when it is matched with a dominant gene. If, however, a child inherits two recessive genes (one from each parent), the particular characteristics

associated with this gene are expressed. When any two members of a pair of genes carry the same genetic instructions, the person carrying those genes is said to be **homozygous** for that particular trait. When the two genes in a pair carry different instructions, the person is **heterozygous** for the trait. One member of a heterozygous pair of genes is the dominant gene.

The concept of genes as dominant or recessive is important in the study of birth defects because some parents who carry defective genes can have healthy children or children who are carriers but are not affected themselves. This concept also explains how outwardly normal parents can give birth to a baby with a defect (Figure 4-1). An individual's particular set of genes is known as a **genotype.** Researchers have localized many genes to specific chromosomes, which is termed **gene mapping.** The availability of these techniques makes an accurate family health history more vital than ever.

KARYOTYPE

Geneticists are able to photograph the nuclei of human cells and enlarge them enough to see the 46 chromosomes, or karyotype. These chromosomes are cut from the picture, matched in pairs, and grouped from large to small. The result is called a **karyogram** (*karyo,* nucleus; *gram,* chart). The karyogram of a normal individual shows 22 pairs of chromosomes called **autosomes.** These chromosomes, which are alike in males and females, direct the development of the individual. An example of an autosomal defect is **Down**

syndrome, also known as trisomy 21 because these individuals have a third, or extra, number 21 chromosome.

The remaining pair of chromosomes are **sex chromosomes.** These differ in males and females, determining gender and secondary sexual characteristics. Defects in sex chromosomes are more prevalent than

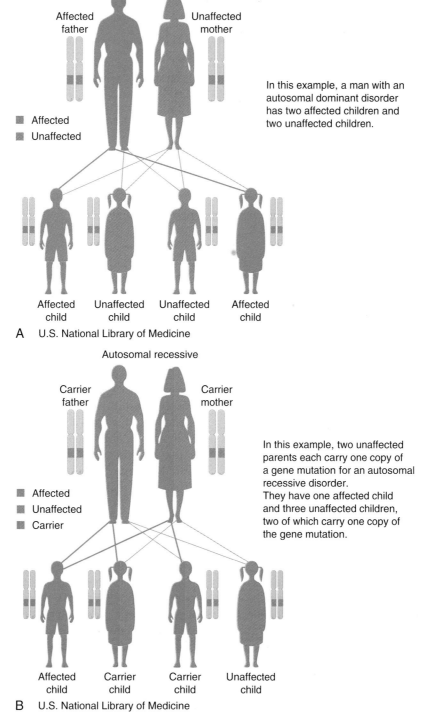

Figure 4-1 Patterns of inheritance. **A,** Dominant inheritance. **B,** Recessive inheritance.

Continued

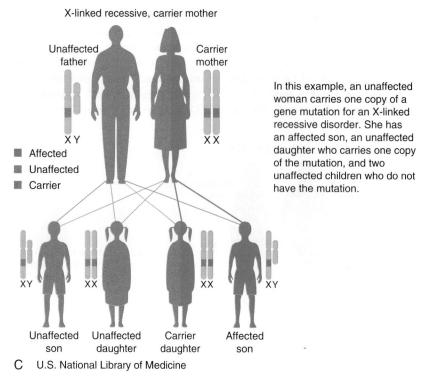

X-linked recessive, carrier mother

Unaffected father

Carrier mother

X Y

X X

■ Affected
■ Unaffected
■ Carrier

In this example, an unaffected woman carries one copy of a gene mutation for an X-linked recessive disorder. She has an affected son, an unaffected daughter who carries one copy of the mutation, and two unaffected children who do not have the mutation.

XY   XX   XX   XY

Unaffected son   Unaffected daughter   Carrier daughter   Affected son

C   U.S. National Library of Medicine

Figure 4-1, cont'd **C,** X-linked inheritance.

Box **4-1**	**Examples of the Genetic Origin of Illnesses and Conditions in Children**

AUTOSOMAL ABNORMALITIES
Down syndrome (trisomy 21)
Edward syndrome (trisomy 18)
Patau syndrome (trisomy 13)
Mosaic trisomy 8 (trisomy 8)

SEX CHROMOSOME ABNORMALITIES
Klinefelter syndrome (XXY)
Double Y syndrome (XYY)
Trisomy X (XXX)
Turner syndrome (XO)

---

those in autosomes and account for a greater variety of abnormal conditions. The Y chromosome is small and apparently carries only the genes for masculinity. The X chromosome is much larger and carries the female genes plus many traits essential to life, such as those that direct various aspects of metabolism, blood formation, color blindness, and defense against bacteria. When the genes that cause a specific condition are known to be carried on the sex chromosomes, the disorder is **sex-linked** (Box 4-1).

Omissions and duplications of chromosomes can occur during **meiosis** (the cell division seen only in sex cells in which the chromosomes divide in half before the cell divides in two). When either a piece of a chromosome or an entire chromosome becomes joined to another chromosome, or when broken segments exchange places, the abnormality is termed a **translocation.**

Mutations, or accidental errors in duplication, rearrangement, or loss of parts of the DNA genetic code, are not completely understood. Once a gene becomes abnormal, the defect is repeated whenever the chromosome on which it appears reproduces itself during normal cell division. Radiation in the form of radiographs, radium, atomic energy, and isotopes can cause mutations. Because a defect may not appear for generations, the amount of radiation to which a person can safely be exposed is difficult to determine. New gene mutations may also occur. A mutation of a gene that directs the production of an enzyme can result in a disruption of the orderly process of metabolism. These biochemical disorders are termed **inborn errors of metabolism.** Without proper direction of the enzymes, harmful chemical products accumulate in the system. If a genetic mistake affects only an unimportant link in the metabolism chain or if the body otherwise compensates, no abnormal symptoms may occur, even though a gene is defective. Some examples of inherited pathologic conditions discussed in this text are cystic fibrosis, sickle cell anemia, and hemophilia.

GENETIC COUNSELING AND RESEARCH

As researchers gather more information concerning the mysteries of the gene, they are able to discover more ways to prevent and treat genetic mishaps. The role of the **genetic counselor** has broadened and taken on greater importance in recent years. Genetic counseling is the process whereby parents and families are counseled regarding the pattern of a gene's transmission and the probability of occurrence or recurrence. Patterns of inheritance are known for hundreds of specific birth defects. Counselors often can suggest laboratory tests to determine whether prospective parents are carriers. A list of genetic counseling services can be obtained from the National Foundation/March of Dimes.

In specific genetic disorders in which a precise enzyme or protein is missing, it is often possible to supply the necessary factor. For example, clotting agents may be given to persons with hemophilia and pancreatic enzymes to those with cystic fibrosis. In other disorders, elimination of an offending substance can correct the problem. This is seen in phenylketonuria, in which the elimination of foods high in phenylalanine can prevent brain damage.

Medical research is on the threshold of important breakthroughs in the understanding and treatment of genetic disorders. The U.S. Human Genome Project, funded by the federal government, is locating DNA on genes. Biochemists can at this time create many of these genes in laboratories. As the genetic code is further deciphered, sending messages to the nuclei of cells and supplying the minute amount of DNA needed to correct a mistake will become possible. Gene therapy replacement is a highly experimental project that holds great potential for diseases that are the result of a defective gene, such as cystic fibrosis.

With the development of new technology, obstetric and pediatric providers are faced with questions about pediatric genetic disorders. The ethical and moral obligations for care of such disorders are a constant issue for providers. Definition of standards of care for those who receive genetic testing and counseling is crucial to this area.

GROWTH AND DEVELOPMENT

Growth generally refers to the processes that result in increases in size, whereas development refers to increases in complexity of form or function. Growth is **orderly** and proceeds from the simple to the more complex. Although orderly, growth is uneven at times. Growth spurts are often followed by plateaus. The periods of most rapid growth are infancy and adolescence. The **rate** of growth varies with the individual child. Each has a timetable that revolves around established norms. Siblings within a family vary in growth and development.

Growth and development are measurable and can be observed and studied. This study is done by comparing height, weight, an increase in vocabulary, the development of physical skills, and other parameters. There are variations in growth within the systems and

subsystems, because not all parts mature at the same time. Skeletal growth approximates whole body growth, whereas the brain, lymph, and reproductive tissues follow distinct and individual sequences.

CLARIFICATION OF TERMS

The stages of growth and development referred to in this chapter are as follows:

Prenatal Life	*Conception to Birth*
Newborn or neonate	Birth to 4 weeks
Infant	4 weeks to 1 year
Toddler	1 to 3 years
Preschool	3 to 6 years
School age	6 to 12 years
Adolescence	12 to 21 years

As *growth* refers to an increase in physical size, measured in inches/centimeters or pounds/kilograms, *development* refers to a progressive increase in the function of the body. The two are inseparable. Maturation (*maturus*, ripe) refers to the total way in which a person grows and develops, as dictated by inheritance. Although maturation is independent of environment, the timing of maturation may be affected by the environment.

CHARACTERISTICS OF GROWTH AND DEVELOPMENT

Directional Patterns

Directional patterns are fundamental to the growth of all humans. Cephalocaudal development proceeds from head to toe (Figure 4-2). The infant is able to raise the head before he or she can sit and gains control of the trunk before walking. The second pattern is proximodistal development, or inner to outer. Development proceeds from the center of the body to the periphery. These patterns occur bilaterally. Development also proceeds from the general to the specific. The infant grasps with the hands before pinching with the fingers.

Height. The newborn infant at birth has an average length of about 20 inches (50 cm). Linear growth is caused mainly by skeletal growth. Growth fluctuates throughout life until maturity is reached. Infancy and puberty are both rapid growth periods. Height is generally a family trait, although exceptions do exist. Good nutrition and general good health are instrumental in promoting linear growth. Height is measured during each well-child conference.

Weight. Weight is another good index of health. The average newborn infant weighs 7 pounds (3.25 kg). The quality of the uterine environment has a bearing on weight. Birth weight usually doubles by 5 to 6 months of age and triples by 1 year of age. After the

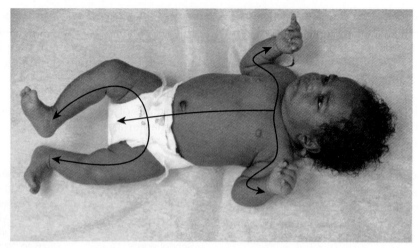

Figure 4-2 The development of muscular control proceeds from head to foot (cephalocaudal) and from the center of the body to its periphery (proximodistal).

first year, weight gain levels off to approximately 4 to 6 pounds (1.81 to 2.72 kg) per year until the pubertal growth spurt. Weight is determined at each office visit. A marked increase or decrease requires further investigation.

Body Proportions. Body proportions differ greatly in the child and adult. The head is the fastest growing portion of the body during fetal life. During infancy, the trunk grows rapidly, and during childhood, lower limb (leg) growth predominates. In adolescence, characteristic male and female proportions develop as childhood fat disappears. Alterations in proportions in the size of the head, trunk, and extremities are characteristic of certain disturbances. Routine measurements of head and chest circumferences are important indices of health. Head circumference need not be measured routinely after 3 years of age.

Metabolic Rate

The metabolic rate in children is higher than in adults. Infants require more calories, minerals, vitamins, and fluid in proportion to weight and height than do adults. Higher metabolic rates are accompanied by increased heat production and increased production of waste products. The body surface area of young children is far greater in relation to body weight than that of the adult. The young child loses relatively more fluid from the pulmonary and integumentary systems.

Bone Growth

Bone growth is one of the best indicators of biological age. Bone age can be determined from radiographic films. In the fetus, bones begin as connective tissue, which later is converted to cartilage. Through ossification, cartilage is converted to bone. The maturity and rate of bone growth vary within individuals; however, the progression remains the same. Growth of the long bones continues until **epiphyseal fusion** occurs. Bone

is constantly synthesized and reabsorbed. In children, bone synthesis is greater than bone destruction. Calcium reserves are stored in the ends of the long bones.

Critical Periods

There appear to be certain periods when environmental events or stimuli have their maximal effect on the child's development. The embryo, for example, is adversely affected during times of rapid cell division. Certain viruses, drugs, and other agents are known to cause congenital anomalies during the first 3 months after conception. It is believed that sensitive periods also occur in respect to bonding, developing a sense of trust during the first year of life, and learning readiness.

Integration of Skills

As the child learns new skills, those skills are combined with ones already mastered. For instance, the child who is learning to walk may sit, pull herself up to a table by grasping it with her hands, balance herself, and take a cautious step. Tomorrow she may take three steps. Children connect and perfect each skill in preparation for learning a more complex one. As a child focuses on a new skill, he or she will not work on any other new skills because the child is not able to cope with several new skills at the same time.

GROWTH STANDARDS

Growth is measured in dimensions such as height, weight, volume, and thickness of tissues. Measurement alone, without any standard of comparison, limits the interpretation of the data. Thus data have been collected and standards developed that make it possible to (1) compare the measurement for any one child with those for other children of the same age, gender, and ideally, race and (2) compare that child's

Table **4-1**	BMI Weight Status Categories and Percentile	
Underweight	Less than 5th percentile
Healthy weight	5th percentile to less than 85th percentile
Overweight	85th percentile to less than 95th percentile
Obese	Equal to or greater than 95th percentile

present measurements with the former rate of growth and pattern of progress. The 2000 Centers for Disease Control and Prevention (CDC) growth charts are recommended for all children in the United States. These charts have been revised with samples of children that include breastfed and formula-fed infants. The new charts include the 14 previous charts (revised) as well as two new charts that show body mass index (BMI)-for-age percentiles. These charts monitor data for infants, children, and adolescents up to age 20 years. They can also be used for low birth-weight infants. Head circumference measurements for infants and children up to age 36 months continue to reflect brain growth and size.

Body mass index (BMI) has been established as a screening tool used to identify body fatness in children and teens. Plotting height and weight measurements on the CDC BMI-for-age growth charts determines a percentile. Percentiles are used to determine a weight status category (Table 4-1). The importance of BMI data has been validated by the American Academy of Pediatrics indicating that children with BMI values of more than 85% have risk factors for cardiovascular disease and should use weight loss or maintenance to achieve a BMI below 85% (Spiotta et al., 2008).

It is important to note that a child whose height or weight falls below the 10th percentile may be normal if the child has shown regular growth in height and weight and has a growth pattern that is comparable with that of the general population. Likewise, children whose height and weight fall in the 75th percentile may need further evaluation if this constitutes a major change from previous measurements (for example, if the child previously was in the 25th percentile). See Appendix C for examples of growth charts, or visit the CDC website (*www.cdc.gov/growthcharts/*).

 Nursing Brief

BMI is a tool that may indicate the need for further assessment. A higher childhood BMI is associated with an increased risk of coronary heart disease in adulthood.

FACTORS THAT INFLUENCE GROWTH AND DEVELOPMENT

Growth and development are influenced by many factors that can have profound effects. While there are many, they can be grouped into genetics and environment.

GENETIC OR HEREDITARY TRAITS

Characteristics derived from our ancestors are determined at the time of conception by countless **genes** within each chromosome. Each gene is made up of a chemical substance called **DNA** that plays an important part in determining inherited characteristics. Examples of these inherited traits are eye color, hair color, and physical resemblances within families. **Gender** may impact development with differences in size and rate of development. Parents often treat boys and girls differently by providing gender-specific toys during play and by having differences in expectations.

ENVIRONMENTAL

The way of life or **culture** affects many areas, including speech, food preferences, family structure, religious orientation, and moral code. Ascertaining cultural beliefs and practices is important in the collection of data for nursing assessment and in providing culturally sensitive nursing care.

 Cultural Considerations

Families of various ethnic groups may collaborate with other practitioners such as folk healers, curandero or curandera, or spiritualists. In the Hispanic culture, major health decisions are made with grandparents and other extended family members. Native Americans may include tribal elders in decisions.

Family structures are a major influence of how a child grows and progresses. The 1990s and early 2000s have seen a great increase in both the number of women working outside the home and the number of women as the head of household. Children may be raised by one parent, by a relative such as the grandparent, or in a foster home (Figure 4-3). The traditional roles of the mother and father have changed, with many parents sharing both child care and household duties.

Many families have both parents working, which may require finding child care. While daycare centers provide the majority of the settings, many children are being cared for in a home setting. When selecting child care, families should be guided in finding an appropriate setting. The daycare setting can provide experiences that enhance the child's development, and some may provide early childhood programs. The health care practices of the daycare setting should be closely

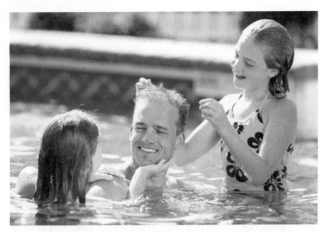

Figure 4-3 A single-parent family may result from divorce, death, or other events.

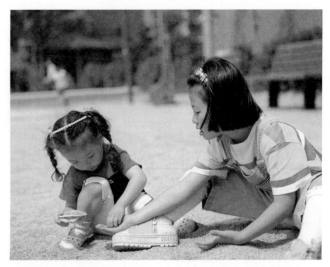

Figure 4-4 Siblings can play important roles in the family. Children who are secure and loved can direct their energies toward positive development.

evaluated as children under the age of 3 have more illnesses than children cared for in their home.

Other family structures that can influence how a child grows and progresses may include homelessness; divorce; blended families; adoption; gay or lesbian families; and latchkey situations. See Chapter 9 for further discussion on these family structures. The family is also more mobile, disrupting the family's support systems and requiring children to change schools and friends.

Many children live in poverty and lack proper nutrition and health care. **Nutrition** may be the most single important influence on growth and development. Inadequate nutrition can have long-lasting effects in all stages of development and may impact the health status of the child. If the socioeconomic level of the family is insufficient, it can impact the ability to provide adequate nutrition, child care, and health care. Because infants and young children experience rapid growth, they require a higher demand for calories. The prenatal health of the mother at the time of conception and the amount and quality of her diet during pregnancy are important for proper fetal development. Maternal infections or diseases may lead to malformations of the fetus.

Parental attitudes and **child-rearing philosophies** develop as a result of the parent's life experiences and impact the child's course of development. Parental finances, education, marital status, and support systems are additional influences impacting parental attitudes. Well-educated parents tend to have a better grasp of the need and ability to provide a rich, safe learning environment. Parents with a lower socioeconomic status may have more difficulty providing a safe, stimulating environment. An uneducated mother may not know the proper methods of cooking foods to preserve nutritional value. She may neglect immunizations and other medical issues. An understanding of growth and development can help parents set realistic goals for their children and themselves. Most home environments are neither completely positive nor completely negative but a mixture. Poverty can be less detrimental to a child in a home where love and affection are present than in a home where there is discord and rejection.

Whether the child is first, middle, or last in **birth order** in the family has a bearing on development. Younger children learn from their older brothers and sisters (Figure 4-4). The motor development of the youngest child in a family may be prolonged because this child tends to be "babied" or may progress quickly as the child tries to keep up with the siblings. An only child may tend to mature faster intellectually but may be slower in motor development because much is done for her or him.

Intelligence, cognitive and emotional, plays an important role in social and mental development. Cognitive intellect is believed to be inherited, and emotional intellect is greatly affected by environment. These factors are related and are at times dependent on each other in the effect on growth and development. They make each person unique. The effect of the family greatly affects the emotional well-being of the child. If a child is ill, physically or emotionally, the developmental processes may be altered. It is imperative that we, as health care providers, not only attend to families' needs, but also take advantage of their strengths and diminish their weaknesses.

Nursing Brief

The family is an important resource for the child and the nurse. Nursing care of children involves caring for the whole family. The nurse will need to have skills to deal with both adults and children.

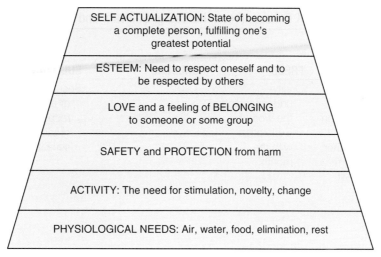

Figure 4-5 Maslow's hierarchy of basic needs.

THEORIES OF DEVELOPMENT

Although no one group of theories can explain all human behavior, each theory can make a useful contribution. Many experts have devoted their lives to understanding why children and families behave as they do. Some, called **systems theorists,** believe that everyone in the family (or system) is affected by everyone else in the family. This theory focuses on relations between and among the various individuals rather than on the individuals themselves. The nurse who relates to the systems theory focuses on caring for the child by caring for the whole family. The family, or system, is seen as protector, educator, resource, and health provider for the child. In turn, the child's health is seen as having an impact on each individual member of the family and on the family as a whole.

Many see human development as a composite of various theories. **Maslow's hierarchy of needs** is depicted in Figure 4-5, and the developmental theories of Erikson, Freud, Kohlberg, Sullivan, and Piaget are presented in Table 4-2. These theorists are discussed here and in later chapters, where their theories relate to the specific age group discussed. Theories provide a framework for the practitioner, but it must be emphasized that humans are not a gathering of isolated parts, even though these parts may be analyzed for research purposes.

PSYCHOSOCIAL DEVELOPMENT

Erik Erikson developed a psychosocial theory that focused on the interrelationship between emotional and physical variables. He used a five-stage approach to his theory. Each stage has a major developmental conflict that needs to be resolved to successfully move to the next stage. Erikson believed that major conflicts are rarely completely resolved but they become less important as other conflicts arise in later stages.

However, he does not explain how outcomes from one stage impact another. Nor does he specify experiences needed to resolve the conflicts. His theory does provide health care providers with a method for assessing developmental conflicts children face. Understanding development can assist health care providers in helping families/caregivers understand the behaviors they can expect to see in their children. It is most important that parents understand that love, approval, and praise are important to children of all ages.

During infancy, trust can be developed by meeting basic needs such as feeding in a timely and appropriate manner. A toddler's independence can be encouraged by maintaining familiar daily routines. Providing opportunities for toddlers to feed or dress themselves promotes independence. Preschoolers' curiosity about their world should be encouraged by exploration and questions. Providing choices, answering questions, and allowing them opportunities to play with equipment (medical) promotes self-satisfaction and broadens their experiences. School-age children use activities to provide them with a feeling of self-worth and value. Opportunities to continue schooling, hobbies, or interacting with peers in a hospital setting can assist with the feeling of accomplishment. Adolescents are seeking to define themselves and gain independence. Encouraging and promoting them to take responsibility for their actions and supporting their choices can enhance their developing identity.

COGNITIVE DEVELOPMENT

Cognition refers to intellectual ability. Children are born with inherited potential, but this must be developed. There are a number of theories as to how learning takes place, with some disagreement as to the roles or importance of inner drives or needs and environmental stimuli. The development of logical thinking and conceptual understanding is a complex process.

Table 4-2   Developmental Theories of Erikson, Freud, Kohlberg, Sullivan, and Piaget

STAGE	ERIKSON	FREUD	KOHLBERG	SULLIVAN	PIAGET (INTELLECTUAL DEVELOPMENT)
Infancy (birth to 1 year)	Trust/mistrust getting Tolerating frustration in small doses Recognizing mother as distinct from others and self	Orality—understanding the world by exploration with the mouth	—	Security, patterns of emotional response, organization of sensation	Sensorimotor stage (birth to 2 years)—at birth responses are limited to reflexes; begins to relate to outside events; concerned by sensations and actions that affect directly
Toddler (1 to 3 years)	Autonomy/shame and doubt Trying out own powers of speech Beginning acceptance of reality versus pleasure principle	Anality—learning to give and take	—	Mastery of space and objects	Preoperational (2 to 7 years)—child is still egocentric; thinks everyone sees world as he or she does Preconceptual (2 to 4 years)—forms general concepts, not yet capable of reasoning
Preschool (3 to 6 years)	Initiative/guilt Questioning Exploring own body and environment Differentiation of genders	Phallic/Oedipal phase—becoming aware of self as sexual being	Preconventional or premoral morality—rules are absolute; breaking rules results in punishment (4 to 7 years)	Speech and conscious need for playmates, interpersonal communication	Perceptual (4 to 7 years)—capable of some reasoning, but can concentrate on only one aspect of a situation at a time
School age (6 to 12 years)	Industry/inferiority Learning to win recognition by producing things Exploring, collecting Learning to relate to own gender	Latency—focusing on peer relations, learning to live in groups and to achieve	Conventional morality—rules are created for the benefit of all; adhering to rules is the right thing to do (7 to 11 years)	Chumship, one-to-one relationship, self-esteem, compassion (homosexuality)	Concrete operations (7 to 11 years)—reasoning is logical but limited to own experience; understands cause and effect
Adolescence (12 to 21 years)	Identity/role diffusion Moving toward heterosexuality Selecting vocation Beginning separation from family Integrating personality (e.g., altruism)	Genitality	Principled morality (autonomous stage; 12 years on)—acceptance of right or wrong on basis of own perceptions of world and personal conscience	Capacity to love, empathy, partnership (heterosexuality)	Formal operational stage (11 to 16 years)—acquires ability to develop abstract concepts; oriented to problem solving

One outstanding authority on cognitive development was Jean Piaget, a Swiss psychologist. He proposed that intellectual maturity is attained through four orderly and distinct stages of development, all of which are interrelated. These stages are **sensorimotor** (up to 2 years), **preoperational** (2 to 7 years), **concrete operations** (7 to 11 years), and **formal operations** (11 to 16 years). The ages are approximate, and each stage builds on the preceding one.

Piaget held that intelligence consists of interaction and coping with the environment. Babies begin their interaction with reflex response. As they grow older, their use of symbolism (particularly language) increases. This gradually shifts to a here-and-now orientation (concrete operations) and finally to a fully abstract comprehension of the world (formal operations). Current theorists have identified inconsistencies in Piaget's theories; however, he remains an important pioneer in the study of intelligence.

MORAL DEVELOPMENT

Lawrence Kohlberg is one of the leading theorists of moral development. Kohlberg's theory is described in three levels, with two stages at each level. In the **preconventional** phase, children operate on a level of obedience to parental authority, and behavior is driven by a wish to avoid punishment. At the **conventional** level, the child is interested in pleasing others, and there is a need to maintain social order in society by maintaining law and order. At the **postconventional** level, moral principles are developed that can be used to solve complex moral and ethical dilemmas. Children pass through and reach these stages at various ages. It is believed that most children begin to develop the stages of the postconventional level only in adolescence and do not fully attain this stage until adulthood.

NURSING IMPLICATIONS OF GROWTH AND DEVELOPMENT

An understanding of growth and development and its predictable nature, including individual variation, has value in the nursing process. Such knowledge provides the basis for the nurse's **anticipatory guidance** to parents. For example, the nurse who knows when the infant is likely to crawl begins to expand teaching on safety precautions. The nurse also incorporates these precautions into nursing care plans in the hospital and in other health care settings.

Age-appropriate care cannot be administered when one does not have an understanding of growth and development. As the nurse explains various aspects of child care to families, the importance of individual differences is stressed. Parents tend to compare their children's development and behavior with those of other children and with information in popular magazine articles. This may relieve their anxiety or cause them to impose impossible expectations and standards. In addition, some parents have had poor role models who influenced their own experiences as children. Lack of knowledge concerning parenting can be recognized by the nurse, and suitable interventions should be implemented.

The nurse who understands that children are born with their own personalities can help frustrated parents cope with a newborn baby who is having difficulty settling into the new environment. During well-child visits, an assessment can determine whether an infant is merely on his or her own timetable or whether a variation from normal exists. The nurse provides **anticipatory guidance** to direct the parent's or caregiver's attention to upcoming events in the child's growth and development. The nurse also recognizes when to intervene to promote wellness or to prevent disease. For example, a brief visit with a caretaker may reveal that the child's immunizations are not up-to-date. Promotion of health can be achieved by educating the expectant mother. Other threats to health may likewise be anticipated. By knowing that specific diseases are prevalent in certain age groups, the nurse maintains a high level of awareness when interacting with these children. This approach, based on knowledge, experience, and effective communication, helps to ensure a higher level of family care.

> **[!] Safety Alert**
>
> The nurse with knowledge of growth and development can identify parents who need assistance with understanding what behaviors can be expected and what safety precautions are appropriate for their child.

Finally, the nurse must understand how to provide nursing care to children of various ages so that their physical, mental, emotional, and spiritual development is enhanced according to their specific needs and comprehension.

Get Ready for the NCLEX® Examination!

Key Points

- The genetic component of a child is based on chromosomes.
- Genetic disorders can result from mutations.
- Prenatal testing can detect some defects.
- Growth occurs in a cephalocaudal direction, which is from head to toe, and proximodistal, which is inner to outer.
- Growth charts are used to assess a child's growth.
- BMI charts identify children who are at risk for cardiovascular disease.
- Factors influencing growth and development are heredity, ethnicity, race, ordinal position in the family, gender, environment, and the family.
- Maslow's hierarchy provides a framework for identifying the priority of basic human needs.

- Theorists of development include Erikson, Freud, Kohlberg, Sullivan, and Piaget.
- Assessment of growth and development identifies the need for anticipatory guidance.

Additional Learning Resources

evolve Go to your Evolve website (*http://evolve.elsevier.com/Price/pediatric/*) for the following FREE learning resources:

- 3-D Animations
- Answer Keys
- Appendixes
- Audio Glossary
- Spanish/English Glossary
- Video Clips

Review Questions for the NCLEX® Examination

1. An individual's particular set of genes is known as a(n):
   1. Autosome
   2. Chromosome
   3. Genotype
   4. Karyotype

2. The infant is able to raise the head before he or she can sit and gains control of the trunk before walking. This is an example of:
   1. Cephalocaudal development
   2. Proximodistal development
   3. Maturational development
   4. Peripheral development

3. The theorist whose hierarchy provides a framework for identifying the priority of basic human needs is:
   1. Erikson
   2. Freud
   3. Kohlberg
   4. Maslow

4. A child has been weighed by the school nurse and BMI is documented to be in the 70th percentile. The nurse is aware that this BMI indicates:
   1. Underweight
   2. Healthy weight
   3. Overweight
   4. Obesity

5. Erikson's stage of industry/inferiority includes: (**Select all that apply.**)
   1. Integrating personality
   2. Exploring
   3. Selecting vocation
   4. Tolerating frustration in small doses
   5. Learning to relate to own gender

The Newborn Infant

Objectives

1. Define the vocabulary terms listed
2. Discuss the importance of airway maintenance in the neonate
3. Identify the range of average measurements in the newborn infant
4. Describe the importance of thermoregulation, particularly in the preterm infant
5. Discuss normal vital signs of the newborn
6. Differentiate AGA, SGA, and LGA infants
7. Differentiate low–birth weight, very low–birth weight, and extremely low–birth weight neonates
8. Describe the APGAR and the Ballard scoring systems
9. Briefly describe three normal reflexes of the neonate (including approximate age of disappearance) and the tests for their appearance
10. Discuss implications and treatment methodologies of jaundice in the newborn
11. List three causes of preterm birth
12. Describe the differences in care for the preterm infant with respiratory distress syndrome and apnea
13. Differentiate hypoglycemia and hypocalcemia
14. List three characteristics of the postterm infant
15. Describe the six neonatal states of the newborn
16. Discuss medications administered to the newborn
17. Discuss the purpose of metabolic screenings
18. Compare and contrast breastfeeding and formula feeding
19. Contrast the techniques of feeding the preterm and the full-term neonate
20. Describe precautions to prevent infection while caring for the newborn
21. Summarize teaching principles of bathing the newborn, providing cord care, and providing circumcision care
22. Discuss ways to help facilitate the maternal-infant bonding process for a preterm neonate
23. Describe discharge teaching needs of the parents

Key Terms

acrocyanosis (ăk-rō-sī-ă-NŌ-sĭs; p. 79)
anuria (ă-NŪ-rē-ā; p. 86)
Apgar score (p. 77)
atelectasis (ă-tĕ-LĔK-tă-sĭs; p. 93)
Auditory Brainstem Response (ABR) (O-dĕ-tōr-ē; p. 84)
bilirubin (bi-li-RŪ-ben; p. 88)
caput succedaneum (KĂP-ĕt sŭk-sĕ-DĀ-nē-ĕm; p. 80)
cephalhematoma (sĕf-ăl-hē-mă-TŌ-mă; p. 80)
circumcision (sĭr-kŭm-sĭzh-ŭn; p. 86)
cold stress (p. 78)
cradle cap (p. 80)
exogenous (ĕk-SĂ-je-nes; p. 93)
fontanels (fŏn-tă-NĔLZ; p. 80)
grunting (p. 93)
high risk (p. 80)
hypospadias (hī-pō-SPĀ-dē-ăs; p. 86)
icterus neonatorum (ĭk-tĕr-ŭs NĒ-ō-nā-tor-ŭm; p. 88)
kernicterus (kĕr-NĬK-tĕr-ŭs; p. 88)
lanugo (lă-NOO-gō; p. 87)
lecithin/sphingomyelin (L/S) ratio (LĔS-ĭ -thĭn/SFĬNG-gō-MĪ-ă-lĭn; p. 93)
macrosomia (măk-rō-SŌ-mē-ă; p. 98)
molding (MŌL-dĭŋ; p. 80)
Moro reflex (MŌR-ō; p. 83)
neonate (NĒ-ō-nāt; p. 77)
neonatal intensive care unit (NICU) (p. 77)
nonshivering thermogenesis (THER-mō-JĔN-ĕ-sĭs; p. 78)
ophthalmia neonatorum (of-THAL-mē-a NĒ-ō-nā-tor-ŭm; p. 100)
previability (prē-VĪ-ă-bĭl-Ĭ-tē; p. 92)
respiratory distress syndrome (RDS) (rĕs-PĬ-ră-tō-rē; p. 93)
rickets (RI-kets; p. 101)
rooting reflex (RÜT-iŋ; p. 82)
thermoregulation (THER-mō-rĕg-ū-LĀ-shŭn; p. 78)
transport team (p. 108)
vernix caseosa (VER-niks KA-sē-ō-sa; p. 87)

INTRODUCTION TO THE NEWLY BORN INFANT

Every parent wants a perfect baby. Reality is, however, that not all babies are born without defects. Birth defects can vary from minor to fatal. Chapter 1 discusses infant mortality. A birth defect is defined as "an abnormality of structure, function, or metabolism (body chemistry) present at birth that results in physical or mental disability or death. Several thousand different birth defects have been identified. Birth defects are the leading cause of death in the first year of life" (March of Dimes, 2006). Birth defects are the cause of death in one of every five infant deaths. The March of Dimes lists three major categories of birth defects: structural/metabolic, congenital infections, and other. Because these disorders include so many conditions, it has been necessary to limit the number discussed in this chapter and to discuss others in relevant areas of the textbook (see the Index for specific conditions).

In 1998, Congress passed the Birth Defects Prevention Act, which provides funding to the Centers for Disease Control and Prevention to collect and analyze data on birth defects, to support research, and to educate the public regarding birth defects. Defects present at birth often involve the skeletal system; limbs may be missing, malformed, or duplicated. Some abnormalities, such as congenital developmental dysplasia of the hip (DDH), are more subtle and require alertness on the part of health care providers to detect them. Inborn errors of metabolism include a number of inherited diseases that affect body chemistry. There may be an absence or a deficiency of a substance necessary for cell metabolism. This is usually an enzyme deficiency. Almost any organ of the body may be damaged. Examples of inborn errors of metabolism include cystic fibrosis and phenylketonuria. In disorders of the blood, there is a reduced or missing blood component or an inability of a component to function adequately. Sickle cell anemia, thalassemia, and hemophilia fall into this group. Chromosomal abnormalities number in the hundreds. Some involve mental retardation, and some are incompatible with life. The newborn infant with Turner syndrome or Klinefelter syndrome may be retarded in physical growth and sexual development. Perinatal damage also has many causes and can be seen in a variety of forms. The most common form is premature birth. Only a few birth defects can be attributed to a single cause; most are thought to result from a combination of environment and heredity.

Some prenatal tests (ultrasound, amniocentesis, and chorionic villus sampling [CVS]) may assist in the diagnosis of certain birth defects before birth. These tests may be helpful in detecting or ruling out a possible birth defect with families that are suspected of having a history of birth defects. Medical therapies, which can be used in the prenatal period, are being developed for some birth defects. Prenatal surgeries also have had some success repairing congenital diaphragmatic hernias and urinary tract blockages. As medical technology improves, new interventions may have positive results for additional defects.

With this understanding in mind, the remainder of the chapter will focus on the "normal" newborn, care of the newborn, and complications that can occur with prematurity. Additional chapters in the text will elaborate on the various systems and disorders that occur from birth through the teenage years.

ADAPTATIONS OF THE NEONATE

When a baby is born, an orderly process of adaptation from fetal life to extrauterine life takes place. All the body systems undergo some change. Respirations are stimulated by chemical changes within the blood and by chilling. Sensory and physical stimuli also appear to play a role in respiratory function. Gentle physical contact is used to provide stimulation to begin breathing. Cold, pain, touch, movement, and light are other stimuli that affect the stimulation of respirations. With the first breath, which initiates the opening of the alveoli, the newborn enters the world of air exchange and begins an independent existence. In addition, this process begins cardiopulmonary interdependence (see Chapter 12). The ability of the neonate to metabolize food is hampered by immaturity of the digestive system, particularly by deficiencies in enzymes from the pancreas and the liver. Although the kidneys are developed structurally, their ability to concentrate urine and maintain fluid balance is limited. This is because of a decreased rate of glomerular flow and limited renal tubular reabsorption. Most neurologic functions are also primitive.

INITIAL EXAM OF THE NEWBORN INFANT

AIRWAY

Regardless of the site of delivery (home, birthing room, taxicab), clearing the neonate's airway is an immediate concern. A bulb syringe or suction may be used. Spontaneous breathing should begin within a few seconds. If there are no complications, the newborn is placed on a warming table where care can be given and the newborn's general condition can be observed. The newborn is dried gently to remove excess blood from the face, scalp, and body. This also provides stimulation and decreases the risk of hypothermia. Mothers who are alert are given their child to hold and inspect.

If spontaneous breathing does not occur, resuscitative measures are taken. The need for resuscitation often can be anticipated from the history of the mother's pregnancy, abnormal progression of labor, the size of the neonate, and the difficulty of delivery. Well-trained personnel and properly functioning equipment are imperative. Periodic review of techniques is also necessary. Resuscitation methods are directed toward clearing the airway, providing oxygen, and maintaining circulation. The administration of appropriate drugs, such as naloxone hydrochloride (Narcan), epinephrine, dextrose, or calcium gluconate, may also be warranted. Procedures range from the simple to the more complex. Measures such as tactile stimulation (rubbing the neonate's back), assisted ventilation with bag and mask or endotracheal tube, and chest compressions may be necessary, if the newborn's condition warrants this. The infant is then transferred to the nursery in a bassinet, isolette, or warmer. Assisted breathing via a mechanical ventilator may be necessary in the neonatal intensive care unit (NICU).

UMBILICAL CORD

The umbilical cord, which is attached to the placenta at birth, is cut and clamped by the attending physician. Before the clamp is applied, the cord is inspected to determine that two arteries and one vein are present. A single umbilical artery is often indicative of genitourinary anomalies. The findings are recorded.

Cord blood may be collected at the request of the parents. This is the blood that remains in the umbilical cord and placenta following birth. Cord blood is stored at a blood bank. This blood serves as an abundant source for stem cells, which are genetically distinctive to the newborn. These cells contribute to the development of all tissues, organs, and systems in the body. They can transform into other types of cells in the body and create new growth and development. They may be used one day to help treat problems such as heart disease, cancers, and stroke. Parents need to be aware there is a cost involved for this service.

Nursing Brief

The American Academy of Pediatrics (AAP) encourages parents to donate cord blood to a blood bank for public use. The AAP discourages cord blood donation for later personal or family use, because most of the conditions that could be helped by cord blood stem cells are already present in the infant's cord blood. An exception would be when siblings with a malignant or genetic medical condition may benefit from cord blood transplantation (AAP Policy Statement, 2007).

The cord stump may be painted with a substance to help dry the cord and prevent infection. This dye may cause a temporary purplish discoloration. Parents should not try to rub or wash this off. The cord stump gradually shrinks, turns black, and falls off. This process usually takes 10 to 14 days. Until the umbilical wound is completely healed, the blood vessels of the cord and their extension into the abdomen are potential portals of entry for disease organisms. Redness, odor, or discharge from this area should be reported to the physician. The nurse observes the cord for bleeding, particularly during the first 24 hours.

APGAR SCORING

A system for recording the condition of the neonate and the need for resuscitation was devised by Dr. Virginia Apgar and is currently used in many delivery

Table 5-1   Apgar Scoring System

SIGN	0	1	2
Heart rate	Absent	Slow (less than 100 beats/min.)	Above 100 beats/min.
Respiratory effort	Absent	Slow, irregular	Good; strong cry
Muscle tone	Limp	Some flexion of extremities	Well flexed
Reflex irritability	No response	Grimace	Cry or sneeze
Color	Blue, pale	Body pink, extremities bluish	Completely pink

rooms. The first assessment is made 1 minute after delivery. This generally produces the lowest score. A second evaluation is made after 5 minutes. Table 5-1 shows how to determine the Apgar score. An infant with a score of 8 to 10 is in good condition and needs only routine suction and observation. Infants with a score of 4 to 7 require various forms of intervention and close observation. An infant with a score of 0 to 3 needs resuscitation and care in the NICU. Apgar scores, however, are not the sole indicator used to evaluate the long-term prognosis of a child.

MEASUREMENTS

The newborn is weighed and measured shortly after birth. The length of the average neonate is 19 to 21.5 in (48.25 to 54.5 cm). The weight varies from 6 to 9 lb (2700 to 4000 g). Girls generally weigh a little less than boys. In the first 3 to 5 days after birth, the newborn loses about 7% to 10% of the birth weight. This is from the loss of excess extracellular fluid and meconium and from limited food intake, especially in breastfed infants. The total weight loss for the newborn should not exceed 10%; this amount of weight loss is reflective of dehydration. By the tenth day of life, birth weight should be regained. Weight loss is expected, and parents should not be alarmed by it. For a more accurate assessment of weight, neonates are weighed naked on the same scale at the same time each day.

Head circumference is generally between 33 and 35 cm (13 to 15 in). This measurement may be somewhat less because of the molding process during a vaginal delivery (Figure 5-1). Within 2 to 3 days, it is usually the normal size. Chest circumference is normally 30.5 to 33 cm (12 to 13 in). Head circumference is generally about 2 to 3 cm (1 in) greater than the chest circumference.

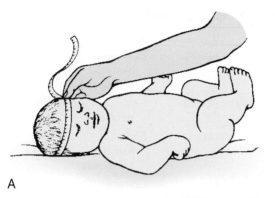

A

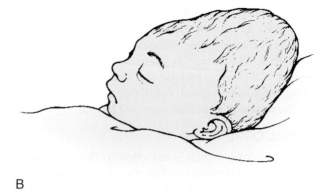

B

FIGURE 5-1 **A,** The circumference of the head is measured with the frontal occipital circumference (FOC). **B,** Molding of the head occurs as the bones of the fetal head overlap at the suture lines to conform to the mother's pelvis.

VITAL SIGNS

Temperature

The most accurate way to determine body temperature is to measure it with a thermometer. The initial temperature of the neonate is generally taken via the axillary route. It is not usually taken rectally because this method could cause perforation of the mucosa. Tympanic thermometers are not as accurate in a newborn. Daily routine temperatures are taken in the axilla. Review the procedure for evaluation of vital signs in Chapter 3.

The neonate has an immature heat-regulating system. Thermoregulation of the neonate (regulation of heat) requires close monitoring. The newborn's temperature falls immediately after birth to about 96° F (35.5° C). Within a few hours, it climbs slowly to a range of 98° F to 99° F (36.6° C to 37.2° C). The body temperature is influenced by the temperature of the room and the number of blankets covering the newborn. The nurse also needs to recognize the possibility of fever or sepsis (temperature could be low) in the newborn and alert the charge nurse or physician immediately.

One of the most critical needs of the infant is control of body temperature. This is especially true if the infant is at high risk. The neonate is at immediate risk for heat loss at the time of delivery. The newborn does not have the ability to produce or conserve heat that an older infant does. A newborn cannot shiver to generate heat. Through a process called nonshivering thermogenesis, brown fat is metabolized to increase metabolic rate and to generate heat. Brown fat is a fat store located in the axillae, between the scapulae, in the mediastinum, around the liver, and down the spine. If not corrected, cold stress can actually cause metabolic and physiologic problems in the neonate such as hypoglycemia (low blood sugar), hypoxia (low oxygenation), and metabolic acidosis.

Immediately after birth, the newborn is thoroughly dried (especially the hair) to eliminate evaporative heat loss and placed uncovered under radiant heat

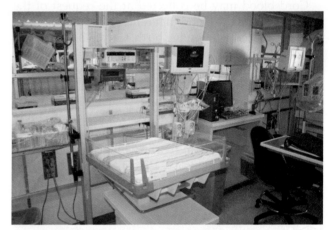

FIGURE 5-2 The radiant warmer prevents heat loss in the newborn. The open nature of the warmer allows health care providers access to the baby from all sides.

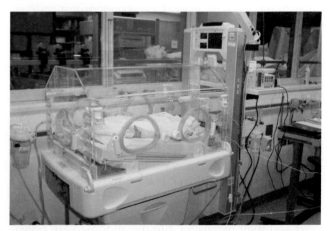

FIGURE 5-3 The isolette ("incubator") provides not only temperature control but protection from external stimuli, drafts, infection, and excess handling.

(Figure 5-2). The premature infant may be placed in the isolette (Figure 5-3). The infant's temperature is maintained at a constant level with a heat-sensitive probe that is taped over a nonbony prominence on either the abdomen or back. This allows the infant to become a thermostat for the radiant warmer. The infant's axillary temperature is also monitored. Overhead radiant warmers have the advantage of providing easier access to the child while maintaining a neutral environment. The nurse should also do the following:

- Prewarm all surfaces that come in contact with the infant.
- Avoid drafts in the room.
- Use discretion in bathing the infant. Regular assessment has a much higher priority than a routine daily bath because of the danger of loss of heat through evaporation.
- Provide a plastic heat shield (vapor shield) for very low–birth weight infants.
- Use knitted caps and booties when the infant is removed from the radiant warmer or isolette.
- Wrap the infant in a blanket if he or she is removed from the radiant warmer or isolette.

If the newborn is placed on the mother's chest, skin-to-skin contact should be maintained. A cap for the newborn prevents heat loss (Figure 5-4). The nurse remains with the mother and the newborn to ensure their safety, to monitor progress, and to ensure that the newborn stays warm. Table 5-2 discusses types of heat loss.

Another sign of the neonate's system immaturity is **acrocyanosis** (*acro*, extremity; *cyanosis*, blue color) or peripheral blueness of the hands and feet. The hands and feet are also cooler than other parts of the body. The neonate has difficulty adapting to changes in temperature. Because heat perception is poor, the newborn must be monitored closely whenever an external heat source, such as a radiant warmer, is used. The newborn should also be wrapped in a blanket.

Heart Rate and Blood Pressure

An apical heart rate should be auscultated for 1 full minute (discussed in Chapter 3) in the newborn, and it can range between 120 and 160 beats per minute.

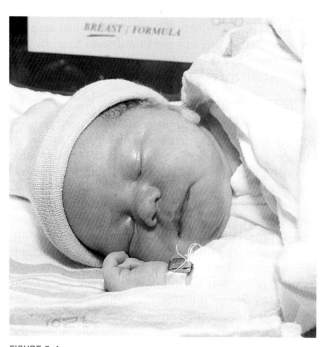

FIGURE 5-4 It is important that the newborn stay warm because heat is easily lost. Note the hat and the identification bracelet.

Table 5-2	Heat Loss in the Neonate		
TYPE OF HEAT LOSS	**MECHANISM**	**CONDITIONS CONTRIBUTING TO HEAT LOSS**	**NURSING INTERVENTIONS**
Evaporation	Heat lost by evaporation of moisture from the skin and with body fluids from mucous membranes	Increased skin permeability, increased respirations, and insensible water loss (25% of heat loss)	Dry quickly after birth/keep infant warm and dry (including head) Change wet diapers/clothing Bathe only after infant's temperature is stable Monitor/support infants experiencing rapid respirations
Conduction	Heat lost to surfaces with direct contact with them	Cool temperature of objects the infant comes into direct contact with	Warm equipment having direct contact with the infant Warm hands before touching the infant Use paper on scale to weigh; use blankets on other surfaces
Convection	Heat lost by air moving over the skin	Drafts and cool air (air conditioning)	Avoid exposure to drafts/cool air Ensure oxygen is warmed and humidified whenever used Transport in isolette
Radiation	Transfer of heat to cooler, solid objects in the environment not in contact with the infant	Cool environment of hospital unit including walls and windows	Keep infant's bed away from outside walls and windows Keep infant clothed with hat; wrap warmly Use temperature probe in isolette to monitor infant's temperature

This rate may increase if the infant is crying and decrease if the infant is sleeping. As a general rule, however, if the pulse is above 180 or drops below 100, the finding should be reported. Blood pressure in the newborn is usually low, and use of the correctly sized cuff is important. The average blood pressure at birth is 80/46 mm Hg.

Respirations

Respirations in the newborn may be irregular and should be counted for 1 full minute. Normal respirations are 40 to 60 breaths per minute and then drop to 30 to 50 breaths per minute after the first 24 hours after birth and are typically shallow and unlabored.

WEIGHT AND GESTATIONAL AGE

Gestational age refers to the actual time from conception to birth that the fetus remains in the uterus. A full-term infant is born between 38 and 42 weeks after conception. Infants born between 34 and 37 weeks are considered *late preterm,* while those born at less than 34 weeks are called *preterm,* and those born at more than 42 weeks are called *postterm.* Infants are considered **appropriate for gestational age (AGA)** if they are born between the 10th and 90th percentiles for weight. This infant has grown at a normal rate, regardless of the time of birth. If the infant is **small for gestational age (SGA)**, below the 10th percentile, the infant has experienced intrauterine growth restriction or delay. In a similar fashion, those infants weighing above the 90th percentile on intrauterine growth curves are referred to as **large for gestational age (LGA)**. Emphasis is placed on the gestational age *and* the level of maturation—preterm, term, and postterm (Figure 5-5). Current data also indicate that intrauterine growth rates are not the same for all babies and that individual factors must be considered.

Prematurity and low birth weight often occur together, and both of these factors are associated with increased neonatal morbidity and mortality. The less a baby weighs at birth, the greater are the risks to life during delivery and immediately thereafter. High-risk infants are also classified according to the following guidelines:

- Low–birth weight (LBW) infant—an infant whose birth weight is less than 2500 g (5.5 lbs), regardless of gestational age
- Very low–birth weight (VLBW) infant—an infant whose birth weight is less than 1500 g (3.3 lbs)
- Extremely low–birth weight (ELBW) infant—an infant whose birth weight is less than 1000 g (2.2 lbs)
- Intrauterine growth restriction (IUGR)—an infant whose intrauterine growth is restricted

MATURITY

Several differences are seen between a premature and a full-term infant. Muscle tone is decreased in the infant who is not full-term. The position that the infant maintains can also indicate low gestational age. When in a prone position, the full-term infant lies with the pelvis high and the knees drawn up under the abdomen. The premature infant that is placed in a prone position lies with the pelvis low and the knees at the side of the abdomen, with the hips flexed. In the supine position, the infant of 28 to 32 weeks' gestational age lies in a froglike position with the lower limbs extended and the hips abducted. The full-term infant in a supine position lies with the limbs strongly flexed. Differences also exist in the hand movement of the infant across the chest to the opposite side of the neck. The reach of an infant of 28 weeks' gestation can extend well past the acromion, whereas the hand of the full-term infant does not go beyond that point. If the hand is put behind the neck to the opposite side, the same difference between the ages is noted. This is called the **scarf sign** (Figure 5-6). The new Ballard scoring system is used to determine gestational age and consists of an evaluation of physical characteristics and neuromuscular tone (see Appendix C).

CHARACTERISTICS OF THE NEWBORN INFANT

HEAD

The newborn infant's head is proportionately large in comparison with the rest of the body because the brain grows rapidly before birth. The head may be out of shape from molding, which occurs as the fetal head conforms to the size and shape of the mother's pelvis. Another condition that can alter the shape of the newborn's head is caput succedaneum, which is edema of the newborn's scalp resulting from pressure against the cervix.

This condition usually clears within 24 to 48 hours. Occasionally, a **hematoma** (*hemato,* blood; *oma,* tumor) protrudes from beneath the scalp. The cephalhematoma takes longer to subside, but it usually clears by the time the infant is 2 to 4 weeks of age (Figure 5-7). Cephalhematoma can increase the risk of hyperbilirubinemia (the additional accumulation of blood increases the number of red blood cells, therefore there is an increased release of bilirubin; refer to section on jaundice).

Some neonates have a large amount of hair that eventually is replaced by new hair. The infant's hair should be washed when the newborn is bathed and then can be brushed into place. Some infants develop cradle cap (seborrheic dermatitis), characterized by yellow, oily, crustlike scales on the scalp and forehead. Using mineral oil to soften the scales, massaging with a soft baby brush, and shampooing the area with a mild shampoo will help eliminate cradle cap.

Fontanels are junctures at the cranial bones that can be felt as soft spots on the cranium of the young infant.

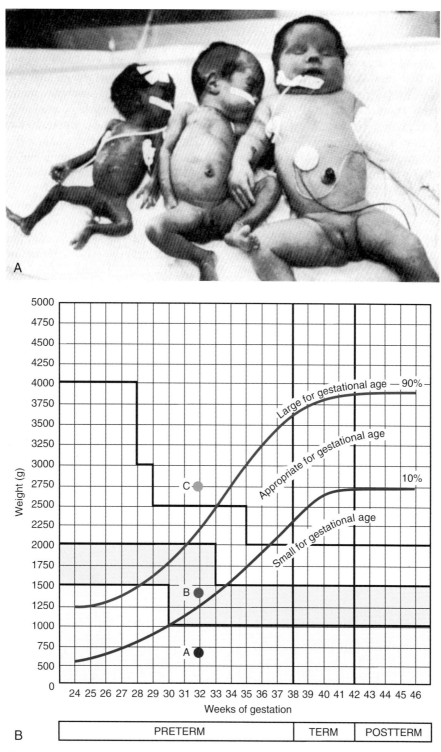

FIGURE 5-5 **A,** Three babies of the same gestational age (32 weeks) weighing 600, 1400, and 2750 g, respectively. **B,** Classification of the newborn infant as indicated by relationship of weight to gestational age. The status of babies of the weights shown in **A** is plotted at 32 weeks (dots *A, B,* and *C*).

Two can be palpated on the neonate's head. The fontanels may be smaller immediately after birth than several days later because of molding. The anterior fontanel is diamond-shaped and located at the junction of the two parietal and the two frontal bones. It usually closes by 12 to 18 months of age (Figure 5-8).

The posterior fontanel is triangular and located between the occipital and the parietal bones. It is much smaller than the anterior fontanel and has usually ossified by the end of the second month. The pulsating of the anterior fontanel may be seen by the nurse. These areas are covered by a tough membrane, and

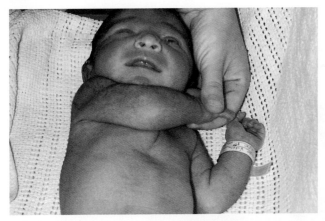

FIGURE 5-6 Examining the newborn baby for maturity. The full-term neonate's elbow resists attempts to be brought farther than the midline of the chest. Little or no resistance is seen in the preterm infant. This is called the scarf sign.

Table 5-3	Neurologic Signs Present at Birth in the Newborn	
REFLEX	**OCCURRENCE**	
Protective Reflexes		
Blink		
Gag		
Cough		
Feeding Reflexes		
Root		
Suck		
Swallow		
Muscle Tone Reflexes	**Age of Disappearance**	
Moro	1-3 mo	
Tonic neck	5-6 mo	
Palmer grasp (hand)	~4 mo	
Plantar grasp (foot)	4-6 mo	
Babinski	Variable—not diagnostic until after 2 yr of age	
Reflexes of Vision	**Age of Appearance**	
Horizontal following	4-6 wk	
Vertical following	2-3 mo	
Blinking to a threat	6-7 mo	

there is little chance of their being injured with ordinary care.

NERVOUS SYSTEM

Reflexes

The nervous system directs most of the body's activity. The neonate can move his or her arms and legs vigorously but cannot control them. The reflexes that a full-term baby is born with, such as blinking, sneezing, gagging, rooting, sucking, and grasping (Figure 5-9 and Table 5-3), help keep the child alive. The **rooting**

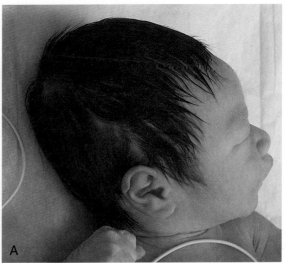

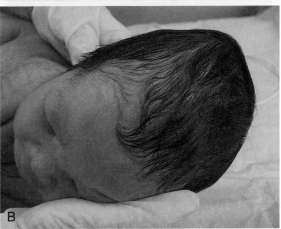

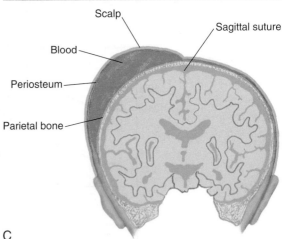

FIGURE 5-7 **A,** Caput succedaneum is an edematous area on the head from pressure against the cervix. It may cross suture lines. **B** and **C,** A cephalhematoma is characterized by bleeding between the bone and its covering, the periosteum. It may occur on one or both sides and does not cross suture lines.

reflex causes the infant to turn the head in the direction of anything that touches the cheek, such as in anticipation of food. The nurse should remember this when helping a mother breastfeed her infant. If the breast touches the infant's cheek, the newborn turns toward

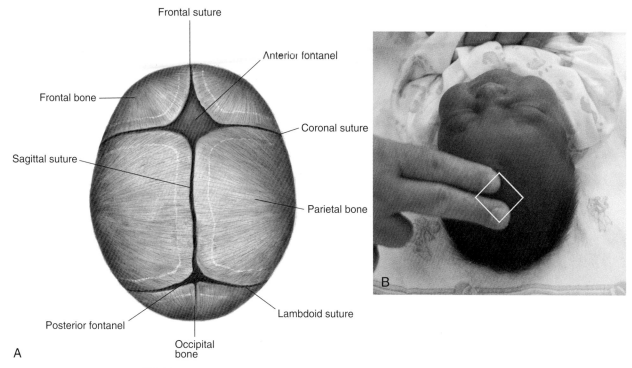

FIGURE 5-8 **A,** Location of sutures and fontanels. **B,** Palpating anterior fontanel.

it to find the nipple. The infant can also cry, swallow, and lift the head slightly when lying on the stomach. If startled, the newborn extends the extremities and then draws the legs up and folds the arms across the chest in an embrace position. The hands open, but the fingers often remain curved. This is normal and is called the Moro reflex (Figure 5-10). Its absence may indicate abnormalities of the nervous system.

The **tonic neck reflex** is a postural reflex that is sometimes assumed by babies while asleep (Figure 5-11). The head is turned to one side, with the arm and leg extended on the same side, whereas the opposite arm and leg are flexed in a "fencing" position. This reflex disappears around the 20th week of life. Prancing movements of the legs, seen when a newborn is held upright on the examining table, are termed the **dancing reflex.**

SENSORY SYSTEM

The neonate can both taste and smell. In fact, the mother's scent appears to stimulate the neonate to smell breast milk and to search for the nipple.

Vision

Although vision is the most poorly developed sense at birth, the neonate can see sizes, shapes, colors, and patterns and is able to fixate points of contrast. The infant shows preference for observing a human face and follows moving objects. Visual stimulation thus becomes an important ingredient in caring for the baby. Auditory toys and contrasted colors attract the

neonate. Sensory overload, of course, should be avoided.

Most newborn infants appear cross-eyed because their eye muscle coordination is not fully developed. After birth and into the first few months of life, the infant's eyes appear to be blue or gray; however, the permanent coloring becomes fixed by the first birthday.

Hearing

Hearing in newborns is thought to be keener than was once believed. Increased response to vocal stimulation, particularly higher-pitched female voices, can be documented. The ears and nose need no special attention, except for cleansing. This can be done during the bath with a soft cloth. Cotton-tipped applicator sticks are dangerous to use and may cause injury if inserted too far into the ear or if the newborn moves suddenly. They should *never* be used for ear wax removal.

Undetected hearing loss can cause a child to develop problems in speech, language, and cognitive development and can also lead to development of behavioral problems. Hearing loss is a common birth defect, occurring in up to 3 per 1000 newborn infants, and needs to be identified as soon as possible. In the past, parental observation and assessment by health care providers have not been reliable in identifying hearing loss in the first year of life. In 2000, the Joint Committee on Infant Hearing (JCIH) recommended universal screening of hearing loss before

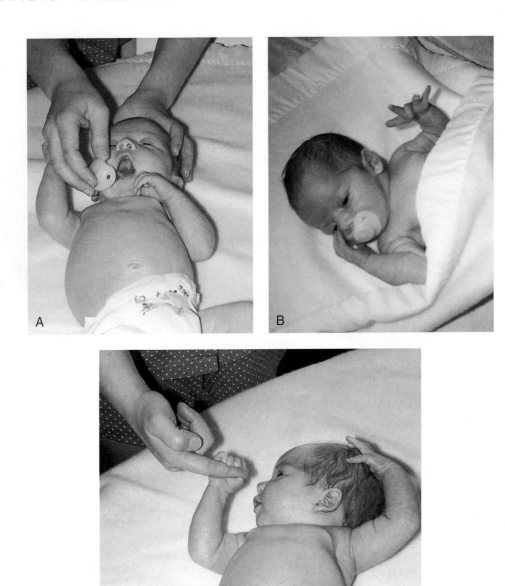

FIGURE 5-9 **A,** Rooting reflex. The infant opens the mouth and turns the head toward the pacifier stimulating the cheek. **B,** Sucking reflex. Vigorous sucking movements are initiated when an object is placed in the infant's mouth. **C,** Grasp reflex (palm). Transverse stimulation of the midpalm leads to a grasp by the infant.

hospital discharge. The automated Auditory Brainstem Response (ABR) screening test as well as the Evoked Otoacoustic Emissions (OAE) screening test detect hearing loss in infants. The detection of hearing loss and early interventions aid the child in achieving academic and social success because they allow for the development of thinking and visual or spoken language skills.

CIRCULATORY AND RESPIRATORY SYSTEM

Before birth, a baby is completely dependent on the mother for all vital functions. The fetus needs oxygen and nourishment to grow. These are supplied through the bloodstream of the mother by way of the placenta and the umbilical cord. The fetus is relieved of the waste products of metabolism through the same route. The lungs are not inflated and are almost completely inactive. The circulatory system is adapted only to life within the uterus. Little blood flows through the pulmonary artery because of natural openings within the heart (foramen ovale) and vessels that close at or shortly after birth. When the umbilical cord is clamped and cut, the lungs take on the function of breathing in oxygen and removing carbon dioxide. The first breath taken helps expand the fluid-filled alveoli in the lungs. The physician assists the first respiration by holding the infant's head down and removing mucus from the

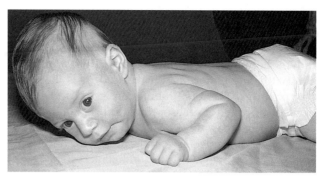

FIGURE 5-12 The newborn is barely able to lift his or her head while lying prone.

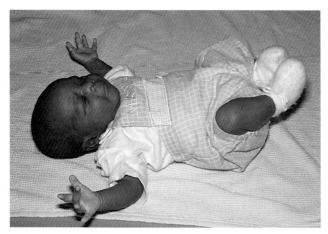

FIGURE 5-10 Moro reflex. Sudden jarring causes extension and abduction of the extremities and spreading of the fingers.

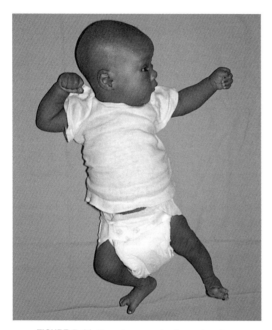

FIGURE 5-11 Spontaneous tonic neck reflex.

passages to the lungs. The newborn's cry should be strong and healthy. The most critical period for the neonate is the first hour of life, when the drastic change from life within the uterus to life outside the uterus takes place.

The nurse refers to the child's chart to review the Apgar score and to determine whether or not there were any particular difficulties during the birth process. The orders left by the doctor are reviewed. The nurse must observe the newborn *very closely.* Respiratory distress may be indicated by the rate and character of respirations, color (the nurse observes the newborn for signs of cyanosis), and overall general behavior. *Any retractions* should be reported

immediately. (See Complications of the Preterm Infant Respiratory System later in this chapter for a discussion on retractions.) Mucus may be seen draining from the nose or mouth. Gentle suctioning with a bulb syringe may also be indicated. See Chapter 3 to review the use of a bulb syringe.

MUSCULOSKELETAL SYSTEM

The bones of the newborn infant are soft because they are made up chiefly of cartilage, with only a small amount of calcium. The skeleton is flexible. The joints are elastic to accommodate passage through the birth canal. Because the bones of the child are easily molded by pressure, the position must be changed frequently. If the baby lies constantly in one position, the bones of the head can become flattened.

Movements and Tremors

Movements of the neonate are random and uncoordinated. The newborn lacks the muscular control to hold the head up (Figure 5-12). The development of muscular control proceeds from head to foot and from the center of the body to the periphery (discussed in Chapter 4). The baby, therefore, holds up the head before sitting erect. In fact, the head and neck muscles are the first ones under control. The legs are small and short and may appear bowed. There should be no limitation of movement. Fingers clenched in a fist should be separated and observed.

Freedom of movement is observed as the baby stretches, sucks, and makes faces. The whole body moves vigorously when the newborn cries. Tremors of the lips and extremities during crying are normal. Constant tremors during sleep, which are accompanied by eye movements and are not related to any particular stimuli, may be pathologic. The morning assessment provides an excellent opportunity for the nurse to inspect and evaluate the newborn's condition. When handled, the infant should not feel limp. General body proportions are noted. Bathing is also an excellent way to provide the neonate with stimulation.

GENITOURINARY SYSTEM

The kidneys function normally at birth but are not fully developed. The glomeruli are small. Renal blood flow is only about one third of that in an adult. The ability to handle fluid load is reduced, as is the excretion of drugs. The renal tubules are short and have a limited capacity for reabsorbing important substances such as glucose, amino acids, phosphate, and bicarbonate. There is a decrease in the ability to concentrate urine and to cope with fluid imbalances. The infant should void within the first 24 to 48 hours after birth. The newborn may void in the delivery room, and it may not be observed. The nurse must keep an accurate record of the frequency of urination. Anuria (absence of voiding), changes in the color of urine, and any unusual findings should be brought to the attention of the physician. The newborn is not sent home unless voiding is observed.

Male Genitalia

The genitals are undeveloped at birth. The testes of the male child descend into the scrotum before birth. Occasionally, they remain in the abdomen or inguinal canal. This condition is called *cryptorchidism* (undescended testes). The prognosis is good with proper surgical treatment.

The penis is covered by a sleeve of skin called the *foreskin* or *prepuce*. After the foreskin separates from the glans, it can be pulled back away from the glans toward the abdomen. This is called *foreskin retraction*. This should never be forced because it can harm the penis and cause pain, bleeding, and tears in the skin. Most boys are able to retract their foreskins by age 5 years. Parents should be taught to wash all the male infant's body parts and not to forcibly retract the foreskin. Parents may be surprised when their baby boy has an erection and should be taught that this is common and has no significance.

Circumcision is the surgical removal of the foreskin. The procedure has been subject to much controversy. Among the risks are infection and hemorrhage. Infants with congenital anomalies of the penis, such as hypospadias (occurs when the opening of the urethra is on the undersurface of the penis), should not be circumcised because the foreskin may be needed for surgery. Studies show that the risk for penile cancer and urinary tract infections are reduced in circumcised men compared with those who are uncircumcised; however, the incidence of such illness is so low that circumcision cannot be justified for prophylaxis (Hirji et al., 2005). There is also new research that indicates male circumcision has proven to be a primary prevention strategy against transmission of HIV (Uys, 2009/2010). A discussion of the pros and cons of this procedure should be included as part of the prenatal and postpartum education. The parents' knowledge and understanding of the procedure of circumcision is necessary because a surgical consent form must be signed before this procedure can be performed.

When circumcision is desired, it is performed after 12 hours of age. This period of time allows the newborn to adjust from the stress of birth and for bonding to begin. The nurse needs to advocate for the use of pain medication for babies undergoing this procedure. Analgesics and/or anesthesia should be prescribed for pain control. For the circumcision procedure, the newborn is restrained on a circumcision board. The foreskin is freed with a probe, an incision is made the length of the foreskin, and a Plastibell, Gomco clamp, or Mogen clamp (rarely used) is used to control blood loss. Excess foreskin is removed with a scalpel or a scissor (Figure 5-13). After this procedure, it is important for the nurse to observe for bleeding, irritation, and voiding. Pain is always assessed as the fifth vital sign.

When a Plastibell is used, a string is tied over a fitted plastic ring beneath the foreskin. As the area heals, the plastic ring drops off in 7 to 10 days after the circumcision. Parents are instructed not to remove the plastic ring prematurely. No special dressing is required, and the newborn may be diapered as usual. Tub bathing may be done after the ring falls off and the circumcision is healed. A dark brown or black line encircling the plastic ring is normal and will disappear when the plastic ring drops off. Parents are instructed to consult their physician if there is increased swelling, the ring has not fallen off within 10 days, the ring has slipped onto the shaft of the penis, or for any other questions/concerns.

When a Mogen or Gomco clamp is used, a dressing with Vaseline (or another petroleum jelly) is used for 24 to 48 hours. Complete healing takes approximately 7 to 10 days.

🌐 Cultural Considerations

The Jewish religious custom of circumcision, comparable to baptism in the Christian faith, is performed on the eighth day after birth if the baby's condition permits. The baby receives his Hebrew name at this time.

Female Genitalia

The female genitals may be slightly swollen after birth. Blood-tinged mucus may be discharged from the vagina 3 to 5 days after birth, which is caused from withdrawal of hormones transmitted from the mother to the fetus. The nurse should clean the vulva from the *urethra to the anus,* with three strokes—right side, left side, and center. A clean cotton ball or clean (different) section of a washcloth is to be used for each stroke to prevent fecal matter from infecting the urinary tract.

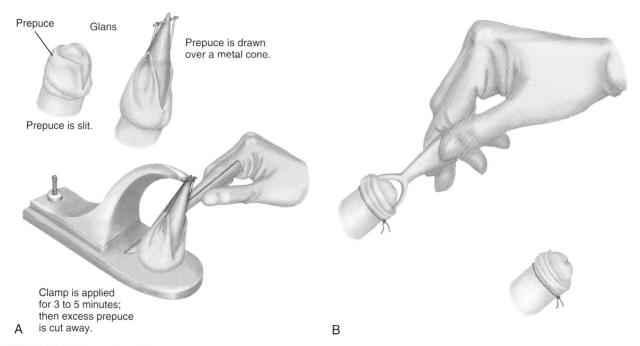

Prepuce   Glans

Prepuce is slit.

Prepuce is drawn over a metal cone.

Clamp is applied for 3 to 5 minutes; then excess prepuce is cut away.

A   B

FIGURE 5-13 **A,** Circumcision with the Gomco (Yellen) clamp. The physician pulls the prepuce over a cone-shaped device that rests against the glans. A clamp is placed around the cone and prepuce and is tightened to provide enough pressure to crush the blood vessels. This prevents bleeding when the prepuce is removed after 3 to 5 minutes. **B,** Circumcision with the Plastibell. The physician places the Plastibell, a plastic ring, over the glans, draws the prepuce over it, and ties a suture around the prepuce and Plastibell. This prevents bleeding when the excess prepuce is removed. The handle is removed, leaving only the ring in place over the glans. The Plastibell ring falls off in 7 to 10 days.

The importance and rationale of cleaning from *front to back* must be emphasized to parents.

INTEGUMENTARY SYSTEM

Skin

The skin of newborn Caucasian babies is red to dark pink in color. The skin of African-American babies may be reddish brown. Infants of Latin descent may appear to have an olive or yellowish tint to the skin. The body is usually covered with fine hair called lanugo, which tends to disappear during the first weeks of life. Lanugo is more evident in premature infants (Figure 5-14). Vernix caseosa, a cheeselike substance that covers the skin of the neonate, is made up of cells and glandular secretions and is thought to protect the skin from infection. White pinpoint pimples caused by obstruction of sebaceous glands may be seen on the nose and chin. These are called **milia** and disappear within a few weeks. **Mongolian spots,** bluish discolorations of the skin, are common in babies of African-American, Latino, Native American, or Mediterranean descent. They are usually found over the sacral and gluteal areas (Figure 5-15). They disappear spontaneously during the first years of life. Be careful not to confuse Mongolian spots with bruises that can occur from child abuse. Pallor or generalized cyanosis is not normal and should be reported.

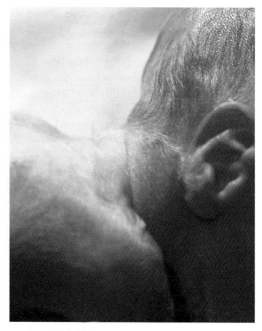

FIGURE 5-14 Lanugo in a premature neonate.

Some hospitals still identify newborn babies with footprints, although many hospitals now have more advanced identification techniques. Footprints may still be used because the skin is so constructed with ridges and grooves that each person has a unique

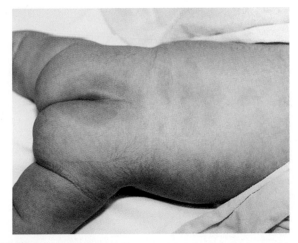

FIGURE 5-15 Mongolian spots are common in dark-skinned children. These bluish skin discolorations should not be confused with bruises.

pattern that never changes. Regardless of hospital policy on identification method, most parents appreciate a copy of the footprint for the baby scrapbook.

Tissue turgor refers to the condition of the skin and indicates how hydrated or dehydrated the newborn is. To test tissue turgor (elasticity), the nurse gently grasps and releases the skin on the chest. It should spring back into place immediately. When the skin remains distended, tissue turgor is termed *poor*.

Desquamation, or peeling of the skin, occurs during the first weeks of life. Skin on the nose, knees, elbows, and toes may break down because of friction from rubbing against the sheets. The area involved should be kept dry, and the newborn's position should be changed frequently. The buttocks also need special attention. A wet diaper should be changed immediately to prevent irritation. The buttocks should be washed and dried well. Parents should be informed that this prevents diaper rash.

JAUNDICE

The liver in the neonate is immature and, as a result, takes longer to start functioning effectively. Physiologic jaundice (also called icterus neonatorum, characterized by a yellow tinge to the skin) is caused by the rapid destruction of excess red blood cells that the newborn no longer needs. This is because the atmosphere contains more oxygen than the amount present during prenatal life. Between the second and fourth day, plasma levels of bilirubin rise from a normal 1 mg/dL to an average of 5 to 6 mg/dL. Physiologic jaundice becomes evident between the third and fifth day of life and lasts for about a week. In the preterm infant, the bilirubin level may be elevated for a longer time and the peak may not occur until the fifth to seventh day. It is necessary to treat physiologic jaundice to prevent kernicterus or **bilirubin encephalopathy**, a syndrome of severe brain damage. Death can also result.

Safety Alert

Erythroblastosis Fetalis

Jaundice on the first day of life is *always* pathologic and should not be confused with physiologic jaundice. *Erythroblastosis fetalis* is a disorder that becomes apparent late in fetal life or soon after birth. This occurs in a sensitized Rh-negative mother who is pregnant with an Rh-positive child. The incidence rate of erythroblastosis fetalis has greatly decreased as a result of the protective administration of Rh antibody (RhoGAM) to women at risk. If an infant is born with this disorder, there are varying degrees of anemia and jaundice. Hyperbilirubinemia occurs, and enlargement of the liver and spleen, with extensive edema may develop. Kernicterus can result. Treatment includes intrauterine transfusions if severe anemia is present. After delivery, phototherapy and exchange transfusion may be required.

Nursing Brief

Infants at less than 38 weeks' gestation, particularly those who are breastfed, are at higher risk of developing hyperbilirubinemia and require closer surveillance and monitoring (American Academy of Pediatrics Practice Parameter Guidelines, 2004).

Treatment and Nursing Care

With the prevalence of early discharges, parents should be instructed about what behaviors they should be alerted to with their new baby. They should be alert to lethargy, hypotonia, a weak suck, and color changes in skin and eyes. If the mother is breastfeeding, she should be evaluated by a lactation consultant or a professional who is experienced with breastfeeding. The mother should understand the importance of follow-up visits with the pediatrician. Phototherapy is the treatment for reducing or preventing rising bilirubin levels related to physiologic jaundice. Phototherapy *for treatment of neonatal hyperbilirubinemia* is initiated based on assessment of risk with the use of an algorithm recommended by the American Academy of Pediatrics (American Academy of Pediatrics Practice Parameter Guidelines, 2004).

Light used in phototherapy changes the bilirubin in the skin into an excretable form (Figure 5-16 and 5-17). Nursing Care Plan 5-1 addresses the nursing care needed by the newborn receiving phototherapy in the hospital.

Community Considerations

Home phototherapy may be ordered on an outpatient basis if the follow-up bilirubin levels are too high. Fiberoptic blankets can be used in place of or in addition to phototherapy lights. The baby is wrapped in the blanket, which is always kept next to the baby's skin. A receiving blanket can be wrapped over the "bili" blanket. The baby can be held for feedings and other activities. The eye patches may still be necessary even if only the blanket is used.

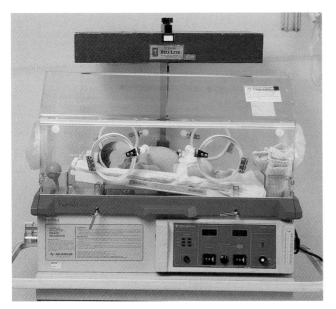

FIGURE 5-16 The infant wears eye patches when receiving phototherapy. The portholes of the isolette facilitate routine infant care.

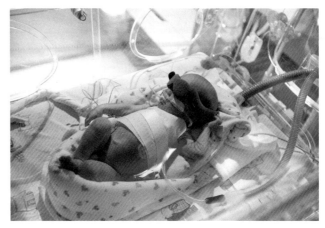

FIGURE 5-17 Phototherapy using a fiberoptic blanket.

GASTROINTESTINAL SYSTEM

Digestion

Breastfed babies may be put to breast on the delivery table to help stimulate milk production and for the psychological benefits of the mother. Bottle-fed babies usually begin their first feeding by 6 hours of age. A baby's hunger is evidenced by crying, restlessness, sucking the fist, and the rooting reflex.

The capacity of the stomach is about 15 to 30 mL at birth and increases about 15 mL each day. It reaches a capacity of 90 mL by 1 week of age. Emptying time for the stomach is 2 to 3 hours, and peristalsis is rapid. A deficiency in pancreatic lipase limits fat absorption. The liver is immature, especially in its ability to conjugate bilirubin, regulate blood sugar, and coagulate blood.

Stools

The normal functions of the gastrointestinal tract begin after birth: food is prepared for absorption into the blood, it is absorbed, and waste products are eliminated. **Meconium,** the first stool, is a mixture of amniotic fluid and secretions of the intestinal glands. It is dark green, thick, and sticky, is passed 8 to 24 hours after birth, and continues for about 3 days. The stools gradually change during the first week. They become loose and are a greenish yellow with mucus. These are called **transitional** stools.

The stools of a breastfed baby are bright yellow, soft, seedy, and pasty. There may be three to six stools a day. With age, the number of stools decreases. The bowel movements of a bottle-fed baby are more solid than those of a breastfed baby. They vary from yellow to light brown and are generally fewer in number. There may be one to four a day at first, but gradually this decreases to one or two a day. The stools are darker when a baby is receiving iron and green when the baby is under the bilirubin lamp. Small, putty-like stools, green watery stools, and bloody stools are abnormal and should be reported. The nursery nurse keeps an accurate record of the number and character of stools each neonate has daily.

Constipation

Constipation refers to the passage of hard, dry stools. Neonates differ in regularity. Some pass a soft stool every other day. This is not constipation. The nurse explains to parents that straining in the newborn period is from undeveloped abdominal musculature. This is normal, and no treatment is necessary.

Hiccups

Hiccups appear frequently in neonates, are normal, and most often disappear spontaneously. Burping the baby may help.

PRETERM INFANTS

Care of the preterm infant is similar to that of the term infant in that the infant is assessed at birth and resuscitation is performed if indicated. Once respiratory function is established, the infant is examined for any other problems that may be present. Routine care may be delayed until the infant is stable. Stabilization of respiration and thermoregulation takes priority over all other types of care. The infant may need to be transferred from a community hospital to the NICU at a larger facility. This may mean immediate separation of the infant from the family unit. Issues of bonding and attachment need to be addressed in such cases.

Parents need guidance throughout the infant's hospitalization to help prepare them for this new experience. They may be disheartened by the unattractive appearance of the premature baby. They may believe

★ **Nursing Care Plan 5-1** **The Neonate Receiving Phototherapy**

NURSING DIAGNOSIS *Nutrition, imbalanced: less than body requirements, related to newborn status and phototherapy*

Goals/Outcome Criteria	Nursing Interventions	Rationales
The infant receives adequate nutrition, as evidenced by: • Weight gain of 0.5 to 1 oz/day • Intake of 2 oz per feeding • Feeds every 3 to 4 hours if on formula • Feeds every 2 to 3 hours if breastfed • Voids at least every 4 hours • Has a stool at least every 24 hours	Weigh and assess the weight daily Feed every 2 to 4 hours Burp halfway through feeding and at the end Record intake Teach parents importance of feeding frequently	Provides data to support that infant is meeting nutritional needs Stomach of a newborn empties in 2 hours if breastfed and in 3 hours if fed formula Allows swallowed air to be expelled, thus increasing the amount of fluid that can be taken and retained Ability to keep accurate record of intake Sharing information increases the parents' ability to participate in care

NURSING DIAGNOSIS *Knowledge, deficient, related to the use of phototherapy*

Goals/Outcome Criteria	Nursing Interventions	Rationales
The parents show an increase in knowledge, as evidenced by: • Understanding the process of jaundice • Demonstrating the ability to care for their infant • Showing positive aspects of bonding every 24 hours	Assess knowledge of parents Give additional information in at least two different forms (e.g., verbal and written) Encourage parent's participation in care of the infant Reassure and praise parent's actions Be aware of parent's level of comfort Provide follow-up	Aids the caregiver in knowing where to begin Use of more than one sense increases the ability to learn new information Allows parents to gradually increase their skills Encourages learning and allows parents to see themselves as successful Allows one to give new information at the parent's level and answer questions Provides opportunity to answer any questions

NURSING DIAGNOSIS *Fluid volume, risk for deficient, related to increased fluid loss through skin and loose stools*

Goals/Outcome Criteria	Nursing Interventions	Rationales
The infant has adequate hydration, as evidenced by: • Good skin turgor • Moist mucous membranes • Less than 10% weight loss • Voiding at least every 4 hours	Assess infant's skin turgor and mucous membranes each shift Weigh daily, record, and report to physician Record voiding and stools	A quick assessment for hydration Weight is a good indicator of the overall hydration status Output of voiding is a good indicator of renal perfusion, which is an indicator of adequate hydration

NURSING DIAGNOSIS *Body temperature, risk for imbalanced, related to phototherapy*

Goals/Outcome Criteria	Nursing Interventions	Rationales
The infant has a normal temperature, as evidenced by: • Temperature between 97.6° F and 99° F axillary • Little or no acrocyanosis • Capillary refill time less than 3 seconds	Assess temperature every 4 hours Record isolette and set temperature Keep skin temperature probe in place Dress the infant and wrap in a blanket for feedings Teach parents the need to maintain infant's temperature	Phototherapy can increase the temperature, and if the environment is not kept warm, the temperature can decrease Oxygen and glucose needs increase when the temperature falls outside the given parameters Shows the infant's need for additional warmth; allows the infant to act as his or her own thermostat Decreases loss of heat from infant to environment Increases parents' understanding of importance of maintaining infant's temperature

⭐ **Nursing Care Plan 5-1**   **The Neonate Receiving Phototherapy—cont'd**

NURSING DIAGNOSIS *Injury, risk for, related to high levels of bilirubin*

Goals/Outcome Criteria	Nursing Interventions	Rationales
The infant is free from neurologic damage, as evidenced by: • No signs of neurologic involvement (lethargy, twitching)	Assess neurologic status of the infant Monitor laboratory reports concerning bilirubin levels Turn off phototherapy lights during collection of blood specimen	Aids in early recognition of any deficits Allows for prompt notification of the physician if bilirubin level exceeds ordered parameters Phototherapy lights can alter bilirubin in specimen tubes and results can be incorrect

NURSING DIAGNOSIS *Injury, risk for, eye damage related to phototherapy*

Goals/Outcome Criteria	Nursing Interventions	Rationales
The infant is free from eye injury, as evidenced by: • No eye discharge • No redness of the eye • No corneal irritation	Apply eye patches over the infant's closed eyes while infant is under the phototherapy light Remove eye patches during feedings Assess eyes for redness, discharge, or irritation at each feeding Check the eye patches frequently to make sure they are in place	Infant's eyes should be closed to decrease the chance of irritation to the eyes and avoid corneal damage Allows eye contact and promotes parental-newborn bonding Provides earliest recognition of a problem; the earlier it is recognized, the earlier it can be treated Infants are active and patches can become displaced

NURSING DIAGNOSIS *Skin integrity, risk for impaired, related to phototherapy*

Goals/Outcome Criteria	Nursing Interventions	Rationales
The infant's skin remains intact, as evidenced by: • The skin being warm, dry, and intact in all areas • Free from any rashes, excoriation, or redness • No burns or breaks in the skin	Assess for any skin irritation at the time of each feeding Use proper phototherapy equipment (Plexiglas cover of the bulbs) Clean the diaper area gently Reposition infant every 2 hours Keep skin clean and dry and do not use powders, lotions, or oils	Phototherapy can be irritating to the thin skin of the newborn Fluorescent bulbs can break, and the Plexiglas cover protects the infant from any exposure to glass Stools are high in bilirubin, frequent, and loose; these factors can be irritating to the perineal area Increases exposure of body surface to the phototherapy lights Although the skin may become dry while the infant is receiving phototherapy, items (e.g., oils) can lead to burning of the skin

Critical Thinking Questions
1. What is the best way to manage a mother who is crying as she stands looking at her baby under the phototherapy lights and feels she is to blame for her baby turning "yellow"?
2. The mother has expressed concern about her ability to care for her new baby. How can you involve the mother in the care of the baby?

that they are to blame for the baby's condition and may fear that the baby will die but are unable to express their feelings. They need time to look at and touch the baby and to begin to see this child as uniquely their own (Figure 5-18). This touch and immediate human contact are vital for the infant as well.

Premature birth deprives the neonate of the complete benefits of intrauterine life. The skin is transparent and loose. Superficial veins may be seen beneath the abdomen and scalp. There is a lack of subcutaneous fat, and fine hair called lanugo covers the forehead, shoulders, and arms. The cheeselike vernix caseosa, seen in more mature infants, is absent. The extremities appear short, and the abdomen protrudes. The nails are short. The genitals are small. In female premature infants, the labia majora may be open and the clitoris evident.

The causes of prematurity are numerous, but in many instances, the cause is unknown (Box 5-1). Adequate prenatal care to prevent preterm birth is

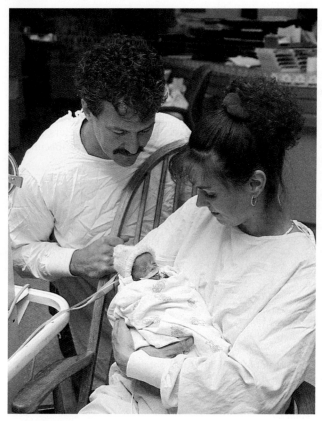

FIGURE 5-18 Parents need time to bond with their premature infant. They are taught that it is important to maintain warmth whenever the infant is removed from the radiant warmer. Note the knitted hat.

Table 5-4	Nursing Observations in Care of Preterm Infants
CHARACTERISTICS	**OBSERVATIONS**
Color	Pallor, cyanosis, jaundice
Respirations	Regularity, apnea, sternal retractions, labored breathing, grunting
Pulse	Rate and regularity
Abdomen	Distention
Stools	Frequency, color, consistency
Skin	Rashes, irritations, pustules, edema, birthmarks
Cord	Discharge, odor, redness
Eyes	Discharge
Feeding	Sucking ability, vomiting or regurgitation, degree of satisfaction
Mucous membranes	Dryness of lips and mouth, signs of thrush
Voiding	Initial, frequency (1-2 mL/kg/hr is normal)
Fontanels	Sunken or bulging
General activity	Increase or decrease in movements, lethargy, twitching, frequency and quality of cry, hyperactivity

Box 5-1	Factors Commonly Associated with Low–Birth Weight (LBW) Infants

- Previous LBW delivery
- Low socioeconomic status
- Low level of maternal education
- Maternal age below 16 and above 35
- Frequent pregnancies with short time between pregnancies
- Cigarette smoking
- Alcohol and/or illicit drug use
- Physical and/or psychological stress
- Maternal health issues such as malnutrition, diabetes mellitus, poor weight gain
- Pregnancy hazards such as pregnancy-induced hypertension, premature rupture of the membranes, placenta previa
- Unmarried status
- African-American race

extremely important. Inadequate prenatal care can result in low–birth weight infants and premature delivery. Many of these premature infants are born into families who already have socioeconomic problems. The presence of parents in special care nurseries is encouraged and commonplace. This encourages bonding and attachment. The parents may not be prepared to handle the additional strain caused by a preterm infant. Parent aides and other types of home support and assistance are vital, particularly because current studies indicate a correlation between high-risk births and child abuse and neglect.

The physician examines the premature baby on a regular basis and writes specific orders concerning treatment and nursing care. The physician also relies on the assessment done by the NICU nurses and must be notified of any significant changes in the baby's condition. The experienced NICU nurse observes and charts care and treatment with great accuracy. Table 5-4 lists *general* observations to serve as a guide in premature infant care. All abnormal findings and/or sudden changes require interventions and should be reported immediately.

COMPLICATIONS OF THE PRETERM INFANT (RESPIRATORY SYSTEM)

Important structural changes occur in the fetal lungs during the second half of pregnancy. The alveoli, or air sacs, enlarge, bringing them closer to the capillaries in the lungs. Failure of the alveoli to enlarge leads to many deaths, which are attributed to previability (*pre,* before; *vita,* life). In addition, the muscles that move the chest are not fully developed, the abdomen is distended and causes pressure on the diaphragm, stimulation of the respiratory center in the brain is immature, and the gag and cough reflexes are weak because of inadequate nerve supply. Surfactant (a chemical in the lungs that helps inflate alveoli) also may be deficient.

ATELECTASIS

The lungs are collapsed during fetal life. Their failure to expand after birth is known as atelectasis. Although some lung expansion must take place with the first breath, full development may not occur until several days later. **Primary atelectasis,** in which the alveoli fail to expand, may occur in preterm infants, infants of mothers who are oversedated before delivery, and infants with damage to the respiratory center in the brain. **Secondary atelectasis** occurs when the lungs collapse after they have once inflated. This may be caused by viral infections, pulmonary disease, aspirated foreign material, or a mucus plug.

Signs and Symptoms

Symptoms vary with the cause and extent of the atelectasis. The infant exhibits irregular, rapid respirations. These may be accompanied by respiratory grunting and flaring of the nostrils. The skin is typically cyanotic and mottled. Tachycardia is generally present. Intercostal and substernal retractions may be noticeable (Figure 5-19). These symptoms cause the infant to tire, and hypoxemia increases. Radiographs showing increased density, sometimes involving both lungs, confirm the diagnosis. The prognosis depends on the general condition of the baby and the cause.

Treatment

Treatment depends on the cause of the collapse. Frequent changes in position (as permitted) and oxygen therapy may be beneficial. Positioning should enhance full lung expansion, and clothing should not be binding. The semi-Fowler's position may facilitate lung expansion. Oxygen must be warmed and humidified. Mechanical ventilation may be required. These babies are usually treated in the NICU. Nursing care should involve close observation for changes in respiratory status.

RESPIRATORY DISTRESS SYNDROME

Respiratory distress syndrome (RDS), formerly known as *hyaline membrane disease*, is a common disorder in infants of very low birth weight. Because of the immaturity of the lungs, there is decreased gas exchange. This, together with pulmonary structural immaturity, results in absolute or functional deficiency of surfactant. Surfactant reduces the surface tension in the lung and allows for easy expansion of the lung, preventing the collapse of the alveoli during expiration. Without surfactant, the alveoli must be reexpanded with each breath so as to allow adequate gas exchange to occur. As a result, the infant uses all available energy to breathe. In the absence of adequate oxygenation, there is decreased or no production of surfactant.

Signs and Symptoms

Signs of RDS may develop at birth in the premature infant. The more premature the infant and the less the infant weighs at birth, the more likely the incidence of respiratory distress. Manifestations of RDS include tachypnea, nasal flaring, cyanosis, intercostal and sternal retractions, and grunting. Infants with severe RDS develop apnea and respiratory failure and need mechanical ventilation.

Treatment

The best approach to treating RDS is to prevent prematurity. This is done through prenatal care. If a problem arises and the fetus must be delivered prematurely, the treatment may involve, if there is enough time, increasing the production of surfactant. If this is not possible, the infant can be given artificial surfactant after birth, which is described below.

In the event that there is time, and delivery is not necessary for at least 2 to 3 days, amniocentesis is done to determine the maturity of the fetus. A test called the lecithin/sphingomyelin (L/S) ratio can be used to detect insufficient amounts of surfactant. If insufficient amounts are found, it is possible to speed up the production of surfactant by giving the mother multiple injections of a corticosteroid such as betamethasone or dexamethasone. Administration 1 or 2 days before delivery may reduce the chance of RDS developing.

Surfactant replacement therapy is being done for very low–birth weight infants and also for infants who show evidence of respiratory distress during the first 24 hours of life. An exogenous synthetic form of surfactant or natural form of surfactant is administered directly into the infant's endotracheal tube. This acts directly on the lungs. Surfactant should be administered only in the NICU, with adequate support of a neonatologist, NICU nurses, and respiratory therapists.

Surfactant has been beneficial in the treatment of RDS. In infants treated with surfactant, there has been an improvement in gas exchange, a reduction in ventilatory pressures, and improved appearance of the lungs on chest radiographs. However, surfactant has not been shown to reduce the incidence of **bronchopulmonary dysplasia (BPD),** which can be a chronic lung problem. BPD is discussed in Chapter 11. Complications of surfactant therapy include transient hypoxia, bradycardia, and hypotension; blockage of the endotracheal tube; and pulmonary hemorrhage (Kliegman et al., 2007).

Additional treatment of RDS includes respiratory support ranging from nasal continuous positive airway

Grade   0   1   2

CHEST/ABDOMINAL MOVEMENT

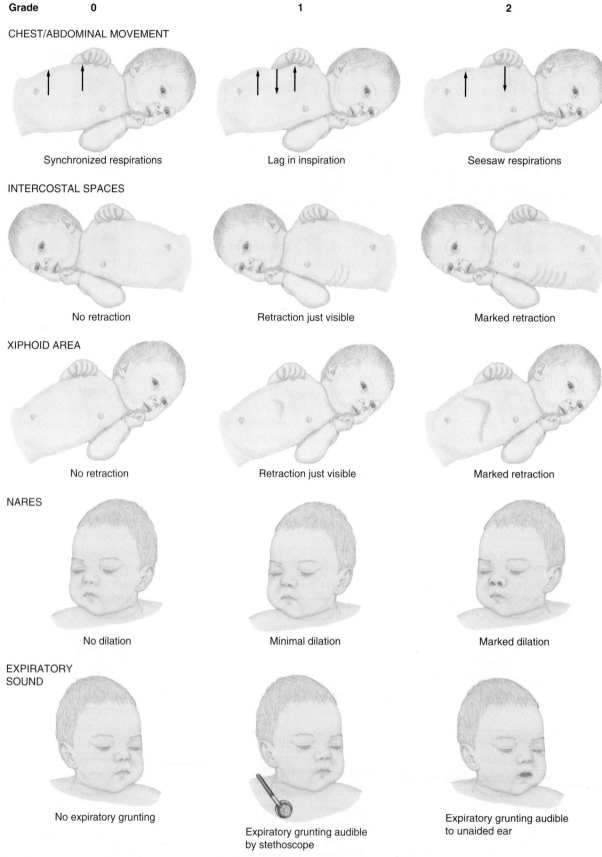

Synchronized respirations   Lag in inspiration   Seesaw respirations

INTERCOSTAL SPACES

No retraction   Retraction just visible   Marked retraction

XIPHOID AREA

No retraction   Retraction just visible   Marked retraction

NARES

No dilation   Minimal dilation   Marked dilation

EXPIRATORY SOUND

No expiratory grunting   Expiratory grunting audible by stethoscope   Expiratory grunting audible to unaided ear

FIGURE 5-19 Indicators of respiratory distress in the neonate.

pressure (NCPAP) to aggressive support with conventional mechanical ventilation or high-frequency ventilation, particularly high-frequency oscillation (Soll and Pfister, 2006). High-frequency oscillation provides effective oxygenation by controlling both inspiration and expiration, resulting in improved carbon dioxide elimination and reduced gas trapping (Boyd and Costarino, 2006).

APNEA

Apnea in the preterm infant is fairly common. Premature infants have periods of rapid respirations, followed by very slow breathing and then a period of no apparent respirations. Apnea is defined as the cessation of breathing for 20 or more seconds. This may be accompanied by bradycardia (fewer than 100 heart beats per minute in infants) and cyanosis. Apnea in the term infant requires diagnostic evaluation. Causes may include sepsis, pneumonia, or intraventricular hemorrhage (Kliegman et al., 2007).

Nursing Care

Apnea monitors, usually set at 20 seconds, help alert nurses to a cessation of respirations. This does not remove the nurse's responsibility to observe the infant for signs of respiratory distress. If the monitor alarm sounds, the nurse should *first* assess the infant for signs of distress, color, and respirations. Because of loose leads and other mechanical causes, it is not unusual for the monitor to emit false alarms. If an apneic spell has occurred, the nurse can gently rub the infant's chest or back. If stimulation fails, the nurse should suction the nose and oropharynx and reposition the infant's head by raising it to a "sniffing" position. If breathing still does not begin, the infant should be ventilated via an Ambu bag.

Infants who experience periods of apnea because of immaturity may be placed on a medication such as caffeine or theophylline to stimulate the central nervous system (CNS) (Schmidt, 2006). Stimulation of the breathing center in the CNS improves the rhythm of breathing. Nursing care includes monitoring the blood levels of these medications because toxicity can occur.

Infants known to have apneic spells often go home on monitors. Before discharge from the hospital, parents are educated about the use of home monitors. It is also imperative that the parents or the caregivers of these infants learn cardiopulmonary resuscitation (CPR) and demonstrate proficiency in CPR before discharge from the hospital.

Nursing Brief

Caregivers of infants being discharged with home monitoring should have a clear understanding that the purpose of monitoring is to alert caregivers to apnea episodes and *not* to prevent sudden infant death.

COMPLICATIONS OF THE PRETERM INFANT (INFECTION)

SEPSIS

Sepsis or *septicemia* refers to a generalized infection in the bloodstream. All neonates are at risk for developing sepsis, but preterm infants are especially vulnerable. Newborns up to 1 month of age with an infection may have sepsis neonatorum. The infant has diminished immunity, and usually there is no local inflammatory response at the site of infection. This makes the signs and symptoms vague. Blood, urine, and cerebral spinal fluid (CSF) cultures are obtained in an attempt to determine the organism causing the infection.

Signs and Symptoms

Manifestations of sepsis are often vague, and the diagnosis is sometimes based on an infant "not looking right." All the body systems may be affected by sepsis. Sepsis is infection manifested by tachypnea, tachycardia, and poor feeding in newborns and infants (Lin and Carcillo, 2006). Some of the more common manifestations include hypothermia, temperature instability, color changes, and changes in activity. Table 5-5 shows the responses of the different systems to sepsis.

Nursing Care

Prevention of sepsis is the goal of the nurse when caring for a preterm infant. Good hand hygiene is

Table 5-5 Clinical Manifestations of Neonatal Sepsis

SYSTEM	SIGNS AND SYMPTOMS
Integumentary	Temperature instability (may be increased, decreased, or both) Rash
Cardiovascular	Tachycardia Decreased perfusion, capillary refill Hypotension Cyanosis, pallor, or mottling
Gastrointestinal	Feeds poorly Abdominal distention Vomiting Diarrhea
Respiratory	Nasal flaring, retractions, grunting Tachypnea Cyanosis Apnea
Central nervous	Lethargy Irritability Hypotonia Seizures (late sign)
Hematopoietic	Jaundice (late sign) Hepatomegaly, splenomegaly (late signs) Petechiae, purpura (late signs) Anemia (late sign)

imperative before and after handling the baby or the equipment used in the infant's care. Nurses caring for infants in the NICU adhere to standard precautions when handling the infant or touching any objects in the baby's environment. The infant should be observed before handling in order to note any changes in behavior and activities. A thermoregulated environment is provided to conserve energy. Isolation guidelines are used to prevent the spread of infection to other neonates.

Treatment

Infants with sepsis are treated with intravenous antimicrobials. Standard precautions (see Appendix B) are to be followed. These neonates are closely observed for changes in color, vital signs, neurologic status, and general condition.

COMPLICATIONS OF THE PRETERM INFANT (GASTROINTESTINAL SYSTEM)

NECROTIZING ENTEROCOLITIS

Necrotizing enterocolitis (NEC) is an acute inflammatory disease of the bowel that occurs more often in preterm and other high-risk infants. The exact cause is uncertain, but there seems to be a relationship among intestinal ischemia, bacteria in the area, and the ingestion of formula. Several medications have also been implicated in the cause of NEC. Studies have shown that there is less incidence of NEC among babies whose diet included breast milk; research has also shown that probiotics reduce the risk of disease (Caplan, 2009).

Signs and Symptoms

Early signs of NEC, such as temperature instability, apnea, and bradycardia, are difficult to differentiate from those of other diseases, especially septicemia. More specific manifestations include a distended abdomen, emesis that contains bile, blood in the stool, and diarrhea. Bowel loops may be seen or felt on the abdomen. Onset often occurs between 4 and 10 days after the initiation of feedings. Radiographic findings show a sausage-shaped dilation of the intestine. The bowel wall is described as having a *bubbly* appearance. This is from air in the submucosal surfaces of the bowel (Hockenberry and Wilson, 2007). Necrosis can occur. The bowel may require surgical resection, possibly resulting in a colostomy, ileostomy, or jejunostomy.

Nursing Care

Early recognition of the signs and symptoms of NEC aids in early treatment. Abdominal distention should be monitored by consistent abdominal circumference measurements. Temperatures should not be taken rectally because of the danger of perforation.

Transmission to other infants must be prevented. Strict hand hygiene and other infection-control measures are implemented. The infant will have a nasogastric tube to decompress the abdomen (relieve abdominal distention) and receive intravenous antimicrobials. Monitoring of laboratory values is required. The use of parenteral nutrition may be necessary to allow the bowel to rest. The nurse monitors vital signs and reports any abnormal findings. Orders for resuming feedings are followed closely.

COMPLICATIONS OF THE PRETERM INFANT (METABOLISM)

HYPOGLYCEMIA

The preterm infant has not remained in the uterus long enough to have sufficient supplies of fat or glycogen to mobilize glucose. Infants born to mothers with diabetes, SGA infants, and infants having trouble maintaining oxygenation levels or temperature are all at risk for hypoglycemia.

Signs and Symptoms

In addition to the obvious low glucose level, determined in the plasma or blood, the nurse should watch for other manifestations of hypoglycemia. These include feeding difficulty, hunger, lethargy, apnea, irregular respiratory effort, cyanosis, a weak and high-pitched cry, jitteriness, twitching, eye rolling, and seizures.

Nursing Care

Nursing care primarily involves identifying signs and symptoms that might indicate the presence of hypoglycemia. The nurse should also control the thermal environment so that the infant does not have to expend extra energy adjusting to a cold environment. Feeding the infant also aids in preventing hypoglycemia. When feedings alone cannot maintain blood glucose concentrations at levels greater than 50 mg/dL, intravenous glucose should be started (Kliegman et al., 2007).

HYPOCALCEMIA

Hypocalcemia (*hypo*, below; *calcemia*, calcium in the blood) is also seen in preterm infants and sick neonates. Calcium is transported across the placenta throughout pregnancy, but particularly during the third trimester. Early birth can result in babies with lower than normal serum calcium levels. Other stressors, such as perinatal asphyxia, trauma, or diabetes in the mother, may predispose the newborn infant to hypocalcemia.

Signs, Symptoms, and Treatment

Early neonatal hypocalcemia is seen in the first 2 or 3 days of life and is usually temporary. Symptoms include muscle cramps, tetany (muscle twitching or hand spasm), weakness, paresthesia, laryngospasm (high-pitched crowing sound), or seizure-like activity. Late hypocalcemia usually appears about 1 week to 1 month after birth. It results when babies are fed unmodified cow's milk, which depresses the activity of the parathyroid glands. This condition, occasionally referred to as *neonatal tetany*, is rare in developed countries, where commercial formula or human milk is used to feed the newborn. Serum calcium levels are monitored in all high-risk neonates. Normal levels range from 7.0 to 8.5 mg/dL. Hypocalcemia is treated by early feedings and calcium supplements when possible. Intravenous administration of 10% calcium gluconate may be necessary.

COMPLICATIONS OF THE PRETERM INFANT (SENSORY)

RETINOPATHY OF PREMATURITY

Retinopathy of prematurity (ROP) may result in blindness in preterm infants. This disorder was once thought to be caused by the toxic effect of oxygen on the developing blood vessels of the premature infant's retina. Other causes have since been implicated. ROP is now believed to be a complex disease of prematurity that has multiple causes such as hyperoxemia, hypoxemia, acidosis, sepsis, and shock. Infants that weigh less than 1500 g and/or have a gestational age of 28 weeks or less should be screened for ROP. Screening should begin when the infant is 4 to 6 weeks of age by an experienced ophthalmologist (Chiang and Flynn, 2006).

Treatment and Nursing Care

Prevention is the primary goal. Pediatric ophthalmologists can treat ROP with **laser** surgery or occasionally with **cryotherapy** (the therapeutic use of cold). The incidence rate may be reduced by decreasing constant bright environmental light and stimuli and by decreasing or avoiding events that cause fluctuations in blood pressure and oxygenation (Hockenberry and Wilson, 2007). Careful monitoring of oxygenation is an important nursing measure related to prevention.

COMPLICATIONS OF THE PRETERM INFANT (NEUROLOGY)

INTRAVENTRICULAR HEMORRHAGE (IVH)

Hemorrhage into and around the ventricles in the brain can occur in the premature infant. While intraventricular bleeding may be asymptomatic, sudden deterioration can result if the bleed is large. Apnea, seizures, and a bulging fontanel are signs of an IVH. Long-term neurologic deficits can result, as can death.

Treatment and Nursing Care

Ultrasound is used to diagnose IVH; grading 1 to 4 determines the severity (grade 4 is the most severe). Ventilatory support, maintaining acid-base balance, seizure control, and maintaining oxygenation are essential. Nursing care is based on preventing increased cerebral blood pressure by avoiding pain, unnecessary stimulation, suctioning, and hypoxia. The head of the bed is usually elevated slightly while the head is maintained in a midline position. Close monitoring is required.

ADDITIONAL HIGH-RISK CONSIDERATIONS

THE POSTTERM INFANT

The newborn baby is considered postterm if a pregnancy goes beyond 42 weeks. This is a great psychological strain on both the mother and the other members of the family, who are eagerly awaiting the birth of the baby. What causes postmaturity is not yet clear; however, it is known that the placenta does not function adequately as it ages. This could result in fetal distress, and the infant may exhibit such problems as hypoxia or meconium aspiration. Very large neonates, such as those of mothers with diabetes, are not necessarily postmature but are instead larger than normal because of rapid growth before delivery.

The mortality rate of the newborn who is delivered after 42 weeks' gestation is higher than that of a newborn delivered at term. The greatest risk for this infant is during the labor process.

The postterm infant is long and thin and looks as though he or she has lost weight. The skin is loose, especially about the thighs and buttocks. There is little downy hair (lanugo) or vernix caseosa. Loss of this cheese-like protection leaves the skin dry; it cracks and peels and is almost parchment-like in texture. The nails are long and may be stained with meconium. The baby has a good head of hair and looks alert. Many postmature babies have few adverse effects from the delay, but they still need careful observation in the nursery.

When it is determined that a pregnancy is past 40 weeks, the well-being of the mother and infant are determined by special tests. The course that is taken is determined by the results of the tests. A cesarean section is performed if there is evidence of fetal distress or a risk to the mother.

MECONIUM ASPIRATION SYNDROME

Aspiration of meconium, which is the fecal material that is sometimes released during the birthing process and therefore is in the amniotic fluid, is sometimes seen in the term or postterm newborn infant. It signals that the fetus was in distress while in utero. This intrauterine stress causes relaxing of the infant's anal sphincter and passage of meconium into the amniotic fluid. Aspiration of meconium may occur with the first breath. This results in small airway obstruction, manifested by tachypnea, hypoxia, retractions, grunting respirations, and cyanosis. Respiratory distress may be immediate or delayed, and pneumothorax may result. If the course is mild, improvement may occur within 48 hours. If the aspiration is severe, respiratory failure can occur very rapidly.

TREATMENT

Immediate suctioning of the nasopharynx and oropharynx at birth is indicated. A chest radiograph may show coarse, patchy intensities. Atelectasis sometimes occurs. Infants with respiratory distress are transferred to the NICU for close observation. These infants are treated with intravenous fluids, systemic antimicrobials, exogenous (artificial) surfactant administration, and possible ventilatory support (Hockenberry and Wilson, 2007).

INFANTS OF MOTHERS WITH DIABETES

The successful regulation of diabetes has led to increasing numbers of women with diabetes bearing children. These infants are considered at high risk because they were exposed to high levels of maternal glucose before birth. The pancreas of the fetus responds by producing more insulin, which is an important regulator of fetal growth and metabolism. This is believed to account for the large size of these babies. **Macrosomia** (*macro*, large; *soma*, body) has been considered a classic symptom of babies of mothers with diabetes. Delivery may be difficult because of the infant's large size. The baby's face is large and puffy, resembling that of a child on steroids. These infants are also candidates for problems such as perinatal asphyxia, birth trauma, polycythemia, hyperbilirubinemia, RDS, and other complications. It is imperative that these babies be born in centers where there is expert supervision or be transferred to a regional care center shortly after birth. Nursing care includes initiating feedings early after birth, monitoring blood glucose levels closely, monitoring vital signs, and close evaluation of the infant's overall condition.

INFANT BEHAVIOR

INFANT ACTIVITY

REACTIVITY

After delivery, the vigorous neonate exhibits a characteristic pattern of activities. These patterns are termed the **first and second periods of reactivity.** During the first period, which lasts for about 30 minutes after birth, the neonate is awake and active. The heart and respiratory rates are rapid. There is grimacing, sucking movements, and random motor activity. This is usually followed by a period of rest that lasts from 2 to 4 hours. At this time, the neonate is disinterested in sucking and stimulation. On awakening, there is a second period of reactivity. This second period of reactivity occurs between 2 to 6 hours of age and is when the neonate's responsiveness returns. Periods of apnea may be seen, and there is an increase in mucus. The color of the newborn infant may vary at times between mildly mottled, pink, and pale. Bowel sounds become audible, and meconium stools are passed. The second period of reactivity can either be brief or last up to several hours. After this period, the newborn becomes relatively stable.

SLEEP

The newborn sleeps approximately 15 to 20 hours a day. As the neonate matures, there is a gradual change in the quantity and quality of sleep. Differentiation between active and quiet sleep is based primarily on whether **rapid eye movement** (REM) occurs. The sleep of a newborn infant consists of approximately 50% REM sleep, as opposed to only 20% in a 5-year-old child. During REM sleep, respirations are rapid and more irregular, movements of the eye are evident beneath the eyelid, and movements of the limbs and mouth may be seen. Premature infants have an even higher proportion of REM sleep than babies born at term. Investigators theorize that REM sleep may be an internal stimulus to the higher brain centers at a time when external stimulation is minimal because of only brief periods of arousal.

Positioning the infant during sleep is an important aspect of care. In 1992, the American Academy of Pediatrics (AAP) recommended that infants be placed on their backs (supine) to sleep to reduce the incidence of sudden infant death syndrome (SIDS). SIDS has been reduced by more than 50% since the "Back to Sleep" campaign began (NIH, 2005). It is strongly recommended by the AAP that infants not be placed in the prone position, which is on their abdomen. The prone position has the highest incidence rate for correlation with SIDS. Although many parents fear choking in the supine position, studies have shown that this is not the case. The AAP Policy Statement (2005, reaffirmed 2009) also stresses the need to avoid soft bedding and soft objects in the infant's sleeping environment, the hazards of adults sleeping with an infant in the same bed, the SIDS risk reduction associated with having infants sleep in the same room as adults, the importance of educating secondary caregivers, using light clothing for sleep, avoiding secondhand smoke, and the benefit of using a pacifier when putting the infant to sleep. Giving a pacifier at the time of sleep significantly reduces the risk for SIDS (Burke, 2006). Finally, sleeping on the side as a reasonable

Table 5-6 Behavioral States of the Newborn

STATE	DESCRIPTION
Quiet sleep	Regular respirations Very few body movements Deep sleep
Active sleep	REM Respirations irregular and primarily abdominal Some body movements
Drowsiness	Transitional state between sleep and awake states Fluttering eyelids If eyes open, they have a glassy appearance Irregular respirations Facial grimacing Variable motor activity
Quiet alert	Regular respirations Minimal movements Eyes bright and shiny Can look at the caregiver Most productive state for bonding
Active awake	Increased movements Increased irritability Fussiness
Crying	Intense, rhythmic crying Accompanied by increased motor activity

alternative to fully supine sleeping is no longer recommended.

NEONATAL STATES

Behavioral states of the newborn have been studied since 1966. In the 1980s, Dr. T. Berry Brazelton described the following six states: (1) quiet sleep, (2) active sleep, (3) drowsiness, (4) quiet alert, (5) active awake, and (6) crying. These states are a reflection of the newborn's ability to react to the environment and a reflection of the ability of the central nervous system to adjust to stimuli (Table 5-6).

BEHAVIORAL ASSESSMENT

Assessing infant behavior is an important nursing role. Observing how babies respond to stimuli in their environment helps nurses teach parents how to respond to their babies. The **Brazelton Neonatal Behavioral Assessment Scale** (http://www.brazelton-institute.com/intro.html) has increased our understanding of the neonate's capabilities. Among other things, the scale measures the inherent neurologic capacities of the neonate and responses to selected stimuli. Areas tested include alertness, response to visual and auditory stimuli, motor coordination, level of excitement, and organizational processes in response to stress. The Brazelton Neonatal Behavioral Assessment Scale is of particular value during the newborn period; it is used to describe the emerging personality of the baby and includes evaluation of infant reflexes, general activity, alertness, orientation to spoken voice, and response to visual stimuli.

CARE OF THE NEWBORN INFANT

IDENTIFYING THE NEONATE

Proper identification of the newborn is ensured by placing wristbands with preprinted, matching numbers on the newborn, the mother, and the father or significant other. This is done in the delivery room. The AAP recommends that two identical identification bands be placed on the infant. Bracelets are usually placed on the wrist and ankle. The neonate loses weight after birth, so the bracelets must be snug. Hospitals today often take a color photograph of the infant soon after birth for identification purposes. The National Center for Missing and Exploited Children (2009) also recommends foot-printing the infant and storing a sample of the infant cord blood until at least the day after discharge. A full physical assessment along with a description of the infant needs to appear in the medical chart. Finally, electronic security tags are placed on the infant, if such a system is being used. These devices trigger an alarm in the event that they exit the maternity unit. In case a newborn is abducted, hospitals have an emergency code to secure elevators and exits of the building. Some hospitals will "lock down" in the event of a security breach. Employees in all areas are aware of the code name for a newborn abduction and can assist in identifying and delaying the departure of any suspicious person.

Security issues have played a major part in the care of the newborn infant. Parents must be assured that their newborn is safe and secure whenever the infant is not in their care. They also need to be taught the security guidelines. Nursery and postpartum nurses must follow established protocols when removing the newborn from the parents. These nurses also need to wear appropriate identification badges. Many of these are now complete with staff picture and are color-coded according to the area in which the nurse works. When the newborn is returned to the parents, identification bands are again checked to reestablish security. Identification is reaffirmed on admission to the nursery and before transferring the infant to any other location. Infants are *always* transported by bassinet and are never carried by hospital staff.

MEDICATION ADMINISTRATION AND SCREENING TESTS

Vitamin K (AquaMephyton) is administered within 1 hour after birth to promote blood clotting and prevent hemorrhage in the neonate. A mild vitamin K deficiency is not unusual in newborns and is common in preterm infants. The neonate's intestinal flora is sterile at birth, and, as a result, the newborn is unable to synthesize vitamin K. A normal intestinal flora is established after birth. Vitamin K is administered intramuscularly into the lateral aspect of the thigh or the ventrogluteal site.

All infants should receive the first dose of hepatitis B vaccine soon after birth and before hospital discharge. The hepatitis B vaccine is administered intramuscularly into the lateral aspect of the thigh or ventrogluteal site. This immunization is the first in the *series* of three hepatitis B injections that the infant receives. Hepatitis B is further discussed in Chapter 18.

A 0.5% erythromycin ointment is instilled in the neonate's eyes to prevent ophthalmia neonatorum (Figure 5-20). Ointment needs to be administered within 1 hour after birth. Mild inflammation may occur, and any discharge from the eyes should be reported.

Blood work such as a hematocrit determination and a glucose recording may be indicated if the newborn is having difficulty adjusting to the environment. Screening tests for metabolic conditions that, if left untreated, could lead to conditions such as mental retardation are done after birth. In the United States, all states require **newborn** screening for metabolic disorders; however, states vary on requirements. Phenylketonuria (PKU), hypothyroidism, galactosemia, and hemoglobinopathies are commonly screened. States may screen for additional disorders such as maple syrup urine disease, cystic fibrosis, and congenital adrenal hyperplasia.

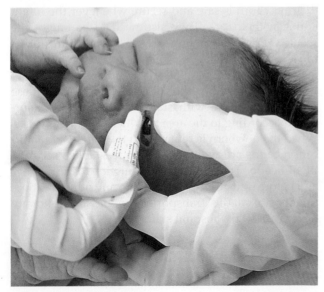

FIGURE 5-20 A ribbon of ointment is administered into each conjunctival sac to prevent infective conjunctivitis of the newborn.

- **Phenylketonuria (PKU):** A genetic metabolic disorder that can result in mental retardation if left untreated. No signs and symptoms are usually present at birth. Treatment consists of a low-phenylalanine diet; foods high in protein are also avoided.
- **Hypothyroidism:** A condition in which the thyroid gland does not produce sufficient thyroid hormone; can result in mental retardation, growth delay, lack of activity, feeding problems, and abnormal facial appearance if untreated. Signs and symptoms may include skin mottling, a large fontanel, a large tongue, hypotonia, slow reflexes, and a distended abdomen; may be asymptomatic (McKinney et al., 2009). Treatment consists of lifelong thyroid hormone replacement (levothyroxine).
- **Galactosemia:** Condition in which infants cannot properly digest milk or sugar; can result in mental retardation, cataracts, liver disease, or even death if untreated. Signs and symptoms include intrauterine growth retardation and hypoglycemia; vomiting and diarrhea occur after feedings. Treatment is a lifelong lactose-restricted diet.
- **Hemoglobinopathies:** Conditions such as sickle cell anemia, which can result in serious complications or infections if untreated. Sickle cell anemia is discussed in Chapter 21.

With the current trend toward early discharge of mothers and newborns, it is imperative that parents understand the importance of possible follow-up screening and keep the scheduled laboratory appointment.

NUTRITION

BREASTFEEDING ADVANTAGES

The nurse can play an important role in teaching, supporting, and encouraging the nursing mother. Breast milk provides immunologic, nutritional, and psychosocial advantages. Compared with cow's milk, breast milk contains more iron, sugar, vitamins A and C, and niacin. Breast milk has less protein and calcium than cow's milk, but the amounts present are better utilized by the baby. Breast milk is more digestible because its fat globules are smaller, and it is free from bacteria. It provides the baby with greater immunity to certain childhood/adult onset diseases including insulin-dependent diabetes, allergies, asthma, lymphoma, ulcerative colitis, and adult-onset hypertension. It also has potential protective effect against SIDS, and there is decreased incidence or severity of gastrointestinal and respiratory infections, otitis media, meningitis, urinary tract infections, and necrotizing enterocolitis (Association of Women's Health, Obstetric and Neonatal Nurses, position statements reaffirmed 2007). Breastfed babies are less prone to intestinal upsets. In

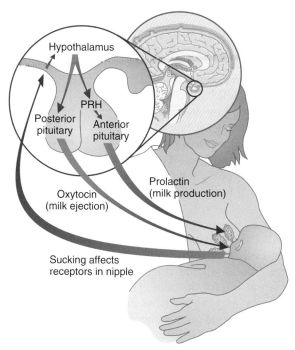

FIGURE 5-21 Milk release during breastfeeding.

brief, the quality of the mother's milk is suited to the needs of the baby. Many physicians and breastfeeding support groups encourage breastfeeding for the first year of life.

Practical factors in favor of breast milk include the fact that it saves time and money. It is also delivered to the newborn in the proper temperature and quantity; the more frequently a woman nurses, the more breast milk is produced (Figure 5-21). Breast milk provides the newborn with the most recommended nutrition, and it aids the mother physically. As the baby nurses, the mother's uterus contracts, thus hastening its return to a normal size and shape. Furthermore, mothers receive emotional satisfaction, and bonds of attachment are enhanced during feeding.

Breast milk can be stored in the refrigerator for up to 72 hours after pumping and 24 hours after thawing. It can be stored in a separate door freezer for 3 months after pumping and in a deep freezer 6 months. Frozen breast milk should be thawed under warm running water and not in the microwave. Thawed breast milk should never be refrozen.

In order to prevent rickets and vitamin D deficiency, 400 international units of oral vitamin D daily are recommended for breastfed infants, beginning the first few days of life. This should continue unless the infant is weaned to at least 1 L/day or 1 qt/day of vitamin D-fortified formula or whole milk. Whole milk should not be used until after 12 months of age (Wagner et al., 2008).

Although the nurse must keep in mind that breastfeeding is highly recommended, the individual choice of the mother should be respected. Ensuring that the baby receives the best nutrition available is always the ultimate goal.

CONTRAINDICATIONS TO BREASTFEEDING

Breastfeeding is contraindicated in infants with galactosemia and in mothers with active tuberculosis, septicemia, breast cancer, malaria, typhoid fever, substance abuse, and severe neuroses or psychoses (Kliegman et al., 2007). Mothers who are HIV-positive should not breastfeed, even if they are in relatively good health because the virus can be passed through breast milk. Certainly, the mother who has a personal preference not to breastfeed should not be forced to do so.

Occasionally, elevated levels of bilirubin occur in the breastfed infant. This is known as *breast milk jaundice*. If breastfeeding is continued, bilirubin gradually decreases; if breastfeeding is discontinued, levels fall rapidly. If breastfeeding is then resumed, bilirubin levels do not increase significantly. Phototherapy may be beneficial (Kliegman et al., 2007).

Nursing Brief

If a pacifier is used, instruct parents to obtain the type that is of one-piece construction to prevent choking. Pacifiers should not be tied around the neonate's neck. To avoid nipple confusion, some practitioners still recommend that breastfeeding be well established (1 month) before introducing a pacifier.

TECHNIQUE OF BREASTFEEDING

In the establishment of lactation, the mother's milk goes through three stages: colostrum, transitional milk, and mature milk. Colostrum secretion is watery and yellowish, begins early in pregnancy, increases, and may last for several days after delivery. Transitional milk replaces colostrum after 2 to 4 days and lasts until about 2 weeks postpartum, when mature breast milk is present. The neonate is generally put to breast immediately or shortly after delivery. Current research supports this practice because it appears to increase early maternal-infant attachment, increase milk production, and decrease the chances of engorgement. The sucking of the neonate stimulates the production of milk. The let-down reflex, by which the milk is squeezed into the large ducts and nipples, is stimulated by the infant's sucking or sometimes even by the baby's crying. The mother feels a vague tingling sensation in her breasts when this occurs. If she is tense or tired, this feeling can be inhibited. The crying infant does not usually stimulate the let-down reflex until the mother has been conditioned to the infant's crying. Supplemental nursery feedings should be avoided in favor of more frequent nursing. Most difficulties are eliminated if the mother has a good fluid intake, an ample diet with extra milk, an adequate vitamin intake, and moderate rest and exercise. Factors to be emphasized are depicted in the Home Care Considerations box.

Home Care Considerations

Summary of Breastfeeding Instructions for the Mother

INFORMATION	RATIONALE
1. Wash hands before proceeding; wash nipples with warm water, no soap.	Prevents infection of the newborn and breast.
2. Position options: • Comfortably seated in chair with back and arm support (baby in football position). • Side-lying with pillow beneath head, arm above head. • Mother needs to experiment initially to find most comfortable positions for her. • Entire body of infant turned to mother's breast.	Alternating positions facilitates breast emptying and prevents sore nipples.
3. Stroke baby's cheek with nipple.	Infant will use rooting reflex, and will turn toward nipple.
4. Baby's mouth should cover entire or large amount of areola.	Compresses ducts, lessens tension on nipples.
5. Initially, both breasts are used; the first side for about 10 minutes; on the other, breastfeed for unlimited time (at least another 10 minutes).	Allows for let-down on the first breast.
6. After the milk supply has come in, the baby can nurse 10 to 20 minutes at the first breast, then the other breast if necessary. Alternate breasts with each feed.	Allows baby to get the high-fat, calorie-rich hind milk. Nursing at second breast increases milk production.
7. Retract breast tissue from baby's nose during sucking.	Baby releases nipple if unable to breathe.
8. Break suction by placing finger in corner of baby's mouth.	Removing baby in this way prevents irritation to nipples.
9. The neonate is nursed shortly after birth and approximately every 2 to 3 hours thereafter.	Initial feedings provide colostrum; establishing a pattern helps baby develop own schedule.
10. Burp baby after each breast and after feeding.	Rids stomach of air bubbles, reduces regurgitation.

POSSIBLE PROBLEMS WITH BREASTFEEDING

Although many women nurse successfully with few problems, some concerns include the neonate who does not eat well, sore and cracked nipples, and breast engorgement. Some babies do not seem to nurse vigorously and fall asleep after 5 minutes only to wake again when they are put in their crib. The mother can first try shifting the baby to the other breast. Babies can obtain a major portion of what is in the breast after 5 minutes of nursing. With further sucking, a second let-down occurs, which supplies the newborn with milk that is higher in fat.

There are several remedies for sore and cracked nipples. It is important to instruct mothers to be certain that the baby takes a large amount of the areola into the mouth when sucking. To accomplish this, the mother slides all the fingers under the breast to lift and support it for the baby. The thumb is placed above the areola, and the breast is moved so that the nipple lightly tickles the baby's lower lip. The baby is brought to the breast, *not* the breast to the baby. Time limits on each breast are no longer thought to prevent nipple soreness. Positioning of the newborn is more effective in decreasing nipple soreness than is limiting the time at the breast. When breaking suction before removing the infant from the breast, the mother should insert a finger into the infant's mouth beside the nipple. Frequent nursing provides continued stimulation of the breast and relieves fullness. After breastfeeding is established, the mother should continue feeding on the first side as long as the infant nurses vigorously, then burp the baby, and then continue on the other breast.

The nipples and areola should be washed with water and then allowed to dry thoroughly. Airing the nipples and applying a small amount of expressed breast milk to the areola has been found to be successful in the treatment of cracked or sore nipples. Ointments specific for breast care may be used to help reduce irritation. It is also important to keep breast pads dry to decrease contamination.

Breast engorgement may occur in the first week of nursing or if a feeding is missed. The breasts become swollen, firm, and tender, and there is less nipple protrusion. Prevention consists of emptying at least one breast at each feeding. The nurse also instructs the mother to purchase a well-fitting nursing bra and to wear it 24 hours a day. Treatment consists of breast massage during feedings, which aids in the release of oxytocin, which causes the let-down reflex. Also, frequent feedings (every 2 to 3 hours) are helpful in emptying the breasts at each feeding. It may be necessary to soften the areola region first by hand expression of milk if the nipple is too hard to get into the baby's mouth. Warm, moist compresses or a warm shower before feeding may also provide relief. Ice packs may be applied between feedings.

Community Considerations

With many mothers being discharged within 48 hours or less after delivery, resources such as the La Leche League can be helpful *(www.lalecheleague.org)*. Lactation consultants from the hospital are also a great resource and readily available to answer questions.

BOTTLE FEEDING

Newborn babies whose mothers choose to bottle feed their infants are given formula. Modern research has made such feedings safe and nutritionally adequate. The composition of formulas is designed to closely resemble breast milk.

Studies have indicated that babies tolerate cool or room-temperature formula equally as well as formula that has been heated slightly. If room-temperature formula is used, there is no chance of burns from overheated bottles; also, time and energy are conserved. Bottles should never be warmed in the microwave, because these ovens heat unevenly, formula can get too hot, and burns can result. Bottles are best heated under warm running water.

The mother or nurse needs to be relaxed and comfortable when feeding the neonate (Figure 5-22). The newborn's head and back are supported in the crook of the arm. Propping the bottle deprives the baby of the pleasure of being held and loved. It is also dangerous because the baby may choke if the flow of milk is too rapid. Milk can also pool in the pharynx, resulting in middle ear infections. A baby's natural tendency to push the tongue out when the nipple is placed in the mouth (the tongue retrusion reflex) should not be taken as an indication that the infant is not hungry.

USE OF FORMULA

There are many types of infant formulas to choose from. Most formulas are made from cow's milk, such as Enfamil and Similac. Other formulas such as Pro-Sobee and Isomil are soy based and are good for babies who have trouble digesting cow's milk formulas. LactoFree is a lactose-free formula intended for babies who cannot digest lactose. Other formulas are hypoallergenic or protein hydrolysate formulas such as Nutramigen, Pregestimil, or Alimentum. These formulas may be used if babies do not tolerate cow's milk or soy formulas. Health care professionals will recommend iron-fortified formulas unless there is a contraindication.

Expense governs the choice of formula for many families. In general, the more convenient, the higher the cost. Basically, prepared formulas come in three forms: (1) ready to use in cans (use as-is without dilution); (2) in concentrated form (dilute with an equal amount of water); and (3) in powdered form (1 scoop of powdered formula for every 2 ounces of water). Cold tap water may be mixed with concentrated formula or powder if the water is from an uncontaminated source (allow the water to run for about 2 minutes before collecting). Parents may prefer to purchase purified water designated for this purpose.

In homes with dishwashers, the high temperature of the water used in the dishwasher is excellent for cleaning the bottles and nipples. Regardless of the method used, all bottles, nipples, and other utensils must be thoroughly cleaned. Bottles and nipples are scrubbed with a bottle brush in hot, soapy water and rinsed well in hot, clear water. Water is squeezed through nipple holes during washing and rinsing. Bottles are placed upside down on a rack to drain. Check package inserts on sterilizing bottles and nipples for first-time use.

Many babies tolerate room temperature or cool formula. If the bottle needs to be warmed, it can be placed under warm running water. Leftover formula should not be rewarmed for future feedings because bacteria thrive at room temperature. This can be avoided by filling the bottle with the approximate amount the baby generally drinks.

TECHNIQUE OF BOTTLE FEEDING

The following points should be observed when feeding the baby by bottle:

1. Change the baby's diaper if needed.
2. Wash hands.
3. Hold the baby unless doing so is contraindicated. If the baby cannot be removed from the crib, sit by the baby and elevate the head and shoulders (unless contraindicated).

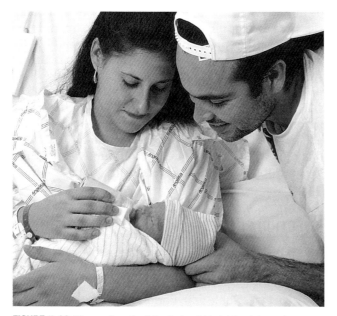

FIGURE 5-22 The mother (or father) should hold the infant close during feeding. Hold the bottle so that the baby receives formula and not air.

4. Use of a burp cloth (clean diaper, bib, or towel) under the baby's chin is helpful.

5. Observe the kind and amount of formula in the bottle.

6. Let a few drops of formula fall on the inner aspect of your wrist to test (only necessary if it was warmed).

    a. Temperature should be warm but not hot.

    b. Size of nipple hole: Formula should drop but not flow in a steady stream. If the holes are too small, the weak baby tires and fails to finish the feeding. If they are too large, the baby may choke or miss the satisfaction received from sucking.

7. Do not contaminate the nipple.

8. Hold the bottle so that the nipple is full of formula. This prevents the baby from swallowing air.

9. Burp the baby halfway through the feeding and at the end of the feeding with one of the following methods:

    a. Place a diaper or small towel over your shoulder. Place the baby firmly against your shoulder and gently pat his or her back.

    b. Place the baby in a sitting position. Put a towel beneath his or her chin. Support the baby's chest and head with one hand. Gently rub the baby's back with the other hand.

10. The feeding should take 15 to 20 minutes. A newborn will take approximately 2 to 3 ounces of formula every 3 to 4 hours for the first few weeks, progressing to 4 ounces every 4 hours by the end of the first month. Do not hurry the baby or force the baby to eat too much.

11. Leave the baby clean and dry. Place the baby who is *awake* on the right side to promote digestion (Figure 5-23). Remember, however, that babies should *sleep on their backs*.

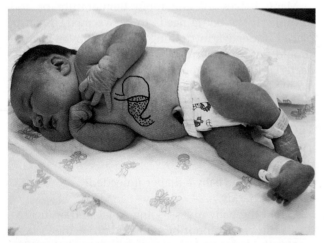

FIGURE 5-23 Right side-lying position after feeding while awake. Supine positioning is recommended during sleep.

12. In the hospital, chart the amount of formula offered, the amount taken and retained, any regurgitation or vomiting, how the formula was taken, and whether or not the baby appeared satisfied after the feeding. (Note that regurgitation is an overflow of milk that occurs shortly after feeding, whereas vomiting means bringing up a more substantial amount of partially digested milk.)

NUTRITION AND THE PRETERM INFANT

Feeding of the preterm infant may be done by mouth (orally), by gavage (feeding by tube), or by parenteral methods (intravenously). Sick and very premature infants are usually given intravenous fluids. Parenteral feeding given intravenously through a catheter passed into the umbilical vein may be started shortly after delivery. They may receive **total parenteral nutrition (TPN)** if they cannot tolerate oral or gavage feedings. TPN includes nutrients essential to meet their nutritional needs.

Preterm infants younger than 32 to 34 weeks' gestation are usually fed through a nasal or gastric tube (gavage) because of their immature suck and swallow reflexes. As the infant matures and becomes stronger, nipple and gavage feedings may be alternated. The nurse observes the infant's suck and swallow reflexes, weight gain, and lack of respiratory distress to determine whether nipple feeding is being tolerated. Breast milk that has been expressed and stored properly or formula may be fed to the infant when ordered. Breast milk has many advantages over commercial formula. Benefits include prevention of infection and a reduction in the rate and severity of NEC.

Special small and soft nipples are available for the small infant. The feeding should take no longer than 30 minutes. Feeding for longer periods uses more calories than are supplied by the feeding. The infant is fed in a semisitting position and burped frequently. After the feeding, the infant may be placed on his or her right side with the head slightly raised if awake. This position facilitates emptying of the stomach.

Fluid intake is recorded carefully. The nurse reports the number of voids and observes for signs of edema. The hydration needs of the child are reviewed daily on the basis of intake, output, weight, and general appearance. Blood chemistries are reviewed regularly.

INFECTION PREVENTION

Infections that are relatively harmless to an adult may be fatal to the newborn infant. Symptoms are often subtle in the early stages, the recognition of which can be crucial (see Table 5-5). Portals of entry are the respiratory tract, the gastrointestinal tract, the genitourinary tract, and breaks in the skin. The portals of exit are the same as those just mentioned, and the organisms are in the excretions from the various systems: sneezes, sputum, vomitus, feces, saliva, urine, and discharges from the skin and mucous membranes. Nursery standards are developed and enforced by various professional agencies such as the AAP, hospital accreditation boards, and local health agencies. Provisions governing space, control of temperature and humidity, lighting, and safety from fire and other hazards are considered. Each newborn infant has his or her own bassinet/crib, bath equipment, and linen supply. Any shared equipment is sterilized after each use.

 Nursing Brief

Advise parents to limit the neonate's exposure to crowds during the early weeks of life. Family and friends who visit need to wash their hands before holding the newborn.

Nursery personnel wear scrub uniforms. Nails are kept short and clean. Artificial nails are not permitted because they harbor bacteria. A nurse who has a fever, skin infection, or gastrointestinal disease should not work in the nursery. Because many hospitals have open visiting, all visitors should be cautioned not to come if they are sick. Annual flu shots are often required of employees working in the nursery or NICU.

HAND HYGIENE

The most effective procedure used in the prevention of infections is **proper hand hygiene.** The nurse must conscientiously wash and rinse the hands and forearms before and after caring for each newborn or handling equipment. Hand hygiene before care protects the newborn, and hand hygiene after care protects the nurse. Although most organisms are transmitted by direct contact, some are capable of remaining alive for a time outside the body and may be transferred indirectly by articles. Personnel entering the newborn nursery initially scrub their hands with soap and water. Parents and relatives should be taught the importance of this simple but highly effective procedure.

 Nursing Brief

When washing hands, make sure the water flows from the least to the most contaminated area (keep hands lowered). Use friction and rub well between the fingers and around the nails. Wash hands, wrists, and forearms for a minimum of 10 to 15 seconds. If there is no foot pedal, turn the faucet off with a clean paper towel.

CARE OF THE PATIENT UNIT

A baby in the newborn nursery is usually placed in a small, transparent bassinet) equipped with a drawer that can be pulled out (holds the newborn's linens and supplies). Supplies in the newborn's crib should be used only for that newborn. By following this practice, the rate of cross-contamination can be reduced. The head of the newborn's crib should be considered the clean area. This is where the bulb suction should be placed. The bottom of the crib is less clean, so that is where soiled diapers should be placed until they can be removed from the crib.

The newborn infant in the hospital may wear a hospital shirt and diaper and should be wrapped in at least one blanket, or may wear clothes from home. Remind parents to wash new baby clothing before it is worn (see Clothing the Baby). Be sure the baby remains warm enough. *Remember that babies are transported in their bassinet; they are never carried. Anyone carrying an infant in a hallway should be questioned.*

SIGNS AND SYMPTOMS OF INFECTION

The following signs and symptoms of infection in newborns and infants should not only be recognized and reported to the charge nurse but taught to parents as well:

- Temperature above 100° F (37.8° C) or below 97° F (36° C)
- Refusal to take nourishment
- Rashes or skin lesions
- Loose, watery stools
- Discharge from eyes, nose, or umbilicus
- Vomiting
- Lethargy or irritability
- Others, as indicated in Table 5-5

The ill newborn is isolated from other newborns. If warranted, the baby will be placed in the NICU with specific isolation guidelines.

ONGOING CARE

BATHING THE BABY

After the newborn's temperature and vital signs have become stable, the newborn receives his or her first bath. This is an excellent time to observe the naked newborn infant. Always bathe the baby in a warm area. Bath water should be approximately 38° C (100° F). Special attention must be given to areas of the skin that come in contact with each other because chafing may occur. These areas are on the neck, behind the ears, in the axillae, and in the groin. They should be dried well to prevent evaporative heat loss. Because powder can be irritating to the respiratory tract, it is not used in the hospital and parents are discouraged from using it at home. Lotions and the type of soap used vary with each institution. The newborn is then dressed in a diaper and a shirt and wrapped in blankets and placed in a bassinet. The procedure for bathing the newborn infant is described in Chapter 3.

Nursing Brief

Emphasize flexibility in the timing of the bath. Stress the need to gather all materials beforehand to avoid leaving the neonate unattended or chilled. The nurse attempts to help parents relax by emphasizing that there is nothing difficult about bathing a baby.

CLOTHING THE BABY

Parents should be taught that babies should be dressed as other family members are dressed. They do not need an extra blanket or extra clothing unless they are in a cool environment. New parents should prewash all of the baby's clothes, linens, and washable accessories in a mild detergent before they are used. Clothes should be easy to put on and take off. Safety should always be kept in mind.

CORD CARE
Patient Teaching
- The cord clamp is removed once the end of the cord is dry and crisp, usually about 24 hours after birth.
- Parents need to check for redness, odor, swelling, or any drainage and should report any of these symptoms to the physician.
- Dry cord care is preferred; nothing needs to be used around the base of the cord in order for it to heal. Wash with soap and water (some practitioners recommend sterile water only) if it becomes dirty, and then dry it with a clean cloth.
- The diaper should be folded below the cord to keep it dry and free from urine contamination.
- Until the cord falls off (10 to 14 days), parents should only sponge-bathe their baby.

POSITION AND SKIN CARE FOR THE PREMATURE INFANT

Developmental positioning in the preterm infant is vital to decreasing the risks of atelectasis and possible positional/orthopedic deformities. It is always important to *gently* change the positions of preterm and high-risk infants. Changing the baby's position also prevents pressure breakdowns on the delicate skin. The supine position requires support of the head, trunk, and extremities. Positioning aids or blankets are used to maintain positioning. The prone position may also need positioning aids to keep babies properly aligned. The prone position is used when the infant is awake.

The delicate skin of the preterm infant also requires close monitoring. The skin is easily excoriated. Caution must be used with any products used on the skin; adhesives can adhere to the skin surface so well that damage can occur when these are removed. If such a breakdown should occur, the area is exposed to the air and treatment is done as prescribed by the physician.

FAMILY RELATIONS
GETTING ACQUAINTED

The nurse can play an important role in helping the new parents make the transition to parenthood. If the parents have attended parenting classes, they know more of what to expect as they begin their new roles. Regardless, having the nurse spend time with the new family is invaluable. The nurse calls the baby by name, encourages holding the baby *en face*, discusses particular behavior patterns, and points out unique characteristics that help enhance the bonding process (Figure 5-24). This is especially important if the baby differs from the parents' perceived "fantasy child" in terms of gender, physical attributes, or health. Nursing assessment includes the observation of specific parenting behavior, such as the amount of affection shown to the baby, the level or lack of interest in the child, and the amount of time spent interacting with the baby. In addition, the nurse should look for the amount of stimulation and the amount of physical and eye-to-eye contact that occurs between the parents and the child. The extent to which the parents encourage the involvement of siblings and grandparents is also noteworthy in assessing the attachment process. This information provides a basis for nursing intervention that may serve to foster positive family relationships.

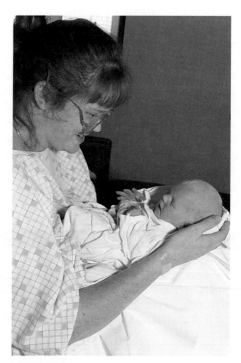

FIGURE 5-24 The mother demonstrates the *en face* position as she becomes acquainted with her newborn. She positions her infant so that their faces are aligned, aiding the eye contact that is important in the bonding process.

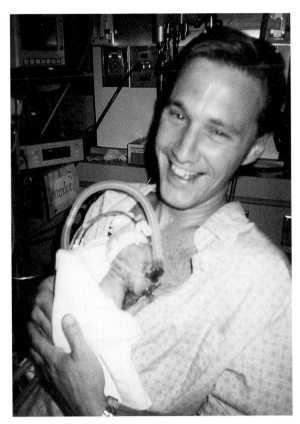

FIGURE 5-25 This father is providing kangaroo care to his preterm infant.

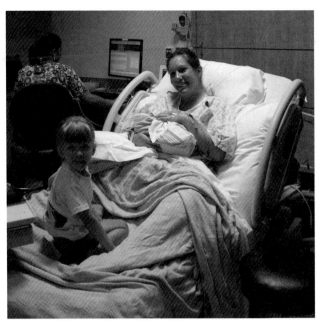

FIGURE 5-26 It is important that siblings be involved when there is a new baby in the family.

BONDING/ATTACHMENT

Although the terms **bonding** or **attachment** are sometimes used interchangeably, they actually have different meanings. Bonding is thought to occur soon after birth, and attachment occurs gradually during the first year of the infant's life. Maternal attachment behaviors include gazing at, kissing, touching, and holding the infant *en face,* along with talking to the infant in a higher-pitched voice than normal. The father is included in the bonding process, as are other family members. The nurse can point out various behaviors of the neonate, encourage eye contact, and provide periods of privacy for the couple.

Kangaroo care, or skin-to-skin contact, has been advocated for fostering intimacy and attachment between premature infants and their mothers or fathers. In this situation, the infant wears only a diaper while the parent holds the infant semi-upright, against his or her skin. The parent covers the infant with his or her own clothing so as to facilitate temperature stability (Figure 5-25). Monitoring temperature remains important.

SIBLINGS

Brothers and sisters (siblings) are less likely to regard a new baby as an intruder or a rival if they are made to feel that the baby is theirs as well as their parent's baby. If the other children feel wanted, accepted, and cherished, their jealousy of the newborn baby will be minimized.

Classes to help siblings prepare for a new baby are held in most hospitals. Questions are answered and a tour of appropriate areas given. These classes help the staff become acquainted with the rest of the family before delivery and enable them to directly involve the siblings. Siblings will enjoy visiting the new baby in the hospital and will have many questions about the new baby, even if the parents have tried to prepare them ahead of time (Figure 5-26).

Siblings of preterm infants may have a difficult time understanding the complexities of the care involved with their new brother or sister. They also may not understand the worry their parents are experiencing. Children need to be prepared for a visit to the NICU if the hospital policies allow such visitation. Such practice, however, may prove beneficial to all family members.

SPIRITUAL CARE

If the condition of a neonate is poor, parents who are Christians may wish to have the baby baptized. The minister or priest should be notified. Parents of other religious affiliations may have special requests or rituals as well. Occasionally, parents attach small pins or medals to the baby's blankets or clothing. The nurse must be extremely careful not to lose these items because they are probably of great sentimental and/or religious value to the parents, particularly if the baby dies. See Chapter 22 for further discussion.

TRANSPORTATION OF THE HIGH-RISK NEONATE

If a hospital is not equipped to care for a high-risk neonate, transportation to a facility that can care for these infants is necessary. Transportation of the high-risk neonate requires organization and the expertise of a special team. Successful transport depends on several factors. First, anticipating the need for the transport is vital. The infant must be stabilized before transport. Preparing and educating the parents is also extremely important. Many hospitals with an NICU have a special transport team that includes a nurse, a respiratory therapist, and sometimes a neonatologist. Baseline data, such as vital signs and blood work (blood gas and glucose levels), are obtained. The neonate is weighed if this is not contraindicated. Copies of all records are made. This includes the baby's record, the mother's prenatal history and delivery record, and pertinent admission data. A transport incubator is provided for warmth. Batteries in all equipment are kept fully charged.

The parents are shown the baby before the departure. If they are unable to hold the infant because of the infant's condition, the transport isolette is wheeled to the mother's bedside so she may observe and touch the baby. On occasion, a mother is unable to see her baby because of her own unstable condition. Such situations require special empathy from nursing personnel.

Once the baby has arrived at the receiving hospital, the parents should be contacted by telephone. It is also thoughtful if the receiving hospital personnel provide feedback to the hospital personnel who initiated the transport, letting them know the results of their efforts.

 Community Considerations

S.T.A.B.L.E. (sugar and safe care, temperature, airway, blood pressure, lab work, and emotional support) is a program that was developed to meet the educational needs of health care providers who must deliver important stabilization care to the neonate (www.stableprogram.com/contact.php).

DISCHARGE TEACHING

Discharge planning should begin at the baby's birth. Parents may experience anxiety when they take their infant home. They may question their ability to care for their infant who has been receiving specialized care. Involve the newborn's parents as much as possible in the daily care. This allows them to have some degree of comfort in the infant's care before being dismissed from the hospital. They need to be confident in routine infant care and any special care the infant requires. Instructions in preventing infection should be a priority teaching goal. Follow-up visits should be scheduled and any home health care needs identified and met. The nurse should stress the importance of well-baby examinations and immunizations for the infant.

If the infant was preterm, rooming in allows the parents to care for their baby under the supervision and support of the nursery staff. These parents may rely on the NICU staff, their primary care physician, and support groups for follow-up care. Oftentimes home care equipment will need to be ordered and a case manager may prove invaluable to the family for support as well.

PATIENT TEACHING FOR DISCHARGE

- Feeding, bathing, skin care, cord care, elimination
- Recognizing illness, particularly jaundice
- How to take the baby's temperature
- How to contact the baby's doctor
- Safety issues, including proper use of car seat, supine position for sleeping, and maintaining a smoke-free environment
- Follow-up medical care (risk of hyperbilirubinemia, well-child care, immunizations)
- Support groups offered by hospitals for new parents
- Home care equipment such as oxygen, apnea monitors, possibly even ventilators for preterm infants

 Community Considerations

Newborns leaving the hospital should be placed in an approved car seat. The seat should be placed in the back seat of the car, facing the rear. Most communities have programs to assist parents in obtaining an approved car seat for their newborn before discharge.

Get Ready for the NCLEX® Examination!

Key Points

- Establishment of respirations begins the newborn's adaptation to extrauterine life.
- The Apgar score, which is done at 1 and 5 minutes after birth, is a quick assessment of the newborn's response to extrauterine life.

- Heat loss is a major consideration in caring for the newborn in the delivery area.
- Gestational age refers to the time the fetus spends in the uterus from conception until birth.
- Reflexes present at birth include protective reflexes, feeding reflexes, and reflexes involving muscle tone.

- The newborn is born with the ability of all the senses to function. These are vision, hearing, tasting, smelling, and feeling.
- Issues of concern for the newborn are respiration, circulatory changes, thermoregulation, and feeding.
- In small preterm infants, the large surface area to body weight ratio causes an increase in the loss of body heat, creating problems related to thermoregulation.
- Physiologic jaundice can result in brain damage and even death if untreated.
- Preterm births can result from many factors, and, in some cases, the cause may not be known.
- In the preterm infant, immaturity of all body systems, especially the respiratory system, is of concern in care and treatment.
- The immaturity of the immune system and the stress put on the immune system in high-risk conditions puts preterm newborns at risk for sepsis.
- The quiet alert state is most conducive for bonding.
- Placing babies to bed on their backs has reduced the incidence of SIDS.
- Newborns need to be properly identified before leaving the delivery room or being separated from their mothers.
- Vitamin K and erythromycin eye ointment are medications given to the newborn within 1 hour after birth.
- Breast milk provides nutrition and immunoglobulins, which provide immunologic protection.
- Proper positioning of the newborn at the breast does more to diminish nipple soreness than does limiting the time at the breast.
- Nutrition issues for high-risk neonates involve their inability to meet the demands of their increased fluid and caloric requirements.
- Hand hygiene is the most effective method to decrease the spread of infections.
- At all times, parents and family need to be considered when caring for the high-risk neonate.
- Discharge teaching is important for all families of newborns, but it is especially important for first-time parents.
- When discharged from the hospital, the newborn needs to be placed in an approved car seat. The car seat must continue to be used at all times when the newborn is transported in a vehicle.

Additional Learning Resources

evolve Go to your Evolve website (*http://evolve.elsevier.com/Price/ pediatric/*) for the following FREE learning resources:

- 3-D Animations
- Answer Keys
- Appendixes
- Audio Glossary
- Spanish/English Glossary
- Video Clips

Review Questions for the NCLEX® Examination

1. When inspecting the umbilical vessels of a newborn, the nurse documents the presence of one vein and one artery. This finding is often indicative of:
   1. Gastrointestinal anomalies
   2. Cardiovascular anomalies
   3. Genitourinary anomalies
   4. Respiratory anomalies

2. An infant with an Apgar score of 4 to 7:
   1. Is in good condition
   2. Requires only routine suction
   3. Needs resuscitation and care in the NICU
   4. Requires close observation

3. Cold stress can cause metabolic and physiologic problems in the neonate such as: (**Select all that apply.**)
   1. Hypoxia
   2. Metabolic acidosis
   3. Hyperglycemia
   4. Infection
   5. Polydipsia

4. A mother reports yellow, oily, crustlike scales on the scalp and forehead of her newborn son. The nurse explains that this condition is known as:
   1. Seborrheic dermatitis
   2. Cephalhematoma
   3. Caput succedaneum
   4. Molding

5. Which of the following statements made by the mother of a newborn would indicate the need for further education?
   1. "I can feed the baby room temperature formula"
   2. "If my baby pushes the nipple of the bottle out with his tongue, it means he is not hungry"
   3. "I should not use the microwave to heat formula"
   4. "Propping the bottle can lead to choking"

Objectives

1. Define the vocabulary terms listed
2. Discuss general characteristics of the infant including reflexes
3. Discuss the nutritional needs of growing infants
4. Describe the physical development of infants from 1 to 12 months
5. Describe the psychosocial development of infants from 1 to 12 months
6. Describe the care and guidance of infants from 1 to 12 months
7. Describe four developmental characteristics of infants that predispose them to certain hazards, for example, "Puts everything into mouth—danger of aspiration"
8. Discuss teething in infancy
9. Describe colic and recommendations for soothing a colicky baby

Key Terms

deciduous teeth (dē-SĬD-ū-ŭs; p. 121)
extrusion reflex (ĕk-STROO-shŭn; p. 119)
grasp reflex (p. 110)
parachute reflex (PAR-e-shüt; p. 110)

pincer grasp (PIN[T]-ser; p. 110)
rooting reflex (p. 119)
weaning (p. 121)

GENERAL CHARACTERISTICS AND DEVELOPMENT

The first year of life is a period of rapid growth and development. Each baby develops at an individual rate. Although growth is continuous, there are slow and rapid periods. **The most common cause for concern about a child is a sudden slowing in any aspect of development that is not typical for that age group.**

The infant is completely dependent on adults during the first months. Behavior is not consistent. For a baby, sucking brings comfort and relief from tensions. The nurse, understanding how important sucking is to the baby, holds the infant during feedings and allows sufficient time to suck. Infants who are warm and comfortable associate food with love. The baby who is fed intravenous fluids or through a G-button should be given added attention and a pacifier, which enables the infant to experience the much needed satisfaction derived from sucking. When the teeth appear, the infant learns to bite and enjoys objects that can be chewed. Gradually, the baby begins to put the fingers into the mouth. Once they can use their hands more skillfully, infants suck their fingers less often because they are able to derive pleasure from other sources.

The grasp reflex (discussed in Chapter 5) occurs when one touches the palms of the infant's hands and

flexion takes place. This reflex disappears at about 3 months. **Prehension,** the ability to grasp objects between the fingers and the opposing thumb, occurs slightly later (at 5 to 6 months) and follows an orderly sequence of development. By 7 to 9 months, the parachute reflex appears. This is a protective arm extension that occurs when an infant is suddenly thrust downward when prone. By 1 year, the pincer grasp, reflecting coordination of index finger and thumb, is well established (Figure 6-1).

Love and security are vital for infants. Babies need continuous affection from their parents. Infants' needs should be met in a loving, consistent manner that enables them to trust the people with whom they interact (Figure 6-2). Parents should be assured that they will not spoil infants if they respond to their needs. Loving adults help infants to build trust and to believe that the world is a good place. This development of a **sense of trust** is key to the development of a healthy personality. A sense of trust is thought to serve as a foundation on which all subsequent tasks are based. The lack of a sense of trust can have a negative effect on the rest of a child's life because the child mistrusts people and regards the world with suspicion.

The constant care of an infant is a strain on even the most exceptional parents. If the father or mother is the full-time caregiver, he or she needs and deserves

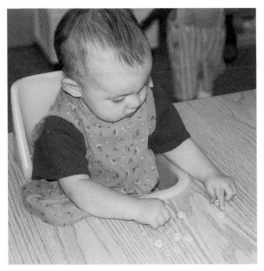

FIGURE 6-1 Pincer grasp. The 12-month-old uses the thumb and index finger to pick up small objects.

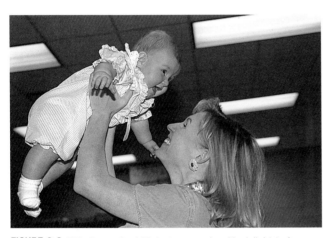

FIGURE 6-2 This 6-month-old infant responds with delight to her mother with a true social smile. Such interactive responses between parent and child promote bonding.

understanding and kind support from the spouse, the relatives at home, and the nurses in the hospital. A short break from the pressures of parenting refreshes parents, renewing their energy and allowing them to enjoy caring for the baby. A trip to the store, a walk with the baby in a stroller, or coffee with neighbors affords stimulation and provides a change of environment for the baby and for the parent. The infant who is left constantly in the crib or playpen and who is not introduced to a variety of learning experiences may become shy and withdrawn. **Sensory stimulation is essential for the development of a baby's thought processes and perceptual abilities.** Exposing babies to sights, sounds, and other stimuli helps the brain to grow. Brain growth is the most critical organic achievement of infancy.

If a mother is unable to room-in with her hospitalized infant, personnel should try to imitate her care

with prompt fulfillment of the infant's physical and emotional needs. In the nursery, the baby who appears hungry should be fed. Wet diapers should be changed as soon as possible, and a crying child should be soothed. The exactness of bathing or feeding the infant is not as important as the way in which it is done. Warmth and affection or the lack thereof are easily recognized by the baby.

 Communication

The nurse can use the time spent caring for an infant to communicate with the child. While feeding, changing the diaper, and bathing, talk softly, sing, touch, and play simple games with the child.

PHYSICAL DEVELOPMENT, SOCIAL BEHAVIOR, CARE, AND GUIDANCE

Table 6-1 is a guide to infant care from the first month to the first year. Some aspects of care, such as safety measures, are important throughout the entire year. The nurse should explain to parents that physical patterns cannot be separated from social patterns and that abrupt changes do not take place with each new month. Like body structures that cannot be separated from their functions, human development cannot be cleanly divided into specific areas. In addition, because no two infants are exactly alike at any given age, the reference provided is just a guide. However, individual variations do range around central norms, which serve as indicators for the evaluation of an infant or child's progress. For instance, although the time of occurrence may vary, an infant's ability to sit without support is still a marker of developmental progress.

HEALTH PROMOTION AND MAINTENANCE

The promotion of health and the prevention of disease during infancy are of the utmost importance and include all measures that improve the physical health and psychosocial adjustment of the child. The concept of periodic health appraisal is not new. In the late 1800s, "milk stations" were established in various localities throughout the United States. These stations' purpose was to reduce the number of deaths from infant diarrhea by providing safe water and milk for babies. Today, skilled health services encompass periodic health appraisal, evaluation of developmental milestones, immunizations, assessment of parent-child interactions, counseling in the developmental processes, identification of families at risk (i.e., for child abuse), health education and anticipatory guidance, referrals to various agencies, follow-up services,

Text continued on page 119

Table **6-1**   Social Behavior, Physical Development, Care, and Guidance for the First 12 Months

AGE/SOCIALIZATION	PHYSICAL DEVELOPMENT	CARE AND GUIDANCE
1 Month Makes small throaty noises; cries when hungry or uncomfortable. 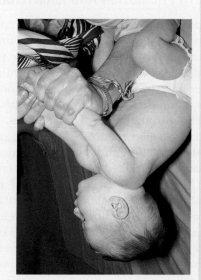	Gains 5 to 7 ounces weekly for the first 6 months; has regained the weight lost after birth; gains about 1 inch in length per month for the first 6 months; head circumference increases by 1.5 cm (½ inch) monthly for the first 6 months. Lifts head slightly when placed on stomach; pushes with toes; turns head to the side when prone; head wobbles. Head lag when pulled from lying to sitting position (provide support to head when holding infant). Obligatory nose breather. Clenches fists; grasp reflexes are strong. Stares at surroundings.	Sleep: Place "back" to sleep; use firm, tight-fitting mattress in crib with bars spaced so baby's head cannot be caught in between; raise crib rails; use no pillow or blanket; sleeps 20 hours. May use monitor system. Nutrition: Breast milk every 2 to 3 hours or iron-fortified formula every 4 hours or as directed by health care provider; burp often; 400 international units/day of Vitamin D Hiccups: Are normal and require no treatment. Immunization: May receive second dose of Hepatitis B vaccine. Exercise: Provide fresh air, but do not allow to overheat; no sunscreen if younger than 6 months of age; avoid exposure to large crowds; provide colorful hanging toys for sensory stimulation.
2 Months Smiles in response to mother's voice. Knows crying brings attention. 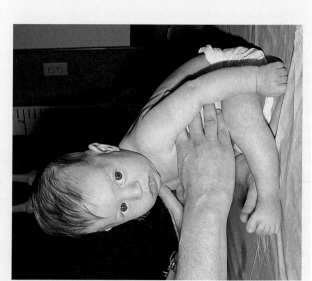	Posterior fontanel closes. Tears appear. Can hold head erect in midposition; follows moving light with eyes. Grasp reflex is fading; can hold a rattle briefly. Legs are active. Needs assistance to maintain upright position.	Sleep: Develops own pattern; may sleep from feeding to feeding; guidelines follow 1 month old. Nutrition: Increasing amount of breast milk or formula with Vitamin D supplement. Immunization: See the Evolve Appendix. Exercise: Provide safe, flat place for baby to kick and be active; *never leave alone on raised surface.* Provide tummy time.

Continued

3 Months

Can wait a few minutes for attention; enjoys responding to people.

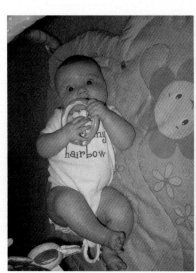

Primitive reflexes fading; stares at hands; reaches for objects but misses them; carries hand to mouth; holds rattle.

Can follow an object from right to left and up and down; supports head steady.

Nutrition: Same as 1 to 2 months; amount of feeding has increased.

Exercise: May have short play periods; enjoys playing with hands and tummy time.

4 Months

Coos, chuckles, gurgles, laughs aloud; makes consonant sounds "n," "k," "g," "p," and "b." Responds to others; likes an audience.

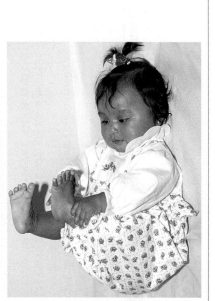

Weighs about 13 to 14 pounds. Lifts head and shoulders when on abdomen and looks around. Turns from back to side; sits with support. Begins to reach for objects; coordination between eye and body movements.

Moves head, arms, and shoulders when excited; extends legs and partly sustains the weight when held upright. May play with feet and put toes in mouth.

Rooting, Moro, extrusion, and tonic neck reflexes are no longer present. Little head lag.

Drooling apparent; can breathe when nose is obstructed.

Sleep: 8 to 10 hours at night; stirs about in crib. Sleeps through ordinary household noises.

Nutrition: Continue breast milk or formula; may begin rice cereal.

Immunization: See the Evolve Appendix.

Exercise: Plays with hand rattles and dangling toys; may use playpen or safe area on floor when rolling safely is possible.

Table 6-1   Social Behavior, Physical Development, Care, and Guidance for the First 12 Months—cont'd

AGE/SOCIALIZATION	PHYSICAL DEVELOPMENT	CARE AND GUIDANCE
5 Months "Talks" to self. Seems to know whether persons are familiar or unfamiliar. Discovers parts of the body; enjoys water play *(never leave alone in water)*; tries to hold own bottle.	Sits with support; holds head well. Grasps preferred objects; puts everything into the mouth. *Be sure toys have no small, removable parts.* Plays with toes. Shows signs of tooth eruption.	Sleep: Takes two to three naps a day. Nutrition: Breast milk or formula; may have started cereal. Exercise: Provide space for movement and rolling; makes jumping motions when held upright in lap. Safety: The infant rides facing the rear of the vehicle, in the middle of the back seat. The infant seat is secured with the seat belt or latch system, and straps on the car seat adjust to accommodate the growing baby. When children reach the highest weight or length allowed by the manufacturer of their infant-only seat, they should continue to ride rear-facing in a convertible seat until age 2 (American Academy of Pediatrics, 2010).

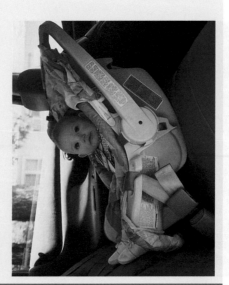

6 Months

Shows increased interest in surrounding world. Babbles and squeals; wakes up happy.

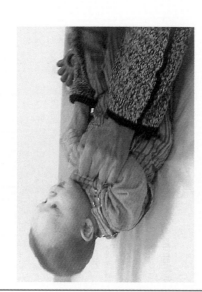

Doubles in birth weight; gains 3 to 5 ounces per week during next 6 months.

Grows about ½ inch per month for the next 6 months.

Head circumferences increases ½ cm (¼ inch) per month for the second 6 months.

Turns completely over. Pulls self to sitting position using hands for support and stability. No head lag is present; easily lifts head, chest, and upper abdomen and can bear weight on the hands.

Nutrition: Begin rice cereal fortified with iron if has not yet been started. Sucks food from spoon. Chewing more mature; approximates lips to rim of cup; bangs table with spoon.

Immunization: See the Evolve Appendix

Safety: Remove toxic plants from baby's reach. *Babyproof house if not done yet (electrical plugs and cabinet locks are essential).*

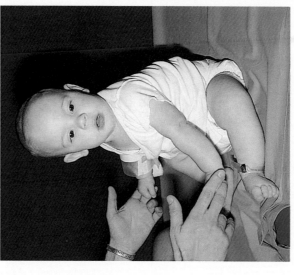

7 Months

Shifts moods easily; shows fear of strangers. Responds to own name.

Two lower teeth appear (central incisors). Begins to crawl. Moves forward, using chest, head, arms; legs drag. Can grasp objects more easily; transfers objects from one hand to the other.

Appears interested in standing; holds adult's hands and bounces actively while standing. Struggles when being dressed.

Sleep: Sleeps 11 to 13 hours at night. Fretfulness as a result of teething may appear; this is generalized by a lack of appetite and wakefulness during the night. Soothing to return to sleep may be necessary.

Nutrition: Anticipates spoon feeding. May add vegetables and fruits to diet. Add finger foods such as toast or zwieback. Add new foods slowly, one at a time.

Continued

Table 6-1   Social Behavior, Physical Development, Care, and Guidance for the First 12 Months—cont'd

AGE/SOCIALIZATION	PHYSICAL DEVELOPMENT	CARE AND GUIDANCE
8 Months Plays pat-a-cake; amuses self a little longer. Reserved with strangers. Impatient, especially when food is prepared. Rides in stroller. Enjoys jump chair, stuffed toys, or toys that squeak or rattle.	Sits steadily alone. Uses index finger and thumb as pincers. Pokes at objects. Enjoys dropping articles into a cup and emptying it. 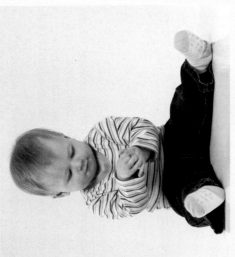	Sleep: Takes two naps a day. Safety: Remain with baby at all times during bath; protect from chewing paint from window sills or old furniture. Paint containing lead can be poisonous. Close doors to ovens, dishwashers, washing machines, dryers, and refrigerators. Do not leave standing water in tub, buckets, and so forth.
9 Months Tries to imitate sounds (e.g., says "ba-ba" for bye-bye); cries if scolded. Drops food from high chair at mealtime. Is busy most of the day exploring surroundings; distract from areas of danger. Avoid spankings and "no" to keep child out of harm's way.	Shows preference for the use of one hand; can raise self to a sitting position. Holds bottle. Creeps; carries trunk of body above floor but parallel to it. More advanced than crawling. 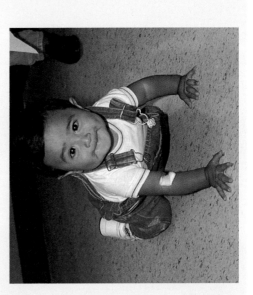	Nutrition: Introduce chopped and mashed foods. Place highchair in area of kitchen where floor is easy to clean. Use unbreakable dishes. Allow baby to pick up pieces of food by hand and put them into the mouth. *Always be alert for signs of choking.* Safety: Know the nationwide toll-free number for poison control (1-800-222-1222). Program it into cell phones, and post it on refrigerators or in specific locations for babysitters. Avoid tablecloths with overhangs that the baby can reach.

Continued

10 Months

Knows name; plays simple games such as peek-a-boo; feeds self a cookie.

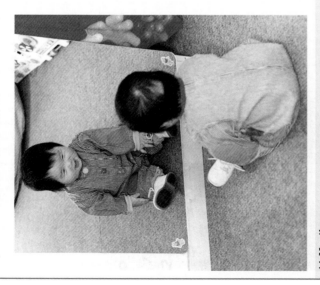

Pulls self to a standing position. Walks around the furniture while holding on to it. Throws toys to the floor for a parent to pick up. Cries when they are not returned. Says "dada" and "mama" with meaning. Understands "bye bye.". Infants this age enjoy their own image.

Sleep: Avoid strenuous play before bedtime. A night-light is convenient for the parent and makes the surroundings more familiar. Pajamas with feet keep the baby warm at night. May cry out in sleep without waking.
Nutrition: Takes juice and water from cup. Solid foods in general are taken well.

11 Months

Understands simple directions. Is impatient when held. Shakes head for "no."

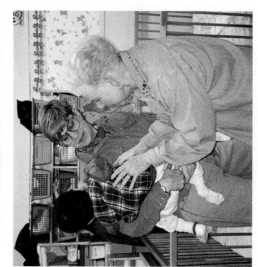

Stands upright holding on to an adult's hands. May begin taking steps on own. Enjoys playing with empty dish and spoon after meals. Greets parents in morning with excited jargon. Older infants fear strangers and cling to parents.

Exercise: Plays with toys in tub. Enjoys gross-motor activity. Kicks and pulls self up. Enjoys blowing bubbles or attempting.
Safety: *Do not use baby walkers.* Be sure stairs have baby gates if not done so already.

Table 6-1 Social Behavior, Physical Development, Care, and Guidance for the First 12 Months—cont'd

AGE/SOCIALIZATION	PHYSICAL DEVELOPMENT	CARE AND GUIDANCE
12 Months Friendly; repeats acts that elicit a response. Recognizes "no-no." Enjoys rhythmic music. Shows emotions such as fear, anger, and jealousy. Reacts to these emotions from adults. Plays with food.	Pulse 100 to 140 beats/min. Respirations 20 to 40 breaths/min. Triples birth weight. Stands alone for short periods; may walk. Puts arm through sleeve when dressed. Eight teeth (four upper and four lower). Says three to five words besides "dada" and "mama." Understands meaning of several words. Recognizes objects by name. Can imitate animal sounds. At 1 year, infants can easily pull to a standing position. On a slick, hard floor, parents should be near to catch the infant if he or she slips backward while trying to pull up.	Nutrition: Gradually add egg white, fish, orange juice, wheat. Add well-cooked table foods. Interest in eating may begin to dwindle. Sleep: Usually still napping twice a day; may begin one long nap daily. Immunization: See the Evolve Appendix

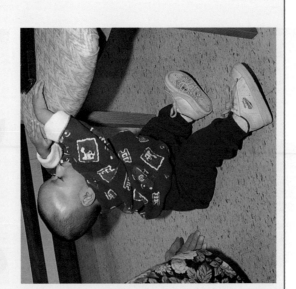

appropriate record keeping, and evaluation and audit by peers. These services are provided in a variety of health settings. However, the kinds and quality of assistance vary. Private group practice, hospital-based clinics, and neighborhood health centers are all examples of different health settings. Chapter 2 discusses this at length.

Infant health care visits should be regular, and a careful health history should be obtained. Growth grids during infancy include measures of weight, length, and head circumference. The reading and recording of growth charts are described in Chapter 3. (See Appendix C for growth charts.) Several developmental screening tests may be used as well. One such test is the Denver II Test (found in Appendix D). This test is used to evaluate social, fine-motor, language, and gross-motor abilities from birth to 6 years.

The physical examination is adapted to the needs of the infant. Routine assessment of hearing and vision is an integral part of the examination. Loud noises in the newborn period should precipitate the startle or Moro reflex. Hearing should be tested before dismissal from the hospital where the infant was born. As the infant grows, hearing can be assessed by his or her response to sounds. Vision is assessed mainly through light perception. The examiner shines a penlight into the baby's eyes and notes blinking, following to midline, and other responses. Laboratory tests are performed according to hospital policy. Newborn screening is completed (see Chapter 5).

NUTRITION COUNSELING OF PARENTS

The nutrient needs of infants reflect rates of growth, energy expended in activity, basal metabolic needs, and the interaction of nutrients consumed. The baby is born with a rooting reflex, which assists in finding the nipple. The suck is rather immature because of the small mouth. There is a forward-and-backward movement of the tongue. As the infant grows, neural maturation of the cheeks and tongue enables advancement to a more mature sucking pattern that uses negative pressure to obtain milk. This occurs around the third or fourth month of age. At about this time, the extrusion reflex (protrusion), which pushes food out of the mouth to prevent intake of inappropriate food, disappears. The digestive system continues to mature. By 6 months, the digestive system is able to handle more complex nutrients and is less susceptible to food allergens. By 12 months, the stomach has expanded from 10 to 20 mL at birth to 200 mL. This increase enables the infant to consume more food at less frequent intervals. At first, most babies dislike spoon-feeding. In the beginning, they try to grasp the spoon. This gradually progresses until the child is able to scoop a little food, although the child still spills most of the contents. As the pincer grasp becomes more developed, the baby is able to pick up food with the fingers and place it in the mouth. By 2 years, the child has mastered spoon-feeding (Figure 6-3).

Parents have many concerns about feeding their infant during the first year of life. This is a time when parents are receptive to receiving nutritional education; as a result, the nurse should look for opportunities to provide sound nutritional information. It is important for the nurse to assess parental knowledge; infant development, behavior, and readiness; parent-child interactions; and cultural and ethnic practices. Nutrition care plans based on developmental levels assist parents in recognizing changes in feeding patterns. One means of assessing adequate intake is to determine whether the infant has gained 4 to 7 ounces per week for the first 6 months. Adequate hydration is evident by the infant having at least six wet diapers per day. After the feeding, the infant should fall asleep and have several hours of uninterrupted sleep. Continued monitoring of weight, height, and skinfold thickness determines whether or not the infant's diet is adequate. This can easily be done during the periodic well-baby examinations. Parents should be assured that although intake is rarely constant, varying in quantity and quality, most children do eat enough to grow normally.

Infants need more calories, protein, minerals, and vitamins in proportion to their weight than do adults. Compared with an adult, the normal infant needs approximately three times more energy to maintain rapid growth and development. Breast milk and infant formula provide the young infant calories needed for growth and development. Human milk is the best food for infants. It contains the ideal balance of nutrients in a readily digestible form (see Chapter 5). Iron-fortified infant formulas are recommended if the infant is formula fed. If an infant cannot tolerate milk-based formulas, soy protein–based formulas are available. These formulas are nutritionally sound and safe alternatives to cow's milk–based formulas. For the first year of life, infants should remain on human milk or iron-fortified formula. Whole cow's milk is not recommended for infants of less than 1 year of age because (1) it may create a potential for intolerance of whole milk protein; (2) an increased incidence rate of iron-deficiency anemia is associated with the intake of whole cow's milk; (3) the metabolism of whole cow's milk is difficult for the gastrointestinal tract; and (4) the high level of resulting solutes, which need to be excreted, places stress on the renal system.

Solid Foods

At about 4 to 6 months of age, solids are introduced. This introduction is based on the developmental readiness and the nutrient needs of the infant. Foods selected can either be commercial or home-prepared.

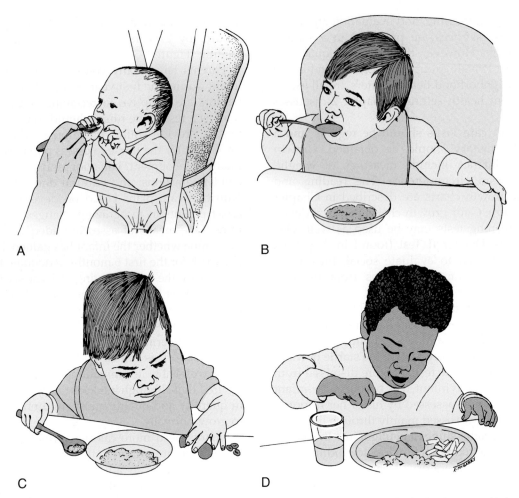

FIGURE 6-3 Development of feeding skills in infants and toddlers. **A,** At 7 months, the child shows beginning involvement with feeding and reaching for the spoon. **B,** At 9 months, the child is beginning to use the spoon independently, although there is difficulty in keeping food on it. **C,** The 9-month-old shows a refined pincer grasp to pick up food. **D,** The 2-year-old is much more skillful at self-feeding and has the ability to both rotate the wrist and elevate the elbow to keep food on the spoon.

The Home Care Considerations box shows the sequence in which foods are added. Rice cereal is recommended as the first solid food because it is less allergenic than others. Three tablespoons of iron-fortified cereal mixed with breast milk or formula provide 7 mg of iron (more than half the daily requirement). Offer only small amounts at first (1 teaspoonful). Place food on the back of the infant's tongue. The consistency and amounts of solid foods are gradually increased as the infant becomes more familiar with them. *Never* mix cereal with formula in a bottle. The baby's spoon should have a long handle, and the body of the spoon should be small and shallow. Cereal is usually followed by fruits and vegetables (some parents like to introduce vegetables before fruits) and then meat. New foods should be introduced one at a time, with 4 to 7 days between each new food. This makes determination of food allergies easier if an intolerance is present.

🏠 Home Care Considerations

Guidelines for Introduction of Foods

1. Introduce iron-fortified baby rice cereal at about 4 to 6 months of age.
2. Add pureed vegetables and fruits, one at a time, at about 7 to 8 months (starting with vegetables may help to increase acceptance by the infant not yet exposed to the sweet taste of fruits).
3. Add pureed meats at about 8 to 9 months.
4. Add juice when the infant is old enough to drink from a cup, at about 9 months.
5. Add foods with more texture and finger foods at about 9 months (chopped meats, crackers, and so on).
6. Add allergenic foods, such as egg whites (or whole eggs), whole milk, wheat products, and orange juice, after 1 year (especially important for the infant with a family history of allergies or asthma).

Modified from Peckenpaugh, N. (2007). *Nutrition essentials and diet therapy* (10th ed.). St. Louis: Elsevier.

No scientific evidence supports the belief that cereal helps babies sleep through the night. Cereal should not be started before 4 to 6 months of age.

If the baby refuses a certain food, omit it temporarily. Keep mealtime pleasant. Let infants try new foods; they may like foods that the parent does not care to eat. Do not introduce new foods when the baby is ill. The amount of food consumed varies with each child. Fruit juices are generally offered by about 9 months of age, when the infant begins to drink from a cup. An exception to this is the addition of orange juice. If family members have known allergies, orange juice is withheld until the baby is 1 year old. Other highly allergenic foods that may be delayed include fish, nuts, strawberries, chocolate, and egg whites.

When the baby first begins to learn to drink from a cup, a spouted plastic cup can be helpful. Dilute the juice initially, and then gradually increase the quantity to 3 to 4 ounces per day. The directions for preparing baby food at home are provided in the Home Care Considerations box. Baby food can be prepared in a food grinder, blender, or food mill or by mashing the food until it is the desired texture.

Home Care Considerations

Directions for Home Preparation of Infant Foods

1. Select fresh, high-quality fruits, vegetables, or meats.
2. Be sure that all utensils, including cutting boards, grinder, knives, and the like, are thoroughly cleaned.
3. Wash hands before preparing the food.
4. Clean, wash, and trim the food in as little water as possible.
5. Cook the foods until tender in as little water as possible. Avoid overcooking, which may destroy heat-sensitive nutrients.
6. Do not add salt. Add sugar sparingly. Do not add honey or corn syrup to food intended for infants younger than 1 year of age. (Botulism spores have been reported in honey and corn syrup, and young infants do not have the immune capacity to resist this infection.)
7. Add enough water for the food to be easily pureed.
8. Strain or puree the food with an electric blender, a food mill, a baby food grinder, or a kitchen strainer.
9. Pour puree into an ice cube tray and freeze.
10. When the food is frozen hard, remove the cubes and store in freezer bags.
11. When ready to serve, defrost and heat in a serving container the amount of food to be consumed at a single feeding.

From Mahan, L.K., and Escott-Stump, S. (2007). *Krause's food, nutrition, and diet therapy* (12th ed.). Philadelphia: Elsevier.

The infant's height and weight should progress at approximately the same rate. Variations may result from illness, malabsorption, psychological factors, overfeeding, and underfeeding. It is important to ascertain feeding procedures and practices regularly and to repeat essential information as indicated.

Buying, Storing, and Serving Food

Baby foods stored in jars are vacuum-packed. When a jar is opened, a definite "pop" sound should be heard as the vacuum seal is broken. Also check the expiration date of the product. Dates are usually found on the caps of jars and on the sides of cereal and bakery items. Unopened jars of baby food and juices should be stored in a dry, cool place. Transfer food to a serving dish. Do not feed the infant from the jar or return leftovers to the jar because saliva may turn certain foods to liquid by digesting them in the jar. Unused portions may be stored in the refrigerator in the original jar. Special precautions should be taken to prevent burning when warming food in the microwave. When food is heated in the microwave, check its temperature because sometimes the food heats unevenly. Test all warmed foods. This can be done by tasting or by dropping a portion of a warmed liquid on the parent's inner wrist.

WEANING FROM THE BREAST

Weaning is usually influenced by the mother's decision to discontinue breastfeeding or the infant's desire to breastfeed less often. Weaning is done gradually over several days or weeks. Weaning should start with daytime feedings; however, it should not be done during the first feeding of the day or the nighttime feeding. The experience should be made as pleasurable as possible for both the mother and the infant, which helps compensate for the loss of satisfaction from sucking. Weaning should not be attempted when the baby is ill. The mother can decrease her fluid consumption and the number of infant feedings and limit the time of the feeding to assist in decreasing her milk supply. Weaning from the breast is a changing point in the infant's life, and efforts should be made to make this experience as comfortable and as pleasurable as possible. Weaning is usually completed by age 1 to 2 years, although in some cultures it may continue longer.

TEETH

Deciduous Teeth

The development of the 20 deciduous teeth, or baby teeth, begins around the fifth month of intrauterine life. The health and diet of the expectant mother affect their soundness. The 20 baby teeth erupt during the first 2 ½ years of life, beginning around the sixth month. It is a normal process and is generally accompanied by little or no discomfort. However, in healthy infants, there are wide individual differences in tooth eruption.

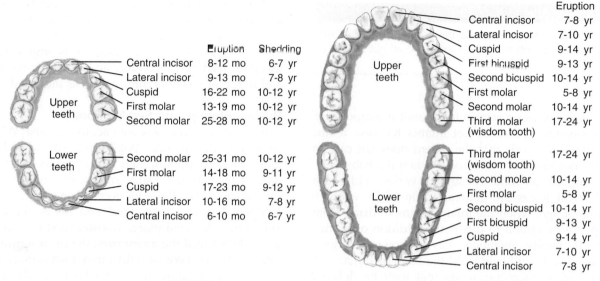

FIGURE 6-4 Eruption of permanent and deciduous teeth.

A delay in teething is significant if other forms of immaturity or illness are present. The physician evaluates the process of teething during the baby's regular health checkups. The first tooth generally appears around the seventh month. The 1-year-old has about six teeth, four upper and two lower. The order in which the teeth appear is almost always the same (Figure 6-4). They are shed in about the same order in which they appear; that is, the lower central incisors first and so forth.

Teething During Infancy

Teething refers to eruption of the crown of the tooth through the periodontal membrane. The gums may be red, swollen, and sensitive. The normal appearance of saliva and drooling at 4 months is frequently attributed to teething. However, drooling is more the result of the maturing of the salivary glands than teething. The first (deciduous) teeth act as a guide for the proper positioning of the secondary teeth. Teething does not cause infection, yet, at this time, the infant's maternal antibody supply is low, making the child more prone to infection. The infant may be fussy and may wake during the night. Teething does not cause fever, nor is it responsible for respiratory tract infections, rashes, or diarrhea. Cold appears to soothe inflamed gums. A cool washcloth, a hard rubber teething ring, or a teething pretzel may bring relief. Acetaminophen or ibuprofen is useful when discomfort is clearly related to the teeth; however, ibuprofen is not given to infants less than 6 months of age.

Good oral hygiene at this age consists of gently wiping the gums and teeth with gauze or a clean washcloth every day. Calcium, phosphorus, vitamins C and D, and fluoride help ensure healthy teeth. Avoid bottle mouth caries, which can occur when an infant is regularly put to bed with a bottle of milk or sweetened juice. Sugar pools within the oral cavity, causing severe decay. It is seen most often in children between the ages of 18 months and 3 years. Eliminating the bedtime bottle or substituting water is recommended. A condition similar to nursing bottle caries is also seen in breastfed babies, particularly in infants who nurse at will throughout the night. To prevent this, nocturnal nursing and frequent intermittent night feedings after the age of 1 year should be discouraged.

An additional cause of erosion of dental enamel is repeated exposure to gastric acids. This is now being recognized in infants with gastroesophageal reflux who are old enough to have teeth and also in teenagers with bulimia. When the effects of gastric acid are recognized early, the teeth can be protected with an acrylic sealant. In addition, parents need to be taught the tooth-decaying effects of refined sugars, particularly those that are sticky and remain in the mouth for long periods of time.

COLIC

Also known as *paroxysmal abdominal pain*, colic is often manifested by crying, usually at the same time each day, with the infant's legs drawn up toward the abdomen. Many parents describe the infant as acting as though they have "gas." Colic usually disappears by 3 months of age but can strain the parent's relationship with the infant. Dietary changes may be investigated by the health care provider; these changes may be of some help. Drugs, including sedatives, antispasmodics, antihistamines, and antiflatulents may help. Sometimes positional changes, including placing the infant prone over a hot water bottle or heating pad, are beneficial. Use of a pacifier, massaging the infant's abdomen, placing the infant in a wind-up swing, going for a walk outdoors, going for a ride in the car, burping frequently with feeds, and rocking may all be beneficial. Parents should never smoke near an infant. Avoiding overstimulation and emotional stress may also be helpful. Parents need to be reassured that their baby will "outgrow" their colicky phase and need an outlet for their own emotions. Parents must be reminded to never shake a baby and that sometimes relief from a second caregiver can give them the break that they need when caring for a crying infant.

Get Ready for the NCLEX® Examination!

Key Points

- The first year of life involves many changes for both the infant and the family.
- Love and security are special needs of the infant.
- Stimulation of all the senses is an essential element in growth and development.
- Well-child visits are important to ensure promotion of health and prevention of disease.
- Recommended health care visits for the well infant begin soon after dismissal from the hospital, usually during the first two weeks of life and then at 1 month, 2 months, 4 months, 6 months, 9 months, and 12 months.
- An adequate diet allows for proper growth and development.
- As the infant grows and develops, solid foods are introduced.
- As the diet of the infant changes, the needs for breastfeeding and formula also change.
- Weaning from the breast is a big turning point for the mother and the infant, and both individuals need to be considered during the process.
- There are 20 deciduous teeth. Teething begins around 5 to 7 months of age and continues until about 2½ years of age.
- Colic can test the patience of a new parent; many interventions can be tried to calm the crying baby.

Additional Learning Resources

evolve Go to your Evolve website (http://evolve.elsevier.com/Price/pediatric/) for the following FREE learning resources:
- 3-D Animations
- Answer Keys
- Appendixes
- Audio Glossary
- Spanish/English Glossary
- Video Clips

Review Questions for the NCLEX® Examination

1. Which of the following situations would be considered the **most** cause for concern regarding infant development?
   1. A 2-month-old who requires assistance to maintain an upright position
   2. A 12-month-old who is not yet walking independently
   3. A 5-month-old with poor head and neck control
   4. An 8-month-old who uses the index finger and thumb as pincers

2. Whole cow's milk is not recommended for infants younger than 1 year of age because it: (**Select all that apply.**)
   1. Can be difficult to metabolize in the gastrointestinal tract
   2. Places stress on the renal system
   3. Potentially creates an intolerance of whole milk protein
   4. Increases the risk of infection
   5. Can lead to impaired skin integrity

3. When educating parents regarding proper nutrition for their infant, the nurse relays that juice can be added to the diet at approximately:
   1. 2 months of age
   2. 4 months of age
   3. 6 months of age
   4. 9 months of age

4. The 1-year-old child can be expected to have:
   1. Two teeth
   2. Four teeth
   3. Six teeth
   4. Eight teeth

5. All of the following are true regarding infant colic **except:**
   1. Colic usually disappears by 1 month of age.
   2. Overstimulation should be avoided.
   3. Antispasmodics may be of some help.
   4. Use of a pacifier may be beneficial.

Objectives

1. Define the vocabulary terms listed
2. Describe the physical and psychosocial development of children from 1 to 3 years of age, listing age-specific events and guidance when appropriate
3. Discuss how adults can help small children combat their fears
4. Identify five strategies that aid in meeting a toddler's nutritional needs
5. Identify the principles of toilet training (bowel and bladder) that assist in guiding parents' efforts to provide toilet independence
6. Discuss questions to use in evaluation of daycare centers
7. Discuss the use of car seats for toddlers
8. Identify four potential safety hazards specific to the toddler and anticipatory guidance for caretakers in preventing such accidents
9. Discuss care of the child with poisonings (acetaminophen, ibuprofen, aspirin, lead, hydrocarbons, and corrosives)

Key Terms

associative play (e-SŌ-sh-ē-ā-tiv; p. 134)
autonomy (ăw-TAWN-ŏ-mē; p. 126)
baby bottle tooth decay (p. 130)
cariogenic (KĀR-ē-ō-JĚN-ĭk; p. 130)
cooperative play (kō-Ä-p[e]re-a-tiv; p. 134)
corrosive (ke-RŌ-siv; p. 141)
defecation (děf-ĭ-KĀ-shĭn; p. 126)
Denver II (p. 129)
egocentric (Ē-gō-SĚN-trĭk; p. 124)
fluorosis (FLOO-ō-RŌ-sĭs; p. 130)
hydrocarbons (HĪ-drō-cär-bens; p. 141)

hyperpnea (hī-perp-NĒ-ă; p. 143)
negativism (NĔG-ă-tĭv-ĭsm; p. 124)
parallel play (PAR-ě-lel; p. 134)
phagocytosis (făg-ō-sī-TŌ-sĭs; p. 127)
physiologic anorexia (fĭz-ē-ō-LŎJ-ĭk ăn-ŏ-RĔK-sē-ă; p. 131)
pica (PĪ-kă; p. 144)
rickets (RI-kets; p. 131)
ritualism (RI-chū-we-li-sem; p. 124)
tantrum (p. 124)

GENERAL CHARACTERISTICS AND DEVELOPMENT

Children between 1 and 3 years of age are referred to as toddlers. They are able to move about on their own and are no longer completely dependent persons. By 1 year of age, they have generally tripled their birth weight and gained control of their head, hands, and feet. The remarkably rapid growth and development that occurred during infancy begins to slow. The toddler period presents different challenges for parents and children. This chapter discusses what toddlers are like as people and some of the obstacles they face (Table 7-1).

Toddlers are curious explorers who get into everything. As each month passes, they gain more control of their bodies. Soon they are walking, running,

jumping, and climbing (Figure 7-1). They enjoy repeating these new skills, and with practice, they become less clumsy and awkward. Their desire to touch, taste, smell, and smear leads them into trouble. They quickly discover that much of their conduct alarms their parents. Unlike when they were infants, toddlers find that their parents no longer accept their actions willingly and without question. Toddlers cannot understand the need for restrictions, and, as a result, they revolt. Temper tantrums are common, and behavior is not consistent. Negativism is reflected in unreasonable behavior and by saying "no" frequently. Ritualism is characteristic of toddlers. By making simple tasks into rituals, they increase their sense of security and self-mastery. Dawdling serves essentially the same purpose, and egocentric thinking predominates.

Table 7-1	Summary of Toddler Growth and Development				
AGE	**PHYSICAL**	**GROSS-MOTOR**	**FINE-MOTOR**	**VOCALIZATION**	**SOCIALIZATION**
15 months	Steady growth in height and weight Head circumference,48 cm (19 in) Weight, 11 kg (24 lb) Height, 78.7 cm (31 in)	Walks without help Cannot throw a ball without falling	Builds tower of two cubes Releases a pellet into a narrow-necked bottle Uses cup well	Says four to six words, including names Understands simple commands Uses "no" while agreeing to request	Less likely to fear strangers Begins to imitate parents, such as cleaning house Has temper tantrums Kisses and hugs parents
18 months	Physiologic anorexia from decreased growth needs Anterior fontanel closed Physiologically able to control sphincters	Runs clumsily, falls often Walks up stairs with one hand held Throws ball overhand without falling Pulls and pushes toys	Builds tower of three to four cubes Turns pages of a book two or three at a time	Says 10 or more words Points to a common object, including two to three body parts	Takes off shoes and socks; unzips Beginning awareness of "my" toy, and so on. May develop dependency on transitional object such as blanket
24 months	Head circumference, 49.5 to 50 cm (19 to 20 in) Chest circumference exceeds head circumference Usual weight gain is 1.8 to 2.7 kg (4 to 6 lb) Usual gain in height is 10 to 12.5 cm (4.5 to 5 in) Adult height, approximately double height at 2 years May have achieved readiness for beginning control of bowel and bladder Primary dentition (16 teeth)	Goes up and down stairs alone with two feet on each step Runs fairly well, with wide stance Picks up object without falling Kicks ball forward without overbalancing	Builds tower of six to seven cubes Aligns two or more cubes like a train Turns pages of book one at a time In drawing, imitates vertical and circular strokes Turns doorknob and unscrews lid	Has vocabulary of approximately 300 words Uses two-word and three-word phrases Says "I," "me," "you" Understands directional commands Gives first name; refers to self by name Verbalizes need for toileting, food, or drink Talks incessantly	Stage of parallel play Has sustained attention span Temper tantrums decreasing Pulls people to show them something Increased independence from mother Dresses self in simple clothing
30 months	Birth weight quadrupled Primary dentition (20 teeth) completed May have daytime bowel and bladder control	Jumps with both feet Jumps from chair or step Stands on one foot momentarily Takes a few steps on tiptoe	Builds tower of eight cubes Good hand-finger coordination Draws cross	Gives first and last name Refers to self by appropriate pronoun Uses plurals Names one color	Separates more easily from mother Helps put things away Begins to notice gender differences; knows own gender May attend to toilet needs without help except for wiping

Modified from Hockenberry, M., and Wilson, D. (2007). *Wong's nursing care of infants and children* (8th ed.). St. Louis: Elsevier.

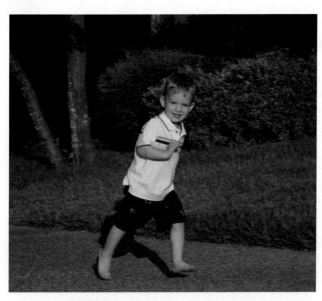

FIGURE 7-1 Older toddlers run with ease.

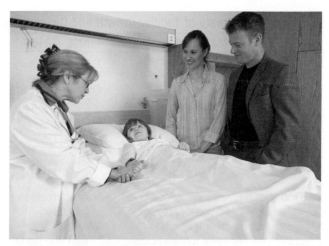

FIGURE 7-2 The hospital can be frightening to a toddler. A parent's presence is often reassuring.

 ## DEVELOPMENTAL TASKS

The developmental tasks seen during this period are based on a continuum of trust established during infancy. Physicians and nurse practitioners can readily focus on age-related tasks at the toddler's well-visit. Toddlers are now ready to give up total dependence. They become autonomous and seek independence (see discussion on Erikson in Chapter 4). They begin to differentiate themselves from others, particularly from their mother. They learn to delay gratification and to incorporate rudiments of socially acceptable behavior as determined by the limits of their family's culture. Important self-regulatory functions include toilet independence, eating, sleeping, and perfection of newfound physical skills.

Separation continues to be a major issue with this age group. Toddlers are beginning to separate somewhat from their parents but can tolerate only brief periods of independence and still remain very interested in knowing where their parents are (Figure 7-2). Their greatest fear is separation from their parents. They need to be reassured that when their parents leave, they will return. The younger toddler might exhibit night waking as a response to fear of separation. This same child might use a transitional object (blanket, toy) for consolation when separated from the parent. By 2 years of age, the child still gets upset when separated from the parents, although not as much as before. The nurse should be reminded that separation fears are increased when a child is under stress. So the hospitalized child needs to be supported if the parents are unable to stay. Parents should never "sneak out" on a child. Mastering separation is a normal developmental process. The gradual control of these activities provides toddlers with a sense of mastery and contributes to their positive self-concept.

Erik Erikson (in his theory on psychosocial development) defines the developmental task of the toddler age as learning autonomy versus shame or doubt. Toddlers need to be encouraged to become independent, and the caregiver should not do everything for them. The toddler who is happy and is allowed gradually increasing independence also develops a sense of security.

Lawrence Kohlberg (in his theory on moral development) believes that the toddler begins to formulate a sense of right and wrong but obeys only because the parent tells the toddler to. Moral development continues throughout childhood.

Sigmund Freud (in his theory on personality development) described the toddler as being in the "anal phase" because elimination has taken on a new meaning. The child learns in this phase to control urination and defecation.

PHYSICAL GROWTH

Certain physical changes foster the growth process. Weight gain slows to about 4 to 6 pounds (1.81 to 2.72 kg) per year, and height increases about 5 inches (12 cm) per year during the toddler period. Toddlers' bodies change proportions. Legs and arms lengthen from ossification and growth in the epiphyseal areas of the long bones. The trunk and head grow more slowly. The growth of the brain decelerates. The increase in head circumference during infancy is 4 inches (10 cm). During the second year, the increase is only 1 inch (2.5 cm). Chest circumference continues to increase. Head circumference equals chest circumference at 6 months to 1 year of age. The size and strength of muscle fibers increase. Myelination of the spinal cord is practically complete by 2 years of age, allowing for control of anal and urethral sphincters. Respirations are still mainly abdominal but shift to thoracic as the child approaches school age. The stomach capacity increases to the point where the child can eat three meals a day. Appetite decreases, but it remains important that the toddler get adequate intake of all nutrients. (Nutrition is discussed later in this chapter.)

The toddler is more capable of maintaining a stable body temperature than is the infant. The shivering process in which the capillaries constrict or dilate in response to body temperature has matured. The skin becomes tough as the epidermis and dermis bond more tightly, protecting the child from fluid loss, infection, and irritation. The defense mechanisms of the skin and blood, particularly **phagocytosis**, are working more effectively than during infancy. The lymphatic tissues of the adenoids and tonsils enlarge during this period. Eruption of deciduous teeth continues. By 3 years of age, all 20 deciduous teeth are generally present (see Chapter 6).

The senses of toddlers do not function independently of one another or of their motor abilities. Two-year-old toddlers reach, grasp, inspect, smell, taste, and study objects with their eyes. Their attention becomes centered on those characteristics of their surroundings that capture their interest. They can correlate sight with sound, as in the ringing of a bell. Binocular vision is well-established by 15 months of age. By 2 years of age, visual acuity is about 20/40. Memory strengthens; toddlers can compare present events with stored knowledge. They assimilate information through trial-and-error plus repetition. They try alternative methods of accomplishing a goal. Thought processes advance, preparing the way for more complex mental operations. Language development parallels cognitive growth. The increase in the level of comprehension is particularly striking and exceeds their verbalization. (Language development is discussed later in this chapter.)

GUIDANCE AND DISCIPLINE

Toddlers' emotions fluctuate greatly. They show ambivalence. They love one minute and hate the next. They cry, kick, and slap when they decide to play outdoors longer than the parent wants and then turn around and kiss that same parent for giving them a drink of water. It may be difficult for parents to understand these mood swings. Toddlers are usually trying to assert their independence. It may be best to ignore this behavior as long as children are not hurting themselves or someone else. After the tantrum, parents should divert toddlers to some pleasant activity. Table 7-2 summarizes behavior problems that may occur during early childhood, causes of those problems, and parenting tips for correcting the problems.

One of the objectives in the management of toddlers is to help them establish limits for themselves and to find socially acceptable outlets for their behavior. Parents who direct all their child's activities cannot expect the toddler to develop self-confidence or autonomy.

Rituals play an important part in toddlers' ability to achieve independence. They provide them with known routines and people and places to come back to for support and security. Children's rituals (as at bedtime) should be incorporated into the hospital routine.

💬 Communication

Whenever possible, children should be given choices: "Would you like to take your medicine from a medicine cup or from the syringe?" or "Would you like Mommy to put the medicine in your mouth?" Never say, "Do you want to take your medicine?" If the child replies "no," the nurse has created a communication block.

Toddlers need a certain amount of discipline. They get into many situations that are "over their head." When adults make a firm decision for them, the problem is at least for the time being resolved. Children feel secure because parents have helped them escape from their own primitive natures. There is controversy concerning spanking children. A time-out period is effective (Figure 7-3). The general rule is 1

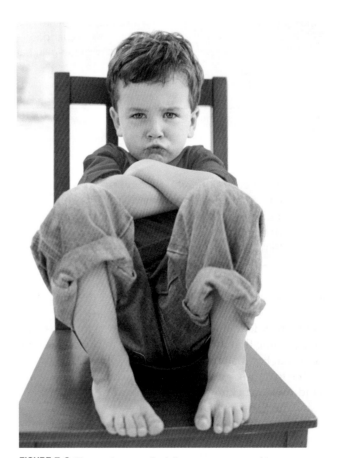

FIGURE 7-3 Time outs are a disciplinary measure used to remove the child from an activity and allow him or her to calm down and consider what was wrong in his or her actions.

Table **7-2**   Behavior Problems of Toddlers

BEHAVIOR	CAUSES	PARENTING TIPS FOR CORRECTING BEHAVIOR
Biting	Teeth are established. Child wants attention; child is angry.	Establish "no biting" rule. Firmly tell child "no" while looking straight in the eye. Suggest alternative safe behavior. Put child in time out. Never bite your child for biting someone else.
Bedtime resistance or refusal	Child does not want to go to bed or stay in his or her bedroom; child has already established history of being allowed to sleep with parent.	A child should stay in his or her own bed at night; explain rules for this. Establish a pleasant bedtime routine. Escort child back to bed.
Physical fighting and spitting	Children fight when angry or jealous. They see other children or people on television act this way.	Establish "no hitting" rule because it does not solve problems. Teach children "Spitting doesn't look nice." Tell child to handle with words; ignore bullies. Use time out. Never hit your child for hitting someone else. Praise friendly behavior.
Nightmares	Relate to developmental challenges (toddlers fear separation from parents).	Reassure and cuddle child. Provide night light, leave door open. Talk about the dream during the day. Avoid frightening movies or television programs (applies more to older children).
Night terrors	These inherited disorders involve dreams during deep sleep from which it is difficult to awaken.	Sleep deprivation may contribute to these; have child take afternoon nap or at least "quiet time." Comfort and reassure child during night terror.
Temper tantrums	Child is angry (may be precipitated by wanting something but not getting it).	Ignore child but monitor safety. Take child to his or her room for 2 to 5 min. Avoid spanking (conveys you are out of control).
Sibling quarrels	Occurs because of nature of being siblings. Quarrel over possessions, and so on. Want to gain parents' attention.	Encourage them to settle their own arguments; if children come to you, keep an open mind when resolving and avoid getting in the middle. Intervene if argument gets too loud. Do not permit hitting. Avoid showing favoritism. Praise cooperative behavior.

Modified from Schmitt, B. (2010). *Discipline basics.* ©2010 RelayHealth and/or its affiliates. All rights reserved.

minute per year of the child's age, up to 5 minutes. Time out can change almost any disruptive childhood behavior and is most effective if the child is older than 2 years of age.

Children, like adults, seek approval. *Time-in* refers to the positive interactions and feedback children receive when they are not misbehaving. Teach parents to catch their children being good! Providing this approval is effective and helps increase their self-confidence. Take the positive approach as much as you can. Assume that the toddler is going to be good rather than bad. For instance, "Thank you, Johnny, for giving me the matches," will make the matches arrive in your hand more quickly than saying in a threatening tone, "Give me those matches right now."

Positive parenting steps also include spending time alone with the toddler, praising the toddler for good behavior ("You were such a good boy to help put your toys away"), and making the child feel safe and secure through discipline and love.

 Nursing Brief

Caregivers need to provide safe areas for the toddler to explore. They need to watch carefully before saying no.

COMMUNICATION

Language Development

At about the end of the first year, the baby has begun vocalizing words such as "bye-bye," "ma-ma," and "da-da." When toddlers see a happy response to these sounds, they repeat them. This is true throughout the toddler period. For small children to want to learn to talk, they must have an appreciative audience. At first, children refer to animals by the sounds the animals make. For example, before saying "dog," toddlers repeat "bow-wow." Soon they can say short phrases, such as "daddy gone car." The 2-year-old can speak in simple two-word noun-verb sentences. Three-year-olds generally speak in three-word sentences, and so on. Toddlers respond also to tone of voice and facial expression. If an adult sounds threatening, toddlers may answer "no" and then "no" again in a louder voice. Toddlers also use "no" to express their developing autonomy. It is good to remember that toddlers who talk remarkably well and understand more than they say still cannot comprehend much of adult conversation. Sometimes when adults forget this, they scold the child merely for being too young to understand what is requested of them. Imagine yourself being punished in a foreign country because you are unable to speak or understand the language well enough to defend yourself. Adults who show empathy to small children can help minimize their frustrations. A guideline for vocalization appears in Table 7-1.

Toddlers who have just learned to walk may practically give up repeating words because they are so overjoyed at being able to get about independently. As soon as their initial fascination becomes less pronounced, they take up speech again. Delayed speech does not necessarily indicate that a child is mentally slow. The temperament and personality of the child and the family play an important role. No two toddlers have the same vocabulary at the same age; however, generalities are found in language development. If a parent is concerned about a child's delayed speech, it can be discussed with the pediatrician during one of the child's routine physical examinations. This allows the concern to be evaluated in light of the child's total physical growth and development. Late talkers may be perfectly normal children who prefer listening to active participation.

Developmental norms in the use of language have been established. One widely used tool is the Denver II (see Appendix D), a revision of the Denver Developmental Screening Test (DDST). This test is used to assess the developmental status of children during their first 6 years. It evaluates according to four categories: personal-social, fine-motor–adaptive, language, and gross-motor. It is neither an intelligence test nor a neurologic test. A low score merely indicates a need for further evaluation. The test is designed for both professionals and paraprofessionals to use, and because it is a standardized test, proper administration and interpretation are crucial. Specific instructions for administering the test, scoring of the results, and a further description of the test are included in a manual that may be purchased from the publisher.

Communicating with Toddlers

Adults must keep their everyday conversation with small children simple. Offering them too many choices confuses them. When talking to a toddler, adults should position themselves so that they are at eye level with the child. In this way, adults seem less overwhelming. This is of particular importance when the child is in a fear-provoking environment such as the hospital.

Adults should also use the "I message" when communicating with a child. Saying "I feel angry when you hit your sister" does not blame or criticize in the way that "You are a bad boy to hit your sister" does. "Bad" also demoralizes the child and makes him or her feel guilty. This can leave a lasting impression.

HEALTH PROMOTION AND MAINTENANCE

DAILY CARE

Toddlers need proper nutrition, plenty of fresh air and exercise, and sufficient rest. They also need structure and routine. By the time a child is a toddler, the mother has usually found it easier to give the bath in the evening rather than in midmorning. A flexible schedule organized around the needs of the entire household is best. This routine, however, can vary during the summer months because outdoor water play may make a tub bath optional. Parents may need to be reminded to never leave a toddler alone in the bathtub because at this age drowning and burns from hot water are still a concern.

The clothing of toddlers should be simple and easy for them to put on and take off. Pants with elastic waists are convenient for them to pull down when they go to the toilet. All clothing must be fairly loose to provide freedom of movement for jumping and other strenuous activities. Children should wear shoes with flexible soles. Tennis shoes are good choices once children are walking well. Shoes should fit the shape of the foot and be ½ inch longer than the big toe. The heels must fit securely. Children should wear their usual shoes at their periodic checkups because these show how the shoes have been worn, which indicates to the doctor how the children are using their bodies. Parents need to check the fit every few months because shoe size changes frequently as toddlers grow.

In the summer months, children may sunburn quickly and should be protected by sunglasses that are 99% UV protection, and by clothing/sunscreen so as to prevent future skin damage. Sunscreen should be applied at least 30 minutes before going outside and be reapplied every 2 hours. Sunscreen should be used even on cloudy days. The SPF (sun protection factor) should be at least 15, and the UV protection should be "broad-spectrum" (American Academy of Pediatrics, 2010).

Sleep needs gradually decrease as children grow older. For example, they may enter toddlerhood sleeping 12 hours a night with 2 daytime naps. By the time they reach the preschool years, this amount may decrease to 8 hours of sleep at night and 1 nap. Establishing a routine for bedtime and naptime is also helpful advice. Parents may need advice on how to get

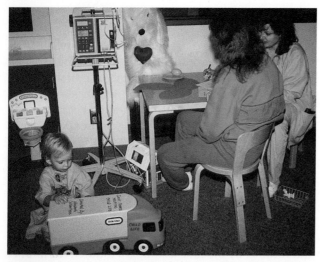

FIGURE 7-4 A child's play area should have furniture adapted to his or her size.

the child out of the crib and into a regular bed. During the adjustment period, be sure there is a railing or chair placed next to the bed at night. The toddler's mattress should be firm.

Adapt the toddler's environment accordingly. The chair and play table should be adjusted to their size (Figure 7-4). In some cases, this can be easily accomplished by placing a few magazines in the seat of the chair. A sturdy, small stool placed in the bathroom allows a toddler to stand at the proper height for brushing the teeth. These simple actions help to promote independence.

DENTAL HEALTH

By the time they are 30 months, most toddlers have a complete set of 20 deciduous teeth. An easy way to remember how many teeth young children should have is the age of the toddler in months minus 6. This approximation is a helpful rule to teach parents. Care of the toddler's teeth begins in infancy when teeth begin to erupt. Parents need to realize that access to a bottle of milk or juice exposes tiny teeth to hours of sugary acids that can cause severe damage (baby bottle tooth decay). The Health Promotion box lists important reminders for dental health.

🏃 Health Promotion

Care of the Teeth

- Encourage fruits, protein foods, and calcium-rich foods.
- Promote low-cariogenic snack foods.
- Avoid sucking on lollipops and chewing sugary gum.
- Examine labels for sugar content (e.g., cereals).
- Avoid using the bottle as a daytime or nighttime pacifier.
- Encourage toddlers to drink from a cup instead of a bottle.

Good dental health is essential to the growing child. Attractive, healthy teeth promote self-esteem and contribute to physical well-being. Today techniques are available to prevent dental problems in most children. Unfortunately, many poor children seldom visit the dentist's office. More children today are uninsured for health services than in earlier years. When parents have limited income, they fall behind in dental health practice. These factors have an impact on preventive and acute health care. Nurses must realize that although most middle-class children see their dentist regularly, tooth decay is still rampant among the poor. Nurses can play an important role in decay detection, nutrition education, and teaching oral hygiene. They also can direct parents to dental clinics (and dental schools) serving low-income clientele.

Prevention of dental problems consists of good nutrition (a diet high in calcium, phosphorus, and appropriate vitamins), proper brushing and flossing of the teeth, and regular dental care. It is also important after 6 months of age to administer fluoride by mouth. City water typically contains fluoride. The recommended level according to the American Dental Association is 0.7 to 1.2 parts fluoride per million parts water. Local testing can determine whether the content is adequate. Fluoride supplements can be given if water levels are not sufficient. Supplements should be given until about 12 years of age, when the last permanent tooth erupts.

The 2-year-old enjoys putting toothpaste on a brush. However, the use of too much toothpaste must be avoided; only a small amount (pea-sized) is necessary. Check with the child's dentist or physician before using toothpaste. Toothpaste with fluoride is not usually recommended for children younger than 2 years of age. Children can ingest fluoride from toothpaste, leading to a total fluoride intake higher than recommended. Too much fluoride can cause fluorosis, or mottling of the teeth. In addition, during brushing, allow the toddler to experience and handle frustration. Technique improves with practice. To ensure effectiveness, parents need to assist the child until school age. Teeth should be brushed at least twice daily.

The American Academy of Pediatric Dentistry and the American Dental Association recommend that children see a dentist when the first tooth erupts but no later than 12 months of age. When the child visits the dentist, the visit includes an examination of teeth, gum tissue, and bone structure. It also includes educating parents about proper nutrition, feeding patterns, tooth-cleaning procedures, and fluoride treatments.

NUTRITION COUNSELING

A toddler's need for food is not as great as that of an infant. This is because, despite an increased activity level, a toddler's growth is not as rapid. Often the growth patterns for toddlers are described as steplike because of periodic growth spurts. Children need an adequate protein intake to meet maintenance needs and to provide for optimal growth. The protein is provided mainly by milk, other dairy products, meat, and eggs. Milk should be limited to 2 to 3 cups per day (16 to 24 ounces). Whole milk is recommended until 2 years of age because the fat content of regular milk is needed for brain growth. After 2 years of age, children can be given low-fat or skim milk. Too few solid foods can lead to dietary deficiencies of iron. Children between 1 and 3 years of age are high-risk candidates for anemia. Drinking too much milk satiates their appetite and decreases their intake of solid foods that are rich in iron.

Fruit juice should not be introduced into the diet before 6 months of age and should be limited to 4 to 6 ounces per day for children 1 to 6 years of age. It should not be given at bedtime and should not be given in a bottle. High intake of juice can contribute to diarrhea, overnutrition or undernutrition, and the development of dental caries (American Academy of Pediatrics, Policy Statement, 2001, 2007).

Vitamins and minerals are necessary for normal growth and development. Insufficient intake can result in impaired growth and deficiency diseases. Calcium is needed for adequate mineralization and maintenance of growing bone; vitamin D is needed for calcium absorption, regulating blood levels of calcium, and promoting bone and teeth mineralization (Peckenpaugh, 2007). Playing indoors can promote rickets, because of less exposure to sunshine. Health care providers need to be alert for Vitamin D deficiencies.

The child who is healthy does not need vitamin supplementation; a balanced diet consisting of a variety of foods is more likely than a vitamin preparation to supply all the necessary nutrients for growth. Vitamin and mineral supplements can help infants and toddlers with special nutrient needs or marginal intake achieve adequate balance. A well-nourished toddler shows steady proportional gains on height and weight charts and has good bone and tooth development.

The toddler is noted for having a fluctuating appetite and strong food preferences. Physiologic anorexia is a phenomenon of toddlerhood that occurs because of decreased appetite and decreased nutritional need. These children have appetite fluctuations and may show a preference for one particular food for a period of time. Remind parents that any nutritious food can be eaten at any meal: for example, soup for breakfast, eggs for supper. Serving size is important. Servings that are too large are discouraged because they can overwhelm the child and lead to later overeating problems. Generally, a toddler will eat one fourth to one third of an adult portion. A quiet time before meals provides an opportunity for the child to wind down. Toddlers may refuse to eat because they are fatigued or because they are not particularly hungry. They may

eat one food with vigor one week and refuse it completely the next. A flexible schedule designed to meet the needs of the toddler and those of the rest of the family must be worked out by the individual family. Forcing toddlers to eat only creates further difficulties. They are quick to sense parental frustration and may then use mealtime as a tool to obtain attention by behaving poorly and refusing to eat. Discipline and arguments during mealtime only upset everyone's digestion. Two or three healthy snacks during the day help to ensure a balanced diet.

Toddlers are fond of ritual. This is frequently seen at mealtime. They may want a particular dish, glass, and bib. It is best to go along with these wishes, as long as they do not become too pronounced. These rituals give them a sense of security and, in the long run, saves time and energy for the adult.

Toddlers have a brief attention span. They may be able to sit still for only about 15 minutes. They may try to stand in the highchair or wander away from the table. If they have eaten a fair amount of the meal, excuse them; otherwise, distraction of some type is necessary. Some restaurants that cater to families provide crayons and a special place mat to keep the small child occupied until adults finish their dinners. In the hospital, the toddler who is fed in a highchair needs to have the safety straps and tray secured. The nurse also needs to remain with the child while he or she is in the chair.

Toddlers are at risk for choking on foods such as grapes, hot dogs, and raw vegetables. Injury prevention can be achieved by simply cutting foods into small pieces or thin strips and cooking raw vegetables until slightly soft. All food portions should be small and separated. Foods should be served at moderate temperatures. Candy, cake, and soda between meals should be avoided. Offer a variety of foods, and try to plan contrast in colors and textures. Finger foods such as crackers or cereal can be introduced at 8 to 10 months of age. Toddlers will continue to eat finger foods and can begin using a spoon at 12 months. By 15 months, many are feeding themselves.

Health promotion for nutrition and toddlers includes the following:
• Provide plenty of vegetables, fruits, and whole-grain foods.
• Serve milk at mealtime.
• Provide lean meats, poultry, fish, lentils, and beans for protein.
• Limit consumption of sugar and saturated fat.
• Limit drinking sugar-sweetened beverages.

MyPyramid was introduced by the U.S. Department of Agriculture in 2005 to encourage people to make healthy food choices and to be active every day (Figure 7-5). Healthy food choices include emphasis on fruits, vegetables, whole grains, and fat-free or low-fat milk and milk products. Lean meat, poultry, fish,

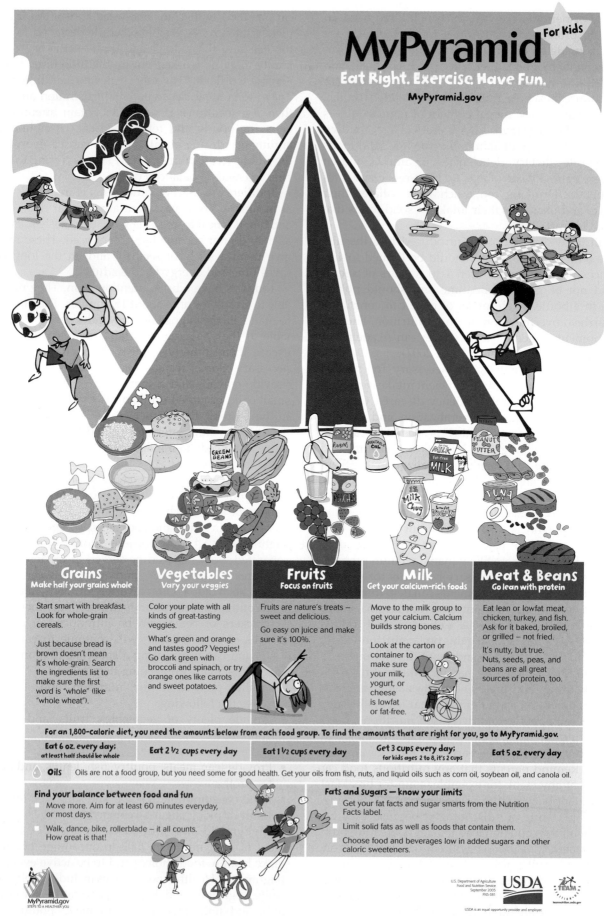

FIGURE 7-5 The U.S. Department of Agriculture's new MyPyramid (*www.mypyramid.gov/*) symbolizes a personalized approach to healthy eating and physical activity. MyPyramid for Kids is adapted for 6- to 11-year-olds. My Pyramid for Preschoolers is used for 2- to 5-year-olds.

beans, eggs, and nuts are also promoted. The diet should be low in saturated fats, trans fats, cholesterol, salt, and added sugars. Parents should follow the guidelines of the pyramid by placing greater emphasis on the grains, fruits/vegetables, and milk products—the food groups that have wider color stripes. The wider base of the stripe stands for foods with little or no solid fats or added sugars. The narrower top area represents foods containing more added sugars or solid fats. The more active someone is, the more of these foods can fit into their diet. According to the guidelines, 2- and 3-year-olds require from 1000 to 1400 calories, depending on whether their lifestyle is sedentary or active. The guidelines then discuss how many servings of each group are required to meet the calorie level. For example, a child requiring 1000 calories per day would need 1 cup each of fruits and vegetables, 3 ounces of grains, 2 ounces of meat/beans, 2 cups of milk, 3 teaspoons of oil, and a discretionary calorie allowance of 165 calories.

Nursing Brief

The customized *MyPyramid Plan for Preschoolers* (ages 2 to 5) provides parents a customized eating plan for their preschooler, based on the child's age, gender, and physical activity level. It also includes links to information about each food group, snacks, beverages, salt, and "extras" *(www.mypyramid.gov/preschoolers/Plan/index.html).*

Children like colorful dishes, which must be made of an unbreakable substance. Washable plastic bibs and place mats are convenient. Protect the floor around the highchair with newspapers. Silverware should be small enough so that it can be handled easily. Adjust seating equipment so that the child is comfortable and maintains good posture. Allow children to eat outdoors if weather permits. A picnic is enjoyable at any age (Figure 7-6).

TOILET INDEPENDENCE

There are many approaches to toilet training. Much depends on the temperament of the individual child and the person guiding him or her. Readiness is important. Voluntary control of anal and urethral sphincters occurs at about 18 to 24 months. If the child wakes up dry in the morning or after a nap, this is an indication of maturity. Children must also be able to communicate in some fashion that they are wet or need to urinate or defecate. They must be willing to sit on the potty for at least 5 to 10 minutes. The parent can place the child on the potty chair or toilet at regular intervals, such as when the child wakes up in the morning, after naps, before meals, and at bedtime. Toddlers seek approval and like to imitate the actions of their parents. They wander into the bathroom and are curious about what is taking place there. If parents feel that their

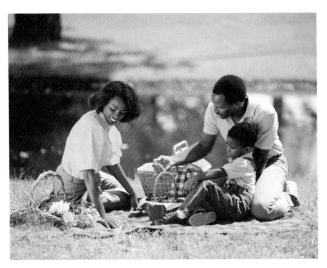

FIGURE 7-6 Children enjoy picnics. Keep servings small and nutritious.

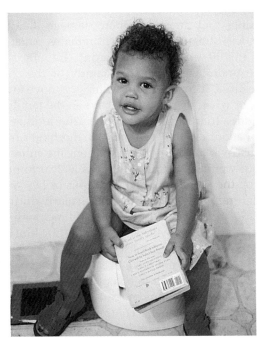

FIGURE 7-7 No set rules exist for toilet training. The nurse can help parents understand that both physical readiness and psychological readiness are necessary for success.

child will respond to training at this time, they might first put the toddler in training pants (e.g., Pull-Ups). These can be removed quickly and easily, and the child becomes more aware of being wet. The use of a child's potty chair or a device that attaches to an adult seat is a matter of personal preference. A potty chair may make a toddler feel more secure because it is smaller-sized (Figure 7-7). The child's feet should touch the floor. The child needs time to become accustomed to this new piece of equipment. Toddlers may want to climb in and out of it and drag it about before they actually try to use it. If a potty seat is not available, a child can sit on a regular toilet facing the toilet tank back. This sitting in reverse gives the child a greater feeling of security.

Bowel training is generally attempted first; however, some toddlers become bladder-trained during the day because they enjoy listening to the "tinkle" in the potty. If toddlers have bowel movements at the same time each day, they may progress fairly rapidly. Do not leave them on the potty chair or toilet for more than 5 to 10 minutes at a time.

If a child's bowel movements are not regular, it might be good to delay training for a while because the toddler resents being constantly interrupted from play and taken to the bathroom. Toddlers generally enjoy having a parent remain with them during the procedure. Most parents find some phase of toilet training discouraging. Perhaps it is because some parents work at it too hard. They think of it as an obstacle that they must overcome rather than a normal process that the toddler easily masters when ready. Spankings and threats do more damage than good. Life is less stressful if the parent remains patient and keeps this new adventure pleasant. Training should not be undertaken when the family or the child is under stress, such as during an illness, a move to a new home, or when there is a new baby in the family.

Bladder training is begun when the toddler stays dry for about 2 hours at a time. One morning a mother may discover that her toddler has gone the entire night without wetting. At this point, it is logical to put the child on the potty chair and praise his or her success. Bladder training varies widely, particularly during the night. Restricting fluids before bedtime may help. Getting the child up half asleep and putting him or her on the potty chair accomplishes little.

If the child does not seem to catch on after a couple of weeks, parents need to accept that the child is not ready yet and they should not make the child feel bad. It is perfectly acceptable to continue to use diapers and then to try again after a month or so.

Most children continue to have occasional accidents until 4 or 5 years of age. If the toddler has a mishap, parents should accept it as a matter of course and merely change the child's clothes. When adults show continuous affection toward their children and accept the bad and the good days, everyone benefits.

> ### 🏠 Nursing Brief
>
> Nurses can help parents identify readiness for toilet independence.

The word that toddlers use to signal their need to defecate or urinate should be one that is recognized by others besides the immediate family. Sometimes, a parent may forget to inform the babysitter or the nursery school teacher of the word that the child uses.

This causes children unnecessary frustration because no one can understand what they are trying to say.

Toddlers who are toilet-trained at home should continue to use the potty in the hospital setting. They may be embarrassed if they have "accidents." Nurses regularly consult parents about their child's habits so as to make young patients feel more at home. Attentive nurses quickly respond to a toddler's pleas and consider whether or not the child needs to urinate. Although regression in bowel and bladder control is common during hospitalization, personnel often contribute to this regression by not taking the time to investigate children's needs.

PLAY

Toddlers spend much of the day playing. In this way they develop coordination, which contributes to physical well-being. Play also contributes to mental health by bringing relief from emotional tension. At first, toddlers enjoy **parallel play**, playing near other children but not with them (Figure 7-8). This is the beginning of socialization. Gradually, as they learn to communicate more easily and become more skilled in handling toys, **associative play** occurs (Figure 7-9). Children then learn **cooperative play**. They learn to give and take and begin to sense moral values of right and wrong. Play also has educational value. Toddlers learn continuously as they explore, and they delight in having many new play experiences.

It takes time for small children to learn to share. They clutch their toys, shouting "Mine!" Once in a while, they voluntarily offer a toy to a playmate. Parents should not force toddlers to share their possessions. This comes at a later stage of development. If they are constantly corrected for hoarding, they may eventually give up their toys when they are supervised but then seldom share when left to their own devices.

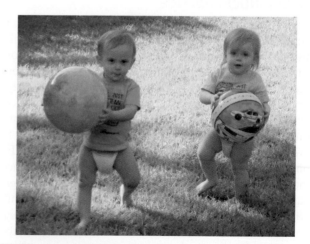

FIGURE 7-8 During parallel play, children may play side by side but do not influence each other's play activities.

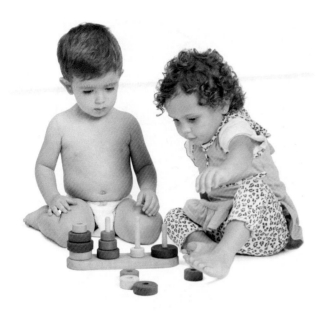

FIGURE 7-9 Associative play begins as toddlers approach the preschool years. Socialization is becoming important.

Toddlers need adult supervision during play, especially when other children are involved. The oldest in the group must be distracted from pushing, hugging, and directing the play of others. The youngest child needs protection from being bullied. Toddlers feel secure when they know they will be rescued from alarming experiences. It is unfair to expect them to rise to situations beyond their capabilities.

The type of toy the toddler selects for play depends on age. The young toddler is content with pots and pans from the mother's kitchen and enjoys repeating acts such as removing clothespins from a bucket and replacing them. The toddler likes certain books and looks at the same pictures over and over again. Some children become attached to a certain stuffed toy or blanket. Two-year-olds like to unlace their shoes and remove them frequently. They are fond of water play and may resent being removed from the tub. They enjoy playing in a sandbox, scribbling with a crayon, and prancing to rhythmic music. It is not long until toddlers discover the stairs. Most small children start going up the stairs on all fours. As children become more accomplished in walking upright, they shift to the method of placing one foot on the stairs and drawing the other foot up to it, supporting themselves with the handrail. Eventually they can climb the stairs by using their feet alternately, as in walking.

Toddlers like puppets, puzzles, stuffed animals, and clay or Play-Doh. They enjoy imitative toys (lawnmowers, carpenter kits, housekeeping toys)—anything that looks like what their parents use. In addition, toys do not need to be expensive. Toddlers need to use their imaginations when they play.

Toys that can be pedaled, such as a tricycle, should be adapted to the size of the child. Wind-up toys, as a rule, cannot be fully enjoyed by toddlers because they cannot manipulate them by themselves. Objects that can be pushed or pulled delight the small child. Toys with small, removable parts are dangerous because of the risk for aspiration. As a rule, toys should be larger than the size of a toddler's fist. See Chapter 8 for further discussion on play.

DAYCARE

Daycare has become a way of life for many children younger than 6 years of age. For school-age children, it also provides before-school and after-school care. More mothers are not only working, but also returning to work sooner after their children are born. Today most mothers of childbearing age work at least part time outside the home. It is clear that alternative methods of child care are necessary. These arrangements must meet families' personal preferences, cultural perspectives, and financial and special needs. Parents must take an active role in ensuring high-quality care. Nurses need to serve as resource persons and family advocates because finding adequate daycare can be stressful.

There are basically two types of child care: home-based and center-based. In home-based care, caregivers either give care in their own homes or come to the home of the child. These caregivers may be relatives, neighbors, friends, or those who have advertised their services. There is little research available on these types of private arrangements and few standards of quality control. With registered family homes, there are minimum standards published at the state and national levels.

Community Considerations

The Maternal and Child Health Bureau has established the National Resource Center for Health and Safety in Child Care and Early Education (*http://nrckids.org/providers.htm*). The "State Licensing and Regulation Information" link lists child care licensure regulations.

Center-based care providers care for several children at once. These centers are usually private businesses run for profit. They too are subject to state regulations regarding physical makeup, number of children per caretaker, education of personnel, and so on. Child care centers run by businesses for their employees are becoming common. Sick-child care centers are also available in some areas for children who have minor illnesses that would prevent them from attending conventional types of daycare. Often these centers are located in hospitals that provide pediatric services. Parents need to determine their child's

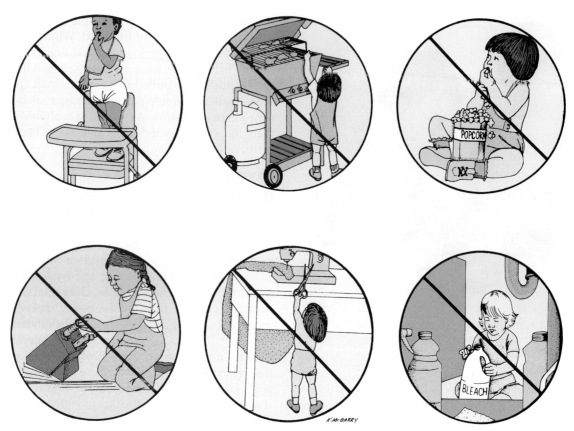

K.McGARRY

FIGURE 7-10 Safety measures should be taken to protect toddlers from these household hazards.

needs when choosing daycare. The philosophy of the center and the attitudes of the caregivers need to be evaluated. Parents should also consider the precautions taken by the daycare center to prevent disease transmission. The fewer the number of children to be cared for, the lower the incidence of infectious disease. Inspection and monitoring of child care facilities in terms of health (physical and mental) and safety standards are paramount. Parents should inquire whether the center is licensed and what the staff members' qualifications are. Additional criteria for evaluating a daycare center are similar to those discussed for preschools or nursery schools.

Ideally, all future daycare programs might include comprehensive health services and health education programs. Health care resources would be readily available to children, and the concept would tremendously increase the access of small children to health care.

INJURY PREVENTION

Accidents kill and cripple more children than any human disease and are the leading cause of childhood deaths. Although we do not have a preventive weapon,

we do have a defensive one. This is knowledge. If parents understand their child's activities at certain ages, they can take the necessary precautions and prevent many serious injuries. For example, when statistics indicate that poisonings or burns are particularly prevalent at a specific age, parents can take measures to guard against them. It is also important to consider the developmental level of the child. Some children developmentally do not match their age chronologically.

Most accidents occur in or near the home (Figure 7-10). Toddlers are especially vulnerable because they have a natural curiosity for investigating their environment. Specific toddler behaviors as well as injury prevention measures are noted in the Health Promotion box. Parents must allow them some natural experiences, which teach them to look out for their own safety. They should also strive to teach toddlers what is and what is not safe. Toddlers are at the highest risk for accidents involving motor vehicles, drowning, and burns. Many of these accidents are preventable; parents and caregivers need to become aware of these dangers, which are directly related to toddlers' ability to be mobile, their need for independence, their lack of knowledge of danger, and their curiosity.

Health Promotion

Injury Prevention—Toddlers

HAZARD	BEHAVIORAL CHARACTERISTIC	PREVENTIVE MEASURE
Motor vehicle accidents	Impulsive and unable to delay gratification, egocentric; has increased mobility	Use car safety seats. Caution children not to run from behind parked cars or snow banks. Hold toddler's hand when crossing the street. Never allow child to ride on/never carry on a tractor or riding mower. Supervise tricycle riding; allow toddler to ride as a passenger on adult bike only with special seat and helmet. Do not allow children to play in a car or leave them alone in it. Do not allow children to ride in the back of open trucks. Drivers must look carefully in front of and behind vehicles before accelerating. Teach children what areas are safe for playing. Watch children younger than 3 years of age at all times. Teach children never to run into the street after a ball and never to ride toys in the street.
Burns	Fascinated by fire Can reach articles inaccessible to the infant	Teach the child the meaning of "hot." Install smoke detectors. Put matches and cigarettes out of reach and sight. Turn handles of cooking utensils toward the back of the stove. Avoid scalding; do not leave the bathroom when hot water is being drawn or after the tub is filled. Treat burns with cool water; call doctor or emergency number. Teach child to turn on "cold" first. Avoid tablecloths that overhang. Keep appliances such as coffee pots, electric frying pans, and food processors out of reach. Test food and fluids heated in microwave ovens to ensure that portions are evenly warmed and not too hot. Keep hot foods and liquids out of reach; never carry such items around a child. Beware of hot barbecue grills. Never smoke near a child. Use snug fireplace screens. Teach child to stop, drop, and roll until fire is extinguished. Devise a fire escape plan, and practice what to do in case of a fire in your home. Mark children's rooms to alert firemen in an emergency.
Falls	Likes to explore different parts of the house Can open doors and lean out open windows. Depth perception is immature. Capabilities change quickly. May seem grown up but still requires constant supervision at home and on the playground.	Never underestimate climbing ability. Never leave alone on changing table, and so on. Use safety straps. Teach children how to go up and come down stairs when they show a readiness for this task. Fasten crib sides securely, and leave them up when child is in the crib. Lock basement doors, use safety knobs, or use gates at top and bottom of stairs. Mop spilled water from the floor immediately. Avoid use of baby walkers. Keep scissors and other pointed objects away from the toddler's reach. Use window screens or guards that cannot be pushed out. Fill in under playground equipment with sand or other soft material.
Suffocation and choking	Explores with senses, likes to bite on and taste things Eats on the run	Do not allow small children to play with deflated balloons because they can be sucked into windpipes. Keep powders out of reach; do not use when changing child's diaper. Inspect toys for loose parts. Remove small objects, such as coins, buttons, and pins, from children's reach. Store toys in a toy box without a dropping lid. Avoid popcorn, nuts, small hard candies, chewing gum, and hard vegetables.

Continued

Health Promotion—cont'd

HAZARD	BEHAVIORAL CHARACTERISTIC	PREVENTIVE MEASURE
		Cut food into small pieces.
		Debone fish and chicken.
		Learn Heimlich maneuver.
		Inspect width of crib slats (should be no more than 2⅜ inches apart).
		Keep plastic bags away from small children; do not use as a mattress cover.
		Use a snug-fitting, firm mattress; children should sleep in their own bed.
		Turn on his or her side if vomiting.
		Avoid night clothes and play clothes with drawstring necks; do not allow cords near crib.
		Discard old refrigerators (have door removed).
		Be sure pack-and-plays (playards) have sturdy sides.
Poisoning	Ingenuity increases, can open most containers	Store household detergents and cleaning supplies out of reach; install safety latches on cabinets.
	Increased mobility gives child access to cupboards, medicine cabinets, bedside stands, and interior of closets.	Do not put chemicals or other potentially harmful substances into food or beverage containers; store in separate cabinets.
		Keep medicines in a locked cabinet; put them away immediately after using them.
	Looks at and touches everything	Use child-resistant caps and packaging.
		Dispose of old medications.
	Learns by trial and error	Follow physician's directions when administering medication.
		Do not allow one child to give another child medication.
		Do not refer to pills as "candy."
		Keep mouthwash away from small children to avoid potential alcohol poisoning.
		Keep telephone number of poison control center available.
		Wash fruits and vegetables before eating.
		Obtain name of any new plant purchased and record.
		Alert family of location of poisonous plants on or around property.
Injuries from firearms	Often curious and lacks safety awareness	Do not keep guns in the house.
		Unload and lock away all firearms separate from ammunition.
Cuts	Very active	Pad sharp corners of furniture (and fireplaces).
		Use safety latches on drawers.
		Never allow children to play near running lawnmowers or power tools.
Drowning	Lacks depth perception	Watch child continuously while at the beach or near a pool or pond (including frozen ponds or lakes in winter).
	Does not realize danger	Empty wading pools when child has finished playing.
	Loves water play	Cover wells securely.
		Never allow child to swim unsupervised.
		Wear recommended life jackets in boats.
		Begin teaching water safety early.
		Lock fences surrounding swimming pools. Supervise hot tubs; be aware that a young child can drown in an inch or two of water.
Electrical shock	Pokes and probes with fingers	Cover electrical outlets.
		Cap unused sockets with safety plugs.
		Water conducts electricity; teach child who is wet not to touch electrical appliances; keep appliances out of reach.
Animal bites	Immature judgment	Teach child to avoid stray animals.
		Do not allow toddler to abuse household pets.
		Supervise closely; do not allow child to play near a pet that is eating or has a bone.
General		Keep first aid chart and emergency numbers handy.
		Know location and how to access local emergency care system.
		Become trained in child and infant CPR.

Vacations and relocations, which place small children in strange environments, are also potentially dangerous. Discussing potential hazards in the home and reviewing the locations of those hazards can be helpful for the parents. Emphasize that the kitchen and bathroom are the two most dangerous rooms in the house as far as accidents are concerned. A discussion of the neighborhood environment, such as playgrounds, may also be relevant. Nurses can demonstrate safety measures to children and their families. This is most effectively done by good example. Measures pertinent to the pediatric unit are discussed in Chapter 2. Nurses in the community often can contribute indirectly to the welfare of others by the example they set and by being aware of emergency medical facilities available in the community.

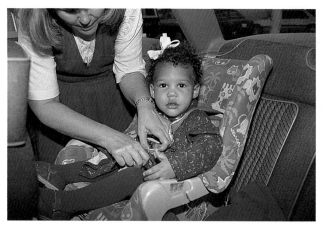

FIGURE 7-11 When a child reaches age 2, he or she can use a forward-facing convertible seat with a full harness. The safety straps should fit snugly. The seat should be placed in the back seat, ideally in the middle.

 Community Considerations

Nurses in clinics and schools need to promote safety through anticipatory guidance.

The federal government and concerned private agencies have attempted to regulate some of the variables surrounding certain accidents. A few examples are the use of nonflammable material for children's sleepwear, childproof caps on medicine bottles and certain household products, and the establishment of maximum temperatures for home hot water heaters. The U.S. Consumer Product Safety Commission has established regulations for crib slats, locks and latches, and mattress size and thickness.

CAR SAFETY SEATS

Motor vehicle accidents are the number one cause of childhood death from injury after 1 year of age. Laws have been passed in all states requiring infants and small children to be restrained while riding in automobiles (Figure 7-11). Children younger than 1 year of age and less than 20 pounds should be in rear-facing car seats, placed in the middle of the back seat of the automobile. These seats should be reclined at a 45-degree angle to receive full protective benefit. When children reach the highest weight or length allowed by the manufacturer of the infant-only seats, they should continue to ride rear-facing in a convertible seat until age 2 (AAP Policy Statement, 2011). When they outgrow the rear-facing seat, they should use a forward-facing seat with a full harness as long as they fit. Forward-facing only seats can be used with a harness for children who weigh up to 40 to 80 pounds (depending on the model). Combination seats with a harness can be used forward-facing with a harness for children who weigh up to 40 to 80 pounds or without the harness as a booster (up to 80 to 100 pounds). Booster seats are used for older children who have outgrown their forward-facing car seats. (American Academy of Pediatrics, Car Safety Seats: Information for Families for 2010). Belt-positioning booster seats are to be used until children have reached 4 feet 9 inches tall and are between 8 and 12 years of age (AAP Policy Statement, 2011). Children age 12 years and younger should *never* ride in the front seat where there is an active airbag. All child seat restraints must follow standards established by the Federal Motor Vehicle Safety Department. Installment guidelines come with the automobile and the car seat. Many hospitals also have car seat installation checks that are free to the public. This service should be recommended for parents with young children, especially for first-time parents. Unfortunately, many parents still do not understand the importance of the proper use of safety seats. This is an essential area of patient teaching and begins with the first ride home from the hospital. Most hospitals have a car seat loan program and mandate the use of car seats for any young child leaving the hospital.

 Community Considerations

SafetyBeltSafe U.S.A. (*www.carseat.org*) is a national child safety seat resource that offers a help line, materials, training, recall lists, and answers to questions. Car seat installation should always be verified by a certified car seat technician.

Legislation mandating car seats has reduced the risk for injury while toddlers are in cars. However, toddlers remain at risk for being hit by a car while playing in their own driveways. Before drivers start the car, they must be aware of any nearby children and pay attention to the children's locations.

FIRE AND BURN PREVENTION

New homes are required to have smoke detectors. Consumers who live in older homes and apartment complexes are also encouraged to install them. Various other safety codes are mandatory for public buildings, with additional measures required for buildings that are specifically for the disabled. The problems of surveillance and upkeep are, nevertheless, considerable. Many children live in substandard housing with little supervision. The education of parents is of monumental importance in decreasing death and disability.

Scald burns are the most common type of burn injury in children. Toddlers can pull liquids down on themselves by tugging at tablecloths, cords, and handles. Parents need to watch for toddlers underfoot, especially when working in the kitchen. Knobs, handles, and cords should be placed out of the child's reach. The temperature of the water coming from the hot water faucet should be monitored. Hot water heaters should be set no higher than 120° F to prevent scald burns. Small children can turn on the hot water while playing in the bathtub or while playing with the knobs. Always teach toddlers to turn on the cold water first.

Matches and lighters can cause devastating accidents. They should be stored out of reach of children. Parents should teach children the dangers of playing with them. Electrical outlets should have safety guards so as to prevent harm.

DROWNING

Anyone who cares for children should be aware of the danger posed by any standing body of water. This includes bathtubs, toilets, swimming pools, hot tubs, and even small containers holding water. Parents should be instructed *never* to turn their back on a child, whether in a tub or standing near a body of water. Turning their back could result in tragedy. All parents should be trained in CPR.

CHOKING

Choking is a concern with the young child. They do not understand that they should not put small items in their mouths. Coins, pins, removable toy parts, deflated balloons, and hard foods are common causes of choking. Nuts, popcorn, and hard candy should never be given to young children. Abdominal thrusts (Heimlich maneuver) are the treatment of choice for the conscious choking person older than 1 year of age (Figure 7-12). Recall that with conscious infants younger than 1 year of age, back slaps and chest thrusts are used to dislodge the object (Figure 7-13). Specific instructions on how to relieve a foreign body airway obstruction are taught in a CPR class.

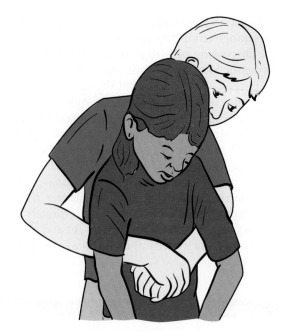

FIGURE 7-12 Abdominal thrusts (the Heimlich maneuver) are used for choking victims older than 1 year of age.

PLAYGROUNDS AND FALLS

Playground injuries are another cause for concern. The toddler loves to run and climb and often disregards the danger associated with these activities. Children should be taught how to safely play when on playground equipment or riding toys.

For prevention of falls, doors, windows, and gates should be kept closed or guarded with a screen. When the child begins to climb out of the crib, parents should consider moving the child to a bed.

POISONINGS

Because toddlers are naturally curious and particularly mobile, they are prone to accessing places and items that are dangerous. Poisoning incidents are a particular risk for young children. With their natural curiosity and new-found mobility, toddlers can find and swallow plant leaves, cleaning materials, medication, and anything else that catches their attention. All potentially dangerous substances should be placed out of the child's reach. A lock should be attached. Although most medications now have a safety cap, many children have been able to remove these caps. Parents should have the nearest poison control center number readily available and should always call this number *first* before treating the child (Figure 7-14).

PREVENTION

Nurses play a major role in the prevention of poisoning in children. As nurses use their knowledge of growth and development in teaching anticipatory guidance, they must focus the attention of the parent

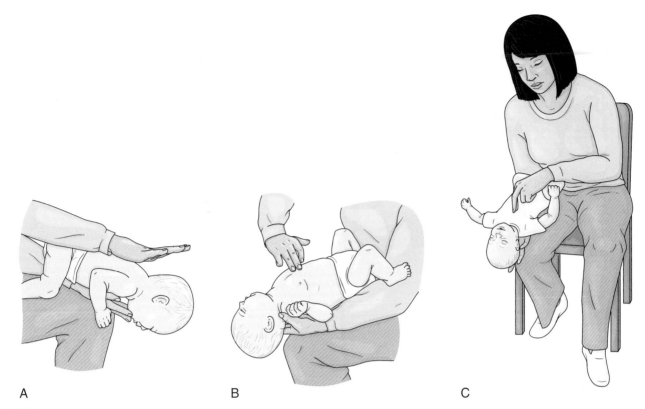

A   B   C

FIGURE 7-13 Infants up to 1 year of age who are choking are positioned with the head lower than the trunk. Back slaps are initiated **(A)**, followed by chest thrusts **(B)**. Both may be performed while seated; chest thrusts are shown here **(C)**.

on the dangers of each age. Children are naturally curious, and as they become mobile, they can climb and reach any hiding place.

Syrup of ipecac is no longer used. From the Brazilian plant *caephalis ipecacuanha,* this over-the-counter medicine was kept in the medicine cabinets of families for years. Its purpose was to induce vomiting after a poisoning, when recommended by the Poison Control Center. Concern over misuse and controversy over exactly how effective this medicine really was are the reasons home use is no longer recommended.

Community Considerations

Teach parents that the American Association of Poison Control Centers' nationwide poison control hot line is 800-222-1222.

Emergency Care

Most poisonings can be managed in the home with the advice of the poison control center. If a child is not breathing after ingesting a poison, EMS (911) should be called. When a poisoned child is brought to the emergency department, certain steps should be taken. The nurse initially assesses the child for any signs of either impending or current respiratory or cardiac distress (ABCs). Cardiorespiratory support is initiated if needed.

Removal of toxins has historically been done with the use of emesis with syrup of ipecac, gastric lavage, and activated charcoal. Gastric lavage is now rarely used. There is little, if any, benefit when performed beyond 30 minutes after ingestion. The child requires a protected airway, a large-diameter tube that will facilitate passage of gastric contents, and possibly sedation. According to Kliegman and colleagues (2007), lavage should only be used in older children, specifically in poisonings involving iron, calcium channel blockers, lithium, and tricyclic antidepressants. Activated charcoal use has increased since its effectiveness has been proven. It binds with most poisonous compounds; exceptions are metals, ethanol, caustics, and many hydrocarbons (Burg et al., 2006).

Depending on the poison, the nurse can anticipate the need for follow-up tests or treatments (e.g., electrolyte studies, IVs, temperature control measures, cardiac monitoring, respiratory treatments, and dialysis). When the child has ingested a corrosive substance such as toilet cleaner or bleach, tissue injury can interfere with breathing or swallowing. Corrosives should be diluted with water or milk; vomiting should never be induced. Vomiting redamages the mucosa. Some children need a tracheostomy to maintain an airway. Children with esophageal strictures may need a permanent gastrostomy. Hydrocarbons such as gasoline or paint thinner cause gagging, choking, coughing,

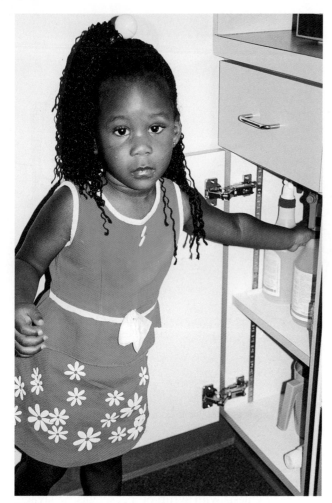

FIGURE 7-14 Children can easily discover poisons that are not in childproof cabinets.

Table 7-3		Stages in the Clinical Course of Acetaminophen Toxicity
STAGE	**TIME AFTER INGESTION**	**CHARACTERISTICS**
I	0.5-24 hr	Anorexia, nausea, vomiting, malaise, pallor, diaphoresis
II	24-48 hr	Resolution of above; upper quadrant abdominal pain and tenderness; elevated bilirubin, prothrombin time, hepatic enzymes; oliguria
III	72-96 hr	Peak liver function abnormalities; anorexia, nausea, vomiting, malaise may reappear
IV	4 days to 2 wk	Resolution of hepatic dysfunction or complete liver failure

From Kliegman, R., Behrman, R., Jenson, H., et al. (2007). *Nelson textbook of pediatrics* (18th ed.). Philadelphia: Saunders.

ACETAMINOPHEN POISONING

Description
Acetaminophen (Tylenol) has become the most common drug poisoning in children. Because acetaminophen is readily found in the medicine cabinet, children are accidentally ingesting this medication. Acetaminophen poisoning occurs from acute ingestion, not long-term overdose as may be seen in aspirin toxicity. Acetaminophen is metabolized in the liver. Therefore hepatic damage is the major concern. Children younger than 6 years of age are much less likely to have significant toxic effects from acetaminophen ingestion than are older children and adults (Kliegman et al., 2007).

Signs and Symptoms
Four stages occur in the clinical course of acetaminophen poisoning (Table 7-3). Signs and symptoms may be vague, and the diagnosis may be delayed. Most children recover if treated promptly and correctly. Death may result if treatment is delayed in severe overdosage.

Treatment and Nursing Care
N-acetylcysteine (Mucomyst) is the antidote and is given as soon as possible after ingestion but may be started 24 to 36 hours after ingestion in severe cases. It is administered according to the serum acetaminophen level. Active charcoal absorbs acetaminophen and should be given within 1 to 2 hours of ingestion (Kliegman et al., 2007).

If the antidote is given, the nurse assists and supports the child in taking the offensive-smelling Mucomyst (smells like rotten eggs). It may be given with

and vomiting. The immediate danger is aspiration, and the nurse should observe for respiratory symptoms such as tachypnea and cyanosis. Changes in sensorium can also occur. Inducing emesis is also contraindicated with hydrocarbon ingestion. Gastric lavage is generally not performed because of the aspiration risk. Chemical pneumonia is treated with high humidity, oxygen, hydration, and antimicrobials for secondary infection (Hockenberry and Wilson, 2007).

The Family
The nurse should give special attention to the family. The parents may feel guilty and blame themselves for the child's condition. The nurse must not reinforce this belief through either verbal or nonverbal communication. The parents should be kept informed about their child's condition, allowed to be with the child if at all possible, and given a chance to vent their feelings. The nurse should listen to them and support them through this difficult period. Preventive teaching should not be done until the acute stage has passed.

nasogastric tube or mixed with a carbonated drink. N-acetylcysteine may also be given intravenously (IV); however, there is a higher incidence of anaphylaxis. Vital signs are monitored, intake and output are observed and recorded, and laboratory results (particularly liver functions) are monitored and reported if abnormal.

SALICYLATE POISONING

Description

Because of the risk of Reye syndrome, aspirin should not be given to children unless recommended by a physician. Although salicylate poisoning has decreased since childhood fever has been treated more often with acetaminophen, it is still a problem. Aspirin is used by adults in most homes and often is stored carelessly on a bedside stand or in a mother's purse. This drug acts rapidly but is excreted slowly. Aspirin toxicity can occur from a single toxic-level ingestion or from repeated small therapeutic doses. Salicylates are also an ingredient in some over-the-counter antihistamines and decongestants. Pepto-Bismol *(bismuth subsalicylate)* even contains salicylate. Parents should be taught to read the labels and to use caution when giving these drugs.

Signs and Symptoms

The symptoms of salicylate poisoning vary depending on whether the toxicity is from an acute or chronic ingestion. The peak action occurs about 1 to 2 hours after a single toxic dose. Poisoning may manifest with ringing in the ears, dizziness, anorexia, sweating, nausea, vomiting, and diarrhea. Hyperpnea, faster and deeper respirations, is an early symptom of more serious trouble. This is because the respiratory center is stimulated by the drug. When carbon dioxide is eliminated, respiratory alkalosis quickly follows. Dehydration, metabolic acidosis, high fever, convulsions, and coma may follow. Bleeding is sometimes seen because excessive levels of aspirin inhibit the formation of prothrombin, which is necessary for normal blood clotting. Hypokalemia often accompanies this condition because salicylates directly affect the renal tubular mechanism.

Treatment and Nursing Care

There is no specific antidote for salicylate poisoning; therefore treatment is aimed at gastric emptying, preventing further absorption, and relieving the child's symptoms. Activated charcoal is important in the treatment. A blood sample is taken to detect the level of salicylate poisoning and to determine electrolyte and blood gas status. Urine pH and output are monitored frequently. The doctor may request that the child be admitted to the hospital for observation. The child's vital signs are closely observed and recorded. When IV fluids are necessary to correct electrolyte imbalance and rid the body of toxins, the child's intake and output of fluid are charted hourly.

Vitamin K may be administered to correct bleeding tendencies. IV infusions of fluids with sodium bicarbonate and potassium help correct imbalances. With severe intoxication, dialysis may be necessary. As with acetaminophen poisoning, the psychological needs of the family are a top priority.

IBUPROFEN POISONING

Ibuprofen (Motrin, Advil) is commonly used as an analgesic and antipyretic. Seizures and coma can occur with toxic levels. Nausea, vomiting, epigastric pain, drowsiness, lethargy, and ataxia (unsteady gait) are common effects of overdosage. Renal function studies and acid-base balance need to be monitored with ingestion of large doses. This is treated with activated charcoal.

LEAD POISONING (PLUMBISM)

Description

Lead poisoning results when a child repeatedly ingests or absorbs substances containing lead. Because of public awareness and health concerns, lead content from gasoline, paints and ceramic products, caulking, and pipe solder has been dramatically reduced in recent years. Children may, however, be exposed to lead through the use of health care products or folk remedies that contain lead, such as azarcon and greta (which are use for upset stomach) and pay-looah (which is used for rash or fever).

Another major source of lead in the environment is soil contaminated with lead (usually paint from a deteriorating house), ingestion of paint chips, or inhalation of paint dust from lead-painted surfaces. In addition, lead solder was used in house plumbing in some sections of the country until 1978. The lead leached into the drinking water in these homes. The highest prevalence of lead poisoning is among inner-city, underprivileged children who live in deteriorating pre-1970s housing containing lead-paint surfaces.

Lead poisoning is more common in the summer months. Children chew on windowsills and stair rails. They ingest flakes of paint, putty, or crumbled plaster. They play outside in soil contaminated with lead. Food, particularly fruit juices consumed from improperly glazed earthenware, is another source.

 Cultural Considerations

Lead poisoning among Mexican Americans may be caused by azarcon, a bright orange powder containing approximately 93.5% lead. This folk remedy is given for diarrhea. Another folk remedy containing lead used for diarrhea among Mexican Americans is greta, a yellow-orange powder.

Signs and Symptoms

Lead exposure can affect unborn children. Harmful effects include premature births, smaller babies, decreased mental ability and learning difficulties in children, and reduced growth in young children. Children may also develop anemia, stomachaches, and muscle weakness. Radiographs of the long bones may show deposits of lead.

The child's history might reveal pica. This is a condition in which a child has an unusual appetite, eating a variety of things that most persons consider unpalatable, such as sand, grass, wool, glass, plaster, coal, animal droppings, and paint from furniture. This tendency is sometimes seen in children with mental health disorders. An underlying nutritional disturbance and family dysfunction may also account for it.

Treatment and Nursing Care

Preventing lead poisoning is foremost. Lead paint should not be used on children's toys or furniture. Instead use paint that is marked for indoor use. Close observation of children in this age group also acts as a deterrent. The nurse and the parents should provide safe objects such as a teething ring or washcloth for the toddler to suck and chew on during the oral stage of development; this meets the normal sucking and chewing needs.

The Centers for Disease Control and Prevention (CDC) recommends that children who may be exposed to lead have their blood tested. The CDC considers children to have an elevated level of lead if the amount of lead in the blood is at least 10 mcg/dL. Medical evaluation and environmental investigation and remediation should be done for all children with blood lead levels equal to or greater than 20 mcg/dL. Medical treatment may be necessary in children if the lead concentration in blood is greater than 45 mcg/dL.

The treatment approach selected for the child and parent depends on the result of the blood lead test. In addition to more frequent screening, educational materials that describe how lead exposure can be decreased in the home and environment may be the only intervention necessary. In some cases, a professional environmental assessment is warranted. The child should not remain in any home where renovations involving lead paint are taking place.

Treatment is generally initiated in the child with moderate-to-severe lead poisoning (blood lead level greater than 45 mcg/dL). Reducing the concentration of lead in the tissues and blood becomes important when levels get this high. First, the child is removed from the source of lead and is closely supervised. Family members should also be tested. Chelating agents that render the lead nontoxic and allow it to be excreted in the urine are given. All chelating agents can have potentially serious side effects. Calcium disodium edetate (CaEDTA) and British antilewisite (BAL) are the two most commonly used drugs. CaEDTA may be given either with a deep intramuscular injection or with an IV drip. BAL is given with a deep intramuscular injection. Succimer, an oral chelating agent, can be used for children with blood lead levels of 45 to 69 mcg/dL. The child may need repeated courses of chelating therapy before normal lead levels return.

The prognosis depends on the degree and duration of the lead ingestion. Some children do not have any residual effects; others may have severe encephalopathy.

The nurse should stress the importance of continued treatment to prevent the recurrence of lead poisoning symptoms. Infectious disease in these youngsters must be treated promptly to avoid reactivation of the process. Parents are taught to be suspicious of changes in the disposition of their child. Siblings and playmates should also be screened. All residents should be removed from homes being de-leaded to avoid exposure. Parents living in apartments owned by uncooperative landlords may need assistance in relating to the housing authority. Appropriate literature and explanations are provided at the "therapeutic moment" and thereafter.

Nursing Care Is Symptomatic. Unnecessary handling of the child is avoided to prevent stimulating the central nervous system. Injection sites are rotated, and the skin is evaluated for thickness of fibrous lumps. Therapeutic syringe play is advised. Observation and charting of seizures are critical. Indications of respiratory distress are reported immediately. The services of the public health nurse are valuable in investigating the physical and emotional environment of the child and in continuing the education of the parents.

Get Ready for the NCLEX® Examination!

Key Points

- Toddlers are developmentally ready to give up total dependence and seek autonomy and independence.
- Weight gain slows as body proportions change.
- Thought processes and language development become more advanced.
- Daily care becomes easier as toddlers become more independent.
- Good dental health becomes essential; routine dental care is established.
- Physiologic anorexia occurs; appetite fluctuations are best managed by providing nourishing foods and snacks.

- Toilet training occurs when the child becomes physically able, can communicate the need, and has patience to sit on the potty.
- Play is the work of the child; toddlers enjoy parallel play.
- Daycare is a part of many toddlers' lives; parents need to visit daycare facilities and evaluate the philosophy of the center and the attitudes of the caregivers.
- Accidents are the leading cause of death in childhood; safety precautions must be upheld at all times by all toddler caregivers.
- Parents feel guilty when their child is admitted to the hospital because of a poisoning.
- Lead poisoning is treated with chelating agents when levels reach 45 mcg/dL and above.

Additional Learning Resources

Ɛvolve Go to your Evolve website (*http://evolve.elsevier.com/Price/ pediatric/*) for the following FREE learning resources:
- 3-D Animations
- Answer Keys
- Appendixes
- Audio Glossary
- Spanish/English Glossary
- Video Clips

Review Questions for the NCLEX® Examination

1. A child's birth weight is 7 pounds 8 ounces. By 1 year of age, the nurse can expect this child's weight to be approximately:
   1. 14 pounds
   2. 15 pounds
   3. 20 pounds
   4. 23 pounds

2. Sigmund Freud described the toddler as being in the:
   1. Oral phase
   2. Anal phase
   3. Latent phase
   4. Phallic phase

3. The Denver II is a test used to assess children during their first 6 years. It evaluates according to the following categories: (**Select all that apply.**)
   1. Nutritional
   2. Personal-social
   3. Cognitive
   4. Fine-motor–adaptive
   5. Language
   6. Gross-motor

4. A 2-year-old child that primarily plays indoors it at risk for:
   1. Rickets
   2. Physiologic anorexia
   3. Anemia
   4. Fluorosis

5. Treatment for salicylate poisoning involves:
   1. Administration of Mucomyst
   2. Provision of syrup of ipecac
   3. Gastric emptying
   4. Medicating with calcium disodium edetate

The Preschool Child

Objectives

1. Define the vocabulary terms listed
2. Describe the physical and psychosocial development of children from 3 to 5 years of age, listing age-specific events and guidance when appropriate
3. Describe the characteristics of a good preschool facility
4. Discuss the value of play in the life of a child

5. Designate two toys suitable for the preschool child, and provide the rationale for each choice
6. Identify the developmental characteristics that predispose the preschool child to certain accidents, and suggest methods of prevention for each type of accident

Key Terms

animism (ĂN-ĭ-mĭsm; p. 148)
artificialism (ĂR-tĭ-FĬSH-ăl-ĭsm; p. 148)
centering (p. 148)
domestic mimicry (MĬM-ĭk-RĒ; p. 148)

egocentrism (Ē-gō-SĔN-trĭsm; p. 146)
modeling (p. 152)
play therapy (p. 158)

GENERAL CHARACTERISTICS AND DEVELOPMENT

The child from 3 to 5 years of age is often referred to as the preschool child. This period is marked by a slowing down in the child's growth. By 1 year, infants have tripled their birth weight, whereas by the age of 6 years, these same children have only doubled their 1-year weight. For instance, the boy who weighs 20 pounds on his first birthday will probably weigh about 40 pounds on his fifth. Weight gain during the preschool years is about 5 pounds per year. The child between 3 and 5 years of age grows taller and loses the chubbiness that is seen during the toddler period. Height increases approximately 2.5 to 3 inches per year. Appetite fluctuates widely. The normal pulse rate is 90 to 110 beats per minute. The respiration rate during relaxation is about 20 breaths per minute. The systolic blood pressure is about 92 to 95 mm Hg; the diastolic blood pressure is about 56 mm Hg. By the preschool years, at least 90% of brain growth is achieved and handedness begins to become apparent. A summary of preschooler growth and development is presented in Table 8-1.

Preschool children have good control of their muscles and participate in vigorous play activities. As each year passes, they become more adept at using old skills. They can swing and jump higher. Their gait resembles that of an adult. They are quicker, and compared with toddlers, they have more confidence in

themselves. Although preschool children may seem more or less quiet and steady with respect to physical development, certain difficulties do arise from an increase in independence, social participation, interaction, and cognitive ability.

THEORIES OF DEVELOPMENT

The thinking of the preschool child is unique. Piaget called this period the preoperational phase. This phase comprises the ages of 2 to 7 years and is divided into two stages: the preconceptual stage, from 2 to 4 years; and the intuitive thought stage, from 4 to 7 years. The increasing development of language and symbolic functioning is important in the preconceptual stage. Symbolic functioning can be seen when children play and pretend that an empty box is a fort; this creates a mental image, which stands for something that is not there.

Preoperational thinking also implies that children cannot think in terms of operations, or the ability to logically manipulate objects in relation to each other. They base their reasoning on what they see and hear. They also believe they have magical powers that can cause events to occur. For example, a child might wish that someone or something would die. If the death does occur, the child feels at fault because of the "bad" thought that made it happen.

Another characteristic of this period is egocentrism, a type of thinking in which children have difficulty

Table 8-1	Summary of Preschooler Growth and Development				
AGE	**PHYSICAL**	**GROSS-MOTOR**	**FINE-MOTOR**	**VOCALIZATION**	**SOCIALIZATION**
3 years	Usual weight gain of 1.8 to 2.7 kg (4 to 6 pounds) Average weight of 14.6 kg (32 pounds) Usual gain in height of 7.5 cm (3 inches) Average height of 95 cm (37.25 inches) May have achieved night-time control of bowel and bladder	Rides tricycle Jumps off bottom step Stands on one foot for a few seconds Goes up stairs using alternate feet; may come down using both feet on step Broad jumps May try to dance; balance may not be adequate	Builds tower of 9 to 10 cubes Adeptly places small pellets in narrow-necked bottle Copies a circle, imitates a cross, names what has been drawn; cannot draw a stick figure but may make circle with facial features	Has vocabulary of approximately 900 words Uses complete sentences of 3 to 4 words Repeats sentence of 6 syllables Asks many questions Begins to sing songs	Dresses self almost completely Has increased attention span Feeds self completely; can prepare simple meals, such as cold cereal and milk Can help to set table May have fears (of dark or going to bed) Knows own gender and gender of others Play is parallel and associative; begins to learn simple games but often follows own rules; begins to share
4 years	Growth rate is similar to that of previous year Average weight of 16.7 kg (36.75 pounds) Average height of 103 cm (40.5 inches) Length at birth is doubled Maximum potential for development of amblyopia	Skips and hops on one foot Catches ball; throws ball overhand Walks down stairs using alternate footing	Uses scissors successfully Can lace shoes Copies a square, traces a cross and diamond, adds 3 parts to stick figure	Has vocabulary of 1500 words or more Uses sentences of 4 to 5 words Questioning is at peak Tells exaggerated stories Knows simple songs May be mildly profane if associates with older children Names one or more colors	Very independent Tends to be selfish and impatient Aggressive physically and verbally Takes pride in accomplishments Has mood swings Shows off dramatically, enjoys entertaining others Still has many fears Play is associative; imaginary playmates are common Sexual exploration and curiosity shown through play, such as being "doctor" or "nurse"
5 years	Average weight of 18.7 kg (41.25 pounds) Average height of 110 cm (43.25 inches) Eruption of permanent dentition may begin Handedness is established (approximately 90% are right-handed)	Skips and hops on alternate feet Throws and catches ball well Jumps rope Skates with good balance Walks backward with heel to toe Jumps from height of 12 inches Balances on alternate feet with eyes closed	Ties shoelaces Uses scissors, simple tools, and pencil well Copies a diamond and triangle; adds 7 to 9 parts to stick figure; prints a few letters, numbers, or words, such as first name	Has vocabulary of approximately 2100 words Uses sentences of 6 to 8 words Names coins Names 4 or more colors Knows names of days of week, months, and other time-associated words	Less rebellious and quarrelsome More settled and eager to get down to business Independent but trustworthy; not foolhardy; more responsible Has fewer fears; relies on outer authority to control world Eager to do things right and to please; tries to "live by the rules"; has better manners Cares for self with only occasional assistance Play is associative; tries to follow rules but may cheat to avoid losing

Modified from Hockenberry, M., and Wilson, D. (2007). *Wong's nursing care of infants and children* (8th ed.). St. Louis: Mosby.

Table **8-2**   **The Nature of Early Childhood Thought**

SAMPLE QUESTION	TYPICAL ANSWER
Ecocentrism	
Why does the sun shine?	To keep me warm.
Why is there snow?	For me to play in.
Why is grass green?	Because that is my favorite color.
What are television sets for?	To watch my favorite shows and cartoons.
Animism	
Why do trees have leaves?	To keep them warm.
Why do stars twinkle?	Because they are happy and cheerful.
Why does the sun move in the sky?	To follow children and hear what they say.
Where do boats go at night?	They sleep like we do.
Artificialism	
What causes rain?	Someone emptying a watering can.
Why is the sky blue?	It has been painted.
What is the wind?	A man blowing.
What causes thunder?	A man grumbling.

From Helms, D., and Turner, J. (1978). *Exploring child behavior: basic principles* (p. 447). Philadelphia: Saunders, with permission.

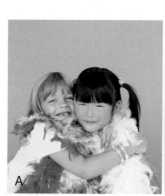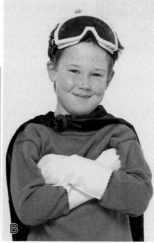

FIGURE **8-1** The preschooler has a vivid imagination and enjoys playing "dress-up."

seeing any point of view other than their own. Children's knowledge and understanding are restricted to their own limited experiences, and, as a result, misconceptions arise. One of these misconceptions is animism. This is a tendency to attribute life to inanimate objects. Another is artificialism, the idea that the world and everything in it is created by human beings (Table 8-2).

Evolving from preconceptual thinking to intuitive thinking involves a shift from egocentric thought to a social awareness and ability to consider another's point of view. This is considered to be closely associated with superego or conscience development.

Another distinctive characteristic of intuitive thinking is centering, the tendency to concentrate on a single outstanding characteristic of an object while excluding its other features. With time and experience, more mature conceptual awareness is established. The process is highly complex, and the implications for practical application are numerous. In addition, through intuitive thinking, play becomes more socialized and words are used to express ideas and thoughts.

According to Erik Erikson's theories, preschoolers acquire a sense of initiative. They believe learning is fun and try new activities and experiences. Conflict arises when initiative is criticized or punished; then they develop a sense of guilt. This guilt can carry over later in life and affect their ability to make decisions or solve problems.

It is important to provide preschoolers exposure to a wide variety of experiences and play materials to enhance their learning. They need to be allowed to play with finger paints, build sand castles, play with clay, and engage in activities that enhance their imaginations.

Preschoolers enjoy dressing up and pretending to be real and make-believe characters (Figure 8-1). They love to imitate people around them and often mimic what they see their parents doing. Playing "store" or "office" or doing household chores such as "lawn mowing" or "doing the dishes" are activities that preschoolers enjoy. Toy companies manufacture many toys that encourage the preschooler to engage in this domestic mimicry.

Lawrence Kohlberg emphasized moral development and moral judgment. Preschoolers are at a preconceptual stage of moral development. Young children learn whether an action is good or bad depending on whether the action is rewarded or punished. Preschool children progress to a stage where they can carry out actions to satisfy their own needs but not society's in general. They do something for another if that person does something for them.

Children at this age are just beginning to learn right from wrong. Spiritual development is strongly linked to development of the conscience (Hockenberry and Wilson, 2007). The preschooler is just beginning to understand spiritual matters. Rudimentary knowledge is provided by parents or significant others. Their concrete thinking allows them to perceive God as an imaginary friend. Children this age enjoy hearing Bible stories and reciting simple prayers. If hospitalized, saying prayers as part of their routine can actually help with the stressors of hospitalization.

Sigmund Freud developed a psychosexual theory with the concept that sexual energy is focused on certain body parts at certain ages. He felt that unmet needs in stages of development could cause later conflicts. While there is criticism of his theory, it does explore emotional development and has provided the basis for other theorists such as Erikson. Freud felt that during the preschool age, the child's focus is on the genital area. The child also is working out emotional relationships with the parent, which is the foundation for the child learning to relate to the opposite sex.

PHYSICAL, PSYCHOSOCIAL, AND COGNITIVE DEVELOPMENT

THE 3-YEAR-OLD

Most 3-year-olds are a delight to their parents. They are helpful and can participate in simple household chores. They obtain articles on request and return them to the proper place. Three-year-olds come very close to the ideal picture that parents have in mind of their child. They are living proof that their parents' guidance during the "terrible twos" has been rewarded. Temper tantrums are less frequent, and, in general, the 3-year-old is a pretty good youngster. Of course, they are still their individual selves, but they seem to be able to direct and control their primitive instincts better than before. They can help dress and undress themselves, use the toilet, and wash their hands. They eat independently, and their table manners have improved.

The 3-year-old talks in longer sentences and can express thoughts such as "What are you doing?" or "Where is Daddy?" They also provide more company to their parents because they can verbally share their experiences with them. They are imaginative, talk to their toys, and imitate what they see about them. Soon they begin to make friends outside the immediate family. They can now converse with playmates and find satisfaction in joining with their activities. Three-year-olds do not play cooperatively for long periods of time, but at least it's a start. Through associative play, they begin to share with other children; playing with other children their own age teaches them socialization skills. Much of their play still consists of watching others, but now if they have the need, they can offer verbal advice. They can ask others to "come out and play." If 3-year-olds are placed in a strange situation with children they do not know, they commonly revert to parallel play because it is more comfortable.

At this time, there is a change in the relationship between the child and the family. Preschoolers begin to find enjoyment away from Mom and Dad. However, they want them to be right there when needed. They begin to lose some of their interest in their mother, who up to this time has been more or less their total world. Their father's prestige begins to increase. Romantic attachment to the parent of the opposite gender is seen during this period. Johnny wants to "marry Mommy"

when he grows up. They also begin to identify themselves with the parent of the same gender. This behavior reflects Freud's beliefs.

Preschool children have more fears than the infant or the older child. Some of the many causes of this are increased intelligence, which enables them to recognize potential dangers; the development of memory; and graded independence, which brings them into contact with many new situations. While toddlers are not afraid of walking in the street because they do not know any better, preschool children realize that trucks can injure them, and therefore they worry about crossing the street. This type of fear is well founded, but many others are not. The fear of bodily harm is particularly peculiar to this stage. They have poorly defined body boundaries and become fearful with intrusive procedures. They are fearful that a minor cut will allow their "insides to spill out." Band-Aids become a necessity to prevent everything from coming out. The little boy who discovers that his baby sister is made differently worries that perhaps she has been injured. He wonders if this will happen to him. Masturbation is common during this stage as children attempt to reassure themselves that they are all right. Other common fears include fear of animals, fear of the dark, and fear of strangers.

Preschool children become angry when others attempt to take their possessions. They grab, slap, and hang on to them for dear life. They become very distraught if toys do not work the way they should. They resent being disturbed from play. They are sensitive, and their feelings are easily hurt. It is good to bear in mind that much of the disturbing social behavior seen during this time is normal and necessary to the children's total pattern of development.

 Communication

Preschool children sometimes believe that they are being punished for something they thought or did. Thus when a painful procedure is performed on the child, the nurse might say, "I am sorry that it hurt when I put the needle in your arm. I did that so we can give you medicine to make you feel better, not to hurt or punish you."

THE 4-YEAR-OLD

Four is a stormy age. Children are not as eager or willing as they were at 3 years of age. They also are more aggressive and like to show off. They are eager to let others know that they are superior and are prone to pick on their playmates. They often take sides and make life difficult for any child who does not measure up to their standards. Four-year-olds are boisterous, tattle on others, and may begin to swear if they are around children or adults who use profanity. Personal family activities are repeated with an amazing sense of recall, but they still forget where they left their bicycle. At this age, children become interested in how old they are and want to know the exact age of each playmate. It bolsters their ego to know that they are older than someone else in the group. Their ego is also bolstered by being a "big brother" or "big sister" to a younger sibling. They are able to help care for and protect them. The relationship of one person to another interests them as well. For example, Timmy is not only a brother but also is Daddy's son.

Four-year-olds can use scissors successfully. They can lace their shoes and do simple buttons (Figure 8-2).

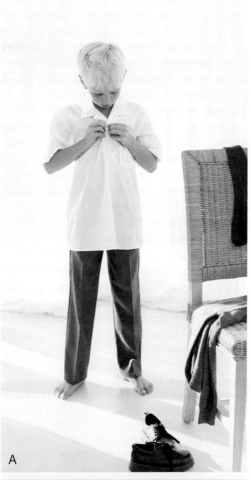
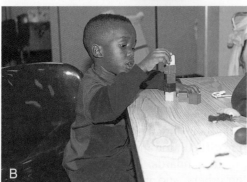

FIGURE 8-2 The child progressively achieves mastery of fine-motor skills and cognitive abilities, such as **(A)** buttoning clothes and **(B)** stacking blocks.

Vocabulary has increased to about 1500 words. They run simple errands and can play with others for longer periods of time. Many feats are done for a purpose. For instance, they no longer run just for the sake of running. Instead, they run to get someplace or to see something. They are imaginative and like to pretend they are firefighters or cowboys. Much of their play time is spent pretending. They may even have an imaginary friend. The friend may "exist" until the child starts school. They also begin to prefer playing with friends of the same gender rather than with those of the opposite gender.

The preschool child enjoys simple toys. They love to color pictures and have mastered the use of large crayons (Figure 8-3). Raw materials are more appealing than toys that are ready-made. An old cardboard box that can be moved about and climbed into is more fun than a dollhouse with tiny furniture. A box of sand or colored pebbles can be made into roads and mountains. A small mirror becomes a lake. "Dress up" becomes more dramatic, especially with the 4-year-old. Parents should avoid showering their children with ready-made toys. Instead they can select materials that are absorbing and that stimulate the child's imagination.

Stories that interest young children depict their daily experiences. If the story has a simple plot, it must

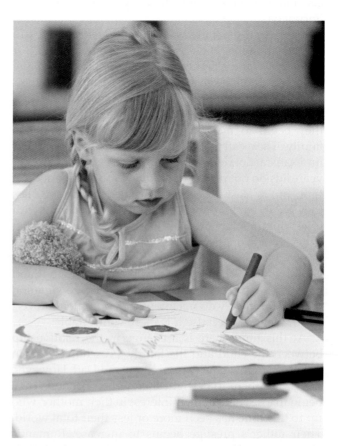

FIGURE 8-3 The preschooler enjoys coloring. Preschoolers often play cooperatively.

be related to what they understand to hold their interest. They also enjoy music; they like songs that they can march around to and simple instruments that they can shake or bang. Make up a song about their daily life, and watch their reaction.

Children's curiosity concerning sex continues to heighten. It is common for children of this age to take down their pants in front of friends of the opposite gender. They discuss their differences with their friends. It is important that parents provide simple explanations when sexual questions are asked. Older children who are more sensitive about their bodies should be told that this is a natural curiosity among small children. This may help to get rid of any guilt feelings that they might have, particularly if they also participated in similar activities during the preschool period. Children are as matter-of-fact about these investigations as they would be about any other learning experience and are easily distracted to more socially acceptable forms of behavior.

Between 3 and 4 years of age, children begin to wonder about death and dying. They may be the hero who shoots the bad guy dead, or they may witness a situation in which an animal is killed. Their questions are very direct: "What is dead? Will I die?" There are no set answers to these inquiries. Preschoolers may see death as a kind of sleep. They may not believe that the dead person no longer breathes or eats. They cannot understand the true concept of death. The religion of the family plays an important role regarding the interpretations of this complex phenomenon.

Usually young children realize that others die but do not relate this to themselves. If they continue to pursue the question of whether or not they will die, parents should be casual and reassure them that people do not generally die until they have lived a long and happy life. Of course, as they grow older, they will discover that sometimes children do die. The underlying idea, nevertheless, is to encourage questions as they appear and gradually help them accept the truth without undue fear. See Chapter 22 for further discussion on end-of-life issues.

THE 5-YEAR-OLD

Five is a comfortable age. Children are more responsible, enjoy doing what is expected of them, have more patience, and like to finish what they start. Five-year-olds are serious about what they can and cannot do. They talk constantly and are inquisitive about the environment. They have a vocabulary of about 2100 words. They want to do things right. They also seek answers to their questions and go to those who they think are knowledgeable. Five-year-olds can begin to play games governed by rules. They are less fearful because they feel that their environment is controlled by authorities. The worries they do have are not as

profound as they were at an earlier age. They may play with and talk to a best friend.

The physical growth of 5-year olds is not particularly outstanding. Their height may increase 2 to 3 inches, and they may gain 3 to 6 pounds. The variations in height and weight of a group of 5-year-olds are remarkable. They may begin to lose their deciduous teeth at this time. They can simultaneously run and play games, jump three or four steps at once, and tell a penny from a nickel or a dime. They like games with numbers or letters. They can name the days of the week and can understand what a weeklong vacation is. They usually can print their first name.

Five-year-olds can ride a tricycle around the playground with speed and dexterity. With training wheels, they also can begin riding two-wheelers as well. They can use a hammer to pound nails. Adults should encourage them to develop motor skills. Adults should not continually remind them to "be careful" because this practice enables children to compete with others during the school-age period and increases confidence in their own abilities. As with any age level, children should not be scorned for failure or for not measuring up to adult standards. Overdirection by solicitous adults is damaging. Children must learn to do tasks themselves for the experience to be satisfying.

The amount and type of television programs that parents allow preschool children to watch is a topic of current discussion. The American Academy of Pediatrics (AAP, 2001) discourages children younger than 2 years of age from watching television and encourages interactive activities that promote brain growth. Additionally, a recommendation for children older than 2 years of age is to limit television viewing to 1 to 2 hours of quality programs per day. Five-year-olds have better comprehension and may spend a great deal of time watching television. The plan of management differs for each family. Whatever is decided needs to be discussed with the children. Television should not be allowed to interfere with good health habits, such as regular sleep, meals, and physical activity. Most parents find that children do not insist on watching television if there is something better to do.

GUIDING THE PRESCHOOL CHILD

DISCIPLINE AND SETTING LIMITS

Much has been written on the subject of discipline, which over time has changed considerably. Today authorities place a great deal of importance on the development of a continuous, warm relationship between the child and the parents. This, they believe, helps prevent many problems.

Discipline and punishment are not one and the same: "Discipline includes all methods that are used to change behavior. Punishment is a very specific procedure that is used to decrease behavior that will be described under basic principles" (Larsen and Tentis, 2003). Children need to have limits set on their behavior. Setting limits makes them feel secure, protects them from danger, and relieves them from making decisions that they may be too young to understand. Expectations, however, must be appropriate to the age and understanding of the child. Parents need to encourage children to make acceptable choices. Children who are taught acceptable behavior have more friends and feel better about themselves. They live more enjoyably within the neighborhood and society. The manner in which discipline or limit setting is carried out varies from culture to culture. It also varies among different socioeconomic groups. Individual differences occur among families, between parents, and according to the characteristics of each child. The purpose of discipline is to teach and to gradually shift control from parents to the child, that is, to promote self-discipline. The Health Promotion box lists discipline techniques.

 Health Promotion

Discipline for Young Children

- Establish rules for safety by 8 months of age
- Explain rules clearly and concretely ("Don't push your brother")
- State acceptable behavior ("Walk, don't run")
- Do not constantly criticize and ignore unimportant behavior
- Use rules that are fair and attainable for the child's age
- Apply rules consistently
- Logical consequences occur as a result of misbehavior (removal of possession or privilege)

From Schmitt, B. (2010). Discipline basics. Pediatric Advisor. McKesson Corporation. Retrieved from *www.nursingconsult.com/das/patient/view/2019.3656-2.*

Timing and Time Out

Most researchers agree that to be effective, discipline must be given at the time the incident occurs. It should also be adapted to the seriousness of the infraction. The child's self-worth must always be considered. Warning the preschool child who appears to be getting into trouble may be helpful. Too many warnings without follow-up, however, lead to ineffectiveness. Spankings, for the most part, are not productive. The child associates the fury of the parents with the pain rather than the wrong deed because anger is the predominant factor in the situation. In addition, the parent serves as a role model for aggression. Whether a parent is affectionate, warm, or cold (uncaring) also plays a role in the effectiveness of child rearing. Time-out periods (discussed in Chapter 7), such as sitting for 5 minutes in a chair or corner, are one alternative to inappropriate behavior. Parents need to be taught to

resist using power and authority for its own sake. As the child understands more, privileges can be withheld. The reasons for such actions should be carefully explained.

Rewarding Positive Behavior

Rewarding the child for good behavior is a positive and effective method of discipline. This can be done by the use of hugs, smiles, tone of voice, and praise. Praise can always be tied to the act: "Thank you, Sara, for picking up your toys." The encouragement of positive behavior eliminates many of the undesirable effects of punishment.

Consistency and Modeling

Consistency is difficult for parents. However, they should try to be consistent as much as possible. Consistency must exist between parents and within each parent. It is suggested that parents establish a general style in terms of what, when, how, and to what degree punishment is appropriate to misconduct. Parents who are lax or erratic in their discipline and alternate such procedures with punishment have children who experience increased behavioral difficulties. The influence of modeling, or good example, has been widely explored. Such studies show that adult models significantly influence the education of children. Children identify and imitate adult behavior, both verbal and nonverbal. Parents who are aggressive and repeatedly lose control demonstrate the power of action over words. Those who communicate, show respect and encouragement, and use appropriate limit-setting serve as more positive role models. Finally, parents need assistance in reviewing their own childhood in regard to parental discipline to recognize destructive patterns that they may be exhibiting.

Spanking

The American Academy of Pediatrics has made the following statement regarding spanking: "Because of the negative consequences of spanking and because it has been demonstrated to be no more effective than other approaches for managing undesired behavior in children, the American Academy of Pediatrics recommends that parents be encouraged and assisted in developing methods other than spanking in response to undesired behavior" (AAP Policy Statement, 2004). The role of the nurse is to encourage parents to use other forms of discipline with their children. By explaining the use of timing, time out, consistency, modeling, and so on, parents become empowered and can make positive choices when raising their children.

BAD LANGUAGE

Parents express astonishment at the words that flow from the mouths of their sweet little children during the preschool period. Bad language is inevitable. Caretakers should suppress their desire to emphatically shout their disapproval. The small child delights in attention, and it does not matter, unfortunately, whether this attention is good or bad. Swearing at this age is not particularly meaningful because children are merely imitating what they hear and it does not have any real significance to them. They use swearing as a way of identifying themselves with the older children in the neighborhood and to shock adults. One mother dealt with this problem by saying, "Johnny, Mommy does not mind if you hear or know what that word means, but we do not use it in our home any more than you would think of going outdoors without your clothes on." Johnny felt free to discuss what he heard with his mother, and shortly thereafter his interest was taken up by other subjects.

JEALOUSY AND SIBLING RIVALRY

Jealousy is a normal response to actual, supposed, or threatened loss of affection. Children or adults may feel insecure in their relationship with the person they love. The closer children are to their mothers, the greater their fear of losing mother. Young children may envy a new baby. They love the sibling but at the same time resent its presence. They cannot understand the turmoil that is taking place within themselves. Jealousy of a new baby is strongest in children younger than 5 years of age and is shown in various ways. Children may be aggressive and may bite or pinch. They may be rather discreet and hug and kiss the baby with a determined look on their faces. Another common situation occurs when children attempt to identify with the baby. They may revert to something they outgrew such as thumb sucking or bedwetting. Some 4-year-olds even try the bottle, but it is usually a big disappointment to them.

Preschool children may be jealous of the attention that their mother gives their father. They may also envy the children they play with if those children have bigger and better toys than they do. There is less jealousy in only children because they are the center of attention and have only a minimum of rivals. Children of varied ages in one family are apt to feel that the younger ones are "pets" or that the older ones have more special privileges. These feelings of sibling rivalry present new challenges for the parents.

Parents can help reduce jealousy with the early management of individual occurrences. Preparing young children for the arrival of the new baby lessens the blow. They should not be made to think that they are being crowded. If the new baby is going to occupy their crib, it is best to get older children happily settled in a large bed before the baby is born. Children should feel that they are helping with the care of the infant. Parents can inflate their ego from time to time by reminding them of the many activities they can do that the new baby cannot. Parents also need to attend to the older child's needs first if both children have needs at the same time (Anderson, 2006). If it is convenient, the new baby is given a bath or feeding while the older child is asleep. In this way, the older sibling avoids one of the occasions on which the mother shows the newborn infant affection for a relatively long period of time. Special time should also be spent with the older child while the new baby is asleep. Some people believe that giving the child a pet to care for at this time helps. Many hospitals offer sibling courses that assist parents in helping the child to overcome jealousy.

If the child indicates an intention to hit the baby or another child, the children must be separated. It is important to remember that the one who has caused or is about to cause the injury needs as much, if not more, attention than the victim. Aggressiveness similar to this is seen when the child is made to share toys. It is even more difficult to learn to share the mother, so the child must be given time to adjust to the new situation. Children should be assured that they are loved but should also be told that they are not allowed to injure others. Use of the "I message" is helpful when correcting this type of behavior: "I feel angry that you hit your brother (or sister), and hitting is not allowed because it can hurt people."

THUMB SUCKING

From 1914 to 1921, the U.S. Children's Bureau pamphlet entitled *Infant Care* cautioned mothers that thumb sucking would deform the mouth and cause drooling. Today we recognize that thumb sucking is an instinctual behavioral pattern that can be considered normal. It is often used as a comforting measure and does not necessarily mean the child is insecure. Finger sucking or thumb sucking does not have a detrimental effect on the teeth as long as the habit is discontinued before the second teeth have erupted. Most children give up the habit by the time they reach school age, although they may regress during periods of stress or fatigue. Management includes education and support of the parents so as to relieve their anxiety and to help prevent secondary emotional problems in their children. The child who is trying to stop thumb sucking is given praise and encouragement.

MASTURBATION

Masturbation is normal behavior in both genders during the preschool years. The child experiences pleasurable sensations, which lead to repetition of the behavior. However, if masturbation is "excessive" or demonstrates "extreme modesty" or involves "acting out of sexual intercourse" or "mimicry of adult seductive behavior," the possibility of sexual abuse must be explored (Kleigman et al., 2007).

Education of the parents consists of assuring them that this behavior is normal and not harmful to the child, who is merely curious about sexuality. The cultural and moral background of the family must be considered when assessing the degree of discomfort in relation to this experience. A history of the time and place of masturbation and the parental response is helpful. Punitive reactions are discouraged because these can be potentially harmful to the child. Parents are advised to try to ignore the behavior and to distract the child with some other activity. If the parent calls unnecessary attention to this behavior, the child's anxiety level and masturbation activity may increase. The child needs to know that masturbation is not acceptable in public; however, this must be accomplished in a nonthreatening manner. Children who masturbate excessively and who have experienced a great deal of disruption in their lives may benefit from ongoing counseling.

LANGUAGE AND SPEECH IMPAIRMENT

The child communicates through speech and language skills. Speech is defined as the utterance of vocal sounds conveying ideas; language is a defined set of characters that, when used alone or in combinations, form a meaningful set of words and symbols that are used for communication.

Parents need to be aware of delays in language development as the child matures. Most children say 10 words by 18 months, 50 words and two-word phrases by 24 months, and so on. Language delay is often a symptom of a larger developmental disorder. Possible causes include hearing loss, mental retardation, learning disabilities, severe emotional disturbances, and certain genetic or organic problems. It is important to recognize milestone achievements. Any signs of problems in language or speech development need to be evaluated (Table 8-3).

Speech impairment can include articulation problems (distorting consonants or omitting consonants), voice disorders (deviations in pitch, loudness, or quality), and rhythm disorders (stuttering and stammering). Stuttering is the involuntary repetition of words or speech sounds, whereas stammering includes an involuntary pause in the formation of words. Speech therapy may be necessary for each of these problems. Remember to provide support to families as well.

HEALTH PROMOTION AND MAINTENANCE

DAILY CARE

Preschoolers are able to provide self-care almost totally, especially as they reach 5 years of age. They like to do things for themselves. Simple clothes make it easy for them to dress. A hook on the door within easy reach is

Table 8-3	Warning Signs of Speech or Language Disorders
AGE RANGE	**SIGNS**
First 12 months	Does not coo by 6 months Does not turn to voice sounds by 6 months Does not babble by 10 months Does not respond to own name by 12 months Does not use gestures such as waving "bye-bye" by 12 months
12 to 24 months	Does not use at least 35 to 50 words by 2 years Does not use two-word utterances by 2 years Does not imitate words or actions by 2 years Does not follow simple instructions by 2 years
24 to 36 months	Does not combine words into short phrases/sentences by 3 years Frequent expression of frustration in communicative situations Does not interact or play with others Unable to understand and answer simple questions
4 years	Unable to be understood by people outside of family Cannot retell simple stories or recall recent events clearly Sentences seem unorganized, with a lot of errors

Modified from Carey, W., Crocker, A., Elias, E., et al. (2009). *Developmental-behavioral pediatrics* (4th ed.). Philadelphia: Saunders.

helpful. They should dress and undress themselves as much as they can. A simple hairstyle is easily managed by the preschooler. Mother or father can assist with daily care but should not take over. Preschoolers may still need supervision with hygiene and may need to be reminded to use the toilet from time to time. Some 3-year-olds may still need assistance to get up onto the seat. A stool kept next to the bathroom sink enables them to wash their hands. They need to be reminded to do this after use of the toilet.

Brushing teeth still needs supervision. Children must be reminded to brush their teeth regularly. Parents still need to check that all tooth surfaces are cleaned, and they should floss the child's teeth. The child needs to visit a dentist regularly, at least every 6 months. Children generally have all 20 of their deciduous teeth by 3 years of age. The first dental visit should have occurred by the first birthday. The deciduous teeth are important for the proper formation of the permanent teeth and should not be neglected. The child's diet should continue to emphasize milk, vegetables, and fruits. Excess sweets, which contribute to dental decay, are restricted. The child should still drink fluoridated water or receive a prescribed oral fluoride supplement.

Preschool children need simple, nourishing meals, prepared with foods according to the basic food groups (see MyPyramid, Figure 7-5). Like toddlers, preschoolers do not like foods mixed together. They also have varying interest in food, and their appetites go up and down. Preschoolers require about 1600 kcal/day for a moderately active child (U.S. Department of Agriculture, 2005). It is also important to provide protein, calcium, iron, and plenty of vitamins A and C. Continue to limit juice intake to 4 to 6 ounces per day. Too much juice can provide excess kilocalories or limit milk intake. Their appetites fluctuate, and they should not be bribed, scolded, or coaxed. Encourage children to try different foods as they get older. If they did not like it in the past, they may like it now. Focus positively instead of negatively. Mealtimes should be happy. Parents who use good table manners set an example. Appropriate eating utensils should be introduced to promote independent feeding.

 Health Promotion

Cultural Nutritional Difference

Health care professionals need to understand:
- The variety of culture traditions that relate to food as well as food practices within and among cultures.
- Different cultures view body weight differently and may view excessive weight as healthy.

Preschool children need periods of active play both indoors and outdoors. Parents who see that their children are having a particularly good time should ask themselves whether it is necessary to interrupt them right at that moment. When children have verbal arguments, parents should avoid rushing in to defend their child. Growth can be painful, but children need to do it at their own rate.

Sleep habits at this time vary. Toward the end of this stage, children may balk at taking a nap. Instead of insisting that they sleep, parents should see that they engage in something interesting but restful, such as reading a story together or playing with a simple puzzle. They need an opportunity to relax. Bedtime rituals are still important, and children may use these to put off going to bed. In addition, preschool children may wake up frightened during the night. Everyday items in the bedroom become frightening at night because of the child's imagination. Parents should attend to their needs and reassure them that they are safe and that the parents are close by. A night-light may be helpful. If the children continue waking up and are usually frightened, parents should talk to the doctor during one of the checkups. Children of this age should

have a complete physical examination each year. Booster injections of various immunizations are given when required.

 Community Considerations

Bright Futures (*www.brightfutures.org*) is a national health promotion initiative that provides an array of publications to health care clinicians and families. One such publication is an activity book (also available in Spanish) that teaches young children about health and safety. Children can color, draw, fill in the blanks, tell stories, and talk about staying healthy and being safe. They learn about nutrition, fitness, self-expression, safety, and oral health.

PRESCHOOL

The change from home to preschool or nursery school is a big step toward independence. At this age, the child is adjusting to the outside world and to the family group. Some children have the complicating factor of a new baby in the house. The child also finds at this time that parents are beginning to expect more in regard to neatness and cooperative play with others. A good preschool provides the child with opportunities to get rid of some pent-up emotions with room to run and shout and a variety of toys to explore. Children are not as emotionally involved with the teacher as they are with their parents, so they may be more willing to express their negative and positive feelings. The teacher expects the child to become more independent by deciding what materials to play with and with whom to play. Children begin to take responsibility for their own belongings.

Children are accepted into preschools between 2 and 5 years of age. Most sessions last about 3 hours. This may be a child's first exposure to different cultures. A good nursery school should challenge the child's imagination and creativity (Figure 8-4). It

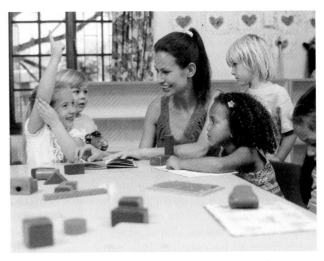

FIGURE 8-4 In the preschool setting, children are exposed to a variety of activities to enhance development of multiple intelligences.

should also attempt to acquaint children with the new social world in such a way that it adds to their security and increases independence. Parents can help with the transition to daycare or preschool attendance by having the child take a family picture, favorite toy, or stuffed animal for comfort. Always discuss the experience at the end of the day, and ask the teacher for feedback as well. The Health Promotion box provides some daycare or preschool guidelines.

Health Promotion

Child Care Guidelines

Parents who are considering preschool for their child should evaluate the following factors:
- Are the teachers trained in CPR?
- How many children are there per teacher?
- Are the teachers prepared in early childhood education?
- Are the physical facilities adequate?
- What is the cost? Is the child ready for preschool?
- Parents should also visit the school and talk with the person in charge before the child starts the program. They may also wish to talk with parents whose children are attending the program. Parents should feel free to drop in to a daycare or preschool *at any time* unannounced.

An opportunity to visit a preschool can be a rewarding experience if nurses use their powers of observation. When observing an individual child, nurses should compare him or her with others in the age group and not merely with one other child. The types of behavior to be observed are outlined in Box 8-1.

PLAY IN HEALTH AND ILLNESS

VALUE OF PLAY

It has often been said that play is the work of children. Investigations stress the importance of play to both the well and the sick child's physical, mental, emotional, and social development. Children climbing on a jungle gym develop coordination of muscles and exercise all parts of the body. They use up energy and develop feelings of self-confidence. Their imaginations may take them to a jungle where they are swinging from limb to limb. They mentally face fears and solve problems that would be much more trying, if not impossible, in reality. They communicate with the other children and take a further step in the development of moral values, such as learning to take one's turn and learning consideration for others. Other types of play help them learn colors, shapes, sizes, and textures and teach them to be creative. This natural and readily available outlet must be tapped by institutional personnel. Preschool children may be unfamiliar with

Box 8-1   Observing the Preschool Child

Objective: To observe the behavioral characteristics of the preschool child

Watch for and evaluate the following in terms of a child's security and independence:

PHYSICAL DEVELOPMENT
Ability to walk, run, jump, use play equipment
General health: easily fatigued, and so on

EMOTIONAL DEVELOPMENT
Easily excited
Whines, cries frequently
Evidence of temper tantrums
Persistence in a task
Aggressive
Shy
Reaction to failure

SOCIAL DEVELOPMENT
Talkative
Quiet
Plays with others
Plays near others
Special friends
Tends to lead
Tends to follow
Friendly toward other children and adults
Ability to share
Ability to take turns
Behavior when an object or attention of the teacher is desired

DEGREE OF INDEPENDENCE
Removing coat, hat, boots; putting them away
Attending to toilet needs
Getting a drink
Amount of time going from one activity to another
Dependence on adult suggestions and help

RELAXATION
Relaxes during rest periods
Sits and listens to stories
Is restless, in constant motion

SPECIFIC ROUTINES
Music period: Sings, plays games
Snacks: Eats lunch, takes other children's food, wanders about, disturbs others, plays with food
Free play period: Toys preferred, amount of skill using hands, span of interest, evidence of destructive play, plays with others or alone, has imaginary friend

every facet of the hospital, but they know how to play, and playing is a good way for the nurse to establish rapport with them.

THE NURSE'S ROLE

Some hospitals have well-established Child Life programs supervised by play therapists. Play experience may be included during the nurse's education. It is not necessary to be an expert in manual dexterity, art, or music. To be of assistance, one must be able to understand the needs of the child. Play is not just the responsibility of those who are assigned to it, nor is it confined to certain times or shifts.

Many factors are involved in providing suitable play for children of various ages in the hospital. The child's state of health has to be considered. This determines the amount of activity in which the child can participate. The nurse can provide many activities that relieve stress and provide enjoyment for the child on bed rest. Overstimulation, nevertheless, is hazardous for the severely ill child, such as the child with a heart disorder, because he or she needs to conserve strength. Nurses should always be on guard for signs of fatigue or pain in a child and should use their judgment accordingly. Basically, toys should be safe, durable, and suited to the child's developmental level. Children love to go to the hospital playroom. If they are unable (e.g., during isolation), toys may be brought to their rooms. Proper cleaning per hospital policy is required of any toy used by any child in the hospital before it is returned to the playroom or used by other children.

Health Promotion

Choosing Toys

AGE	TOYS	GENERAL CONSIDERATIONS
Infant	Soft stuffed animals and dolls Cradle gym Soft balls Bath toys Rattles Pots and pans	Likes to pat and hug. Toys should be brightly colored, of different textures, washable. Large enough so that they cannot be aspirated. Smooth edges. Attention span is short. Looks at, reaches, grabs, chews.
Toddler	Nest of blocks Push-pull toys Dolls Toy telephone Rocking horse or chair Wooden pegs and hammer Cloth books Pots and pans Ball	May have favorite toy. Enjoys exploring drawers and closets. Likes to place things in containers and dump them out. Parallel play. May injure others.
Preschooler	Crayons Simple puzzles Paints with large brushes Finger paints Dolls Dishes, housekeeping equipment Sandbox, playground equipment Floating boats for water play Trucks Horns, drums, simple musical instruments Books about familiar circumstances CDs; audiocassettes	Shifts from solitary to parallel to beginning cooperative play. Exchanges ideas with others. Active play: climbs, runs, and hammers. Imitative play: firefighter, teacher. Imaginative play: Let's pretend. Creative and dramatic play. Toys that do not require fine hand coordination. Games that teach safety in everyday life.
School age	Dolls and doll house Toy housewares Handicrafts Jump rope Skates Construction sets Trains Dress-up materials Table games Books for self-reading Bicycles Puppets Music Video games/computer games	Attention span increases. Play is more organized, more competitive. Interested in hobbies or collections of things.

Continued

Health Promotion—cont'd

AGE	TOYS	GENERAL CONSIDERATIONS
Convalescent child	(Many toys previously listed are also applicable.) Telephone Easy puzzles Large beads to string Tape player Goldfish bowl Miniature autos, trains, dolls, farm animals Stick'ems, paper dolls Hand puppets Lap blackboard Alphabet boards Cutouts VCR or DVD player; videos or DVDs to watch	Play should not require a great expenditure of energy. Offer a wide variety because the child's interest span is decreased. Consider bed limitation. Toys should not require long, continuous focusing of eyes. Consider toys that are a little easier than those liked when well. Pay attention to special interests of individual child.

Toys should not be sharp or have parts that can be easily removed and swallowed. Too many toys at one time confuse the child. Complicated toys are frustrating and disappointing. Well-selected toys, such as balls, blocks, and dolls, are useful throughout the years. Three-year-olds participate in simple games, and four-year-olds have longer attention spans and can participate in group activities. Preschoolers of all ages enjoy coloring and "reading" books. Each child needs sufficient time to complete the activity. In general, quiet play should precede meals and bedtime for both the well and the sick child.

The nurse can utilize play as distraction during routine and painful procedures with nursery rhymes, stories, nonsense games, songs, or finger play. Simple crafts can utilize materials found on the hospital unit, such as tongue depressors, tape, or bits of cotton. An older child may find making a scrapbook, storybook, or diary about the hospital experience rewarding. Games such as scavenger hunts on the nursing unit can assist in encouraging ambulation.

Music can be provided by radio or tape, CD, or MP3 player. Most hospitals have VCRs/DVDs and video and computer games available, as well as a supply of children's media. Drawing materials, finger paints, and modeling clay foster expression and creativity. They require merely a flat surface such as the over-bed table and the particular medium, and even the bedridden child can participate in messy projects. Many hospitals now provide Internet access, which can allow older children to correspond with friends by e-mail.

Nurses can encourage children to play together in the hospital if their condition warrants. Children need playmates to promote social development. Children who are ambulatory can visit other children in the playroom. The 1-year-old plays near other children. The 2-year-old grabs, pushes, and cannot share but in an individual way acknowledges other children. The older preschool child shows a beginning readiness for cooperative play. The ability to play with others increases during the school years and in late elementary years; girls prefer to play with girls, and boys prefer to play with boys. This preference changes during adolescence. It is important for children of all ages to socialize as much as possible with other children while in the hospital.

OTHER ASPECTS OF PLAY
Therapeutic Play
Play and toys can have a therapeutic value. A musical instrument such as the clarinet promotes flexion and extension of the fingers. Blowing bubbles is an excellent prerequisite for speech therapy or improving pulmonary function. Child life therapists supervise such activities. They should leave specific instructions if they wish their work reinforced on the unit.

The nurse can ask the child to draw a picture or make up a story; this can provide the nurse with insight to fears the child may be experiencing. What children *say* about what they draw can also be important in understanding a child's concerns and is an important communication technique (Driessnack, 2006).

Play Therapy
Play therapy is a technique used by psychotherapists to evaluate problems that require psychotherapy. Young children can express their concerns, fears, and developmental issues in a safe setting using whatever articles or activities he or she chooses. Other types of therapy that can be used include behavior, family, or group therapy.

Art Therapy
Art has been defined by Elinor Ulman as "the meeting ground of the world inside and the world outside." Art therapy is a process that is useful in communicating with children and adults. It is becoming more

widely used. The art therapist is specially trained to assist children to express their feelings through drawings, clay, and other media. Some hospitals with inpatient mental health units have art therapy departments.

Role of the Nurse

The nurse who is with a child daily can describe his or her behavior. This is helpful if the child has emotional or social problems. It is important to describe good and poor behavior, conversations that you may feel are pertinent, and the relationships with other children in the hospital. What is the approach to play? Do they join in freely or linger outside the group? Do they prefer active or quiet activities? Do they seem to be able to tolerate frustrations? Can they talk with their playmates and communicate their ideas? What kind of attention span do they have? This type of charting is meaningful and should be used to describe the activities of pediatric patients so they may be better understood.

INJURY PREVENTION

Accidents are still a major threat during the years from 3 to 5. Preschoolers need to follow the same injury prevention guidelines as toddlers. (See the Health Promotion box titled Injury Prevention—Toddlers in Chapter 7.) At this age, children may also suffer injuries from a bad fall. Preschool children hurtle up and down stairs. They climb trees and stand up on swings. They play hard with their toys, particularly those they can mount. Stairways must be kept free from clutter. When buying toys, parents must be sure the toys are sturdy and can take a beating. Preschool children should *never* be asked to do anything that is potentially dangerous, such as carry a glass container or sharp knife to the kitchen sink.

Automobiles continue to be a threat. The use of car seats or booster seats needs to be enforced (depending on age and weight; see Chapter 7). Children should be taught where they can safely ride their tricycles. Once they begin to ride a two-wheeler, they need to wear a helmet every time they use the bike. This prevents brain injury and even death. They also need to be taught where they can safely play. For example, they should not be allowed to use a sled on streets that are not blocked off for this purpose. They must not play in or around the car. Whether they are asleep or awake, children this age must *never* be left alone in the car. In an attempt to "drive like Mommy," they can quickly set a car into motion. Accidents also have been caused by children left in cars who find matches or play with the cigarette lighter. When crossing a street or when in a parking lot, they need to hold hands with a grownup. They should not operate an electronic garage door.

The potential for drowning is a danger. Do not leave children alone in a bathtub, swimming pool, or near

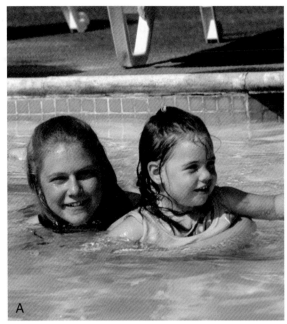

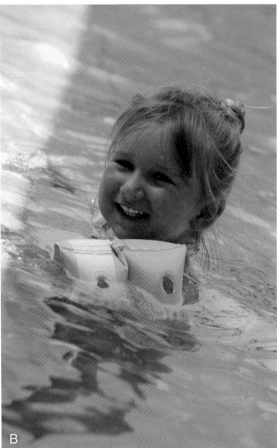

FIGURE 8-5 The preschooler should wear safety equipment while swimming and be accompanied by an adult.

any body of water. They can begin to learn to swim with supervision (Figure 8-5).

Burns that occur at this age are frequently caused by children's experimentation with matches. Children are also intrigued by cigarette lighters. These items are common hazards for this age group; they should be kept well out of reach, and their dangers should be explained.

Poisoning is still a danger. Children try to imitate adults and are apt to sample pills, especially if they smell good or look like candy. Their increased freedom brings them into contact with many interesting containers in the garage or basement. Poisons should *never* be put into used milk cartons or other household containers that would confuse children. Containers should be marked in such a way that the child knows it is a poison.

Trampoline injuries have been on the rise. The American Academy of Pediatrics does not advocate the use of home trampolines and further states that trampolines should not be regarded as play equipment. Trampolines have no place in outdoor playgrounds or in schools for routine physical education (AAP Policy Statement, 2006).

Preschool children should also be taught the dangers of talking to or accepting rides from strangers. They need to know that a stranger is someone they do not know, not just someone who is odd-looking. If they are stopped by a driver, they should run to a house where they know the people. Parents should make it clear to children in preschool that they will *never* send a stranger to see them or to pick them up. Children must know the dangers of playing in lonely places and of accepting gifts from strangers. Children should always know where to go if their mother or father cannot be found.

Preschool children still require a good deal of supervision to protect them from dangers that arise from their immature judgment or social environment.

Get Ready for the NCLEX® Examination!

Key Points

- The preschool period is marked by a slowing of the growth process and more well-developed muscle control.
- Preoperational thinking predominates, and preschoolers base their reasoning on what they see and hear. They also believe they have "magical" powers and can only understand their own viewpoint.
- Preschoolers' sense of initiative empowers them to try new activities and experiences. They still need to be supervised to prevent injury.
- Encouraging positive behavior helps eliminate the undesirable effects of punishment. When necessary, time out is an effective method of discipline.
- Common problems of preschoolers (bad language, jealousy, thumb sucking, masturbation, and enuresis) can be easily dealt with through gentle explanation or correction of behavior and reassurance.
- The attainment of milestones for speech and language needs to be evaluated with the preschooler.
- The older preschooler becomes almost completely independent in dealing with daily care.
- Preschools should be evaluated through parental visits and the evaluation of the facility.
- Play of preschoolers often involves the beginning of cooperative play and imaginative and imitative play.

Additional Learning Resources

evolve Go to your Evolve website (*http://evolve.elsevier.com/Price/pediatric/*) for the following FREE learning resources:
- 3-D Animations
- Answer Keys
- Appendixes
- Audio Glossary
- Spanish/English Glossary
- Video Clips

Review Questions for the NCLEX® Examination

1. A nursing student assesses the vital signs of a hospitalized 4-year-old as follows: pulse rate of 100, respirations of 20 per minute, and blood pressure of 94/56. These values:
   1. Indicate tachycardia
   2. Indicate tachypnea
   3. Indicate hypotension
   4. Are within normal range

2. According to Piaget, the 3-year-old preschool child is in the:
   1. Preconceptual stage
   2. Intuitive thought stage
   3. Stage of industry
   4. Oral stage

3. A preschool child is pretending that the bed is a boat and the rug is the sea. This is an example of:
   1. Egocentrism
   2. Artificialism
   3. Animism
   4. Symbolic functioning

4. The **most appropriate** toys for a preschooler include: (**Select all that apply.**)
   1. Pots and pans
   2. Push-pull toys
   3. Trucks
   4. Jump rope
   5. Finger paints

5. A 5-year-old child usually has a vocabulary of approximately:
   1. 900 words
   2. 1500 words
   3. 2100 words
   4. 3500 words

The School-Age Child

Objectives

1. Define the vocabulary terms listed
2. Describe the physical and psychosocial development of children from 6 to 12 years of age, listing, where appropriate, age-specific events and types of guidance
3. Discuss how to assist parents in preparing a child for school entry
4. List two ways in which school life influences the growing child
5. Identify the positive and negative aspects of television viewing and playing video games
6. Discuss safety issues related to the school-age child
7. Plan a diet that provides adequate nutrition for the school-age child

Key Terms

cyber bullying (p. 169)
latchkey children (p. 172)
latency (p. 162)

myelinization (MĪ-ĕ-lĭ-nĭ-ZĂ-shŭn; p. 161)
sibling rivalry (p. 161)

GENERAL CHARACTERISTICS AND DEVELOPMENT

School-age children between 6 and 12 years of age differ from preschool children in that they are more engrossed in fact than fantasy. They have an ardent thirst for knowledge and accomplishment. They admire teachers and adult companions whom they consider wise. They attempt to use the skills and the knowledge that they obtain to master activities that they enjoy—music, sports, art, and so on. Children in school learn that they must cooperate with others. Participation in group activities increases. Acceptance becomes paramount. The type of acceptance these children receive at home and at school affects the attitudes that they develop about themselves and their roles in life.

Children at this age are aware that their parents are only human and can make mistakes. Conflicts may arise, particularly if what the child learns in school differs from what is practiced at home. Between 6 and 12 years of age, children prefer friends of their own gender. They also prefer the company of their friends to that of their brothers and sisters. They find outward displays of affection by adults embarrassing. Sibling rivalry, intense feelings that can develop when a child feels he or she is competing for parental attention, can develop when a new infant sibling joins the family unit.

PHYSICAL GROWTH

Growth is slow until the spurt, which occurs directly before puberty. Weight gains are more rapid than increases in height. The average gain in weight per year is about 5½ to 7 pounds (2.5 to 3.2 kg). The average yearly increase in height is approximately 2 inches (5.5 cm). Head circumference increases only 2 to 3 cm throughout this entire period. This reflects slowed brain growth with complete brain growth occurring at 10 years of age. Myelinization, the growth process of the myelin sheath around the nerve fiber, is complete by 7 years of age and results in the refinement of fine-motor coordination (Kleigman et al., 2007).

Muscular coordination is improved, and the lymphatic tissues become highly developed. The skeletal bones continue to ossify. The body is supple, and sometimes skeletal growth is more rapid than the growth of muscles and ligaments. The child may appear gangling. There is a noticeable change in facial structure as the jaw lengthens. The sinuses are frequently sites of infection. Sinus headaches may occur. The 6-year molars (the first permanent teeth) erupt. The gastrointestinal tract is more mature. The heart grows slowly and is now smaller in proportion to body size than compared with any other point in time.

The shape of the eye also changes with growth. 20/40 vision is achieved by 3 years of age, 20/30 vision

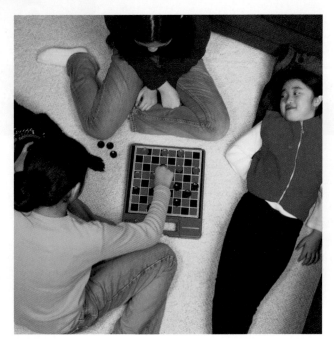

FIGURE 9-1 Competition can be common in the school years. Games can also assist in sharpening a child's cognitive skills.

by 4 years of age, and 20/30 by 5 to 6 years of age. Visual acuity can be measured by 2½ to 3 years of age (Kleigman et al., 2007). The capabilities of the child's sense organs, including hearing, have an important bearing on learning abilities.

The vital signs of the school-age child are similar to those of the adult. Temperature is 98.6° F (37° C), pulse is 60 to 95 beats per minute, and the respiratory rate is 14 to 22 breaths per minute. The systolic blood pressure ranges from 100 to 120 mm Hg, and the diastolic blood pressure ranges from 60 to 75 mm Hg. (See Chapter 3 for further discussion on vital signs.) Boys are slightly taller and somewhat heavier than girls until changes indicating puberty appear. The differences among children are greater at the end of middle childhood than at the beginning.

Language skills continue to develop. School-age children speak in full sentences. They continually add new words to their vocabulary. School-age children may swear to try and impress other children or to express anger. They also delight in the newly found use of humor. In the early school-age years, they delight their parents by telling "knock-knock" jokes.

In evaluating language development, the parent and the nurse should discuss the child's ability to comprehend and use both written and spoken language.

DEVELOPMENTAL THEORIES

According to Piaget's theory of cognitive development, the school-age child thinks and reasons in concrete terms, progressing from inductive to deductive logic. Children at this age learn to comprehend the ideas of conservation and reversibility. Conservation is the ability to recognize two equal quantities regardless of their form. For example, although the same amount of water appears less in a tall glass than in a short glass, the school-age child can determine that it is the same amount of water. Reversibility is the ability to think in either direction. School-age children can take a result and reverse it so as to determine whether it is correct or not. This concept is used in addition and subtraction.

According to Erikson's theories of psychosocial development, the school-age child is in the stage of industry versus inferiority. The child is a worker and producer and wants to accomplish tasks. Competitiveness is common (Figure 9-1). The school-age child's social world is continually expanding, and he or she achieves new competencies. However, without success in this area, they feel inferior. Parents and teachers need to support children in achieving success and developing self-esteem.

Kohlberg's moral development theory describes the school-age child as being at the "conventional level." Rules are the basis for moral judgments, and they must be followed to please others. The school-age child begins to understand what is right and what is wrong. As a result, the child develops a conscience.

Freud believes that at this stage romantic love for the parent of the opposite gender diminishes and that the children start to identify with the parent of the same gender. This is also a period of latency when the child's energy is directed toward cognitive and physical skills. This, however, does not imply a complete lack of sexual activity at this age.

BIOLOGICAL AND PSYCHOSOCIAL DEVELOPMENT

Table 9-1 summarizes growth and development for the various school-age groups.

THE 6-YEAR-OLD

Six-year-old children are bursting with energy and are always on the go. They soon become overtired, and it is necessary to set limits to their activities. Although they like to start tasks, they do not always finish them because their attention span is fairly brief. They tend to be bossy and sometimes rude, but they are sensitive to criticism. Sex investigations begun in earlier years may persist. Their conscience is active, and they find it difficult to make decisions.

One of the most obvious physical changes at this age is the loss of the temporary teeth. The important 6-year molars also erupt. Six-year-old children can jump rope, throw and catch a ball, and tie shoelaces. They perform numerous other feats that require muscle coordination. Their language differs from that of the preschool child. These children use language for a

Table 9-1 Growth and Development During School-Age Years

AGE (YR)	PHYSICAL AND MOTOR	MENTAL	ADAPTIVE	PERSONAL-SOCIAL
6	Growth and weight gain continue slowly Weight: 16 to 23.6 kg (35.5 to 53 lb); height: 106.6 to 123.5 cm (42 to 48 in) Central mandibular incisors erupt Loses first tooth. Gradual increase in dexterity Active age; constant activity Often returns to finger feeding More aware of hand as a tool Likes to draw, print, and color Vision reaches maturity	Develops concept of numbers Counts 13 pennies Knows whether it is morning or afternoon Defines common objects such as fork and chair in terms of their use Obeys triple commands in succession Knows right and left hands Says which is pretty and which is ugly in a series of drawings of faces Describes objects in a picture rather than simply enumerating them Attends first grade	At table, uses knife to spread butter or jam on bread At play, cuts, folds, pastes paper toys, sews crudely if needle is threaded Takes bath without supervision; performs bedtime activities alone Reads from memory; enjoys oral spelling game Likes table games, checkers, simple card games Giggles a lot Sometimes steals money or attractive items Has difficulty owning up to misdeeds Tries out own abilities	Can share and cooperate better Has great need for children of own age Cheats to win Often engages in rough play Often jealous of younger brother or sister Does what adults are seen doing May have occasional temper tantrums Is a boaster Is more independent, probably influence of school Has own way of doing Increases socialization
7	Begins to grow at least 5 cm (2 in) per yr Weight: 17.7 to 30 kg (39 to 66.1 lb); height: 111.8 to 129.7 cm (44 to 51 in) Maxillary central incisors and lateral mandibular incisors erupt More cautious in approaches to new performances Repeats performances to master them Jaw begins to expand to accommodate permanent teeth	Notices that certain parts are missing from pictures Can copy a diamond Repeats three numbers backward Develops concept of time; reads ordinary clock or watch correctly to nearest quarter hour; uses clock for practical purposes Attends the second grade More mechanical in reading; often does not stop at the end of a sentence, skips words such as "it," "the," and "he"	Uses table knife for cutting meat; may need help with tough or difficult pieces Brushes and combs hair acceptably without help May steal Likes to help and have a choice Is less resistant and stubborn	Is becoming a real member of the family group Takes part in group play Boys prefer playing with boys; girls prefer playing with girls Spends a lot of time alone; does not require a lot of companionship

Continued

Table 9-1   Growth and Development During School-Age Years—cont'd

AGE (YR)	PHYSICAL AND MOTOR	MENTAL	ADAPTIVE	PERSONAL-SOCIAL
8 to 9	Continues to grow at 5 cm (2 in) a yr Weight: 19.6 to 39.6 kg (43 to 87 lb); height: 117 to 141.8 cm (46 to 56 in) Lateral incisors (maxillary) and mandibular cuspids erupt Movement fluid; often graceful and poised Always on the go; jumps, chases, skips Increased smoothness and speed in fine-motor control; uses cursive writing Dresses self completely Likes to overdo; hard to quiet down after recess More limber; bones grow faster than ligaments	Gives similarities and differences between two things from memory Counts backward from 20 to 1; understands concept of reversibility Repeats days of the week and months in order; knows the date Describes common objects in detail, not merely their use Makes change out of a quarter Attends third and fourth grades Reads more; may plan to wake up early just to read Reads classic books but also enjoys comics More aware of time; can be relied on to get to school on time Can grasp concepts of parts and whole (fractions) Understands concepts of space, cause and effect Classifies objects by more than one quality; has collections Produces simple paintings or drawings	Makes use of common tools such as hammer, saw, or screwdriver Uses household and sewing utensils Helps with routine household tasks such as dusting, sweeping Assumes responsibility for share of household chores Looks after all of own needs at table Buys useful articles; exercises some choice in making purchases Runs useful errands Likes pictorial magazines Likes school; wants to answer all the questions Is afraid of failing a grade; is ashamed of bad grades Is more critical of self Takes music and sport lessons	Is easy to get along with at home Likes the reward system Dramatizes Is more sociable Is better behaved Is interested in boy-girl relationships but does not admit it Goes about home and community freely, alone or with friends Likes to compete and play games Shows preference in friends and groups Plays mostly with groups of own gender but is beginning to mix Develops modesty Compares self with others Enjoys Scouts, group sports
10 to 12	Weight: 24.3 to 58 kg (54 to 128 lb); height: 127.5 to 162.3 cm (50 to 64 in) Posture is more similar to an adult's; overcomes lordosis Boys: Slow growth in height and rapid weight gain; may become obese in this period Girls: Pubescent changes may begin to appear; body lines soften and round out Remainder of teeth erupt and tend toward full development (except wisdom teeth)	Writes brief stories Attends fifth to seventh grades Writes occasional short letters to friends or relatives on own initiative Uses telephone for practical purposes Responds to magazine, radio, or other advertising Reads for practical information or own enjoyment (stories or library books of adventure or romance or animal stories)	Makes useful articles or does easy repair work Cooks or sews in small way Raises pets Washes and dries own hair Is responsible for a thorough job of cleaning hair, but may need reminding to do so Is sometimes left alone at home for an hour or so Is successful in looking after own needs or those of other children left in his or her care	Loves friends; talks about them constantly Chooses friends more selectively; may have a "best friend" Enjoys conversation Develops beginning interest in opposite gender Is more diplomatic Likes family; family really has meaning Likes mother and wants to please her in many ways Demonstrates affection Likes father who is adored and idolized Respects parents

From Hockenberry, M.J., and Wilson, D. (2007). *Wong's nursing care of infants and children* (8th ed.). St. Louis: Mosby.

purpose rather than for the pure joy of talking. Their vocabulary consists of about 2500 words. They need 11 to 13 hours of sleep a night.

Although 6-year-old children begin to show a preference for associating with children of the same gender, boys and girls do still play together at this age. Certain activities, such as imaginative play, are common to both genders. Most children enjoy collecting objects that catch their fancy, such as leaves, stones, and shells. Play at this time usually reflects events that occur in the immediate environment.

Six-year-old children need time and support to help them adjust to school. If they have nursery school or kindergarten experience, the transition may be more comfortable. Most children go to school expecting the same atmosphere they are accustomed to at home. For example, if parents are critical or overly protective, children automatically assume that the teacher will be too. When the experience at school differs markedly from their expectations, they feel insecure and may be hostile toward the teacher. Parents need to observe children for signs of fatigue and stress. Although they have reached the appropriate age, not all children are ready for school. Children who are ready for school still need time and support from parents and teachers before they can settle down and become completely comfortable in the classroom. At school, the child is also exposed more frequently to infection. Preschool immunizations and a physical examination are indicated.

THE 7-YEAR-OLD

Children at 7 years of age are generally less of a problem than they were at 6 years. It is a quieter age, and the child does not go looking for trouble. Some educators have noted that second graders are the easiest to teach. They set high standards for themselves and for their family, have a good sense of humor, tend to enjoy teasing (wiggle loose teeth to annoy adults), and are a little more modest than they were at an earlier age. They enjoy being active but can also appreciate periods of rest. The second grader may acquire a "crush" on a friend of the opposite gender.

These children know the months and seasons of the year. They also begin to tell time. They have a beginning concept of arithmetic, can count by twos and fives, and know that money is valuable. Their hands are steadier. Interest in God and heaven is heightened.

Active play is still important to both genders (Figure 9-2). The boys are more apt to tease the girls than to participate in such games as jump rope or tag. Both genders enjoy bike riding and table games. Realistic toys, such as dolls that can be bathed and fed or trains that back up and whistle, appeal to the 7-year-old. Comic books are also popular (Figure 9-3). Becoming increasingly independent, these children imagine

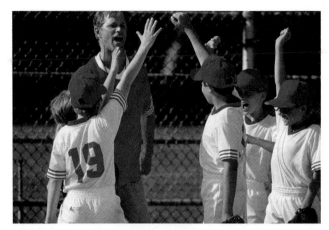

FIGURE 9-2 Organized activities provide both genders with physical and emotional outlets.

themselves accomplishing feats more adventurous than those of their parents.

Stealing

Stealing is one problem that may arise during this age. This is generally a sign that some need of the child is not being met. It may be actual or perceived. In many cases, the child steals only to distribute the loot to neighborhood friends. This may in actuality be an attempt to buy friendship. The children's independence has separated them to a degree from their parents. As a result, if they cannot establish good relationships with their friends, they may feel left out. When children steal something, parents should tell them that they are aware of the fact and should insist on some form of restitution. They should not humiliate the child, but they must make it clear that such actions are not permitted. As always, accept the child but not the deed. Afterward, try to understand the circumstances that are causing such behavior.

THE 8-YEAR-OLD

The 8-year-old wants to do everything and can play alone for longer periods than a 7-year-old. Work is usually creative. Group activities such as Brownies and Cub Scouts are enjoyed, and companions of the same gender are preferred. Group fads begin to appear. Eight-year-olds like to be considered important, particularly by adults. They may behave better for company than for the family. Hero worship is evident.

The arms and hands of the 8-year-old seem to grow faster than the rest of the body. The large and small muscles are better developed, and movements are smoother and more graceful. The child can write rather than only print. The child also understands that a certain number of days must pass before special events, such as Christmas, birthdays, or discharge from the hospital, can occur.

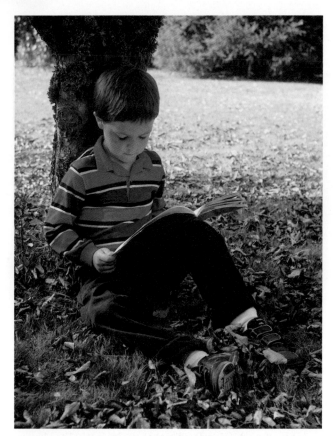

FIGURE 9-3 Reading can become an enjoyable activity. It should be encouraged.

Competitive sports are enjoyed, but the child is generally a poor loser. Long involved arguments occur over decisions made by referees. Wrestling is frequent, and dramatic play is popular. Most children like to be the hero or heroine of their favorite program. Neighborhood secret clubs are organized, and all members must pay strict attention to the rules.

THE 9-YEAR-OLD

The 9-year-old is dependable and is not as restless as the 8-year-old child. More interest is shown in family activities, and more responsibility is assumed for personal belongings and for younger brothers and sisters. Tasks are also more likely to be completed. Children resist adult authority if it does not coincide with their opinions or ideals. They are, however, more able to accept criticism regarding their actions. Individual differences are pronounced.

Worries and mild compulsions are common. Children avoid cracks in the pavement: "Step on a crack, break your mother's back." They realize that these actions are senseless but still feel obliged to repeat them. Nervous habits may also appear and may widely vary; nail biting is one example. The child should not be scolded for such actions because they are caused primarily by tension. Nervous habits usually disappear when home and social life become more relaxed.

Hand-eye coordination is well developed, and manual activities are managed with skill. The child works and plays hard and often becomes overtired. About 10 hours of sleep a night are needed. The permanent teeth are still erupting.

Competitive sports, reading, listening to music, and watching television and movies are popular. Contact sports should be limited to minimize permanent growth-related injuries (Figure 9-4). The child begins to develop interests such as music and may desire to take lessons. Children know the date, can repeat months of the year in order, can multiply, and do simple division. They take care of their bodily needs, and by now table manners have considerably improved.

THE 10-YEAR-OLD

This marks the beginning of the preadolescent years. Girls are more physically mature than boys. The child begins to show self-direction, is courteous to adults, and thinks quite clearly about social problems and prejudices. Although 10-year-olds want to be independent and resent being told what to do, they are receptive to suggestion. The ideas of the group are more important than individual ideas. Interest in sex and sex investigations continue.

Girls are often more poised than boys. Both genders are fairly reliable about household duties. Slang terms are used. The 10-year-old can write for a relatively long period of time and maintains a good writing speed. The child uses fractions and knows numbers over 100. Boys and girls begin to identify themselves with skills that pertain to their particular gender role. There is an intolerance of the opposite gender. The play enjoyed by the 10-year-old is similar to that enjoyed by the 9-year-old. In addition, the child takes more interest in appearance.

THE 11- TO 12-YEAR-OLD

Adjectives that describe this age group include *intense, observant, all-knowing, energetic, meddlesome,* and *argumentative.* This period before the onset of puberty is one of complete disorganization. It may begin earlier in some children than others because the onset and rate of physical maturity greatly vary. Before the end of this period, the hormones of the body begin to influence physical growth. Posture is poor. There are 24 to 26 permanent teeth.

The child has an overabundance of energy and is constantly on the go. Girls become "tomboyish" in their actions. Table manners are a thing of the past, and the refrigerator is constantly emptied. Children this age are less concerned with appearance. They seem to be preoccupied a great deal of the time. This, along with physical activities and numerous anxieties, partially accounts for the decline in school grades. Ability to concentrate decreases and parents complain that the

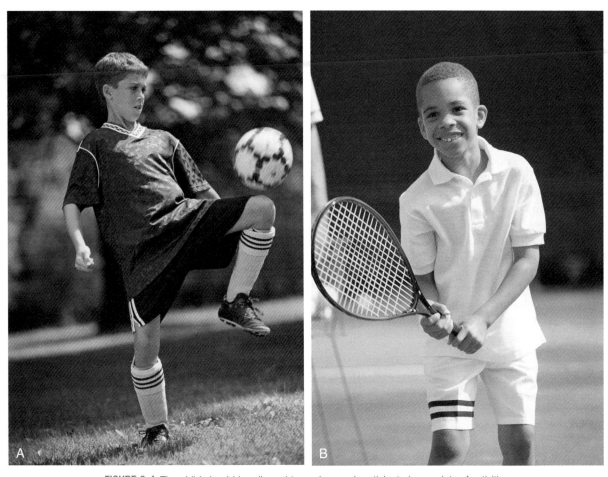

FIGURE 9-4 The child should be allowed to explore and participate in a variety of activities.

children "never hear anything." When asked to do a new task, they moan and groan.

Groups of friends are still important (Figure 9-5). They are not ready to stand alone, but they cannot bear the thought of depending on their parents. They insist that they must overcome their problems without parental help. Their attitude implies, "Can't you see that I'm not a child anymore?"

The older school-age child also begins to see and understand other points of view. Morals and religious ideals become stronger. They begin to play with abstract ideas and become interested in the "whys" of health measures. They understand human reproduction. During prepuberty, they are very much interested in the body and watch for signs of growing up. Girls look forward to menstruation and wearing their first bra. Boys and girls tend to ignore those of the opposite gender, but in reality they are much aware of them. There is a tendency to tease one another. Their descriptions of each other are far from complimentary: "stupid," "crazy," "nerd." Both genders enjoy earning money by doing odd jobs. Preadolescents often seek an adult friend of the same gender to idolize.

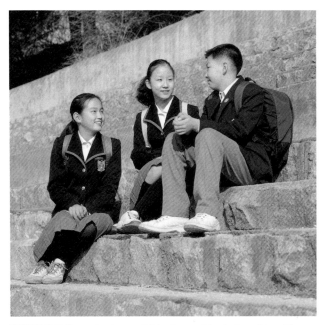

FIGURE 9-5 The school-age child relies on friends for advice. They are not always ready to ask parents to help with problem solving.

Guiding preadolescents is not easy. The primary task of the middle years of childhood is developing social competence. Parents and authority figures need to help children learn how to get along with peers and how to follow group rules. They need to set limits and establish consequences for unacceptable behavior. They also need to monitor television shows, video games, and music lyrics. Parents need to encourage self-discipline and teach young children to respect authority figures. School-age children need freedom within limits and recognition that they are no longer babies. They should know why parents make a decision. They should not be expected to blindly follow household rules. Their conscience enables them to understand and accept reasonable discipline. Constant verbal nagging is ignored. These children should be provided with constructive opportunities that enable them to get rid of pent-up emotions and energies. Their irritating behavior is more easily accepted once one realizes that a good deal of it is indeed "just a phase."

 Community Considerations

Anticipatory guidance at the school-age well checkup includes topics such as sex education, nutrition, physical activity, and injury prevention.

ENVIRONMENTAL INFLUENCES

SCHOOL

Schools have a profound influence on the socialization of children. Children bring to school what they have learned and experienced in the home. Although some children come from healthy intact families that are financially secure, many do not. Children themselves may be physically disabled, developmentally disabled, or abused; others may have a chronic illness (Figure 9-6). Parents may be unemployed or abusers of alcohol or other drugs or may have numerous other physical or stress-related conditions. In addition, children may be unable to verbalize their needs; therefore caretakers must become particularly astute in their observations. Even though children may seem similar, what each one is able to absorb intellectually is directly related to their emotional health and, more often than not, to the emotional health of the family. Schools reflect the social values and the economic standing of the community that supports them. If a community has various ethnic and economic groups, conflicts may appear in the schools. School-age children are exposed to many adults and peers whose values and expectations may be different from what they have experienced. In addition, children can no longer be protected from prejudices regarding beliefs, color, or ethnic background. The teacher becomes an important role model for the child. The child is

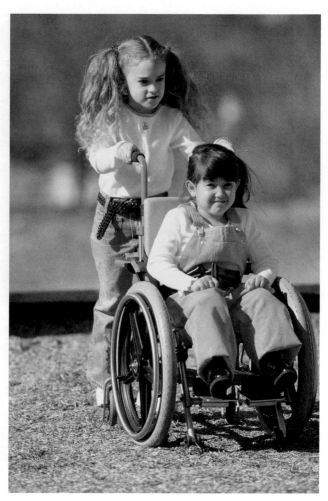

FIGURE 9-6 The school environment can provide the child with the opportunity to interact with children who have different backgrounds. For the child with a chronic condition, school can provide the opportunity to develop social and cognitive skills.

influenced by the teacher and by fellow students. The sensitive nurse can assist parents by affirming the individuality of children. The nurse should encourage parents to tell their children how proud they are of their academic progress.

School can be stressful for children, especially when they are first starting school or are changing schools. In these situations, parents and teachers need to be supportive of the child. It is also important that parents take an active role in their child's education by getting to know the child's teachers, volunteering in the school, and informing the teachers if there are unusual or sudden stressors in the child's life. Children who are starting school should be introduced to the crossing guard if they walk to school or to the bus driver if they ride the bus. Initially, they should also be supervised at the bus stop. School-age children should know their home phone number and address.

By the time a child reaches middle school, anticipatory guidance includes dealing with sex education, peer abuse, organization of time, and the increased hazards of substance abuse. The nurse can assess patterns of communication between the parents and the child and can assist with specific behavioral problems. Parents may have a problem letting go. The nurse can be supportive of their endeavors as long as they are in accordance with the child's maturity. The transition to junior high/middle school generally means multiple classrooms, a series of teachers, and a change of buildings. The child is developing adult characteristics and has new feelings about the body, parents, teachers, and peers. Anticipatory guidance includes a review of normal physiology and how it changes with puberty. Information concerning sexuality is reviewed, and the child is encouraged to ask questions whenever they arise. A warm, ongoing relationship between parents and child helps to provide a safe atmosphere of caring. Adults should develop a heightened awareness for such things as school attendance problems, tardiness, and signs of loneliness or depression. Parents should continue to encourage their children to discuss any school problems and worries with them. It is important to foster the child's ability to communicate with teachers, parents, and other authoritative figures. School-age children need to learn to understand what is right and what is wrong. They also need to learn how to manage anger and resolve conflicts without violence. It is important that parents and children set realistic goals. Adults should periodically ask themselves, "When was the last time this child had a success?" Homework should be the child's responsibility, with minimum assistance from parents.

GENDER

Children may face other problems in school. Research has identified that boys receive more praise than girls. Boys tend to get negative feedback concerning the quality of work such as neatness or spelling. On the other hand, girls get negative feedback about the content of their work. This causes boys to feel that their lack of success is from a lack of effort, and girls feel that their failure is from a lack of ability. Teachers, therefore, need to be more aware of possible biases. They also need to focus their attention on efforts, not gender.

BULLYING

Bullying is a problem for a staggering number of children in elementary and middle schools. A reported 5 million children have been victimized by this behavior. Bullying not only can result in long-term health and mental problems but also can have violent consequences. The U.S. Secret Service Initiative Report (2002) identified several key identifiers for school violence involving firearms. There is no stereotype for the individual, there is a plan of action, the individual usually tells of the plan, and the individual has easy access to a weapon. It was also noted that bullying can be a key factor in triggering the violence.

By being aware of the warning signs, the school nurse may be able to identify a child who is a victim of bullying (see the Community Considerations box). School officials should be involved because bullying usually occurs at school or on the way to and from school. The school environment should be safe for children, and additional adult supervision may be necessary. Both the victim and the bully need help. Victims and their families should be given tools that help them to deal with this problem. Bullies and their families also need to be given tools to help the bully achieve socially acceptable behavior. Children who display aggressive behavior and start bullying at a young age are at high risk for more serious social problems.

? Did You Know?

Warning Behaviors That a Child Is Being Bullied

SOMATIC
Stomach
Insomnia
New-onset enuresis
BEHAVIOR CHANGES
Irritability
Poor concentration
Refusal to attend school
SERIOUS PROBLEMS
School failure
Drug and alcohol abuse
Violence
Self-mutilation

From Scott, J.U., Hague-Armstrong, K., and Downes, K.L. (2003). Teasing and bullying: what can pediatricians do? *Contemp Pediatr, 20*(4), 105-120. Copyright © 2003, Advanstar Medical Economics Health Care, Inc. Reproduced with permission.

Teasing and bullying are serious problems. They need to be recognized, and action must be taken. School officials, health care providers, and parents need to work together to encourage acceptable behavior and healthy socialization. Parents and school officials can find guidelines for dealing with these problems online (*www.bullyproofing.com* and *www. stopbullyingnow.hrsa.gov*).

 Community Considerations

The Internet environment is continually changing. Children are using social networking such as "Facebook" or "Instant Messaging (IM)" instead of chatrooms. **Cyber bullying** or online harassment has increased by 50% from 2001 to 2006. Many children do not alert parents/guardians when an incident occurs. Parents should be more involved with their children's Internet activity (Wolak et al., 2006).

Health Promotion

Guidelines for Parents for Bullying and Teasing

VICTIM	BULLY
Do not overreact; use calm manner	Parents must be aware of the seriousness of the behavior
Listen to the child's perception of the problem	Determine the reason for the child's behavior
Use open-ended question to allow child to tell in his or her own words	Use expression of disappointment rather than anger when dealing with child
Use drawing if child has difficulty communicating	Encourage child's participation in organized, supervised activities
Discuss what makes children be bullies	
Review different options such as conflict resolution using forgiveness, shaking hands	Observe child in play settings
Older children can ignore the teasing event and seek other company	Enforce the philosophy that the parent will not tolerate behavior that hurts other people
Use role playing for practice	Respond to incidents of bullying with negative consequences
Encourage other friendships or organized activities such as clubs or teams	
Praise child who faces up to fears	Encourage discussion of bullying incidents with other individuals who may be involved, such as school officials
Reinforce to the child that the parent will protect him or her	
Parents can talk to witnesses for further information	Teach alternative approaches including negotiating skills
Parents can try to resolve conflict by involving the teaser's/bully's parents	Notice and reward good play behavior
Parents should involve any caregivers responsible for the teaser/bully	Consider mental health counselor if child does not respond or needs further understanding
Parents should approach school officials for incidents that occur on school grounds or function	
Consider group meeting of all involved individuals to resolve problem	
Parents can involve law enforcement	
Support school-sponsored programs that discourage teasing and bullying	

Adapted from Scott, J.U., Hague-Armstrong, K., & Downes, K.L. (2003). Teasing and bullying: what can pediatricians do? *Contemp Pediatr, 20*(4), 105-120. Copyright © 2003, Advanstar Medical Economics Health Care, Inc. Reproduced with permission.

TELEVISION

Television has a powerful influence on children. Television has been called the "great babysitter" of our time. Some complaints regarding children watching television are that (1) it does not challenge the imagination, (2) it interferes with solitude and play, and (3) it promotes materialism and passivity. Also, people portrayed on television are frequently stereotyped.

The American Academy of Pediatrics (AAP, 2009) recommends that parents should not only encourage the careful selection of programs but also watch and discuss the content with their children and adolescents. Parents should also create an "electronic media-free" environment in their children's rooms.

Health Promotion

Television

CONSEQUENCES OF EXCESSIVE TELEVISION

- Displaces active types of recreation
- Interferes with conversation and discussion time
- Discourages reading
- Leads to poorer school performance (if more than 4 hours of television watching per day)
- Discourages exercise
- Affects how a child feels toward life and other people if television shows are violent
- Promotes and encourages material possessions

PARENTAL GUIDELINES FOR POSITIVE TELEVISION VIEWING

- Encourage active recreation.
- Read to children.
- Limit television to 2 hours or less per day ($\frac{1}{2}$ hour if child is doing poorly in school).
- Do not allow television to be used as a distraction or babysitter for preschool children.
- Turn off television during meals.
- Teach critical viewing.
- Teach children to turn off the television at the end of a show.
- Encourage children to watch educational television shows.
- Forbid violent television shows; discuss reality of violence.
- Discuss purpose of commercials.
- Discuss reality and make-believe.
- Set a good example.

Modified from Schmitt, B.D. RelayHealth. Patient Education. Television: reducing the negative impact. MD Consult Web Site. Retrieved June 10, 2010, from *www.mdconsult.com/das/patient/body/204585162-2/0/10068/18586.html*.

VIDEO GAMES

Video games have become the second favorite pastime of children (Figure 9-7). The advantages of video games include the development of eye-hand coordination, visual perception, attention to details, and the interactive component. Children are always using various strategies to win the game.

As the video game industry has grown, the amount of time children spend playing and the level of graphic violence have also increased. Violence in video games can either be fantasy based or human based. Players can be awarded points for killing people or animals. With the improved graphics, these games are very

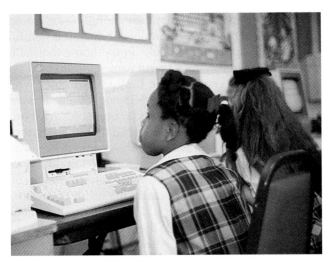

FIGURE 9-7 Children spend several hours per week both at home and school using a computer. Any computer games should be monitored by parents and school officials.

realistic. The violence found in television, video games, and the Internet has decreased the sensitivity to violent actions. Children viewing violence and aggression feel it is normal behavior and begin to imitate it (Marx et al., 2009).

Parents should monitor the ratings of video games. The Entertainment Software Rating Board (ESRB) rates games for computers and home video systems. Parents can find ratings for specific software at their website (*www.esrb.org*).

Health Promotion

CONSEQUENCES OF EXCESSIVE VIDEO GAME PLAYING
- Dominates leisure and study time
- Promotes solitary activity, reducing social interaction with family and friends
- Encourages acceptance of violent behavior in real life
- Leads to fallen grades, inadequate sleep, decrease in outdoor play, and social isolation

PARENTAL GUIDELINES FOR VIDEO GAME PLAYING
- Limit to 2 hours or less per day.
- Encourage games without excessive violence.
- Provide educational games.
- Encourage alternative activities such as physical games, reading.

From Schmitt, B.D. RelayHealth. Patient Education. Video games. MD Consult Web Site. Retrieved June 10, 2010, from *www.mdconsult.com/das/patient/body/204585162-2/0/10068/18906.html*.

PEERS

Peer relationships that form during the school-age years can greatly affect the socialization of the school-age child. Peers can positively and negatively influence school-age children. At this age, children can also be influenced through joining informal "clubs" that have official rules and secret passwords or joining formalized, cooperative groups such as scouts. Older school-age children, especially with limited family interaction or cohesiveness, can be drawn into formal gang activity as it provides a sense of belonging, protection, status, and monetary gain. Gang membership is strongly tied to drug use, sexual activity, violence, and crime. Gangs can have their own subculture with its unique dress style, verbal and nonverbal communication, music, and rituals (Marx et al., 2009). Children need to be taught to walk away if any gang member approaches them. Avoidance is the best policy. Education is crucial in preventing children from becoming involved in gangs.

School-age children need to be wary of peers or other persons offering illegal substances to them. Educational programs such as DARE (Drug Abuse Resistance Education) are taught to school-age children across the country. There have been questions as to the effectiveness versus the cost of the DARE program. There are new programs such as ALERT, LST (Lifeskills Training Program), and SFP (Strengthening Family Program). The goal of these programs is for children and families to gain life skills necessary to becoming responsible citizens.

GUIDANCE

Children who are in school continuously need the understanding of people who are concerned with their care. The types of relationships they have had are reflected in their behavior. They must know that they are wanted and loved. They need to know that their parents are proud of them and of their accomplishments, both in and out of school (Figure 9-8). They need approval, recognition for tasks well done, and a minimum of criticism. They need assistance in recognizing and keeping in touch with their feelings. At this age, they are quite critical of themselves. They need help with self-acceptance. Their judgment improves with age. Their decision-making capabilities need encouragement. For example, a parent can say, "I feel you can make that decision yourself." Some of their decisions reflect their immaturity. If these are life-threatening or may cause injury, it may be necessary for parents to intervene. However, children learn from making minor mistakes. Parents and nurses who empathize with school-age children are able to better understand their views.

Preadolescents want to be accepted by their group; they imitate the group's speech, manner of dress, and actions. Interest in organizations is at its peak. Children enjoy scouting programs and young people's groups affiliated with their religious organization. Parents should encourage such group activities because they are both physically and morally strengthening.

School-age children need time and a place to study. They should have a desk of their own or at least a

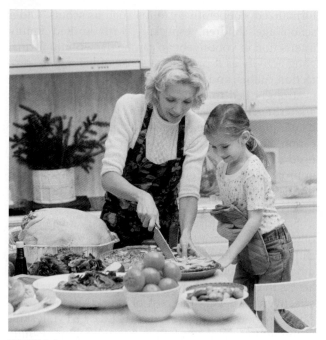

FIGURE 9-8 Learning to cook can be an enjoyable activity for the school-age child. These activities can provide positive accomplishments.

private area of the house where they are able to concentrate. Furniture should be of the proper size; lighting should be adequate. They must learn to take responsibility for their assignments and school supplies and to keep their room orderly. Parents can encourage them by showing an interest in what they are learning, joining parent-teacher organizations, and visiting the teacher periodically. They must also vote on civic matters that benefit the school system in their community.

At this age, an allowance or at least a means of earning money provides children with opportunities to learn the value of money. It takes time and encouragement for them to learn to spend money wisely. These experiences aid in making the school-age child a more responsible person.

SEX EDUCATION

Sexuality refers to the physical, psychological, social, emotional, and spiritual makeup of an individual. Young school-age children are curious about their bodies. This is sometimes evident in their play (doctor or nurse). As children grow and develop, so does their desire for knowledge about male and female roles.

Sex education is a lifelong process. Parents convey their attitudes and feelings about all aspects of life, including sexuality, to the growing child. Teaching is not so much a matter of talking or providing formal instruction as it is a matter of reflecting the whole climate of the home, particularly the respect shown to each family member.

Children's questions about sex should be answered simply and at their level of understanding. It is helpful to have age-appropriate books in the home that help in answering questions. Correct names should be used to describe the genitals. The hospitalized child who says "My penis hurts" is understood by all. Private masturbation is normal and is practiced by both genders at various times throughout their lives. It does not cause acne, blindness, insanity, or impotence. The young boy needs to be prepared for erections and nocturnal emissions ("wet dreams"), which are to be expected and are not necessarily the result of masturbation. The young girl should be prepared for menarche and provided with the necessary articles in anticipation of this event. This is of particular importance to the early maturer because an elementary school may not provide sanitary napkin machines in the restrooms. Both genders are concerned during the school years with the disproportion of their bodies, and they may be self-conscious when undressing. They may compare themselves with their friends. They need reassurance about their feelings concerning their awakening sexuality, which affects their thoughts and behavior.

Sex education programs in the schools are still subject to various group and community pressures. Most are fragmented and provide only basic information about anatomy and physiology with a general discussion of hygiene. If this is the case and if school-age children realize that their parents are uncomfortable with the subject, they turn to their peers, who often supply erroneous and distorted information.

Regardless of their practice setting, nurses can aid in the sex education of parents and children through careful listening and anticipatory guidance. When it is appropriate, they should review normal developmental behavior and provide age-specific information, such as information about masturbation. They can provide families with useful written information that stresses sexuality as a healthy rather than an illness-related concept. Cultural differences should be taken into account during counseling.

 Nursing Brief

When discussing sexuality with the school-age child, it is necessary to identify slang or street terms. Most children hear the terms but may be confused about their meanings.

LATCHKEY CHILDREN

The number of **latchkey children** (children left unsupervised after school) is growing, (Figure 9-9). Many are asked to assume responsibilities that they are not ready to perform. Several factors contribute to this trend, most of which revolve around the changing nature of the family. There has been an increase in single-parent

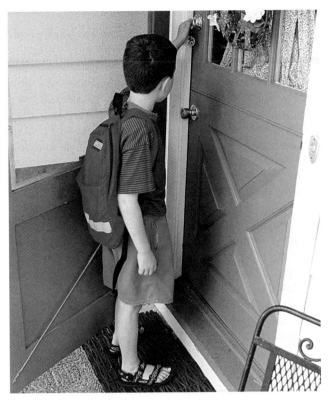

FIGURE 9-9 A child unlocks the door to let himself into his home after school.

SAFETY TIPS FOR LATCHKEY CHILDREN

1. Establish a routine that includes a phone call when the child gets home. The child may call a "telephone friend" if the community offers this service. Incorporate special things into the routine such as a prearranged trip to a friend's house. Be sure the routine includes such things as snack ideas, homework responsibilities, caring for the family pet, or simple household chores to be done. Include allowed activities and those that are not allowed.

2. Teach the child phone numbers, especially his or her own. Include numbers for parents at work, grandparents, neighbors, and emergency numbers. Be sure these are posted. A good location is the refrigerator. Ensure that the child knows his or her address and the correct spellings of parents' names and own name.

3. Be sure the child knows to keep doors locked and never open the door to anyone (unless the child has called the grandparents, neighbor, or emergency number for help).

4. Post and review safety rules and basic first aid. (See Health Promotion Box for safety tips.)

5. Instruct child never to enter the home if the door is ajar or a window is open or broken. Have the child call for help from a neighbor's house.

6. Teach child to tell phone callers that the parent or caregiver is busy; never say the parent or caregiver is not at home.

7. Teach child how to exit the home in case of a fire and to never reenter a burning building. Be sure the child knows what to do for other emergencies, including earthquakes.

8. Discuss with the child the importance of not telling others (including peers) they come home alone after school. Do not display household key in public.

9. Teach child what to do in storms, power outages, and other emergency situations.

10. Be considerate of the child. Parents should always call if they will be late. Praise the child for acting responsibly.

families that are predominantly headed by women and whose income is at or near the poverty level. In addition, the high cost of living may make it necessary for both parents to work to make ends meet. The nuclear family also is often separated geographically from the extended family; therefore relatives are not available for child care.

Latchkey children are at increased risk for accidents because of mischief or immature judgment. They may get into trouble more often than those children who are supervised after school. Studies show that these children are more likely to use alcohol, use other illegal drugs, or commit crimes. They may also show heightened feelings of fear and loneliness. They have fewer opportunities to socialize with friends because they may be instructed to remain alone in the house. It is important that children know where to go and whom to call, such as a neighbor or relative, in case of an emergency.

The Home Care Considerations box shows parental and child guidance for latchkey children. Nurses should be aware of services in their community that are designed to meet the needs of latchkey children. They should provide this information to families. Hotlines have been established in various communities that provide telephone check-in for children and reassurance programs. Nurses can also investigate community after-school services and other programs.

CHILD ABDUCTION

One of parents' greatest fears in raising children is child abduction. There are several categories for missing children, but abduction by a nonfamily member can be the most frightening. Although the number of children abducted by a nonfamily member is smaller than the number taken by a noncustodial family member, the risk for death is higher with a nonfamily member. In the past, children have been taught not to talk to strangers, not to take candy from a stranger, and not to go with a stranger, but perpetrators are finding ways to blur the "stranger" distinction. They can be the child's coach or neighbor. The Internet has provided an additional mode of contact for the perpetrator, who can establish a relationship over a period of time. The topic of strangers should be discussed with the child, and the child should learn to deal with strangers with confidence rather than with fear and avoidance (see Health Promotion Parental Guidelines for Preventing Abductions).

There are commercial devices that parents can use to track their children, such as Ionkids monitors or Wherify watch. These devices can have a global positioning system (GPS), which can identify the location of the child. Cell phones are available that allow the child to contact the parent using a push-button.

 Health Promotion

Parental Guidelines for Preventing Abductions

- Don't let your child go out alone; use the buddy system.
- Always know where your child is and what his or her plans are.
- Teach your child to always say no if feeling uncomfortable.
- Teach your child to know his or her name, address, phone number with area code, and your work number.
- Teach child how to use a pay phone or cell phone and how to contact the emergency number.
- Don't have jackets or t-shirts with your child's name in view.
- Be aware of anyone who pays a great deal of attention to your child.
- Have a current ID kit done on your child (www.pollyklaas.org).

DIVORCE

Divorce is a concern for children of all ages, not just the school-age child. However, unless a divorce is handled carefully, the impact on this particular age group can have serious consequences.

Parents can use the many books available to assist with discussions about divorce. Although younger school-age children may openly show their grief, older school-age children may keep their feelings inside while experiencing deterioration in school performance and peer relationships. Children need to be allowed to express their emotions, and counseling may help them work through their feelings.

Health Promotion

Guidelines for Coping with Divorce

- Provide reassurance that both parents love the child.
- Keep constant as many aspects of the child's world as possible.
- Provide reassurance that the noncustodial parent will visit.
- Find substitutes if the noncustodial parent becomes uninvolved.
- Provide opportunities for the child to discuss painful feelings.
- Clarify that the divorce is final and that the child is not responsible.
- Try to protect the child's positive feelings about both parents.
- Maintain normal discipline in both households.
- Do not argue with the ex-spouse about the child in the child's presence.
- Try to avoid custody disputes.

From Schmitt, B.D. RelayHealth. Patient Education. Divorce: helping children cope. MD Consult Web Site. Retrieved June 10, 2010, from www.mdconsult.com/das/patient/body/204585162-2/0/10068/18593.html.

SAFETY

As children become more mobile, the scope of possible injuries increases. This age group tends to have a high incidence of cuts, abrasions, fractures, strains, and sprains. In addition, although school-age children seek more independence, they often do not have the judgment necessary to ensure safety. They may not be able to judge their own bicycle speed or that of an oncoming car; they may be coerced into playing with matches or a handgun. School-age children (especially boys) enjoy skateboarding and riding various motorized vehicles. Both boys and girls of this age enjoy in-line skating and bicycle riding. Precautions need to be taken with these activities. (See Health Promotion Guidelines for In-Line Skating.) With skateboarding and in-line skating, protective gear must be worn. On a skateboard, the child needs a helmet, protective padding, and wrist guards. Children must be taught to *never* ride in or near traffic. They also need to learn that ramps can be especially dangerous.

Health Promotion

Guidelines for In-Line Skating

- Always wear protective gear.
- Skate under control and leave plenty of room to stop.
- Always skate on the right side of paths and sidewalks; pass on the left.
- Avoid uneven pavement and heavy traffic areas.
- Observe traffic regulations, and yield to pedestrians.

Motorized vehicles (tractors, personal watercraft, mopeds, mini-bikes, all-terrain vehicles, and snowmobiles) are both tempting and dangerous for school-age children. These children often lack the coordination and judgment to avoid crashes. These vehicles achieve high speeds yet provide little protection. The AAP recommends that children not operate these vehicles (AAP, 2007).

Bicycle safety includes the use of a helmet (the same helmet can be used for in-line skating and skateboarding) that meets the standards of the American National Standards Institute (ANSI-approved) or Snell Memorial Foundation (Snell-approved). Bicycle helmets can absorb most of the impact of a crash, thus protecting the head from serious injury (Figure 9-10). Other precautions to take when bicycle riding include obeying all traffic lights and signs, avoiding tricks and double-riding, riding in the same direction as traffic, not wearing headphones when riding, using caution near driveways and alleys, and carrying objects in a backpack or basket. *Never* wear clothing that could become caught in the bicycle chain, *never*

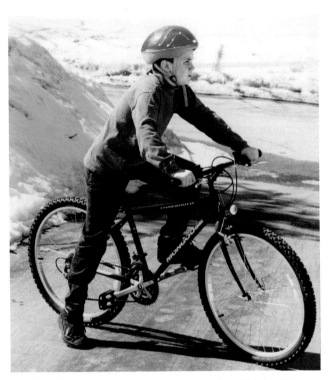

FIGURE 9-10 The right-size bike is important; the child should be able to sit on the bike and place the balls of both feet on the ground. Wearing a protective helmet is mandatory for safe cycling. The helmet should sit on top of the head in a level position with a secure strap. It should not rock side to side or front to back.

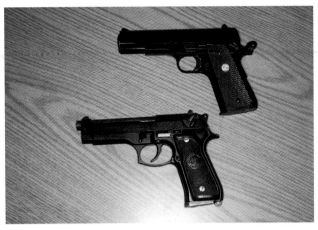

FIGURE 9-11 A child can easily mistake a real handgun for a very realistic looking toy gun, with possible tragic results. Can you identify the real gun? (It is the one on the bottom.)

ride at night, be sure the child's feet touch the ground when sitting on the seat, and always keep the bike in good repair.

Another safety-related area of concern with school-age children is the use of guns. Firearm violence has become a crisis in the United States. By 2003, the leading cause of injury-related deaths was due to firearms. School-age children are curious about and attracted to gun use. They may see it as a symbol of power or superiority. A large number of children are also seriously injured by guns. The AAP supports gun control legislation. They believe handguns, deadly air guns, and assault weapons should be banned. Until then, handgun ammunition should be regulated, restrictions should be placed on handgun ownership, and the number of privately owned handguns should be reduced (AAP, 2004). **Never allow a child access to a gun.** Loaded guns must never be kept in the house or car, ammunition must be locked away in a separate location, and guns should be equipped with trigger locks. Children need to learn that if they ever see a gun in a friend's house, they should not touch it and they should tell their parents. If they ever see a gun at school, they should report it to a teacher or a principal immediately. Children should never use a toy gun that looks so realistic that an adult would not be able to distinguish it from a distance (Figure 9-11).

The Health Promotion box presents a guide for preventing additional injuries and accidents in school-age children.

Health Promotion

Injury Prevention during School-Age Years

DEVELOPMENTAL ABILITIES RELATED TO RISK FOR INJURY	INJURY PREVENTION
	MOTOR VEHICLES
Is increasingly involved in activities away from home Is excited by speed and motion Is easily distracted by environment Can be reasoned with	Educate child regarding proper use of seat belts as a passenger in a vehicle. Maintain discipline as a passenger in a vehicle (e.g., keep arms inside, do not lean against doors or interfere with driver). Remind parents and children that no one should ride in the bed of a pickup truck. Emphasize safe pedestrian behavior. Insist on use of safety apparel (e.g., helmet) where applicable, such as when riding a bicycle, motorcycle, moped, or all-terrain vehicle.

Continued

Health Promotion—cont'd

DEVELOPMENTAL ABILITIES RELATED TO RISK FOR INJURY	INJURY PREVENTION
	DROWNING
Is apt to overdo	Teach child to swim.
May work hard to perfect a skill	Teach basic rules of water safety.
Has cautious, but not fearful, gross-motor actions	Select safe and supervised places to swim.
	Check sufficient water depth for diving.
Likes swimming	Have child swim with a companion.
	Use an approved flotation device in water or boat.
	Advocate for legislation requiring fencing around pools.
	Learn CPR.
	BURNS
Has increasing independence	Make sure smoke detectors are in homes.
Is adventuresome	Set hot water temperatures (120° F to 130° F) to avoid scald burns.
Enjoys trying new things	Instruct child in behavior in areas involving contact with potential burn hazards (e.g., gasoline, matches, bonfires or barbecues, lighter fluid, firecrackers, cigarette lighters, cooking utensils, chemistry sets); avoid climbing or flying kites around high-tension wires.
	Instruct child in proper behavior in the event of fire (e.g., fire drills at home and school).
	Teach child safe cooking (use low heat; avoid any frying; be careful of steam burns, scalds, or exploding foods, especially from microwaving).
	POISONING
Adheres to group rules	Educate child regarding hazards of taking nonprescription drugs and chemicals, including aspirin and alcohol.
May be easily influenced by peers	Teach child to say "no" if offered illegal or dangerous drugs or alcohol.
Has strong allegiance to friends	Keep potentially dangerous products in properly labeled receptacles, preferably locked and out of reach.
	BODILY DAMAGE
Has increased physical skills	Help provide facilities for supervised activities.
Needs strenuous physical activity	Encourage playing in safe places.
Is interested in acquiring new skills and perfecting attained skills	Keep firearms safely locked up except during adult supervision.
	Teach proper care of, use of, and respect for devices with potential danger (power tools, firecrackers).
Is daring and adventurous, especially with peers	Teach children not to tease or surprise dogs, invade their territory, take dogs' toys, or interfere with dogs' feeding.
Frequently plays in hazardous places	Stress eye, ear, or mouth protection when using potentially hazardous objects or devices or when engaged in potentially hazardous sports (e.g., baseball).
Confidence often exceeds physical capacity	Teach safety regarding use of corrective devices (glasses); if child wears contact lenses, monitor duration of wear to prevent corneal damage.
Desires group loyalty, and has strong need for friends' approval	
Attempts hazardous feats	Stress careful selection, use, and maintenance of sports and recreation equipment such as skateboards and in-line skates.
Accompanies friends to potentially hazardous facilities	Emphasize proper conditioning, safe practices, and use of safety equipment for sports or recreational activities.
Delights in physical activity	Caution against engaging in hazardous sports, such as those involving trampolines.
Is likely to overdo	Use safety glass and decals on large glassed areas, such as sliding glass doors.
Growth in height exceeds muscular growth and coordination	Use window guards to prevent falls.
	Teach name, address, and phone number and to ask for help from appropriate people (cashier, security guard, and policeman) if lost; have identification on child (sewn in clothes, inside shoe).
	Teach stranger safety:
	Avoid personalized clothing in public places.
	Caution child to never go with a stranger.
	Have child tell parents if anyone makes child feel uncomfortable in any way.
	Always listen to child's concerns regarding others' behavior.
	Teach child to say "no" when confronted with uncomfortable situations.

From Hockenberry, M.J., and Wilson, D. (2007). *Wong's nursing care of infants and children* (8th ed.). St. Louis: Mosby.

HEALTH PROMOTION AND MAINTENANCE

HEALTH EXAMINATIONS

The yearly preschool physical examination is given in the spring preceding admission. This allows time for correcting any problems that are found. Booster immunizations are given as needed (see Evolve Appendix). Blood pressure, height, and weight must all be evaluated. Ensuring that the child regularly visits the dentist is also part of the examination. Blood cholesterol may be evaluated, especially if the child is at risk (e.g., from heredity).

School-age children need to be evaluated for the amount of exercise they receive. Exercise should be done daily. It can range from bicycle riding to organized team sports. If this is not encouraged, obesity may result as a preteen problem.

School health programs aimed at maintaining and promoting health are provided by most school systems. Nurses and other professionals who take part in such programs can play an important role in counseling parents. They also can help in meeting the needs of disabled children who are enrolled in their schools. A carefully taken health history provides the nurse with much-needed information. Audiograms are done as part of the school health program, as are vision and scoliosis screenings. Deviations from normal in any of these areas require further assessment by the child's physician.

DAILY CARE

School-age children generally provide their own daily care. Teeth should be brushed at least twice daily with a pea-sized amount of fluoridated toothpaste. Drinking water should also contain fluoride. Twice-yearly dental visits should continue. The dentist may evaluate for application of dental sealants.

Children are so active during the day, both physically and mentally, that they soon become exhausted. Children from 6 to 8 years of age average approximately 11 to 13 hours of sleep per night, while the 9- to 12-year-old averages about 10 hours per night. Parents can judge the amount of sleep children need by their behavior. If a child is eating and playing well and keeping up with schoolwork, chances are that the amount of sleep is sufficient.

PLAY

Play is still very much a part of the school-age child's life. It simply takes on a new dimension. During the beginning of this period, play occurs in groups, which are mostly of the same gender. These children still enjoy dolls, cars, and trucks. They ride bicycles and enjoy active games such as hide-and-seek, tag, jump rope, and roller skating. They become involved in sports. Team play has rules and goals. They also enjoy quiet activities and often start collections, play board games or card games, and read books. They enjoy being creative and learning new things. As they get older, school-age children become more independent and peer relationships (discussed earlier in the chapter) become more important.

NUTRITION

The eating habits of school-age children are usually not a problem as long as a variety of nutritious foods are offered. Review the discussion about MyPyramid in Chapter 7 (see Figure 7-5) for the recommended food intake for school-age children. A good breakfast is important. The chief breakfast foods necessary are fruit, cereal, and milk. Eggs add variety. Older school-age children need to have the importance of breakfast stressed because they may decide that breakfast is no longer important or they may feel too rushed in the mornings. Peers may also influence this behavior. Menus centered on nutritional foods are more substantial than those consisting of doughnuts or sweet rolls. Nutritious snacks are also important to provide energy for after-school activities and homework. Good nutrition also prevents problems of obesity that can occur with school-age children.

Depending on individual activity levels, an 8-year-old girl needs approximately 1200 to 1800 calories per day, and boys of the same age need about 1400 to 2000 calories per day. The 12-year-old girl needs 1600 to 2200 calories, whereas 12-year-old boys require about 1800 to 2400 calories, again depending on activity level. The U.S. Department of Agriculture has developed new dietary guidelines, which are available online (*www.mypyrimid.gov*). This site provides information for parents, children, and school officials.

 Community Considerations

The school nurse can work with teachers to provide nutrition instruction in the classroom. Children can participate in learning activities that focus on nutrition education to encourage good habits.

The federal government has established the School Breakfast Program in many areas. The National School Lunch Program has been ongoing. Summer lunch programs are also available in some communities. These lunches must meet certain nutritional standards (the goal is to provide one third of the recommended daily allowance of foods).

Table 9-2   Obesity Staged Action Plan

Stage 1: Prevention Plus protocol	5 or more age-appropriate servings of fruits and vegetables 2 or less hours of television, computer, or video games and no media in sleeping areas 1 hour or more of physical activity No sugar-sweetened beverages Daily breakfast Limit of fast foods
Stage 2: Structured weight management protocol	Organized diet developed by a nutritionist 1 hour or more of physical activity Limit of media screen time to 1 hour or less Improved monitoring of exercise, screen time, or diet by family/patient
Stage 3: Comprehensive multidisciplinary protocol	Eating and activity requirements from Stage 2 Structured behavioral modification techniques including counseling
Stage 4: Tertiary care protocol	Referral to weight management center, which may include medications and surgery when appropriate.

Adapted from Schuman, A.J. (2008). An obesity action plan for children. *Contemp Pediatr, 25*(4), 37-8, 41-2, 45-6.

CHILDHOOD OBESITY

Childhood obesity has become a major health issue with 19% of 6- to 11-year-olds categorized as overweight or obese. Obesity in the childhood years can lead to adult obesity with increased risks of cardiovascular issues and Type 2 diabetes. Hispanic children and African-American girls have the highest incidence of obesity. Parental obesity is the highest predictor of childhood obesity (Kleigman et al., 2007). Management of the overweight child should be aggressive and should begin as early as 2 years of age. BMI, dietary, and activity assessments should be obtained and evaluated. A "staged protocol" approach has been recommended for a child with a BMI greater than or equal to the 85th percentile (Table 9-2).

It is difficult to treat obesity at any age. A team approach including a nutritionist, psychologist or psychiatrist, physician, and nurse should focus on helping the child and the family gain control of this aspect of the child's life.

Get Ready for the NCLEX® Examination!

Key Points

- School-age children are more engrossed in fact than fantasy; they begin to master activities they enjoy and learn they must cooperate with others.
- Growth is slow until just before puberty. Muscular coordination is improved, and vital signs are near those of an adult. Language continues to develop, and school-age children build an impressive vocabulary.
- The school-age child thinks in concrete terms and is in the stage of industry versus inferiority. He or she begins to understand right and wrong and develops a conscience.
- Each age brings out individual differences and personalities. Parents need to understand these differences as their child matures.
- School is an important influence in children's lives. Teachers, parents, and other caregivers need to instill values and help school-age children develop social competencies.
- Teasing and bullying can lead to long-term mental problems. Both the victim and the bully need assistance in handling these situations.

- Television and video game play should be limited. Both can have a detrimental effect on children.
- Peers are also a strong influence on children. Gangs and drugs are real temptations in children's lives; parents, teachers, and other caregivers must educate children to deter these activities.
- Sex education is discussed with the school-age child. Simple, straightforward answers at the child's level of understanding are the best advice for parents.
- Latchkey children need reminders and reassurance to keep them safe after school.
- Child abduction prevention guidelines should be discussed with children based on developmental age.
- Divorce is a problem for school-age children and children of other ages. When divorce occurs, parents need to be honest and provide reassurance to children.
- Safety is also a priority for school-age children. Although they have different types of injuries than do toddlers and preschoolers, school-age children still need supervision and education to prevent injuries.
- Good nutrition based on MyPyramid is important at this age. Children are growing slowly but steadily, and healthy eating habits formed at this age are important later in life.

3. Competitiveness
4. Industry

2. The parents of a 6-year-old child ask how many hours their child should sleep at night. The nurse correctly responds:

1. 6 to 8 hours
2. 8 to 10 hours
3. 11 to 13 hours
4. 13 to 15 hours

2. No sugar-sweetened beverages
3. The elimination of fast foods
4. Structured behavior modification
5. 1 hour or more of physical activity per day

The Adolescent

Objectives

1. Define the key terms listed
2. Identify two major developmental tasks of adolescence
3. Discuss three ways in which youth can help prevent violence
4. Discuss anticipatory guidance for a 15-year-old girl just beginning to date
5. Describe three ways an adolescent can be given responsibility
6. Describe at least five ways a home health care worker can assist in caring for a disabled child
7. Explain three ways parents can be assisted in the skills of parenting adolescents

8. Discuss the strategies for decreasing adolescent pregnancy
9. Discuss how health care workers can assist adolescents in making informed decisions regarding body piercing and tattoos
10. Summarize the nutritional requirements of the adolescent, and cite two factors that may contribute to dietary deficiencies in this age group
11. Discuss the three leading causes of accidents in adolescence, and suggest methods of prevention for each

Key Terms

adolescence (ĂD-ō-LĔS-ĕns; p. 180)
androgens (ĂN-drō-jĕnz; p. 181)
asynchrony (ā-SĬN-krō-nē; p. 181)
estrogens (ĔS-trō-jĕnz; p. 181)
identity (p. 180)

intimacy (p. 180)
menarche (mĕ-NĂR-kē; p. 181)
puberty (PŪ-bĕr-tē; p. 181)
respite care (p. 188)
thelarche (thĕ-LĂR-kē; p. 181)

GENERAL CHARACTERISTICS AND DEVELOPMENT

Adolescence is the period of life that begins with the appearance of secondary sex characteristics and ends with cessation of growth and achievement of emotional maturity. The term comes from the word *adolescere,* meaning "to grow up." For purposes of clarification, adolescence is often divided into early, middle, and late periods. This is because a 13-year-old teenager is very different from an 18-year-old one. Middle adolescence appears to be the time of greatest turmoil for most families. Perhaps one of the most characteristic features of adolescence is its uncertainty. In our culture, it is a period of life that lasts a comparatively long time and involves a great number of adjustments.

Life is never dull with adolescents in the family. The adolescents' surge toward independence becomes more and more pronounced. This makes it practically impossible for them to get along with their parents, who represent authority. When adolescents submit to

their parents' wishes, they feel humiliated and childish. If they revolt, conflicts arise within the family. Parents and teenagers have to weather this storm together and must try to come up with solutions that are more or less acceptable to everyone.

Numerous other factors also account for the restlessness of youth. Adolescents' bodies are rapidly changing, and they experience intense sexual drives. They want to be accepted by society but are not sure how to go about it. Adolescents question life and search to find what psychologists term as their sense of identity: "Who am I?" "What do I want?" Gaining an understanding of self-concept is an important aspect of adolescence. This sense of identity is followed by the intimacy stage, in which teenagers must learn to avoid emotional isolation. Through shared activities such as sports, close friendships, and sexual experiences, they must face their fear of rejection. The older adolescent thinks about the future and is generally idealistic. This age also brings about an increased sophistication in moral reasoning. Thinking also has evolved to abstract reasoning.

BIOLOGICAL DEVELOPMENT

Preadolescence is a short period that immediately precedes adolescence. It is marked by a growth spurt that can begin at 10 years of age for girls and 13 years of age for boys. It is distinguished by puberty, the stage at which the reproductive organs become functional and secondary sex characteristics develop. Both genders produce male hormones, androgens, and female hormones, estrogens, in comparatively equal amounts during childhood. At puberty the hypothalamus of the brain signals the pituitary gland to stimulate other endocrine glands—the adrenals and the ovaries or testes—to secrete their hormones directly into the bloodstream in differing proportions (more androgens in boys and more estrogens in girls).

The age at which puberty takes place varies and is about 2 years earlier in girls than in boys. In both genders, it is preceded by spurts in height and weight. Overall, girls stop growing sooner and have smaller increases in height and weight than boys. During the pubertal growth spurt, weight increases 50%; this varies according to pubertal maturation, degree of adiposity, and size of muscle mass. During puberty, the growth spurt results in a 15% to 20% increase in height.

The adolescent's general appearance tends to be awkward—long-legged and gangling. This growth characteristic is termed asynchrony because different body parts mature at different rates. The sweat glands are very active, and greasy skin and acne are common. Both genders mature earlier, grow taller, and are heavier than adolescents in past generations.

The development of secondary sexual maturation can be assessed using Tanner staging. Stages are based on breast and pubic hair development for girls and genital and pubic hair development for boys (Table 10-1). Development (growth and sexual maturation) is predictable but variable. Tanner staging provides a more accurate assessment of a child's development than chronologic age (James and Ashwill, 2007). In most girls, changes in the breast with the development of a small bud of breast tissue (thelarche) signals the earliest sign of puberty. The average age is 11 years. Menarche (onset of menstrual periods) occurs approximately 2 years afterward. Menarche can range from 10½ to 15 years and still be within normal guidelines. According to Hockenberry and Wilson (2007), girls' peak height velocity occurs at about 12 years of age (6 to 12 months before menarche); girls gain 2 to 8 inches in height and 15 to 55 pounds during adolescence. In addition to secondary sex characteristics becoming

Table 10-1 Sexual Maturation Rating (SMR): Tanner Stages

Boys

STAGE 1	STAGE 2	STAGE 3	STAGE 4	STAGE 5
Pubic hair: none Penis: preadolescent Testes: preadolescent	Pubic hair: slight, long, straight, slightly pigmented at the base of the penis Penis: slight enlargement Testes: enlarged scrotum, pink, slight alteration in texture	Pubic hair: darker in color, starts to curl, small amount Penis: longer Testes: larger	Pubic hair: coarse, curly, similar to adult but less quantity Penis: larger, glans and breadth increase in size Testes: larger, scrotum darker	Pubic hair: adult distribution spread to inner thighs Penis: adult in size and shape Testes: adult

Early puberty: Testes, 9½-13½ yr; penis, 10½-14½ yr; pubic hair, 12-12½ yr

Middle puberty: Testes, 13½-14½ yr; penis, 13½-15 yr; pubic hair, 12½-14½ yr

Late puberty: Testes, 13½-17 yr; penis, 13½-16 yr; pubic hair, 13½-16½ yr

Continued

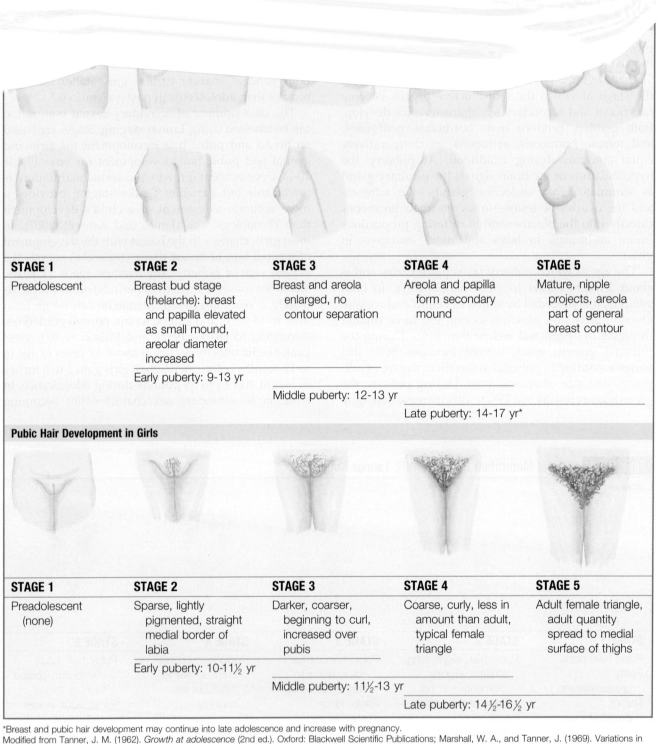

STAGE 1	STAGE 2	STAGE 3	STAGE 4	STAGE 5
Preadolescent	Breast bud stage (thelarche): breast and papilla elevated as small mound, areolar diameter increased	Breast and areola enlarged, no contour separation	Areola and papilla form secondary mound	Mature, nipple projects, areola part of general breast contour
	Early puberty: 9-13 yr			
		Middle puberty: 12-13 yr		
			Late puberty: 14-17 yr*	

Pubic Hair Development in Girls

STAGE 1	STAGE 2	STAGE 3	STAGE 4	STAGE 5
Preadolescent (none)	Sparse, lightly pigmented, straight medial border of labia	Darker, coarser, beginning to curl, increased over pubis	Coarse, curly, less in amount than adult, typical female triangle	Adult female triangle, adult quantity spread to medial surface of thighs
	Early puberty: 10-11½ yr			
		Middle puberty: 11½-13 yr		
			Late puberty: 14½-16½ yr	

*Breast and pubic hair development may continue into late adolescence and increase with pregnancy.
Modified from Tanner, J. M. (1962). *Growth at adolescence* (2nd ed.). Oxford: Blackwell Scientific Publications; Marshall, W. A., and Tanner, J. (1969). Variations in pattern of pubertal changes in girls. *Arch Dis Child*, 44(235), 291-303. Modified with permission from Blackwell Scientific Publications and The BMJ Publishing Group.

more apparent before menarche, fat is deposited in the hips and thighs, causing them to enlarge. Hair grows in the pubic area and underarms. The body reaches its adult measurements about 3 years after the onset of puberty. At this time, the ends of the long bones knit securely to their shafts and further growth can no longer take place.

Although breast cancer is rare in adolescents, this is a time when girls are aware of their bodies and breast self-examination should be introduced. Breast self-examination should be routinely performed beginning at 18 to 21 years of age (Fallat et al., 2008). The American Cancer Society provides various informational pamphlets describing the procedure.

The first sign of puberty in boys is usually the enlargement of the testes, which begins between 9½ and 14 years of age. Ejaculation and the appearance of pubic hair occur approximately 1 year after this. The production of sperm begins between 13½ and 14½ years of age. Complete fertility is not present at this time, but impregnation is possible. According to Hockenberry and Wilson (2007), boys' peak height velocity occurs at around 14 years of age, followed by growth of the testes and penis. The penis elongates and widens, testes enlarge, and scrotum pigment becomes evident. Both axillary and facial hair increase, along with body odor. Voice changes are also noticeable. By late adolescence (17 to 21 years of age), adult genitalia is attained. The male voice deepens, and most linear growth is achieved. Overall, boys gain 4 to 12 inches in height; weight gain is between 15 and 65 pounds during adolescence.

The American Cancer Society recommends that boys examine their testes during or after a hot bath or shower. Each testicle is examined with the index and middle finger of both hands on the underside of the testicle and the thumbs on the top of the testicle. It is normal for one testicle to be larger than the other. The testicles are gently rolled between the thumb and finger. Testicular self-examinations are performed once a month. If a lump is discovered, it should be reported immediately. Males also need to report an abnormal enlargement of a testicle or a heavy feeling in the scrotum. In addition, they should report any pain or discomfort in a testicle or in the scrotum, especially if symptoms last as long as 2 weeks.

 Nursing Brief

Although young girls are often taught breast self-examination, young boys are seldom instructed in the examination of the testes. Boys should also be taught to report enlargement or tenderness of their breasts because males, too, can develop breast cancer.

DEVELOPMENTAL THEORIES

Adolescents are in a period of transition from childhood to adulthood (Table 10-2). Erik Erikson identified the major task of this group as identity formation versus role confusion. At this time, children must determine who they are, where they are going, and how they are getting there. This should not imply that adolescents wait until this stage to develop individuation. The child has been developing autonomy since toddlerhood.

Adolescents want to be people in their own right, and they try out different roles (Figure 10-1). Self-identity (one's view of oneself) fluctuates during this time and is molded by the demands of parents, peers,

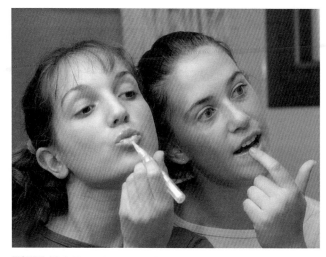

FIGURE 10-1 The adolescent is very concerned about personal appearance. A teenager's self-esteem is influenced by how far body image deviates from the mythical "body ideal."

teachers, and so on. Although gaining a self-identity is an ongoing process, adolescence can be a time that particularly challenges the child's view of self.

As adolescents move toward independence, they begin to separate from the family. Belonging to a group (group identity) becomes essential. Peer influences dominate decisions that relate to appearance, social behavior, and language. Disagreements with parents often revolve around dating, use of the family car, money, chores, school grades, choice of friends, smoking, sex, and the social use of drugs. Parental values and morals are questioned, especially if parents do not practice what they preach. Adults who associate with teenagers should try to create an atmosphere of interest and understanding. A caring environment that sets limits is essential. Adolescence is a little like being on a roller coaster. Parents, nurses, and other adults who interact with adolescents should be reminded that they should remain objective, calm, understanding, and loving.

According to Piaget's theory of cognitive development, development is systematic, sequential, and orderly. Early adolescents are still in the concrete phase of thinking. They take things literally. For instance, assume the nurse asks a young teenager girl, "Have you ever slept with anyone?" The teenager may not perceive this to have anything to do with a vaginal infection or sex. By middle adolescence, the ability to think in abstract terms has increased. Piaget calls this the stage of formal operations. Older adolescents can see a situation from many viewpoints and can imagine or organize unseen or unexperienced possibilities. The failure to develop formal thoughts is cited by some as connected to the failure to develop a high level of moral reasoning. Adolescents who have developed both are most likely to demonstrate a high degree of morality and consistency in their behavior.

Table 10-2 Growth and Development During Adolescence

EARLY ADOLESCENCE (11-14 YR)	MIDDLE ADOLESCENCE (14-17 YR)	LATE ADOLESCENCE (17-20 YR)
Growth		
Rapidly accelerating growth Reaches peak velocity Secondary sex characteristics appear	Growth decelerating in girls Stature reaches 95% of adult height Secondary sex characteristics well-advanced	Physically mature Structure and reproductive growth almost complete
Cognition		
Explores newfound ability for limited abstract thought Clumsy groping for new values and energies Comparison of "normality" with peers of same gender	Developing capacity for abstract thinking Enjoys intellectual powers, often in idealistic terms Concern with philosophic, political, and social problems	Abstract thought established Can perceive and act on long-range operations Able to view problems comprehensively Intellectual and functional identity
Identity		
Preoccupied with rapid body changes Trying out various roles Measurement of attractiveness by acceptance or rejection of peers Conformity to group norms	Modifies body image Very self-centered; increased narcissism Tendency toward inner experience and self-discovery Has a rich fantasy life Idealistic Able to perceive future implications of current behavior and decisions; variable application	Body image and gender-role definition nearly secured Mature sexual identity Phase of consolidation of identity Stability of self-esteem Comfortable with physical growth Social roles defined and articulated
Relationships with Parents		
Defining independence-dependence boundaries Strong desire to remain dependent on parents while trying to detach No major conflicts over parental control	Major conflicts over independence and control Low point in parent-child relationship Greatest push for emancipation; disengagement Final and irreversible emotional detachment from parents; mourning	Emotional and physical separation from parents completed Independence from family with less conflict Emancipation nearly secured
Relationships with Peers		
Seeks peer affiliations to counter instability generated by rapid change Upsurge of close, idealized friendships with members of the same gender Struggle for mastery takes place within peer group	Strong need for identity to affirm self-image Behavioral standards set by peer group Acceptance by peers extremely important—fear of rejection Exploration of ability to attract the opposite gender	Peer group recedes in importance in favor of individual friendship Testing of male-female relationships against possibility of permanent alliance Relationships characterized by giving and sharing
Sexuality		
Self-exploration and evaluation Limited dating, usually group Limited intimacy	Multiple plural relationships Decisive turn toward heterosexuality (or, if homosexual, knows by this time) Exploration of "self-appeal" Feeling of "being in love" Tentative establishment of relationships	Forms stable relationships and attachment to another Growing capacity for mutuality and reciprocity Dating as a male-female pair Intimacy involves commitment rather than exploration and romanticism
Psychological Health		
Wide mood swings Intense daydreaming Anger outwardly expressed with moodiness, temper outbursts, and verbal insults and name-calling	Tendency toward inner experiences; more introspective Tendency to withdraw when upset or feelings are hurt Vacillation of emotions in time and range Feelings of inadequacy common; difficulty in asking for help	More constancy of emotion Anger more apt to be concealed

From Hockenberry, M.J., and Wilson, D. (2007). *Wong's nursing care of infants and children* (8th ed.). St. Louis: Mosby.

Lawrence Kohlberg's theory on moral development places adolescence at a postconventional morality stage. Older adolescents consider others' points of view and consider what rights and values are the best for everyone. They are able to do this because they can engage in abstract thinking. Social responsibility is recognized, and moral decisions can be made.

From the perspective of Sigmund Freud, adolescence is the "genital stage." The adolescent begins to love others and peers. Parents also provide a love that helps set a realistic direction for the teenager. In adolescence, theorists believe, a maturity has developed that sets the stage for adult development. Through support and guidance, nurses can assist children and adolescents through the stages of development necessary to reach that maturity.

SPECIAL NEEDS

PEER RELATIONSHIPS

Adolescent peer groups vary in number, interests, social background, and structure. They may consist of small groups of the same gender or of both genders. In late adolescence, peer groups may be small groups of couples. The young person may belong to one or several groups. The peer group serves as a mirror for "normality" and helps to determine where one fits in. Belonging to a peer group is vitally important to helping the adolescent define the self. Acceptance by one's friends helps decrease the loneliness and the sense of loss that many teenagers experience on the road to adulthood (Figure 10-2).

On the other hand, the social norms and pressures exerted by the group may cause problems (Figure 10-3). The selection of friends and adolescents' allegiance to them may bring about conflicts within the family. Parents need help in understanding that teenagers' exaggerated conformity is a necessary step in moving away from dependence and in obtaining approval from people outside the nuclear family. Failure to develop social competence may produce feelings of inadequacy and low self-esteem.

Nurses can assist the parents through supporting and educating them in the dynamics of this age group. They can direct families to groups such as peer helpers (for the adolescent) and to community educational programs sponsored by various agencies. Organizations such as Parents Without Partners might be another avenue. Nurses must also remember that teenagers who do not belong to the dominant system, such as those from different cultural, social, or economic backgrounds, may see themselves as being quite different from their friends. In such cases, the use of family networks may prove helpful.

CAREER PLANS

Some adolescents enter high school with a definite idea of what they would like to do. Many, however, are unsure of what type of career they want to pursue. To choose a career that he or she is best suited for, the teenager must first know the self and understand what choices are available. What particularly interests him? What is she good at? What are the shortcomings?

By this time, the adolescent has already taken some rather definite steps toward a goal. On completing high school, the choice of high school curriculum and the types of grades received determine eligibility for entrance into college or preparation for a specific vocation (Figure 10-4). Parents should observe the interests of their children and encourage them to take advantage of their particular talents. Whenever possible, a teenager should investigate various fields by talking

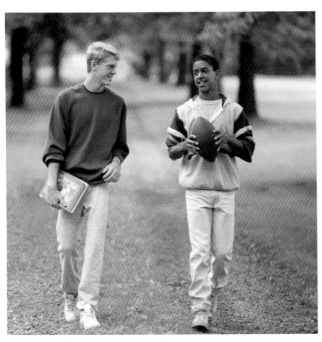

FIGURE 10-2 The peer group is often the adolescent's "safety net" in the search for independence and identity.

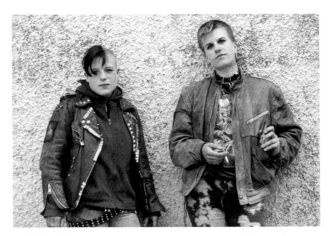

FIGURE 10-3 Peer pressure heavily influences an adolescent's decision to try tobacco, alcohol, and drugs.

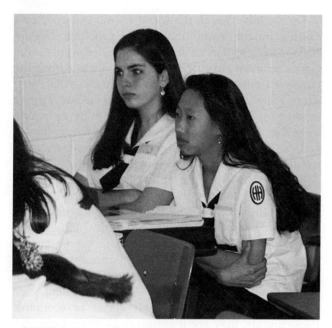

FIGURE 10-4 School is an important part of the adolescent's life.

to people who are involved in them. Valuable information can also be obtained by career exploration, which is available at most colleges and with pamphlets from professional organizations, the government, and other sources. School guidance counselors administer aptitude tests that serve as an additional guide. They also can work with teenagers to expose them to as wide a selection of careers as possible. The final decision must be made by the adolescent. If people are to be happy with their work, they must choose it of their own free will and not because of parental expectations.

Many types of work are open to young women. Although they may choose to marry, many girls are selecting careers that support an independent lifestyle. Women also make up a large proportion of the work force and are being introduced into more nontraditional jobs.

The job market today is extremely competitive—and almost nonexistent for those without skills or education. Unemployment is high among minority groups and in some geographic locales. Although there are numerous causes for this, the individual unable to find a fulfilling job often experiences feelings of hopelessness and decreased self-esteem. Productive employment of young people needs to fit into their total framework of life. It also needs to offer an opportunity for personal growth. Some constructive aspects of employment include building self-esteem, promoting responsibility, testing new skills, constructively channeling energies, providing money for increased independence, engaging young persons in interactions with adults, and allowing them to assume an active rather than a passive role. In contrast, when adolescents are forced to take a job because of economic or personal pressures, they may have to drop out of school. With few skills and no experience, they may remain locked in low-level employment. This is often perpetuated from one generation to the next.

RESPONSIBILITY

Young people look forward to challenges. Parents must watch for ways that they may free their children to take on new responsibilities, which may include a part-time job. Young adolescents must also be taught the value of money. An allowance helps them to learn management. If money is simply handed out as requested, it is more difficult for the adolescent to develop a sense of responsibility regarding finances. Allowances should be increased from time to time to comply with the age and needs of the teenager.

Middle and older adolescents who have jobs can be taught the use of a checkbook and a savings account. Many find satisfaction in being able to purchase their own clothes. If a boy or girl buys a car, he or she soon discovers that it takes money to run and repair it. Experiences such as these provide valuable lessons in finance. A common way of earning money among younger teenagers is babysitting. Many boys and girls begin to babysit at about 12 or 13 years of age. Babysitting courses are valuable because these young people need to be prepared for this important responsibility. Courses are regularly taught by the American Red Cross, Campfire Boys and Girls, and local hospitals. Safe Sitter is an international organization that promotes babysitting skills. Safe Sitter has teaching sites established in all 50 states, as well as in England and Canada.

EMOTIONAL NEEDS

Teenagers worry frequently. They are able to talk about fears that are not too intimate, such as school examinations, how they will look with this or that type of haircut, and so on. They need assistance, however, in getting in touch with their feelings and in sorting out confused feelings. All experts in teenage guidance agree on the importance of keeping the lines of communication open in the family. Providing a confidential accepting atmosphere and using listening skills and awareness of verbal and nonverbal cues are helpful. One of the more difficult aspects of communicating with adolescents is their fluctuating attitude. They may vary from being unconcerned about deadlines to being in a state of panic. They may wish to please but may be overly critical of themselves and their own performance. They may try to control others by being overly talkative. This may come from a desire to demonstrate their competence. Physical symptoms such as stomachaches, headaches, and insomnia surface and disappear periodically. Anxiety over future events, relationships with peers, and meeting others' expectations is also prevalent. Teenagers often experience their parents' pain and feel tremendously responsible for the family's burdens and failures. For many, the image of what a family should be is derived from television. Adolescents who have lifetime handicaps, alcoholic parents, physical or mental illness, or other serious problems such as poverty need the support of the medical community and other community resources.

DAYDREAMS

Adolescents spend a lot of time daydreaming in the solitude of their rooms or during a biology lecture. Most of this is normal and natural for this age group (Figure 10-5). Daydreaming is usually considered harmless if the young person continues usual active pursuits. It also serves several purposes. Adolescence is a lonely, in-between age; daydreaming helps fill the void. Acting out imaginatively what will be said or done in various situations prepares teenagers to deal with others, so when confronted with real scenarios, they are better able to handle and cope with the situation. Daydreams are also a valuable safety valve that allows the expression of strong feelings.

HETEROSEXUAL RELATIONSHIPS

During adolescence, romantic friendships emerge. Special talents and interests influence selection of activities. Social outings to the mall or beach are heavily influenced by the desire to meet members of the opposite gender. Participation in group and individual activities enhances social stature. All adolescents enjoy parties, movies, athletic competitions, and sports. Teen nightclubs and rock concerts are, however, generally reserved for later adolescence.

Adolescents need to meet and become acquainted with members of the opposite gender. Adolescents may start by first admiring from a distance. This is accompanied by daydreams. Gradually, the young person attempts to attract the attention of the person in whom he or she is interested. Competition and rivalry may be keen. A person may date a number of people or merely one. Dates may be frequent or sporadic (Figure 10-6).

The adolescent's cultural background has an influence on patterns of dating. Conflict often arises when

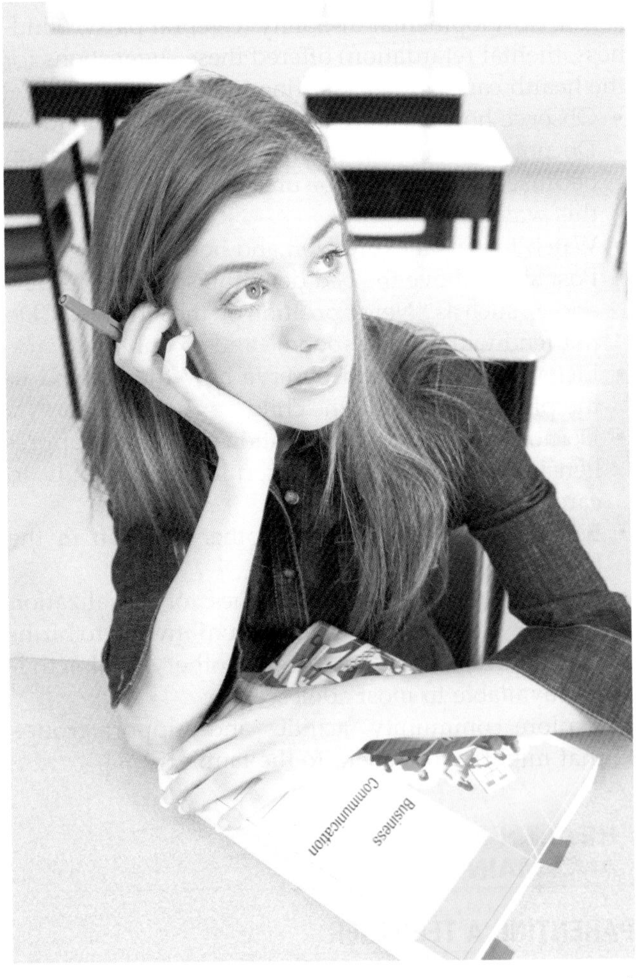

FIGURE 10-5 Adolescents can spend time daydreaming as a normal outlet.

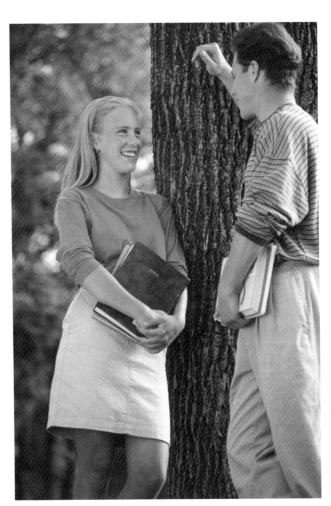

FIGURE 10-6 During adolescence, emerging sexuality is expressed in the development of intimate relationships. Many young couples date on a regular basis and prefer dating only one other person.

the teenager from a different cultural background wants to be independent and quickly adopts American norms of dating while parents insist on strict traditional values. This is particularly noticeable with daughters.

Dating represents one of the early social decision points of growing up. As such, it may become a battleground in the struggle for independence. Parental opposition is often based on unspoken fears of rejection and the adolescent's increased sexual experience or the possibility of pregnancy. Parents may respond by imposing strict restrictions in regard to curfews, chaperones, use of the car, and so on. When these problems are not discussed openly with the young person, the adolescent may react by rebelling, by sexual acting out, or by other means. Often these means are designed to test injunctions of control rather than out of a desire for the sexual act itself.

Date Rape

Teens need to be educated on "date rape." Unfortunately, this can occur simply because boys believe girls want to have sex, even when they say "no." When a girl says "no," her wishes should be respected. If her date does not take "no" for an answer, teenage girls should be taught to shout, scream, fight back, or run away to protect themselves. In addition, teens need to be aware of the effects of Rohypnol, the "date rape drug." Rohypnol is illegally imported into the United States at an alarming rate. The effect of this drug is 10 times stronger than that of Valium. Teens need to learn not only about the effects of this drug but also how to avoid places and situations where it could be used.

CHRONIC ILLNESS/DISABILITY

Chronic illness during adolescence runs counter to developmental needs. Specific programs that foster feelings of security and independence within the limits of the situation are essential. Behavioral problems are lessened when adolescents can verbalize specific concerns with people who are sensitive to their problems. If they feel rejected by and different from peers, they may become depressed. To be in school and to be considered one of the group is important. Hospital school programs for adolescents with long-term hospitalization enable teenagers to keep pace with their classmates and to achieve their educational goals. Recreational programs are also helpful in combating boredom and providing outlets for tension. Peers should be encouraged to spend time with the adolescent who requires long-term hospitalization. Nurses need to help adolescents cope with body image concerns. They must develop an awareness of the teenager's particular fears of forced dependence, bodily invasion, mutilation, rejection, and humiliation, especially within the peer group. The nurse should anticipate a certain amount of reluctance to adhere to hospital regulations, which reflects the adolescent's need for self-determination. Recognizing this as an asset rather than a liability enables the nurse to respond in a constructive manner.

Adolescents who have a developmental disability that affects the intellect or the ability to cope face some unique difficulties. They are often overprotected, unable to break away from supervision, and deprived of necessary peer relationships. The pubertal process with its emerging sexuality becomes a worrisome concern for parents and may precipitate a family crisis. It is becoming more common for hospitals to provide an interdisciplinary team that works to meet the needs of adolescents and their families.

Many adolescents with chronic illnesses or developmental disabilities are assisted at home through home health. Home health agencies, public school districts, and community agencies work together to meet the physical and psychosocial needs of the adolescent. Respite care for parents enables a helper to come into the home to relieve parents of the responsibility of caring for the child for brief periods of time. This enables the parents to shop, transact business affairs, or simply take a much-needed break or vacation.

One mother whose 13-year-old daughter had a severe developmental disability (cerebral palsy, blindness, mental retardation) offered these suggestions for the health care worker assisting in the home:

- Observe how the parents interact with the child.
- Do not wait for the child to cry out for attention because he or she may be unable to communicate in this way.
- Watch for facial expression and body language.
- Post signs above the bed denoting special considerations, such as "Never position on the left side," "Do not feed with plastic spoon," and so on.
- Listen to parents, and observe how they attend to the physical needs of the child.
- Do not be afraid to ask questions or discuss apprehensions you may feel concerning your ability to care for the child.
- Be attuned to the needs of other children in the home.
- Be creative in exploring avenues for socialization because these teenagers are seldom invited to birthday parties, slumber parties, or other social activities available to most adolescents.
- Explore community facilities and support groups that might be of benefit to the family.

HEALTH PROMOTION AND MAINTENANCE

PARENTING A TEENAGER

Adolescence may be one of the greatest parenting challenges. Raising children to be independent and responsible is the goal of all parents. Children should understand that there are house rules and consequences. Children need to understand society's rules and consequences, which will teach responsibility for actions committed outside of the home. Both of these ideas encourage teens to become responsible adults while allowing them to make mistakes and assume responsibility for their actions.

Parents need to be reassured that all parents make mistakes with their children. This may be an excellent time for parents to role-model for their children the ability to say "I'm sorry" or "I made a bad decision." Parents should be encouraged to know their children's friends and parents, become involved in their school and activities, and keep the lines of communication open. They also need to provide their teenager with privacy. Parents need to wait until teenagers are ready and then give them the opportunity to discuss their problems. However, teenagers often end up discussing problems with friends instead. Parents who are experiencing difficulties in parenting may be referred to professional help.

HEALTH EXAMINATIONS

The prevention of illness in this age group, as in all others, is of primary importance. Yearly physical examinations are recommended for healthy adolescents. Immunizations need to be reviewed and updated (see the Evolve Appendix). A menstrual history and gynecologic examination should be a routine part of the assessment of the adolescent girl. With sexually active teenagers, school nurses and other health care practitioners must take an active role in teaching about the prevention of sexually transmitted diseases.

Adolescents are often reluctant to seek health care. This reluctance can be influenced by factors such as perceived availability of confidential services, characteristics of health care providers, geographic access, and financial limitations (Hockenberry et al., 2007). They also feel that nothing will or can go wrong with them and often feel they are invincible. Multiple resources may be the most effective adolescent health promotion effort. School-based clinics, school-linked clinics, physician offices, and community clinics can offer services the adolescent needs for health promotion. It is important that nurses and physicians make adolescents feel comfortable in the waiting room and in the examining room. The physician-patient relationship can be enhanced when a good rapport is established. When facing the issues of the teenage years, adolescents need to be able to turn to a supportive nurse or physician.

The media can also have an impact on the health of the adolescent. The media can offer health promotion messages such as antismoking, antiviolence, and antidrug campaigns. Through these messages, today's

AREAS	FINDINGS
Physical activity and fitness	Number of young people taking part in daily physical education classes has decreased (33%)
Nutrition	Number of young people at risk of being overweight has increased (15.8%)
Tobacco	Number of adolescents reporting smoking has decreased (19.5%); smokeless tobacco use has increased slightly (8.9%)
Alcohol and other drugs	72.5% have tried alcohol; 41.8% have current alcohol use; marijuana use has decreased slightly (36.8%); steroid use has decreased (3.3%)
Mental health and mental disorders	Suicide attempt rates among young people are leveling (16.9%)
Violent and abusive behavior	Number of rapes is 7.4%; homicide rates are increasing; student reporting of weapon carrying at school has decreased (5.6%); physical fighting has decreased (31.5%)
Unintentional injuries	Reported number of young people not wearing seat belts has decreased (9.7%) Number of young people not wearing bicycle helmets has decreased (84.7%)

Table 10-3 Summary of Findings from "Youth Risk Behavior Surveillance, United States—2009"

From Centers for Disease Control and Prevention. (2010). Youth risk behavior surveillance USA—2009. *MMWR, 59*(SS-5), 1-142.

youth can make informed decisions and help maintain good health habits.

Healthy Youth 2020 is a document that outlines the adolescent component of the *Healthy People 2020* objectives. (See Chapter 1 for a discussion on *Healthy People 2020*.) An interim report, "Youth Risk Behavior Surveillance, United States—2009," summarizes some of the findings (Table 10-3). This summary stresses the importance of health promotion among our youth. Nutrition, tobacco, alcohol use, and suicide remain areas that require the attention and educational efforts of health care workers and the community.

SEXUALITY

Sexuality defines the characteristics that make each of us either female or male. A person's sexuality is affected by psychological, biological, and social factors. Because the adolescent is in a period of growth, the various factors of sexuality may be in conflict. The adolescent is not prepared for the responsibility of having a child and yet is biologically capable of reproduction. Adolescents are becoming sexually active at younger ages. Current statistics indicate that 46.8% of adolescents have engaged in intercourse, with girls having a higher rate (CDC, 2006).

The adolescent has an increased need to learn about sexuality. Values must be clarified, and decision-making skills must be evaluated. Although parental involvement in sex education is encouraged, parents often wait until adolescence to talk with their children. In other cases, they might prefer giving others the responsibility of educating their children. Consequently, the adolescent receives information from peers, the media, and other sources that may be incorrect or biased.

If the adolescent receives incorrect information about the body, misconceptions should be identified and teaching should be done regarding menstruation, pregnancy, sexually transmitted diseases, and contraception. Most adolescents do not want to become pregnant, and yet many do not use contraceptives. Adolescents need to be informed about safe sex practices. Contraceptive information needs to be available to prevent pregnancy. Condom information needs to be available to protect against the transmission of HIV and other sexually transmitted diseases. Both boys and girls need to be knowledgeable about protective measures. The school nurse or clinic nurse can often provide this information to adolescents.

Adolescents have fears and concerns that are specific to their sexuality. The girl who is the tallest person in her class is often just as concerned as the boy who is the shortest. Adolescent girls are also concerned about when to wear a bra, when they will begin their menstrual period, and when they will take on the characteristics of a woman. Adolescent boys may be worried because they do not have the height and strength of their peers. There is a wide age range for the physical changes that take place during puberty, and the adolescent needs to be reassured that they are normal. An excellent time to teach normal growth and development to the developing adolescent is at the time of assessment. Nurses can talk about concerns as they examine each part of the child's body. Because there is such a wide variation in the age at which each child develops, nurses should point out to adolescents that they are exactly where they should be for their particular stage of sexual development.

Sex education in public schools tends to concentrate on the physiology of sex, on the reproductive systems, and on sexually transmitted disease. It is usually less informative about the psychological and value aspects of sexuality and the facts concerning contraception. Peers play a major role in providing information on sex. This is because few adolescents can talk freely to their parents about sex (particularly regarding their own sexual behavior and problems). However, sexual values, attitudes, and information are conveyed in less conscious ways by role modeling. In this way, parents serve as an initial source of sex role learning for their daughters and sons. In their sexuality and intimacy, adolescents reflect society's new openness about sexual matters and are inclined to see sexual behavior as a matter of personal choice rather than of morality or law. Parents need to provide factual information.

ADOLESCENT PREGNANCY

While the rate of adolescent pregnancy has declined in the past few years, adolescent's sexual activity continues to increase. Current statistics report that 47.8% of adolescents have engaged in intercourse and 7.1% have had intercourse before the age of 13. Boys, especially African Americans and Hispanics, have a higher rate of activity (CDC, 2008). Many teenage mothers come from economically disadvantaged situations and tend to do poorly in school. They tend to have family situations that they are repeating. Teenage fathers tend to have poor school achievements and are involved with illegal activities (Kliegman et al., 2007).

Teen pregnancies have increased issues with low birth weight that affect perinatal mortality and morbidity. They have a higher incidence of neonatal deaths and infant deaths within the first year of life. The infants have a higher incidence of sudden infant death syndrome. Mothers have a higher incidence of anemia, hypertension and eclampsia, and low maternal weight gain. Teenage mothers have the "highest incidences of violence during pregnancy" (Kliegman et al., 2007). With the increased obesity issues with adolescents, the obese pregnant adolescent creates additional medical issues for the health care providers. It has been documented that almost 50% of pregnant adolescents do not seek prenatal care until at least 12 weeks gestation or later (Aruda, 2007).

Other issues that can become long-term problems for the teenage mother include lack of education. Many of these mothers quit school, which will affect the limits of income for the family. Substance abuse decreases during the pregnancy, but usage reappears after delivery. Many of these mothers are at risk for repeated pregnancies.

Prevention of adolescent pregnancy is a difficult societal issue. While many have fears that sex education will increase teen sexual activity, studies have shown different. Many programs place emphasis on abstinence, while others include contraception. Health care providers need to function in an environment that fosters nonjudgmental support while providing factual information and guidance with their choices. Contraception should be discussed including new options available such as patches, vaginal rings, progestin implants, and progestin-releasing intrauterine devices (Oski, 2009). Sexually transmitted diseases information should be included. These teenage mothers benefit from being connected with community resources such as Women, Infants, and Children (WIC) and Temporary Assistance for Needy Families (TANF).

HOMOSEXUALITY

Homosexual experiences in adolescence are not uncommon. This experimentation is not necessarily a positive prediction of one's sexual preference as an adult. It may merely reflect a desire to explore alternative lifestyles or may arise from curiosity. Homosexuality, although no longer classified as a disease, is nonetheless subject to great controversy. Whether or not the adolescent is homosexual, unspoken suspicions during adolescence can create anxiety and turmoil for the young person and the family. Parents need to accept their child and be supportive. It is also important that nurses remain sensitive to these issues when interacting with homosexual adolescents. Nurses need to be aware of their personal biases to determine their potential effectiveness with this population. Refer adolescents to counseling when they question their sexual orientation and preference.

BODY PIERCINGS AND TATTOOS

Teens and other young people receive body piercing and tattoos because they want to make a "statement" or because they simply feel that it is fashionable and expressive. Ears, navels, tongues, eyebrows, lips, nostrils, nipples, and genitals are all sites used for piercing. Ideally, piercing and tattooing should be performed by an experienced licensed person. Unfortunately, no national regulations exist regarding the piercing or tattooing of minors. Generally, unlicensed uncertified "professionals" perform these procedures. At the very least, new disposable gloves and sterilized or disposable needles must be used to prevent HIV and hepatitis B. There is also a risk for tetanus. The skin at the site of the piercing is inspected regularly for signs of infection or allergic reaction. Jewelry should never be shared. Healing can take anywhere from 8 weeks to more than 1 year when a body part is pierced (Anderson and Martel, 2002). Self-inflicted or friend-inflicted piercing and tattoos should be avoided because improper technique is often used.

It is important that health care workers examine their own feelings regarding these issues and not stereotype or pass judgment when caring for youth with piercing or tattoos. It is also up to health care workers to provide education regarding piercing and tattoos to today's youth and to assist them in making informed decisions.

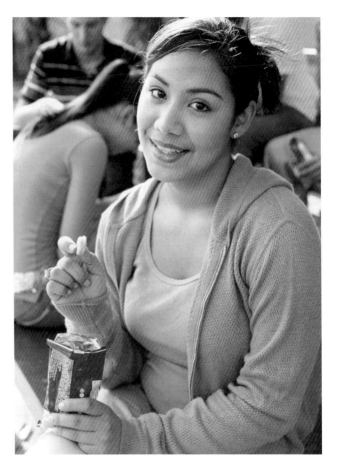

FIGURE 10-7 Snacking on empty calories is common among adolescents.

NUTRITION

Adolescent girls have special nutritional needs. They have fewer caloric requirements than boys do. There is a concern with body image that may lead to anorexia or bulimia. The nurse should emphasize that skipping meals can lead to a decrease in essential nutrients. Encourage physical exercise to maintain body weight and eating nutritious foods that are low in calories such as skim milk and fruits. The adolescent should avoid high-calorie fast foods (Figure 10-7). Besides salad bars, many fast-food chains have added grilled and high-fiber foods to their menus.

Many adolescent boys are concerned with their body image and body building. They should have a well-balanced diet with increased calories. Part of the dietary requirement is proper hydration without the use of supplements.

Overeating can lead to adult obesity. Adolescents who are obese need guidance in weight reduction. They should be instructed to do the following:
- Eat a variety of foods low in calories and high in nutrients.
- Eat less fat and fewer fatty foods.
- Eat less sugar and sweets.

- Eat more fruits, vegetables, and whole grains.
- Increase physical activity.

Teenagers are growing rapidly, and they need foods that provide for the increase in height, body-cell mass, and maturation. Dietary deficiencies are more apt to occur at this age because of the acceleration in growth and increasingly irregular eating patterns. Depending on activity level, 13-year-old girls need approximately 1600 to 2200 calories per day and boys of the same age require 2000 to 2600 calories per day. The 18-year-old female needs 1800 to 2400 calories, whereas 18-year-old males need 2400 to 3200 calories, again depending on activity level. The U.S. Department of Agriculture has developed new food guidelines through the MyPyramid plan (www.mypyramid.gov).

The most noticeable changes in the adolescent's eating habits are skipping meals, an increase in between-meal snacking, and an increase in eating out. Breakfast and lunch are often omitted. Part-time jobs, school activities, and socialization may result in the teenager's eating little or nothing during the day and then catching up in the evening. Fast-food restaurants are inexpensive and quick for the busy adolescent. These foods tend to be high in calories, fat, protein, sugar, and sodium and low in fiber. Most fast-food chains have added salad bars and other healthier foods. These appeal to the diet-conscious teenager and to vegetarians. Carbonated drinks often replace milk, resulting in low intakes of calcium, riboflavin, and vitamins A and D. The few fruits and vegetables eaten provide insufficient fiber.

Nutritional research on this age group is still meager, partly because studies must account not only for age but also for physical maturity. Minerals most apt to be inadequate in the adolescent diet are calcium and iron. Zinc is known to be essential for growth and sexual maturation and is therefore of great importance in adolescence. The retention of zinc increases, especially during the growth spurts, and leads to more efficient use of this nutrient's sources. Good sources of zinc include meat, liver, eggs, and seafood, particularly oysters. Sources for vegetarians include nuts, beans, wheat germ, and cheese. The importance of calcium lies in its key role in bone formation. In both boys and girls, the recommended dietary allowance (RDA) for calcium increases from 800 mg at age 10 years to 1200 to 1500 mg during the growth spurt (American Academy of Pediatrics, 2006). The primary source of calcium is dairy products. The need for iron is increased in both genders at this time. This increased need is caused primarily by increases in muscle mass and blood volume in boys and to a lesser extent in girls. A menstruating woman loses 15 to 30 mg of iron per cycle. Iron absorption varies in individuals. Good sources of iron include liver, poultry, fish, dried beans, vegetables, egg yolk, and enriched breads. Protein needs are increased, particularly during pubertal changes in both genders and for developing muscle mass in boys. Calcium is important for the adolescent because during adolescence 40% to 60% of peak bone mass is developed. Bone mass has relevance for decreasing osteoporosis in later life.

SPORTS AND NUTRITION

The best training diet is one that contains foods from each of the basic food groups in sufficient quantities to meet energy demands and nutrient requirements. There is no evidence that eating large amounts of special foods or nutrients is beneficial in terms of athletic performance. Protein supplements are not necessary and could even be harmful. Sweat losses must be replaced by drinking plenty of fluids during the workout. Carbohydrates should not be used as the sole energy source because they are stored for relatively short spans in the body. Sodium and potassium replacement usually is met by eating a well-balanced diet. Caffeine and alcohol deplete body water and should be avoided. Anabolic steroids, used by some athletes to gain weight and increase strength, are detrimental to bone growth. Iron is particularly necessary for female athletes who may be borderline or deficient in their intake of this mineral. On the day of the event, the athlete is advised to eliminate fiber, fats, and gas-forming foods.

PERSONAL CARE

SLEEP

Sleep requirements vary among individuals. Adolescents may obtain the 8 hours generally suggested but often at irregular hours. Many young people who are employed have to work very late hours, particularly in the summer months. This necessitates sleeping later in the morning. Another trend is for the young person who has worked long hours during the day to try to make up for lost time after work. It would seem that adolescents are either sleeping all the time or burning the candle at both ends! Complaints of fatigue are heard more often at home than elsewhere. The nurse should advise parents to become aware of the young person's sleep patterns. Crankiness, frustration, impatience, accident proneness, and other such behaviors may indicate lack of sleep. Finally, teenagers need to sleep on a bed with a firm mattress, preferably in their own room.

EXERCISE

Exercise has many benefits. Adolescents do not have to participate actively in sports; they can easily exercise by taking a brisk walk, riding a bike, or swimming. Although many teenagers are not athletes, they can benefit from a less sedentary lifestyle. These patterns,

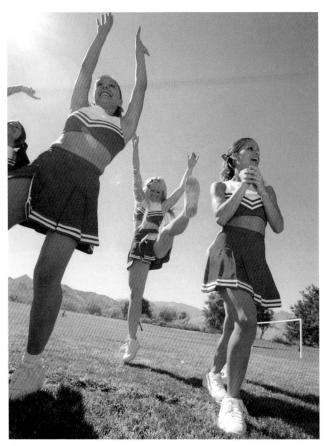

FIGURE 10-8 Cheerleading is an example of an activity that promotes physical fitness and helps the adolescent learn to work with others in a small group.

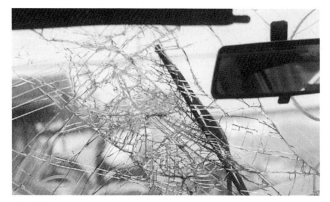

FIGURE 10-9 Accidents involving motor vehicles are a leading cause of injury and death in children and adolescents. Passengers need to have seat belts even if the car has an airbag.

when carried over into adulthood, contribute to good health (Figure 10-8).

PERSONAL HYGIENE

Personal hygiene information is necessary at this time when the body changes of puberty require more frequent bathing and the use of deodorants. The nurse can help the adolescent figure out procedures and the various claims of reliability for products dealing with hair removal, menstrual hygiene, and cosmetics. Nurses need to stress the importance of not sharing razors with friends.

CLOTHING

Clothing is of great interest to the adolescent. Peer influence and the media have a major impact on fashion. How adolescents dress may indicate the peer group to which they belong. Dress varies from very contemporary to conservative, depending on the particular teenager's preferences. Much of this is just for fun and provides for good conversation. The power of television advertising in regard to clothes sales and other commercial messages may be explored.

DENTAL CARE

The prevalence of tooth decay has decreased substantially over the past few years. This is believed to be the result of the widespread use of fluorides, including community fluoridation and the use of dental products containing fluorides. Teenagers, nevertheless, are at risk for dental caries because of inadequate dental maintenance and frequent snacking on sucrose-containing candies and beverages. When dental hygiene is neglected, the period of greatest tooth decay in the permanent teeth is from ages 12 to 18 years. Poor oral hygiene (inadequate brushing, flossing, and rinsing, particularly after meals) fosters the accumulation of plaque and food debris. Missing, aching, or decayed teeth contribute to poor nutrition. Young people with unattractive teeth may have low self-esteem. According to the media, healthy white teeth are synonymous with popularity and sex appeal. A visit to the dentist twice a year is out of reach for many financially strapped young people. For others, it is a low family financial priority. There is a need for more school dental programs and other innovative measures to reach a major proportion of our young people.

SAFETY

The primary danger to the adolescent is the automobile. Road accidents kill and cripple teenagers at alarming rates. Many schools today offer driver training courses as an integral part of the educational program. In these courses, students learn the basic skills of driving, as well as the responsibilities that driving entails. Unfortunately, this does not ensure compliance. Preventing motor vehicle accidents is of utmost importance to every community. Seat belts must be worn every time an adolescent rides in a car (Figure 10-9). No one should ever drink and drive. Students Against Drunk Drivers (SADD) is an organization for youth against drinking and driving. Adolescents who ride motorcycles, motor scooters, or motorized bicycles should know the rules of the road and should wear special safety equipment, such as helmets, for protection. Adolescents must also be told that riding in the back of a pickup truck is dangerous—and possibly fatal.

Homicide is now the second leading cause of death among 15-year-olds to 24-year-olds. Most of these homicides involve firearms. The third leading cause of death among 15-year-olds to 24-year-olds is suicide, which has increased at alarming rates in adolescents over the past several years. Teenagers who do not achieve a sense of identity can experience self-doubt. Loss of relationships and depression can also leave the adolescent vulnerable to suicidal tendencies. It is important for parents and health care workers to be alert for signs of depression or isolation in the adolescent. It is also crucial to work on promoting self-esteem and identity.

Although most adolescents know how to swim, accidents that involve diving into unsafe areas and using alcohol or drugs while playing in the water are not uncommon.

Both accidental and deliberate morbidity and mortality caused by firearms continue to be a major concern during the adolescent period. Regarding handling firearms, this age group is characterized by the feeling of "it couldn't happen to me." Gang-related injuries and deaths often involve the use of firearms. Many adolescents are involved in serious crimes (Figure 10-10), some of which involve guns and violence. Gun control continues to be controversial. At the very least, control must be stringent for this age group. Those who do use firearms legally must be taught to respect the power of firearms and how to use them safely.

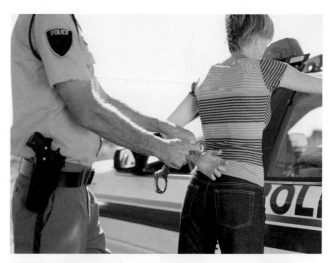

FIGURE 10-10 Increasing numbers of older children and adolescents are involved in serious crimes against persons and property.

Nursing Brief

Boys and girls should both be taught sports injury prevention. Physical conditioning should be emphasized in relation to all intense physical activity (e.g., team sports).

INTERNET SOLICITATION

Children using the home computer is becoming the typical picture of family life. Children and adolescents are spending more time at the computer, for both educational and personal purposes. Internet access allows adolescents to explore topics such as pornography and gambling in the privacy of their home. Reports indicate that 1 million to 2 million adolescents engage in gambling, which can be difficult to monitor and can lead to hidden addictions (Verkler, 2005).

Online predators are able to access unsuspecting children by using chat rooms and instant messaging. With the increasing use of handheld devices, the home computer is not the only mode of contact. Parents need to have an understanding of computers, how to trace websites, and how to use filtering devices. Health care providers need to raise awareness of the potential dangers of Internet access for all ages. The AAP has partnered with Microsoft to offer a free web-based safety service (Windows Live Family Safety Setting), which will provide parents with a tool to control and track Internet access. The service hopes to encourage dialogue between parents and children regarding websites (AAP, 2006).

Health Promotion

Guidelines for Internet Safety

- Never share personal information.
- Never meet with an online contact.
- Discuss with a parent or adult about relationships developed over the Internet.
- Never send a message over the Internet that you would not say in person.

Get Ready for the NCLEX® Examination!

Key Points

- Adolescence begins with the appearance of secondary sex characteristics and ends with cessation of growth and the achievement of emotional maturation.
- Adolescents question life and search for their sense of identity. They seek to understand who they are, where they are going, and how they are getting there.
- It is important in today's society that adolescents learn to develop problem-solving skills and learn to deescalate conflicts.

- Early adolescents are in the concrete phase of thinking; older adolescents develop abstract formal thinking.
- Peer relationships are important in helping adolescents define themselves.
- With increasing maturity comes increasing responsibility. Adolescents need to learn to understand financial management.
- Dating represents one of the early social decision points of growing up.
- Parents need to clarify house rules and consequences; society's rules and consequences teach responsibility outside of the home.
- Annual health examinations are equally important to the adolescent; anticipatory guidance includes nutrition, exercise, and safety.
- Adolescents must come to terms with their own sexuality; this is affected by psychological, biological, and social factors.
- Parents should have an open dialogue with adolescents regarding Internet usage and safety.

Additional Learning Resources

Ǝvolve Go to your Evolve website (*http://evolve.elsevier.com/Price/pediatric/*) for the following FREE learning resources:
- 3-D Animations
- Answer Keys
- Appendixes
- Audio Glossary
- Spanish/English Glossary
- Video Clips

Review Questions for the NCLEX® Examination

1. All of the following are true about Tanner staging **except:**
    1. It provides an accurate assessment of a child's development and chronological age.
    2. It assesses the development of secondary sexual maturation.
    3. Stages are based on breast and pubic hair development for girls.
    4. Stages are based on genital and pubic hair development for boys.

2. Breast self-examination should be routinely performed beginning at age:
    1. 12 to 14 years
    2. 14 to 16 years
    3. 16 to 18 years
    4. 18 to 21 years

3. According to Piaget's theory of cognitive development: (**Select all that apply.**)
    1. Early adolescents can see a situation from many viewpoints.
    2. Middle adolescence is the stage of formal operations.
    3. Older adolescents can imagine unexperienced possibilities.
    4. Moral adolescence is placed at a postconventional morality stage.
    5. Early adolescents take things literally.

4. The second leading cause of death among 15-year-olds to 24-year-olds is:
    1. Motor vehicle accidents
    2. Suicide
    3. Homicide
    4. Neoplasms

5. Which of the following best describes the psychological health of the 17-year-old to 20-year-old?
    1. Wide mood swings
    2. Anger more apt to be concealed
    3. Tendency to withdraw when upset
    4. Intense daydreaming

Objectives

1. Define the vocabulary terms listed
2. List the differences found in the respiratory system of a child, and identify potential risks
3. Develop a teaching plan for the parents of a newborn regarding SIDS prevention
4. Illustrate the anatomic difference in the ear canals of adults and children, and describe the significance of this difference along with nursing care for a child with otitis media
5. Summarize the nursing care for an infant with bronchiolitis

6. Explain the dietary needs for a child with cystic fibrosis
7. Outline the nursing observation and care necessary for a 2-year-old child with croup
8. Describe the nursing care for a child undergoing surgery for removal of tonsils and adenoids
9. Describe the nursing care of the child with asthma, including monitoring of respiratory status, respiratory treatments and medications, and the psychosocial implications of the condition
10. Discuss the important nursing care of a child with tuberculosis

Key Terms

Back to Sleep (p. 197)
hydrocarbons (p. 222)
laryngotracheobronchitis
   (lă-RĬNG-gō-TRĀ-kē-ō brŏn-KĪ-tĭs; p. 207)
meconium ileus (p. 203)
pulmonary function test (PFT) (p. 196)
reactive airway disease (p. 214)

respiratory syncytial virus (RSV) (sĭn-SĬSH-ăl; p. 201)
retractions (p. 196)
stridor (p. 207)
thoracentesis (p. 223)
tripod position (p. 219)
tympanostomy tubes (p. 201)

RESPIRATORY SYSTEM

The respiratory system consists of the nose, pharynx, and larynx (upper respiratory tract) and the trachea, bronchi, and lungs (lower respiratory tract). The respiratory tract continually changes during the first 12 years of a child's life. There are several anatomic differences that predispose children to respiratory difficulties (Box 11-1). This makes respiratory problems common during childhood. Most problems are mild and can be managed at home. Other conditions can be chronic and have an impact on the growth and development of the child. Respiratory distress and failure are the common factors for cardiac arrest in children. Respiratory diseases account for 25% of hospitalizations for children younger than 15 years of age. Pneumonia accounts for 31%, bronchiolitis and bronchitis for 25%, and asthma for 25% of the respiratory diseases (CDC, 2007).

Children with respiratory difficulties have common signs and symptoms that can progress to respiratory failure if not recognized. Assessment findings of the child's respiratory system will vary depending on the age of the child. The nurse must recognize any change in the child's breathing status. Signs and symptoms may include fever, anorexia, vomiting, diarrhea, abdominal pain, nasal blockage, nasal drainage, cough, sore throat, retractions, and abnormal respiratory sounds. Respiratory assessment should be comprehensive and frequent as the status can change rapidly. The assessment should include the guidelines shown in Box 11-2. Retractions can indicate respiratory distress. The severity of respiratory distress can be assessed using the depth and location of the retractions (Figure 11-1).

A variety of diagnostic tests can assist in monitoring respiratory function. Chest x-rays assist in identifying foreign objects or abnormalities in lung tissue. Pulse oximetry is a noninvasive method for measuring oxygen saturation. Pulmonary function test (PFT) and spirometry measure the vital and expiratory capacity.

| Box 11-1 | Pediatric Respiratory Differences |

- Smaller nares and nasopharynx, which can be occluded with edema
- Obligatory nose breathers until 4 weeks of age and are unable to use mouth to breathe
- Small and floppy epiglottis, which can be occluded with edema
- Large tongue, which increases risk for occlusion of airway
- Larynx and glottis are located higher in neck, which increases risk for aspiration
- Trachea is shorter and narrow with flexible cartilage, which can be occluded with edema and neck and head flexion
- Enlarged tonsillar tissue, which increases risk for obstruction
- Underdeveloped respiratory muscles result in poor chest expansion and decreased expiratory lung volume
- Diaphragm and abdominal muscles used for breathing in children under 6 years of age can be impaired by abdominal distention
- Alveoli are underdeveloped and continue to develop until 12 years of age
- Higher metabolic rate, which increases oxygen demands
- Eustachian tubes are horizontal until age 7, which increases the risk of ear infections
- Higher respiratory rate with irregular breathing patterns in infants

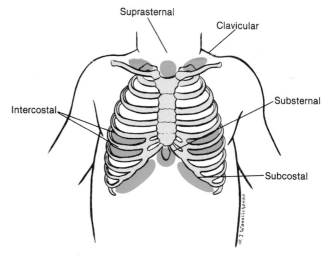

FIGURE 11-1 Retraction sites.

| Box 11-2 | Respiratory Assessment Guidelines |

- Behavior changes such as irritability, restlessness, and level of responsiveness
- Child's position of comfort
- Vital signs including respiratory rate, depth, rhythm, and ease
- Lung sounds including lobe areas, wheezing, crackles, rhonchi, or coarseness
- Respiratory effort including stridor, grunting, retractions (see Figure 11-1), nasal flaring, labored breathing, head bobbing, and tachypnea
- Color of skin and mucous membranes
- Cough including productivity, effort, and noise (barking, musical, croupy)

SUDDEN INFANT DEATH SYNDROME

Sudden infant death syndrome (SIDS) is defined clinically as the sudden, unexpected death of an apparently healthy infant younger than 1 year of age for which a routine autopsy fails to identify the cause. It is also referred to as **crib death** or **cot death**. Although precise data are not available, it is estimated that in the United States, SIDS kills about 3000 infants per year. In industrialized countries, SIDS is one of the leading causes of death in early infancy; the peak incidence is between 2 and 4 months of age. It is more common in low–birth weight babies, in boys, in families with crowded living conditions, and during the winter months. Autopsy may reveal slight respiratory infection or otitis media, petechiae over the pleura, and pulmonary edema. Two clinical features of the disease remain constant: (1) death occurs during sleep, and (2) the infant does not cry or make other sounds of distress. In some cases, the baby is found in one corner of the crib with blood-tinged froth coming from the nose.

Theories concerning the cause of SIDS are numerous. Although there appears to be an increased incidence among siblings, no genetic pattern has been determined. The risk for SIDS is increased in twins.

Many theories concerning cause (e.g., suffocation, aspiration allergy, and hormone deficiency) have been disproved. The exact cause is not known. Some researchers propose that crib death results from an interruption of some basic function in the central or autonomic nervous system that causes apnea. Carotid bodies located in the neck and involved in the control of breathing have been found to be abnormal in victims of SIDS. Current opinion holds that SIDS has more than one cause.

The death rate has continued to decrease, and the focus is on decreasing risk factors that contribute to SIDS. The Back to Sleep program has produced positive results. Co-sleeping has been identified as an increased risk of SIDS even if mothers do not smoke or if they breastfeed. Health care providers should encourage a separate crib or bassinet for sleeping.

| Box 11-3 | Evidence-Based Practice |

Infant Sleeping Position

PROBLEM
Infants discharged from NICU are more likely to be placed in a prone position.

EVIDENCE
Survey of 2300 mothers found 26% did not place 3-month-old in supine position; 42% reported bed sharing at 2 weeks and 27% at 12 months; higher incidence of prone sleeping position with African-American mothers.

Survey of nurses reported that most nurses felt for premature infants a nonsupine sleep position was best during hospitalization. 52% of NICU nurses discussed supine sleeping on discharge. 45% of nurses reported reflux and/or aspiration as reason for nonsupine position (Carrier, 2009).

IMPLICATIONS
Back to Sleep program (BTS) has shown to decrease the incidence of SIDS. Nurses have the opportunity to model and educate families about appropriate sleeping position.

CRITICAL THINKING
Identify practices that would increase the use of supine sleep position for newborns and infants.

 Health Promotion

Guidelines for Prevention of SIDS

- Always place infant on his or her back to sleep, and do **NOT** use side-lying position (see Box 11-3).
- Use a firm sleep surface with a safety-approved crib mattress.
- Keep soft objects and loose bedding out of infant's sleep area.
- Avoid overheating, keeping head uncovered.
- Do not smoke during pregnancy or near babies.
- Avoid co-sleeping, but keep infant's sleep area close. Keep infant's bedroom door open.
- Avoid home respiratory or cardiac monitors used to reduce SIDS risk.
- Avoid devices that claim to maintain sleep position to reduce SIDS.
- Consider offering a clean, dry pacifier (controversial).
- Provide tummy time during awake periods.
- Stress that all care providers for infant follow the guidelines (AAP, 2005).

Cultural Considerations

African-American infants are twice as likely to be put to sleep on their stomachs, and parents may need more instruction (Carrier, 2009).

Babies with **infantile apnea** (also called near-miss infants) and subsequent siblings of babies with SIDS are often monitored at home until they are past the age of danger. Monitors can be leased. Parents are provided with ongoing education and support during this period. Parents are taught cardiopulmonary resuscitation before being discharged.

In dealing with grieving parents after the death of their infant, the nurse must convey some important facts: that the baby died of a disease entity called *SIDS*, that this disease currently cannot be predicted or prevented, and that they are **not** responsible for the child's death. Grieving parents need time to say good-bye to their child. They should be encouraged to hold and rock their infant, shed tears, and assist in burial preparations. This process, not common in the past, is conducive to the resolution of grief (see also Chapter 22). One mother who was denied this experience stated that *5 years later*, while visiting a florist's shop, she noticed a heart-shaped wreath intended for an infant. She unexpectedly burst into tears and wept.

Parents of a child who dies of SIDS experience a great deal of guilt and are catapulted into a totally unexpected bereavement, requiring numerous explanations to relatives and friends. Often needless blame has been placed on one parent by the other or by relatives. The family babysitter and physician may also be targets of attack. Emergency department personnel need to be especially sensitive and supportive during this crisis. There have been occurrences of SIDS for which parents have been charged with child abuse and have even been jailed because of lack of public knowledge about the disease.

Sudden infant death syndrome can occur in the hospital, and many nurses and physicians have personal experience of the suffering that losing a child to SIDS can cause. Group therapy with other parents of SIDS victims is recommended. Two nationally supported organizations are the Compassionate Friends, Inc., and the National Sudden Infant Death Syndrome Foundation. These groups have local chapters in most states.

BRONCHOPULMONARY DYSPLASIA

Bronchopulmonary dysplasia (BPD) is a chronic lung disease that occurs in newborns that are premature or have pulmonary disorders that require mechanical ventilator support with high positive pressure and oxygen. The lung tissue is immature and unable to withstand tissue damage resulting from the required oxygen supplement. The resulting fibrosis and alteration in lung compliance may last from several months to years. Improvements in treatment of low–birth weight preterm infants have increased the incidence of this disorder, and continue to be the primary issue for infants younger than 27 weeks of age (Belcastro,

2004). Newer mechanical ventilators are being used for low birth weight neonates in hopes of decreasing BPD.

Signs and Symptoms

The symptoms of BPD are directly related to the pathophysiology of the disease. Tachypnea, dyspnea, and wheezing can be a result of airway obstruction and increased airway resistance. Increased work of breathing can cause retractions and use of accessory muscles. The infants may display activity intolerance during feedings. They may be irritable and difficult to comfort. Cyanosis may develop during crying spells. Infants who needed intubation for a long period of time may have subglottic stenosis and inspiratory stridor develop. All of the symptoms can be associated with the chronic hypoxia state. The diagnosis is made on the basis of abnormal radiographic findings, signs of respiratory distress, oxygen dependency after 28 days of age, and a history of required mechanical ventilation during the first week of life.

 Nursing Brief

Children in severe respiratory distress should receive nothing by mouth because of the increased workload of breathing and the increased risk for aspiration.

Treatment and Nursing Care

The treatment for infants with BPD is to provide adequate oxygenation and prevent progression of the disease process. Treatment includes oxygen, drug therapy, and nutritional support. Surfactant continues to be included in the course of medical treatment (Askins and Diehl-Jones, 2009). Infants may continue to need oxygen after hospital discharge. These infants do not tolerate excessive or even normal amounts of fluids. They may have problems develop with accumulation of fluids in the lungs that require the use of diuretics. The use of these drugs requires the monitoring of electrolytes and edema. Oral electrolyte supplements may be given. Bronchodilators (albuterol) and steroids may promote improved lung function. These infants are at risk for respiratory infections and should be given RSV-immune globulin (RespiGam) or palivizumab (Synagis) during the RSV season.

Infants with BPD are at high risk for growth failure, and nutrition is an important issue (VanRiper, 2010). They have higher metabolic needs, and providing adequate nutrition without causing respiratory distress can be difficult. Nursing care should be organized to provide periods of rest. Small, frequent feedings and nutritional supplements may be used. The environment should include measures to decrease stimulation.

 Home Care Considerations

The Child with Bronchopulmonary Dysplasia

Advise parents that:
- All caregivers need CPR training.
- House and care should be smoke-free.
- Avoid contact with individuals with colds or fever.
- Avoid crowds.
- Place infant on back to sleep.
- Keep infant's room door open.

Parents may be extremely anxious caring for a child with BPD. All equipment and procedures should be explained in simple terms. Children with tracheostomies can be cared for in the home setting, and home care teaching of the equipment is needed (Figure 11-2). Review care of the child with tracheostomy in Chapter 3. Extended hospitalization can interfere with the development of the normal parent-child relationship and with the normal development of the infant. Parental participation in the infant's care should be encouraged. The family's ability to cope and care for a child with a chronic illness needs to be evaluated as home discharge plans are developed. An adequate period of education may be necessary for the parents to become comfortable with the care required for their child. Families should be referred to social services to assist in providing additional support and to assist in helping the parent gain access to available community services. Parental support groups can be beneficial in providing additional assistance with coping skills necessary for caring for a child with complex care.

OTITIS MEDIA

Otitis media (*ot*, ear; *itis*, inflammation of; *media*, middle) is an inflammation of the middle ear. The middle ear is a tiny cavity in the temporal bone. Its entrance is guarded by the sensitive tympanic membrane, or eardrum, which transmits sound waves

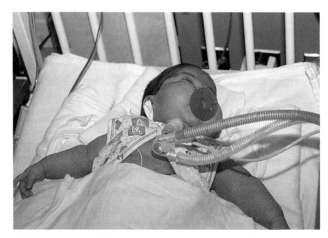

FIGURE 11-2 Humidified oxygen is provided to the child with a tracheostomy.

through the oval window to the inner ear. The inner ear contains the organs of hearing and balance. The middle ear opens into air spaces, or **sinuses**, in the mastoid process of the temporal bone. It is also connected to the throat by a channel called the **eustachian tube**. These structures—the mastoid sinuses, the middle ear, and the eustachian tube—are lined with mucous membranes. As a result, an infection of the throat can easily spread to the middle ear and mastoid. The eustachian tube also protects the middle ear from nasopharyngeal secretions and provides drainage of middle ear secretions into the nasopharynx and equalizes air pressure between the middle ear and the outside atmosphere. These protective functions are diminished when the tubes are blocked. Unequalized air within the ear creates a negative pressure that allows organisms to be swept up into the tube if it opens.

Otitis media may be the result of an upper respiratory tract infection, caused by a variety of organisms. The most common cause of these infections is viral. Bacteria cause the rest of otitis media cases. Of the bacterial cases, 40% to 50% are caused by *Streptococcus pneumoniae,* which is increasingly demonstrating resistance to penicillin. Other common bacteria that cause otitis media are *Haemophilus influenzae* and *Moraxella catarrhalis.* With the use of *H. influenzae* type b vaccine (Hib) as a routine immunization, the number of cases of otitis media caused by this organism has decreased. The addition of the seven-valent *S. pneumoniae* conjugate vaccine to the immunization schedule should also decrease the incidence rate of otitis media caused by this organism (Morris, 2009). Infants are more prone to ear infections because the eustachian tube is shorter, wider, and straighter than in older children and adults. Because babies lie flat for long periods, microorganisms have easy access from the eustachian tube to the middle ear. This is thought by some investigators to be a contributing factor.

There are two types of otitis media. The acute disease is **suppurative** or **purulent otitis media (AOM)**. It is most commonly caused by *S. pneumoniae* and *H. influenzae.* The second type is called **serous** or **nonsuppurative otitis media with effusion (OME)**. The cause is unknown, but it often occurs after an acute episode. OME is the most common cause of hearing loss and hearing impairment in children.

Signs and Symptoms

The symptoms of acute otitis media (AOM) are pain in the ear (often severe), irritability, and interference with hearing. Sucking or chewing has a tendency to increase the pain. Fever, which may run as high as 40° C (104° F), headache, and vomiting may also accompany the illness as may diarrhea. The nurse may suspect an earache in the infant who rubs the ear frequently or pulls at it. The infant may also roll the head from side to side and cry piercingly. The older child

can point to the place that is tender. OME is the result of chronic otitis media. Children may be asymptomatic but may report a feeling of fullness or popping in the ears.

If an abscess forms, the eardrum may rupture as a result and pus may drain from the ear. When this happens, the pressure is relieved and the child is more comfortable.

Complications of an ear infection include hearing loss, mastoiditis, chronic otitis media, and meningitis. These complications are rare with modern treatment. Prevention lies in the prompt treatment of respiratory infections or infected tonsils and adenoids.

Treatment and Nursing Care

The professional who examines the ears first observes their appearance and general hygiene. The lymph nodes about the ear are observed for swelling or tenderness. The child's head is adequately stabilized to prevent injury to the ear canal from sudden, unexpected movement. Excess cerumen or wax in the ear, which may obstruct visibility, is carefully removed. The examiner ensures that no foreign bodies are lodged in the outer canal before inserting the otoscope. To straighten the canal and improve viewing, the ear is pulled **down** and **back** in infants and small children. The ear is pulled **up** and **back** in older children and adults. The physician may also perform a pneumatic otoscopic examination. The ear speculum is used to seal the ear canal, and air is expressed into the canal. The movement or lack of movement of the tympanic membrane is indicative of the degree of fluid behind the membrane. This examination has proven useful in determining the degree of the condition.

New treatment guidelines were released in 2004 by the American Academy of Pediatrics (AAP) (Box 11-4). Treatment included an observation option, pain management, and antimicrobial treatment. Development of resistant strains of bacteria and misuse of antimicrobials assisted in the development of new guidelines. When antimicrobials are used, amoxicillin remains the

---

Box 11-4 **Acute Otitis Media Guidelines**

- Diagnosis of AOM by history, signs, and symptoms
- Assessment of pain and pain management for first 24 to 36 hours
- Optional treatment course of observation for 48 to 72 hours without antibacterial treatment; if child fails to respond within 48 to 72 hours, antibacterial therapy should be started
- Treatment using antibacterial agent; high-dose amoxicillin is recommended
- Encouragement of prevention by reducing risk factors Insufficient evidence to recommend use of complementary and alternative medicine (CAM) (AAP, 2004)

drug of choice, but recurrent infections may require other antimicrobials. Parents are taught to give the entire dose of the antimicrobial even though the child may appear well. Parents will need to understand the new course of treatment using the guidelines and their role in the management of AOM.

Pain control may be needed for the child with AOM. Pain control is achieved using acetaminophen or ibuprofen as prescribed. Antihistamines and decongestants are not effective and may have side effects. Eardrops (Auralgan) may be prescribed to control pain. Warm or cold compresses may be applied to the ear. The child can be placed on the affected side with the ear on top of a hot water bottle (temperature of the water 115° F, or 46° C) or on a heating pad on the low setting. Children should be placed upright to decrease pain. If the ear is draining, the outer canal can be cleaned with sterile water or hydrogen peroxide. Parents should be instructed not to use cotton swabs in the ears.

Nurses need to be aware that environmental factors have been identified that can contribute to the risk for ear infections. Daycare outside the home, parental smoking, and pacifier use has been shown to increase the risk for recurrent otitis media. Breastfeeding for at least 6 months has reduced the risk for AOM. These factors should be discussed with parents.

 Health Promotion

Risks for Otitis Media That Need to Be Discussed with Parents

- Parental smoking
- Excessive pacifier use
- Daycare outside the home

 Community Considerations

Parents may wish to use alternative therapies in the care of their child. Many of the herbal remedies available have not been evaluated for use in the pediatric population. These remedies are not regulated by the U.S. Food and Drug Administration (FDA) and thus may not be as labeled. Homeopathy remedies are regulated. The AAP has not made any recommendation because of insufficient evidence of effectiveness.

 Nursing Brief

Children should be fed in an upright position and should not be put to bed with a bottle.

For children with recurrent AOM or chronic OME, tympanostomy tubes may be effective. The physician performs the procedure by completing a **myringotomy** (*myringo*, eardrum; *otomy*, incision) and inserts a tiny tube into the eardrum. These tubes require surgical placement and special care by the parents. Eventually, the tubes fall out spontaneously.

BRONCHIOLITIS

Bronchiolitis is an inflammation of the small airways. It occurs most often during late autumn through late spring and in children younger than 2 years of age. Bronchiolitis is usually caused by a viral infection. The most common causative organism is the respiratory syncytial virus (RSV). Children are usually exposed through other family members who have symptoms of an upper respiratory tract infection. Children who are at risk for respiratory distress have chronic lung diseases such as bronchopulmonary dysplasia (BPD) or cystic fibrosis (CF).

Inflammation of the bronchioles is associated with obstruction that is caused by edema and accumulation of mucus. There may be partial or complete obstruction. The alveoli are usually not affected. Normal gas exchange in the lung is affected. This leads to hypoxemia.

Signs and Symptoms

The infant first shows signs of a mild upper respiratory infection with rhinorrhea, sneezing, cough, and a low-grade fever. The infant's appetite may be affected. Respiratory distress increases, and rapid breathing and wheezing develop. Bottle feeding may be difficult because of the rapid respiratory rate interfering with sucking and swallowing. As the disease progresses, nasal flaring, retractions, tachypnea (60 to 70 per minute), and cyanosis may occur. Breath sounds may be diminished if the bronchioles are severely obstructed.

Treatment

Mild cases of bronchiolitis can be managed at home. Treatment at home includes increasing the intake of fluids and increasing the humidity in the air. Also useful are antipyretics to control fever. The parents or caregiver should be instructed to bring the child back for reevaluation if any signs of increased respiratory distress occur or if the child's condition worsens.

Indications for hospitalization include an infant younger than 6 months of age, sleeping respiratory rates of 50 to 60 per minute or higher, hypoxemia, apnea, or the inability to tolerate oral feeding.

When the child is hospitalized, intravenous fluids are started to hydrate the child and thin the secretions. The child is placed in an atmosphere of humidified oxygen (mist tent, croupette, or nasal cannula/mask). The goal is to keep oxygen levels at 92% or better with a pulse oximeter. With severe bronchiolitis, the physician may use a bronchodilator and a corticosteroid, but these remain controversial (Zorc, 2010). Antimicrobials may also be used for small or severely ill infants because these infants may be susceptible to a secondary bacterial infection. Fever is controlled with antipyretics. A laboratory study of a nasopharyngeal washing should be done to determine whether the causative organism is RSV. As a precautionary measure for the safety and concern of other children, the infant is placed in contact isolation until RSV has been ruled out.

When the causative organism is RSV, no medications can effectively treat the disease. Ribavirin, antimicrobials, antihistamines, and oral decongestants have been identified as being ineffective for treatment (Zorc, 2010). Medical attention has recently focused on active and passive immunizations. **RSV-immune globulin (RespiGam)** and **palivizumab (Synagis)** have been approved for use with children at high risk. Palivizumab may be preferred because of ease of administration (intramuscular); lack of interference with mumps, measles, and rubella (MMR) vaccine and varicella vaccine; and lack of complications associated with intravenous immune globulin (RespiGam). Monthly administration during RSV season (October to May) is recommended (AAP, 2009).

Nursing Care

Nursing diagnoses for the infant with bronchiolitis include the following:

- Ineffective airway clearance, related to thick mucus
- Impaired gas exchange, related to edema and mucus of the bronchioles
- Deficient fluid volume, related to insensible fluid loss from tachypnea and decreased intake
- Anxiety, related to unfamiliar environment, respiratory distress, and placement in croupette
- Knowledge deficit, related to disease process and treatment

The child with bronchiolitis is monitored closely for signs and symptoms of increasing respiratory distress. Breath sounds, skin color, depth and rate of respirations, and vital signs are assessed. Changes in alertness and increased anxiety can be signs of impending distress. Continuous or intermittent pulse oximetry may be used to monitor the infant's oxygen level.

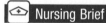 **Nursing Brief**

Infants with a respiratory rate of 60 breaths per minute should have nothing by mouth.

Intravenous fluids are monitored in the acutely ill child. As the child improves, oral fluids are increased and frequent small meals are offered. The child is on intake and output recording, and daily weights are taken. The fontanel and the child's skin turgor are also assessed as indicators of hydration status.

Formula-fed infants may have thickened feeding to improve swallowing dysfunction and to prevent aspiration. Breastfed infants should have more frequent feeding with shorter times. This assists in decreasing the workload of the infant and conserves energy. Nasal secretions should be removed with a bulb syringe before feedings (Allen, 2006).

The child in a mist tent should have the gown and linens changed if they become damp. Also, moisture buildup should be removed from the tubing and the sides of the tent (see Chapter 3 for detailed care of the child in a mist tent). For home care, cold air humidifiers can be used but must be cleaned properly to prevent bacteria or fungal growth.

As always, parents are encouraged to stay with the child. This may be even more important because the child may already be anxious because of respiratory distress. Parents should understand the importance of the child staying in the tent. They should be included in the care and diversional activities for the child.

Preventing the spread of infection is also important. If an infant has RSV, then contact isolation is recommended. RSV is primarily spread by large droplets and fomites. RSV can survive on hands for almost an hour and on hard surfaces up to 24 hours. Health care–associated infections (HAIs) or nosocomial infections can be a serious nursing issue. Hand hygiene is extremely important in all issues of infection. All caregivers, including parents, need to know and apply measures to prevent the spread of infection.

Support of the parents is significant. Most of the infants who are in severe or critical condition are usually young infants or those who have an underlying disease. Their parents may lack confidence when it comes to the care of the infant and need to be supported and reassured in their actions. It can be frightening for them to see their infant so ill. If the infant is admitted to a critical care area, the support of the parents is crucial. Explanations should be given in terms the parents can understand. The family needs information from the physician or the nurse concerning the infant's condition, medications, treatments, and procedures. Plans for all of these issues and discharge information can aid the parents in coping with the situation. Family, friends, and clergy can be a great support for the parents.

CYSTIC FIBROSIS

Cystic fibrosis (CF) is a genetic disorder that results in a multisystem disease involving the cell membrane and the electrolyte and water system of the cell. This disease affects many parts of the body but particularly the lungs and pancreas. It occurs in about 1 in 3000 live births. CF is an inherited congenital disorder. The condition is believed to be inherited as a **Mendelian recessive trait** from both parents. The parents, who are **carriers** of this disease, do not show any symptoms. CF disease results when the two genes for the disease combine during conception. CF affects both genders equally. The survival rate of the children has increased,

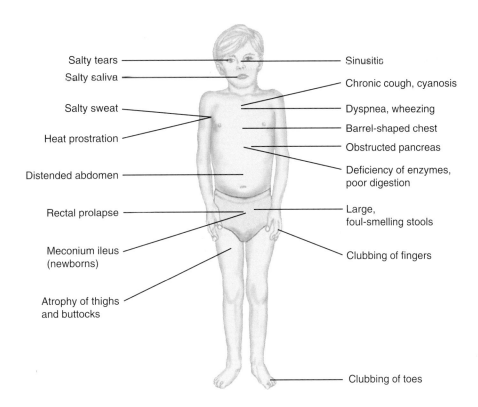

Salty tears — Sinusitis

Salty saliva — Chronic cough, cyanosis

Salty sweat — Dyspnea, wheezing

— Barrel-shaped chest

Heat prostration — Obstructed pancreas

— Deficiency of enzymes,
poor digestion

Distended abdomen —

Rectal prolapse — Large,
foul-smelling stools

Meconium ileus
(newborns) — Clubbing of fingers

Atrophy of thighs
and buttocks —

— Clubbing of toes

FIGURE 11-3 Manifestations of cystic fibrosis.

and many are living into adulthood. Better antimicrobial control of pulmonary infection both at home and during hospitalization and increased numbers of CF centers have contributed to this success.

The gene associated with CF was identified in 1989, and it is now possible to identify healthy individuals who carry the trait. Chromosome 7 is the location of the gene responsible for CF. Sodium and chloride at the cell membrane are controlled by this gene. With a defect in the CF transmembrane regulator (CFTR) protein, secretions become thick and pasty. There are many possible mutations, which helps to explain the various degrees of involvement of the systems: respiratory and GI.

With the ability to identify the CF gene, diagnosis can be assisted with genetic analysis. Caution is noted because of the possibilities of false-positive and false-negative results. Genetic analysis can be used in conjunction with other diagnostic criteria such as the sweat test. New aggressive approaches in treatment have resulted in increasing the life expectancy from less than 10 years to 40 years.

Signs and Symptoms

The major symptoms of CF are manifested in the respiratory tract and the GI tract. The first symptom may be seen in the newborn infant who has a meconium ileus. This condition is seen in approximately 10% to

20% of children who are born with CF. An overview of the manifestations of CF is shown in Figure 11-3.

Lung Involvement. Cystic fibrosis is considered the most serious lung problem in children in the United States. The air passages of the lungs become clogged with mucus. There is widespread obstruction of the bronchioles. It is hard for the child to breathe; expiration is especially difficult. More and more air becomes trapped in the lungs (obstructive emphysema), and small areas of collapse (atelectasis) may occur. Eventually, the chest assumes a barrel shape, with increased diameter across the front and back. The right ventricle of the heart, which supplies the lungs, may become strained and enlarged. Clubbing of the fingers and toes, indicating a chronic lack of oxygen, may be present. *Staphylococcus* and *Pseudomonas* infections can easily occur in the lungs, which provide a suitable medium for these organisms to grow. This causes more thickening of the abnormal secretions, irritates and damages lung tissues, and further increases lung obstruction.

The time of onset of this disease varies. Symptoms may appear weeks, months, or years after birth. In general, the earlier the onset of the disease symptoms, the more severe course of the disease. Symptoms range from mild to severe. Any or all symptoms may be present in varying degrees of severity in one individual. A chronic cough develops that may produce vomiting. Dyspnea, wheezing, and cyanosis may occur. The child is irritable and tires easily. Gradually, there is a change in physical appearance. Chest radiographs reveal widespread infection. Evidence of obstructive emphysema, atelectasis, and **fibrosis** of lung tissue may also be present. The prognosis for survival depends on the extent of lung damage. However, this is only part of the picture because CF also affects the pancreas and sweat glands.

Pancreatic Involvement. The pancreas lies behind the stomach. Some of its cells secrete **pancreatic enzymes** that drain from the pancreatic duct into the duodenum at the same area in which bile enters. Changes occurring in the pancreas are the result of obstruction by thickened secretions that block the flow of pancreatic digestive enzymes. Consequently, foodstuffs, particularly fats and proteins, are not properly used by the body.

In infants, the stools may be loose. Gradually, because of impaired digestion and food absorption, the feces of the child become large, fatty, and foul-smelling. They are usually light in color. In spite of having a good appetite, the infant does not gain weight and may look undernourished. The abdomen becomes distended, and the buttocks and thighs **atrophy** as fat disappears from the main deposit sites. Laboratory test results show a deficiency in pancreatic enzymes (trypsin, lipase, and amylase).

An oral pancreatic extract such as Pancrease is given to the child with each meal and snack to replace the pancreatic enzymes the child's body cannot produce. This medication is considered specific for the disease because it aids in the digestion and absorption of food, thus improving the condition of the stools. If the child is ill and not eating, the medication is withheld.

A presenting condition known as meconium ileus develops after birth when the intestine of the newborn becomes obstructed with abnormally thick meconium while in utero. This is caused by the absence of pancreatic enzymes that normally digest proteins in the meconium. The abnormal, puttylike stool sticks to the walls of the intestine, causing blockage. Vomiting, abdominal distention, and absence of stools lead to the suspicion of intestinal obstruction. Radiographs confirm the diagnosis. The condition is treated surgically. The death rate is high, but the prognosis is more favorable when the obstruction is detected early. Most infants who survive manifest CF. Fortunately, meconium ileus is rare because the pancreatic enzyme deficiency is seldom complete. Nevertheless, the nurse assigned to the nursery must constantly be on guard for suspicious symptoms.

Sweat Glands. The sweat, tears, and saliva of the child with CF become abnormally salty from an increase in sodium and chloride levels. There is also an increase in the potassium level of sweat glands. The normal amount of chloride in sweat is 1 to 60 mEq/L. Higher concentrations are considered specific for the disease. The analysis of sweat is a major aid in the diagnosis of the condition. The **sweat test**, with pilocarpine iontophoresis, is the best diagnostic study. A dilute solution of pilocarpine is applied to the arm, and a weak electrical current is used to stimulate sweating. A positive test should be repeated for confirmation. Because large amounts of salt are lost through perspiration, the child must be observed for heat prostration. Liberal amounts of salt should be given with food, and extra fluids and salt should be provided during hot weather. Infants do not have a lot of sweat; therefore obtaining enough sweat for an accurate test may be difficult. Mothers often report that when they kiss their infants they taste salty.

Complications

Cystic fibrosis is often responsible for **rectal prolapse** in infants and children. This is partly from poor muscle tone in the rectal area and excessive leanness of the buttocks of the child.

As the disease progresses, the liver may become hard, nodular, and enlarged. There may be edema of the extremities. The retina of the eye may hemorrhage, there may be damage to the eye from swelling, and inflammation in part of the optic nerve may occur. **Cor pulmonale** (*cor*, heart; *pulmon*, lung), heart strain from improper lung function, is frequently a cause of death. **Osteoporosis** (*osteo*, bone, pore; *osis*, disease) may occur. When it is caused by CF, the bones become porous because of poor utilization of fat-soluble vitamin D, which is necessary for proper calcium metabolism. There is a deficiency in vitamin A also because the child is unable to absorb the fats from which this vitamin is obtained.

With the extended life expectancy, about 20% or higher of the children develop hyperglycemia and cystic fibrosis–related diabetes (CFRD). Blood sugar control becomes an important objective. With malabsorption and pancreatic insufficiency issues, control becomes challenging. Oral hypoglycemia drugs and insulin may be used. As they become adults, these children can develop the vascular problems seen with the long-term effects of diabetes.

Treatment and Nursing Care

Cystic fibrosis is a chronic condition and must be monitored and maintained daily. The family providers of care need support, as does the child. The care in a regional CF center, where all disciplines are located in one facility, can be extremely helpful because it allows the family to go to one location rather than traveling to several different clinics for care. The CF team can work with the family and the primary care physician to meet the needs of the child and family.

Respiratory Relief. Most new approaches in treatment are focused on the lung. The targeted outcomes are improved airway clearance, thinning of secretions, treatment of infections, and reduction of inflammation. **Antimicrobials** may be given as a preventive measure against respiratory infection; however, this treatment is subject to controversy. Full dosages of antimicrobials are given in an acute infection. The physician determines the particular antimicrobial to be used on the basis of the results of throat and sputum cultures. The route may be oral or intravenous. Intravenous medication may be given via **heparin lock** or, in some cases, a **Broviac catheter** or **implanted port.** This can be used successfully in both inpatient and outpatient settings. The child's respiratory status can be monitored through the pulmonary function test, which indicates the lung's capacity.

Intermittent aerosol therapy is administered to provide medication to the lower respiratory tract and to promote evacuation of secretions. DNase, an enzyme, is administered by inhalation and results in decreasing the viscosity of the sputum. An inhaled antimicrobial, tobramycin (TOBI), is being used as a maintenance prophylactic with chronic *Pseudomonas aeruginosa* to help suppress bacterial growth. Bronchodilators such as Albuterol are used to increase the width of the bronchi, allowing free passage of air into the lungs.

Postural drainage, chest clapping, and breathing exercises are also important. These are performed by the respiratory therapist during hospitalization. When postural drainage and chest clapping are done properly, the secretions in the chest are moved up and out. During latent periods or in mild cases, the child may not raise sputum. This should be explained to the parents so that they do not discontinue this valuable procedure when the child goes home. Instructions may need to be repeated frequently to encourage full cooperation of the parents and child. These procedures should be done after nebulization and at least 1 hour after eating. General exercise is good for the child because it stimulates coughing. Somersaults, headstands, and wheelbarrow play within the child's endurance are therapeutic.

Preventing respiratory tract infections is important. The child should be isolated from individuals and personnel who may harbor infections. The child must be given the necessary immunizations against childhood diseases. Appropriate boosters should be given so that the immunity obtained is kept up to date.

Diet. Adequate nutrition is essential. The diet should be high in calories, as much as 50% more than normal. There should be increased protein and moderate amounts of fat in conjunction with pancreatic extracts. Simple sugars are easy to digest, and banana products are particularly good. Fruits, cottage cheese, vegetables, and lean meats, which are high in protein and low in fat and starches, are recommended. With the improvement of nutritional enzymes, many of these children can tolerate normal to higher amounts of fat in their diet. Enzymes can be adjusted if there is an increased amount of fat in the stool. Extra salt may be provided with pretzels and salted breadsticks and crackers. As the disease progresses, some children will benefit from nighttime feedings with a nasogastric tube or **gastrostomy tube (G-button).** Older children can add supplemental drinks such as Boost or Ensure to increase their calorie input.

Supplements of vitamins A, D, and E in a water-miscible base are given each day in double the recommended dose. Vitamin K may also be given when indicated. Salt tablets may be given to the older child during hot weather. Forcing fluids may be ordered because larger amounts of fluid are lost in the stools. The nurse may be asked to weigh the child daily.

The nurse feeding the infant with CF must be calm and unhurried. The infant may cough, have difficulty breathing, and vomit. Careful burping is necessary to avoid abdominal distention. In general, the appetite is good. Older children need small amounts of food served attractively and frequently. Food piled high on a child's tray is discouraging. The amount of a meal eaten should be compared to what the child normally ingests rather than the amount left on the tray. This practice will decrease a child's appetite being reported as poor. The nurse records the fluid intake at the end of the meal. The child's reaction to new foods and any variations in stools resulting from the food are noted. The food refused and the type, character, and amount of vomiting, if any, are also noted.

 Nursing Brief

Because mealtime is a social time, the nurse should remain with the child if the parents are not present. Try to make the meal more satisfying by giving good companionship mixed with a little encouragement.

General Hygiene. The nurse must pay special attention to the skin of the child with CF. The diaper area should be cleansed after each bowel movement. An ointment to protect the skin is advisable because the character of the stool subjects the diaper area to irritation. The buttocks are exposed to air when a rash occurs. Careful attention to bony areas is necessary to prevent decubitus ulcers. Because the child has little fat and muscle, it is important that the position be changed frequently, especially if the child is weak and cannot get out of bed. This also prevents pneumonia.

The child should wear light clothing to avoid becoming overheated; it should be loose to allow freedom of movement. Good oral hygiene is necessary because the teeth may be in poor condition from dietary deficiencies. Mouth care is given after postural drainage because foul mucus may be raised, leaving an unpleasant taste in the child's mouth.

Long-Term Care. Today the child with a chronic illness spends most of the time at home and is hospitalized mainly for diagnosis, relapses, and complications. Caring for a child with a chronic illness is extremely taxing financially, physically, and emotionally. Somehow the family must distribute their time and energy within the family yet give careful attention to the sick child or, in the case of CF, sometimes children. Questions the family must answer are: How do they keep from spoiling the child? Do they limit the normal activities of the remaining children to spare the sick one? What about birthday parties, camping, Cub Scouts, pets, epidemics at school? What does a trip to the shore or mountains entail? When do the husband and wife find time for themselves? These seemingly overwhelming problems are being faced daily by many people in every community. Parent groups are helpful in promoting exchange of ideas and in providing support. The National Cystic Fibrosis Research Foundation disseminates useful information. The nurse should become familiar with the local chapter to guide parents to reliable sources of information.

Communication

Parents of children with CF need encouragement and reassurance. If you are asked direct questions about the illness, you might say, "Dr. Parker is a fine pediatrician. What did he tell you about Bobby's illness?" This encourages the parents to express themselves and gives you an idea of what the child and parents have been told.

Parents need explicit instructions regarding diet, medication, postural drainage, prevention of infection, rest, and continued medical supervision. Plan teaching periods, and provide printed materials for reinforcement so that parents are not overwhelmed. Many families require the assistance of a social worker to secure funds for equipment and drugs. Parents should be told that help is available as the need arises. The mother, who is usually more directly involved, may benefit from these added hints:

- She needs rest herself; the family must take over some of the responsibilities of the household. Relatives may care for the child periodically so that she can "get away from it all." Respite care is another alternative; it is helpful if she can develop at least one outside interest of her own.
- An alarm clock set for medication time reminds her of this task.
- A downstairs bedroom for the child is preferable.
- Extra spoons and a pitcher of water on the bedside stand save steps.

Emotional Support. The child who is chronically ill may find it hard to accept decreasing activity abilities. The amount and kinds of diversion required vary in CF because the disease affects children of all ages, with variations in severity.

It is believed that children benefit from simple straightforward answers about the illness. An uncomplicated diagram might be helpful. Children who understand why they are being restricted from certain activities are more cooperative. They should know why they must take medications with each meal, use the nebulizer, undergo postural drainage, and so on. They should see and handle the unfamiliar equipment necessary for their care.

The young child may find it difficult to be separated from the parents during hospitalization. Even when the prognosis is grave, a child's courage is sustained if the parents are there. Parents are encouraged to stay with the child when possible. Close contact by mail with school, church, and clubs is important for school-age children. It is helpful for the child to develop an activity at which they are good, such as piano or art. This increases their feeling of worth and provides outlets for emotions. Consideration must be given to ways of fostering love, acceptance, trust, fair play, security, freedom of choice, creativity, and self-identity.

Nurses should learn the child's likes, dislikes, fears, and interests. They should observe them with their families and note the types of relationships that exist. They then can form their own impressions about the child and are not misled by labels given them by those with less understanding. Children have to be allowed to communicate in a manner that is meaningful to them. Sometimes children are able to express feelings; sometimes they are not. Drawing with children may stimulate conversation. It is important that nurses be aware of children's facial expressions, posture, eyes, and how they play. What are they saying to their toys, their playmates? Nurses' observations of children's behavior should be incorporated into nursing care plans.

Nurses and parents must not show undue concern for a child's illness. Overindulging children has a tendency to make them demanding. Children may then exaggerate small problems. The children's impressions of themselves and their illness are determined a good deal by how they feel physically, how the family feels about their condition, and how others behave toward them.

Development of new approaches in treatment has changed the outlook for CF families. Advancements in airway clearance techniques, new medications, gene therapy, and lung transplantation have encouraged optimism toward improvement of lifestyle for the child with CF. The nurse should assist in keeping families informed of new, available therapies (Nursing Care Plan 11-1). As many of these children are living into adulthood, they will need to be transitioned into an adult health care setting.

CROUP

Respiratory infections are common in the pediatric population, especially in children younger than 5 years of age. Children have smaller air passages than adults and experience more narrowing with inflammation. Acute infections of the larynx are common in the toddler. Involvement of other parts of the respiratory tract is frequent. A wide variety of organisms cause croup, but most often the infectious agent is a virus. The child's history is valuable in the diagnosis because

there appears to be a familial tendency. Although it can occur at any age, it is most common in children between 3 months and 6 years of age.

Croup is a nonspecific term applied to a number of conditions, the chief symptom of which is a brassy (croupy) "barking" cough and varying degrees of inspiratory **stridor.** When the larynx is involved, the picture becomes more serious because of possible alterations in respiratory status (e.g., airway obstruction, acute respiratory failure, or hypoxia). Acute spasmodic laryngitis is the milder form of the syndrome. Acute laryngotracheobronchitis is the most common. It is also referred to as **glottic** and **subglottic croup.** Figure 11-4 illustrates croup.

Signs and Symptoms

Croup usually begins with an upper respiratory infection with or without fever. The child begins to develop hoarseness and a harsh, barking, "croupy" cough. As the subglottic area becomes obstructed by edema and exudate, the child develops stridor, a harsh,

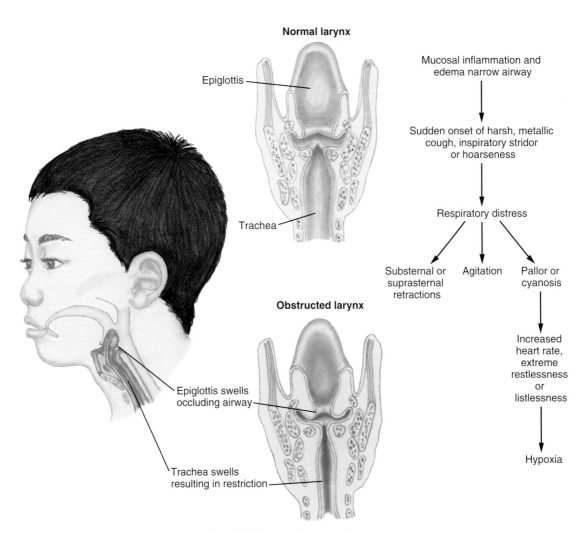

FIGURE 11-4 Pathophysiology of croup.

Nursing Care Plan 11-1 | The Child with Cystic Fibrosis

NURSING DIAGNOSIS *Ineffective airway clearance, related to accumulation of mucus*

Goals/Outcome Criteria	Nursing Interventions	Rationales
The child has improved aeration, as evidenced by: • Absence of dyspnea and tachypnea • Ability to expectorate mucus • Respiratory rate appropriate for age • Heart rate appropriate for age (O2 saturation = 93% on room air)	Assess lung sounds: rate and depth. Assess oxygen saturation. Assess heart rate. Provide adequate hydration. Assist child with aerosol therapy. Assist with chest physiotherapy and postural drainage. Administer medications and explain their use. Teach child the importance of breathing exercises. Monitor the effectiveness of medication and respiratory treatments.	Provides information on how the child is doing. As oxygen is needed, the heart speeds up to help the body compensate. Fluids are needed by the body to help thin secretions. Bronchodilators and an increase in the inspired humidity aid the functioning of the respiratory system and aid in expectorating mucus. Aids in expectorating mucus by dislodging mucous plugs and, with the addition of gravity, aids in removal of mucus from the body. Important for the family to know the effects of the medication and the side effects. Aids in compliance. Breathing exercises increase the body's ability to compensate. The muscles needed to compensate are strengthened. As the child grows and as the body's needs change, adjustments are needed in the course of treatment. It is also important for the family to know how to monitor the effectiveness of the treatment.

NURSING DIAGNOSIS *Imbalanced nutrition, less than body requirements, related to malabsorption from absence of pancreatic enzymes*

Goals/Outcome Criteria	Nursing Interventions	Rationales
The child has adequate nutrition, as evidenced by: • Ability to eat 1½ to 2 times the recommended dietary allowance for age • Weight gain or lack of weight loss • Increase in muscle mass • Maturation in growth and development	Assess baseline nutrition. Administer pancreatic replacement enzymes. Administer water-miscible fat-soluble vitamins. Monitor serum electrolytes. Provide a diet high in calories and proteins and normal in fat. Provide between-meal snacks or supplemental drinks. Monitor caloric count. Teach child and caregiver the importance of daily evaluation of diet. Weigh daily, and record while in the hospital. Monitor and record characteristics of stool. Consult with the dietitian.	Indicates what information is needed for the child and the family. The body lacks the ability to excrete the pancreatic enzymes needed to digest fats and proteins. Fat-soluble vitamins are given in a water-soluble form to aid in the absorption of these vitamins. Electrolytes, particularly sodium, are lost in large amounts during periods of heavy perspiration (fever, hot weather, exercise). Because of the body's inability to absorb nutrients, it is necessary for there to be an abundance. Extra energy is also used by the respiratory system. Adds additional calories and nutrients. A calorie count is needed to ensure that the child is getting the needed calories and nutrients. Allows the family to function in an independent manner; adjustments can be made more easily. Diet and activity can be adjusted according to needs. Because it is difficult for the body to digest fats, the stool record aids in identifying needed adjustments to the diet and medication regimen. A dietitian is an integral part of the team in the treatment and management of the child. A dietitian can provide information for the child and the family and aid them in their selections.

Nursing Care Plan 11-1 The Child with Cystic Fibrosis—cont'd

NURSING DIAGNOSIS *Deficient knowledge, related to the diagnosis and condition of the child*

Goals/Outcome Criteria	Nursing Interventions	Rationales
The parents have an understanding of what is occurring, as evidenced by: • Repeating information correctly that has been given to them • Asking questions • Describing the home care regimen • Discussing the need for medical follow-up • Ability to express fears • Accepting referrals for outside assistance	Assess parents' understanding of the disease process and its future outcome.	Allows the nurse to know where to begin.
	Provide emotional support for the parents and the child.	Parents may find it difficult to deal with all that is going on. Make sure both the parents' and the child's needs are met.
	Allow the parents to ask questions.	Parents may feel overwhelmed by the situation. Make sure they feel comfortable asking questions. If they are not asking questions, use open-ended statements to them.
	Answer questions, or provide parents with resources to answer their questions.	The nurse may not have all the answers to the questions asked, but it is important that resources be used. Find out for the parent or direct the parent where to go (e.g., "That is a good question. Let's write it down so you can ask your doctor when he comes in.").
	Help parents understand and support the child through various activities.	If parents can support the child in the hospital, then they are more likely to be successful in a home setting.
	Encourage parents' participation in the care of the child.	Parents who participate in care can show their concern for the child and feel they are team players in the management of the child.
	Assess the home environment for long-term care.	Allows for home-care plans to be made.
	Initiate referral to aid the parents.	Often, parents need extra resources to meet the needs of this child.
	Teach parents and child the signs and symptoms of respiratory distress.	If these are known, the family can make changes to correct further deterioration. Also knowing what to do is helpful and aids in their independence.
	Consultation or referral with social service.	The family may need additional services, such as financial advice and equipment, and need the aid of a social worker.

NURSING DIAGNOSIS *Risk for infection, related to invasion of respiratory system by bacterial organisms*

Goals/Outcome Criteria	Nursing Interventions	Rationales
The child is free of infection, as evidenced by: • Remaining afebrile • Respiratory rate appropriate for age • Clearing of mucus after regular and routine respiratory treatments • Following proper procedure when doing treatments	Assess vital signs.	Early recognition of changing vital signs alerts nurse to the possibility of an infection.
	Teach the importance of hand hygiene.	Done properly, hand hygiene can decrease the spread of organisms.
	Encourage proper pulmonary hygiene.	By getting rid of mucus and secretions, there is less opportunity for harmful organisms to multiply and spread.
	Teach proper handling and disposal of secretions and sputum.	Helps decrease the possibility of reinfecting the body.
	Teach or review with the child and parents why the pulmonary system is at risk for infection.	Information helps the child and family understand the need to be careful and follow recommendations; aids with compliance in treatment.
	Give reassurance and praise when procedures are done correctly by the child or parents.	Shows that nurse recognizes the child or family has learned and gives them more motivation to learn. The more motivated the child and family are to learn, the more compliant they are in following procedures.
	Provide guidance related to being independent.	Independence increases self-esteem. As learning increases, the child is able to be more independent and self-esteem is greater.

Continued

✦ Nursing Care Plan 11-1   The Child with Cystic Fibrosis—cont'd

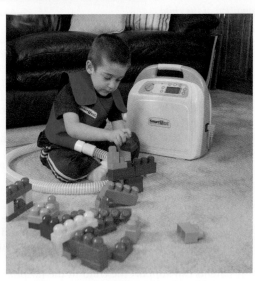

Courtesy of Electromed, Inc. SmartVest

Critical Thinking Snapshot

A newly diagnosed 5-year-old with CF is having difficulties adjusting to the new routines. While he is cooperative with his airway clearance vibration vest, he refuses to take pancreatic enzymes with meals. The mother is frustrated and is threatening the child.

1. What interventions could the nurse use in attempting to obtain compliance with this child?
2. How can the nurse help the mother become more effective in dealing with the situation?

high-pitched sound when breathing. Cough and stridor are usually worse at night. Although croup is alarming to the child and parents because the child is distressed, most cases are mild, and it is not communicable. Signs of pallor, increased respiratory effort, and restlessness indicate that the child should be seen by a physician because respiratory distress is increasing.

Treatment and Nursing Care

Most children can be managed at home. Use of steam from a shower or hot bath in a closed bathroom can often stop the acute respiratory distress and laryngeal spasm. Parents should be instructed to use a cool mist humidifier in the child's room. The machine must be disinfected regularly. Steam vaporizers are usually avoided because of the danger of scalding. Exposure to cold air can relieve stridor. Many a parent has carried a child out into the cold night on the way to the emergency room only to have the child appear quite comfortable when they arrive at the hospital. This may be caused by the colder atmospheric air cooling the upper airway mucosa and decreasing local edema (Kliegman et al., 2007). Clear fluid intake should also be increased to assist with preventing dehydration, preventing thickened secretions, and decreasing a fever.

Children with croup and temperatures above 102.2° F (39° C) should be hospitalized if there is progressive stridor, respiratory distress, or suspected epiglottitis (Kliegman et al., 2007).

The child admitted to the hospital with respiratory distress is anxious and fatigued. A calm, reassuring approach by the nurse can relieve the child's and family's anxiety. As the parents become more relaxed, the child also becomes less apprehensive.

Low-dose oxygen or supplemental oxygen with a nasal cannula or mask might be used if the child is hypoxic. Keeping the mask on a small child can be challenging, while a nasal cannula that is taped to the child's cheek and back may provide a more comfortable route of administration. Helium-oxygen mixtures (heliox) are being used for upper airway obstruction including croup. There are limitations with heliox as it requires greater than 40% oxygen, expense, and complexity of setup. For children who cannot use corticosteroids or epinephrine, this is an effective treatment (Wald, 2010).

Medications used in the treatment of croup include corticosteroids and inhaled racemic epinephrine. Corticosteroids have proved helpful in avoiding intubation in seriously ill children by decreasing subglottic edema. Racemic epinephrine is inhaled via a face mask. It decreases edema by vasoconstriction and provides immediate relief, although this may be temporary. Racemic epinephrine may be repeated in several hours if necessary. A single inhaled dose peaks in 10 to 30 minutes, with an overall duration of 2 hours. **Close observation is necessary because some children may have a relapse, with return of symptoms when the medication effect has worn off.** For this reason, many children who have received racemic epinephrine are admitted to the hospital for observation.

The nurse observes and records temperature, pulse, respirations, and blood pressure, if ordered. Particular attention is given to the type and rate of respirations. The child's color and degree of restlessness and anxiety are also observed. An increase in respiratory distress is reported immediately because complications may arise that necessitate endotracheal intubation or tracheostomy (see Box 11-2, Respiratory Assessment Guidelines). Specific nursing care is indicated in such cases (see Chapter 3 for tracheostomy care).

Administer the child's favorite clear, cool, oral fluids if the child does not have severe respiratory distress. Intravenous (IV) fluids may be started to provide fluid intake and conserve energy. Care should be planned to allow time for uninterrupted rest.

NASOPHARYNGITIS (COMMON COLD)

A cold is the most common infection of the respiratory tract. It is caused by one or a number of viruses, principally the **rhinoviruses.** The spread from one child to another is through sneezing, coughing, and direct contact. Group A beta-hemolytic streptococci is the predominant bacterial offender. Droplets remain suspended in the air and on dust particles for short periods. The infection is transferred mainly during the initial stage. In the second phase of a cold, nasal drainage becomes thicker and purulent. Factors that contribute to the individual's susceptibility include age, state of nutrition, general health, fatigue, and emotional upsets.

As the infant becomes exposed to more children, the number of colds contracted increases. Parents may notice this particularly during the child's first few years of daycare or school because the child has had little opportunity to build up resistance. The older the child, the better he or she is able to resist infection. In temperate climates, the incidence rate of rhinoviral infection peaks in September and again in April or May.

To prevent a cold, avoid exposing children as much as possible to those with this virus. Infants younger than 6 months of age can acquire this infection, so they too must be protected from infected persons. Be sure to provide nourishing foods and see that the child or infant gets sufficient rest.

Signs and Symptoms

The symptoms of a cold in an infant or small child are different from those in an adult (Figure 11-5). Children's air passages are smaller and more easily obstructed. Fever as high as 104° F (40° C) is not uncommon in children younger than 3 years of age. Nasal discharge, irritability, sore throat, cough, and general discomfort are present, and there may be vomiting and diarrhea. The diagnosis is complicated by the fact that many infectious diseases resemble the common cold during their onset. Complications of a cold include bronchitis, pneumonitis, ear infections, and sinusitis.

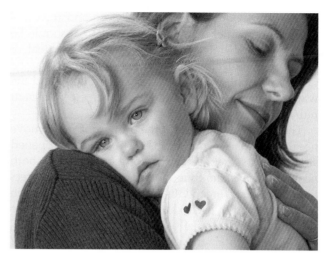

FIGURE 11-5 Common signs and symptoms of a cold include runny nose, red eyes, and fatigue.

Treatment and Nursing Care

There is no cure for the common cold. When a cold is suspected, treatment should be started early. The treatment is designed to relieve the symptoms. Rest, fluids, and proper diet are important. Parents are taught to watch the child for signs of dehydration. If anorexia is present, food should not be forced. The appetite gradually improves as the condition does. When high fever accompanies a cold, the physician must be consulted. Acetaminophen (Tylenol) reduces the temperature, but the correct dosage should be prescribed, particularly in children younger than 1 year of age. Aqueous nosedrops relieve nasal congestion. The infant needs nosedrops mainly before feedings and at bedtime. When drops are instilled 10 to 15 minutes before feedings, the nasal passages are cleared and the infant can suck easily. Each child needs an individual bottle of nosedrops to prevent cross-infection.

 Safety Alert

The FDA recommends that over-the-counter (OTC) cough and cold products **not** be used for infants and children younger than 2 years of age. While review of OTC use for children 2 to 11 years of age is not complete, the FDA strongly suggests that if parents use OTC products, they follow these recommendations:

- Check the "active ingredient" as many medications have more than one
- Take care when giving more than one OTC product as they both may have the same ingredients and an overdose might occur
- Follow directions listed on the label
- Only use measuring instruments made for measuring drugs. Do not use household spoons.
- Do not use OTC products to sedate or make children sleepy (FDA, 2010)

Moist air soothes the inflamed nose and throat. A cold air humidifier is safe and convenient. It should be cleaned and disinfected regularly. If a great deal of moisture is indicated, as for croup, the infant may be taken to a small room, such as the bathroom, and the water faucets can be turned on to create sufficient humidity.

The older child is taught the proper way to remove nasal secretions from the nose. The mouth is opened slightly and secretions are blown gently through both nostrils at the same time. This method prevents infection from being forced into the eustachian tubes. When a large amount of nasal discharge is present, the nurse can apply petroleum jelly to the upper lip to protect it.

In the hospital, the child is isolated with proper isolation restrictions. During the initial stage of the fever, the child is kept in bed. Frequent change of position is necessary. In the home, it is difficult to keep children with a cold away from other members of the family. They must be taught to cover their mouth and nose when sneezing and to wash their hands afterward. Tissues must be properly discarded. The child should stay at home without visitors. Rest, fluids, and adequate nutrition support recovery.

TONSILLITIS AND ADENOIDITIS

The tonsils and adenoids, located in the pharynx, or throat, are made of lymph tissue and act as part of the body's defense mechanism against infection. Group A streptococci are normal flora of the oropharynx and pharynx, and up to 20% of the pediatric population are colonized by this bacteria. However, infectious pathogens such as *Haemophilus influenzae, Staphylococcus aureus, S. pneumoniae, and Moraxella catarrhalis* are also sources of infection. Penicillin is often the drug of choice to treat streptococcal pharyngitis.

The tonsils and adenoids formerly were blamed for causing many assorted illnesses, and for a time it was thought that having them removed was part of growing up. Today, doctors carefully evaluate the need for children to have them removed. A careful physical examination and an evaluation of the child's history are done to rule out other diseases. Enlargement of the tonsils is not sufficient reason for removal. These structures are normally larger in early childhood than in later years. The current trend is to treat the conditions as separate problems, according to individual criteria. Obstructive sleep apnea syndrome, multiple infections, and peritonsillar abscess are indications for tonsillectomy.

Treatment and Nursing Care

The use of antimicrobials during acute infections has reduced the need for surgery. The decision as to whether surgery is necessary is perhaps the single most important factor from a medical standpoint. Ideally, children are beyond toddlerhood when this

surgery is performed. They are better able to understand what is happening, and they are more compliant as a result.

Most children are referred to an ear, nose, and throat specialist when contributing conditions become severe. An acute streptococcal infection should be treated prior to surgery. Surgery is usually performed in day surgery units. New surgical tools are being used for tonsillectomy and adenoidectomy. According to Messner (2003), one such instrument is the ultrasonic dissector coagulator, which uses ultrasonic technology to cut and coagulate tissues at lower temperatures than that used with electrocautery. This ultimately minimizes tissue damage (and possibly, postoperative pain).

Preoperative Care. The child is prepared in advance for surgery. Children need to know that the tonsils are two small lumps located far in the back of the mouth. Because they are causing the throat to be sore (or whatever symptoms the child is experiencing) and are not working properly, they need to be taken out. Reassure children that the doctor will not operate on any other part of the body and that it is all right for the tonsils to come out. Children are also informed that they will receive a special medicine that will make them go to sleep and will keep them asleep until the operation is over. Emphasize that after the operation *they will wake up.* After they wake up, they will be sore for several days, but pretty soon they will feel entirely better. Medical personnel and parents must be alert to the young child's fantasies and anxieties and answer questions honestly and at a level suitable to the age of the child.

Many hospitals have special programs to prepare children for surgery. These programs provide videotapes, prehospitalization tours, and opportunities to handle supplies. Familiarization with equipment and the setting reduces fear. Allowing children hands-on play therapy also minimizes fear (Figure 11-6).

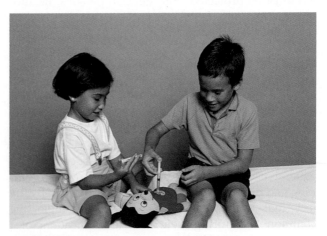

FIGURE 11-6 Playing with syringes provides children with the opportunity to play out fears and concerns.

Children need to know that medical personnel understand their feelings. It is also important that someone they know and trust is close by. Include the child's parents in discussions, and encourage them to stay with the child.

A complete physical examination and urinalysis are performed before surgery. Blood work includes hemoglobin, hematocrit, prothrombin time (PT), and PTT. The latter tests are done because bleeding is anticipated. These procedures are usually performed before admission. The child is inspected for loose teeth and signs of upper respiratory tract infection. It is also important to determine any family bleeding tendencies, any history of chronic illness (such as rheumatic fever), elevations in temperature, and recent exposure to communicable diseases.

Instructions are given to the parents regarding the times to stop eating and drinking before surgery. A preoperative checklist is completed. The nurse checks to see that the child's identification band is securely attached to the wrist. The child should void before going to the operating room. Parents accompany the child to preoperative holding and are encouraged to remain with their child in this area (Figure 11-7).

Many facilities use oral or IV midazolam (Versed) or other preoperative sedation to relax the child before anesthesia induction. Anesthesia induction is usually via inhalation. The child is given a choice of what "flavor" is used.

Many hospitals like to have parents in the recovery room to decrease children's anxiety by providing a familiar face and arms to welcome them when they awaken. Review postoperative procedures with the parents, including what to expect when the child returns to the room (such as color, bleeding, IV fluids, vomiting, and irritability).

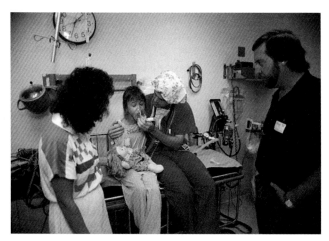

FIGURE 11-7 Parental presence during induction of anesthesia can minimize the child's and parents' anxiety during the preoperative period.

Postoperative Care. Nursing care is focused on providing comfort and minimizing potential bleeding. Immediately after surgery, to facilitate drainage, the child is placed partly on the side and partly on the abdomen (prone), with the knee of the uppermost leg flexed to hold the position. The child is watched carefully for evidence of bleeding. Hemorrhage is the most common postoperative complication. The nurse should not assume that because surgery is minor it does not involve certain risks. Because bleeding after this type of surgery is concealed, the nurse must watch carefully for evidence of hemorrhage (see Did You Know). When bleeding is suspected, packing and sometimes ligation are indicated. Lung abscesses and pneumonia are infrequent complications.

? Did You Know

The Child with Possible Post-Tonsillectomy Bleeding

- Frequent swallowing (a cardinal sign of bleeding)
- Pallor
- Restlessness
- Increased pulse
- Vomiting bright red blood
- Decreasing BP
- Visible blood on careful examination of the throat with a flashlight

An ice collar may be applied for comfort. Some children prefer not to have an ice collar. Most children experience pain and should be medicated. Acetaminophen, with or without codeine, increases comfort and may assist in lessening crying, which can irritate the operative site. Rectal or IV analgesics also may be used.

The child is given fluids intravenously during surgery. It is not uncommon for vomiting to occur. Small amounts of cool, clear liquids are given when the vomiting has ceased. Avoid citrus juices, carbonated drinks, and milk products. Avoid extremely hot or cold fluids as they may irritate the throat. A Popsicle may appeal to the child; however, red juices or Popsicles are not to be given because monitoring for bleeding is an important nursing consideration. If clear liquids are well tolerated, progression to a soft diet is begun. The child is kept quiet for the remainder of the day. A small child may nestle on a parent's lap.

Discharge

Written instructions are given to the parents when the child is discharged. The child should be kept quiet for a few days and should receive nourishing fluids and soft foods. After this, children may continue to take a nap or have a rest period so that they have a sufficient convalescent time. Acetaminophen (Tylenol) may be given to reduce discomfort in the throat. The child needs to be protected from exposure to infections.

Fresh bleeding, chest pain, or persistent cough should be reported to the physician. Although it occurs rarely, bleeding can occur up to 10 days after surgery from tissue sloughing from the healing process (Hockenberry and Wilson, 2007). The doctor may compare this with a "scab" coming off. Earache may follow a tonsillectomy and/or adenoidectomy, and slight fever (99° F to 100° F or 37.2° C to 37.8° C) may occur for 2 or 3 days. A follow-up appointment is made because the surgeon will wish to check the operative site after it has healed. The child usually can resume normal activities within 2 weeks.

● ASTHMA

Asthma is the most common chronic illness in childhood. It is also the leading cause of emergency department visits, hospital admissions, and school absenteeism (Kliegman et al., 2007). Eighty percent of cases of asthma occur before 5 years of age. Asthma is more frequently seen in poor children, partly because they live in old homes with high concentrations of precipitating allergens. School nurses are seeing an increasing number of children with asthma on a daily basis and require a good understanding of the course of treatment for asthma. Nurses are giving inhalation treatments in school; such treatments can help the child manage the condition on a day-to-day basis.

Asthma is a reversible obstruction of the large and small airways caused by mucosal edema, smooth muscle constriction, and thick tenacious mucus. Also known as reactive airway disease, asthma may be precipitated by allergens such as pollens, foods, dust mites, and animal dander, which irritate the airways and initiate bronchoconstriction and the inflammatory process. Asthma may also be triggered by temperature changes, cold air, viral infections, and exercise. One of the major triggers of asthma is exposure to cigarette smoke.

Stress can precipitate an asthma attack or exacerbate the condition. Because asthma is a chronic disease of childhood, the stress on the child and family is important to consider.

Genetic predisposition is the strongest predisposing factor for developing asthma (NAEPP, 2007). Careful management of asthma in children improves the prognosis, and most children do well. Children with severe asthma usually continue to have asthma in adulthood (Kliegman et al., 2007). **Status asthmaticus** is defined as an episode of asthma that does not respond to ordinary therapeutic measures. Hospitalization is necessary, perhaps in the intensive care unit (ICU).

Signs and Symptoms

Symptoms can occur abruptly (e.g., after sudden exposure to cold air or cigarette smoke) or over a period of days (precipitated by upper respiratory infection or mild exposure to an allergen). Initially the child has a tight nonproductive cough. Wheezing, particularly expiratory wheezing, may be audible or heard through a stethoscope. Depending on the severity of the problem, the child can develop signs of increasing respiratory distress (e.g., tachycardia, dyspnea, tachypnea, retractions, pallor). The child might have difficulty talking and appears tired.

Asthma is categorized into four classifications (Table 11-1). Appropriate management of asthma will depend on the symptoms of the child, which determine the classification. These classifications use a sidestep approach for pharmacologic management, control of the environment, and family education. Included in the asthma classifications are impairment and risks, which looks at the effect of asthma on present quality of life and future risks. A baseline measurement of the **peak expiratory flow rate (PEFR),** or the force of expiration from maximum lung inflation, is a component of the classifications. This is done with a special meter, which most children older than 5 years of age can be taught to use successfully. Children determine their personal best PEFR over a 2-week period of testing twice a day (Hockenberry and Wilson, 2007). Then daily (or more frequent) monitoring of PEFR and comparison with the child's personal best can indicate how well the asthma is being controlled.

Oxygen saturation monitoring can help determine the severity of an episode. The child may exhibit elevated eosinophils in a complete blood cell count (CBC) and elevated immunoglobulin E (IgE) levels. Allergy skin tests may reveal precipitating allergens. Chest radiographs can show underlying respiratory infection. Pulmonary function test (PFTs) are used to diagnose and evaluate lung function.

Some school-age children and adolescents have exercise-induced bronchospasm, which often does not indicate underlying asthma. Wheezing, shortness of breath, and chest tightness appear after vigorous exercise. There is bronchoconstriction without underlying inflammation. Treatment of exercise-induced bronchospasm consists of taking an inhaled β-agonist 15 minutes before exercise. Also effective is the use of leukotriene receptor antagonists with exercise-induced asthma. These drugs are more attractive because of the oral route and decrease dependency. The child should avoid exercising in the cold because cold air can precipitate the condition.

Treatment and Nursing Care

The goal of treatment is to appropriately manage the condition so the child can maintain optimal lifestyle and development. The treatment is focused on reducing episodes, minimizing the inflammatory process, decreasing the number of hospitalizations, avoiding precipitating factors, and facilitating normal growth and development. Untreated persistent asthma can

Table 11-1   Classifications of Asthma Severity in Children

| | | INTERMITTENT | | PERSISTENT | | | | | |
| | | | | MILD | | MODERATE | | SEVERE | |
AGES		0-4 YRS	5-11 YRS	0-4 YRS	5-11 YRS	0-4 YRS	5-11 YRS	0-4 YRS	5-11 YRS
Impairment	Symptoms	≤2 days/week		≤2 days/week but not daily		Daily		Through the day	
	Nighttime awakenings	0	≤2x/month	1-2x/month	3-4x/month	3-4x/month	≥1x/week but not nightly	>1x/week	Often 7x/week
	Short-acting β2-agonist use for symptom control	≤2 days/week		>2 days/week but not daily		Daily		Several times per week	
	Interference with normal activity	None		Minor limitation		Some limitation		Extremely limited	
	Lung function		Normal FEV between exacerbations						
	FEV (predicted) or peak flow (personal best)	N/A	>80%	N/A	>80%	N/A	60%-80%	N/A	<60%
	FEV/FVC	N/A	>85%	N/A	>80%	N/A	75%-80%	N/A	<75%
Risk	Exacerbations requiring oral systemic corticosteroids	0-1x/year	≥2 exacerbations in 6 months requiring oral systemic corticosteroids, or ≥4 wheezing episodes/1 year lasting >1 day and risk factors for persistent asthma	≥2x/year	≥2x/year	≥2x/year	≥2x/year	≥2x/year	≥2x/year

Adapted from National Asthma Education and Prevention Program Expert Panel Report 3. (2007). Guidelines for the diagnosis and management of asthma. Bethesda, MD: National Institutes of Health/National Heart, Lung, and Blood Institute. Retrieved July 2, 2010, from www.nhlbi.nih.gov/guidelines/asthma/asthgdln.htm.

lead to permanent and irreversible damage to lung function.

The physician should obtain the child's history in detail. Skin tests may be administered to determine whether allergy is a cause. If so, it is necessary to eliminate the offender, whether it is an environmental agent or a food. Special measures should include reducing dust mites, mold, animal dander, cockroach allergens, and tobacco smoke in the home.

Medications are classified into two categories: long-term medications (controllers) and quick-relief medications (rescuer). Table 11-2 lists the common medications in both categories. The drug of choice for first-time therapy for children older than 5 years of age is inhaled corticosteroids. Quick-relief and long-term medications can be used in combination to manage asthma effectively.

The preferred route of administration for many of these medications is inhalation because it allows the medications to act directly on the airways. Inhalation treatments can be given via nebulizer (Figure 11-8), in which the medication is mixed with normal saline solution and aerosolized; metered-dose inhaler (MDI); or dry powder inhaler (DPI). Bronchodilators can also be given via MDI if the child is able to follow the instructions (Skill 11-1). Most children older than 5 years of age can manage an MDI. Some younger children can use an MDI with an attached spacer device, which directs the medication more precisely and has excellent outcomes. Spacers help reduce infections that can result from the corticosteroids.

Leukotriene modifiers (e.g., Singulair, Accolate) have been useful for the prevention of asthma attacks. They are used in conjunction with corticosteroids and can reduce the level of need for corticosteroids. Singulair is given daily, and Accolate is given twice a day. Omalizumab is an anti-IgE antibody that is administered by subcutaneous injection and is recommended for moderate to severe allergy-related asthma in children 12 years of age or older (NAEPP, 2007).

Nursing Brief

The key to chronic asthma management is long-term control of airway inflammation. Education is the key to reducing underappreciation of the disease, failure to follow treatment guidelines, lack of adherence, and difficulty with inhalation devices.

Children with acute exacerbations of asthma, which require a visit to the doctor's office or emergency room, usually are treated with nebulized albuterol every 20 minutes for 1 hour with oxygen. If the symptoms improve, the child is placed on a daily routine of bronchodilators and short-term oral steroids (3-day to 5-day course). If the child's condition does not resolve and the oxygen saturation is less than 90%, the child should be admitted to the hospital.

On admission, an intravenous solution is started and oxygen is given with nasal prongs, hood, or mask. Nebulized albuterol is continued either continuously or intermittently. Anticholinergic drugs, such as ipratropium bromide, may be added to assist in additional bronchodilation. Currently, aminophylline does not appear to provide additional benefits and is not usually administered. For severe airway obstruction that does not respond to treatment, aminophylline may be administered. Because aminophylline can cause cardiac dysrhythmias, children receiving aminophylline intravenously should be placed on a cardiac monitor during the course of therapy. Intravenous steroids, such as methylprednisolone, are administered to control the inflammatory response. Before discharge, the treatment is changed to oral medication.

Facilitating Optimal Gas Exchange. Place the child in a high Fowler's position. Some children may prefer to have a pillow placed on the over-bed table and to extend their arms over it. This allows maximal use of the accessory muscles of breathing. The child may receive humidified oxygen with mask or cannula. Infants and young children often do better with nasal prongs because they do not feel they are suffocating as they might with a mask. An oxygen mask should not be used if it increases the child's anxiety.

The nurse should organize care to provide for periods of uninterrupted rest. Cuddling and rocking the younger child often reduce distress and promote sleep. Older children can be distracted with quiet music or games.

Vital signs, breath sounds, and a respiratory assessment, which includes oxygen saturation measurement, are done at least every 2 to 4 hours. Children in acute distress are monitored more frequently.

The child may be apprehensive because of the respiratory distress. The nurse should display a calm

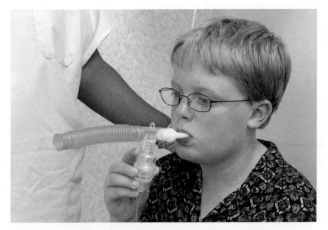
FIGURE 11-8 Appropriate use of a nebulizer involves placing the mouthpiece directly in the mouth. The child is encouraged to breathe normally.

Table 11-2 Asthma Medications

CONTROLLER	TRADE NAME	DOSE FORM	SIDE EFFECTS
Long-Term Control			
Inhaled Corticosteroids (ICS)			
Beclomethasone dipropionate	Beconase, QVAR	MDT, intranasal	Growth retardation, nasal irritation, unpleasant taste, headache; not recommended for children younger than 6 years
Budesonide	Rhinocort, Pulmicort	MDI, intranasal	Growth retardation, nasal irritation, dry mouth; avoid chickenpox exposure
Flunisolide	Aerobid, Nasalide	MDI, intranasal	Growth retardation, gastrointestinal upset, unpleasant taste; not recommended for children younger than 6 years
Fluticasone propionate	Flovent, Flonase	MDI, intranasal	Nausea, vomiting, dizziness, dental problems
Triamcinolone acetonide	Azmacort, Aristocort	MDI, oral, intranasal	Growth retardation, nausea, fatigue, lethargy, dizziness; not recommended for children younger than 6 years
Systemic Corticosteroids			
Methylprednisolone	Medrol, Solu-Medrol	Oral	Mask infection, growth retardation, cushingoid signs, oral thrush
Prednisolone	Prelone, Orapred, Pedipred	Oral	Insomnia, nervousness, mood swings, facial flushing
Prednisone	Sterapred	Oral	Insomnia, heartburn, nervousness, appetite changes, mood swings, nausea, vomiting
Antiinflammatory Agents			
Cromolyn sodium	Intal, Crolom, Nasalcrom	MDI, intranasal, oral	Fatigue, unpleasant taste, tachycardia, headache, rash, nasal congestion
Nedocromil	Tilade	MDI	Headache, unpleasant taste, cough, nausea
Leukotriene Receptor Antagonist (LTRA)			
Zafirlukast	Accolate	Oral, chewable tablet	Headache, nausea, vomiting, dizziness
Montelukast	Singulair	Oral	Headache, flulike symptoms, abdominal pain
Long-Acting β_2-Agonists (LABA)			
Salmeterol	Serevent	MDI, diskhaler	Tachycardia, tremor, nervousness, headache
Theophylline	Slo-bid, Theo-dur	Oral Not used as much	CNS hyperstimulation, seizures
Formoterol	Foradil	MDI	Tremors, dizziness, dysphonia
Immunomodulators (Anti-IgE Antibodies)			
Omalizumab	Xolair	SubQ	Headache
Quick Relief (Rescue)			
Short-Acting β_2-Agonists (SABA)			
Albuterol	Proventil, Ventolin	MDI, syrup, Neb	Tremors, anxiety, insomnia, tachycardia, heartburn, vomiting
Pirbuterol	Maxair	MDI	Tremors, nervousness, hypertension, tachycardia,
Terbutaline	Brethine, Brethaire	MDI, Inject	Tremors, anxiety, insomnia, tachycardia, heartburn, vomiting
Levalbuterol	Xopenex	Neb	Tachycardia, tremor, insomnia, nausea, headache
Systemic Corticosteroids			
Methylprednisolone	Medrol	Oral	Mask infection, growth retardation, cushingoid signs
Prednisolone	Prelone	Oral	Insomnia, nervousness, mood swings, facial flushing
Prednisone	Orasone, Deltasone, Meticorten	Oral	Insomnia, heartburn, nervousness, increased appetite
Anticholinergics			
Ipratropium bromide	Atrovent	MDI	Tachycardia, eye pain, cough, nervousness

Skill 11-1   Use of a Metered-Dose Inhaler

1. Remove cap from MDI and hold canister upright.
2. Shake inhaler canister three or four times.
3. Tilt head back slightly and exhale normally.
4. Position inhaler in one of the following ways:
   - Close lips around mouthpiece of inhaler.
   - Open mouth and hold mouthpiece two finger breadths from mouth.
   - Use a spacer.
5. Start to breathe in slowly, and press down on the inhaler to release the medication as you are inhaling.
6. Continue inhaling slowly and deeply (3 to 5 seconds).
7. Hold breath for a count of 10 (5 to 10 seconds) to allow the medicine to reach the lungs, and then exhale.
8. Wait 1 to 2 minutes, and repeat the puff.
9. Rinse out the mouth with water and spit out, especially when taking an inhaled corticosteroid.

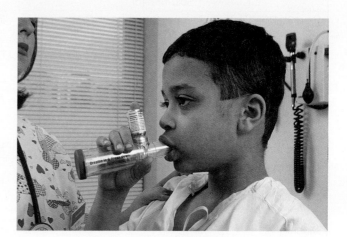

manner and remain with the child during periods of distress. Often, encouraging the child to breathe slowly, or to breathe along with you as you breathe slowly, decreases anxiety and allows for maximum air exchange.

Maintaining Hydration. The child who is hospitalized with asthma should have an intravenous infusion started. If the child is not in acute respiratory distress, clear oral fluids should also be offered. The child's need for fluids is increased because of fluid loss through dyspnea and diaphoresis. The fluids offered should not be cold because these may cause bronchospasm. The child's intake and output are measured and monitored.

Encouraging Self-Care and Asthma Management Skills. Before discharge, the older child and parent are taught self-care. They are taught to recognize early signs of difficulties and personal triggers that can serve as forewarnings of an attack. The importance of

following directions in the administration of medications is stressed as is awareness of side effects. The use of nebulizers or aerosol devices is also taught.

Review the procedure for measuring PEFR (Skill 11-2). Some peak flow meters are colored like traffic lights. These zones should be individualized by the physician for each child. Remind the child to measure PEFR at the same times each day, usually morning/night. If the child does the measurement after taking routine medications, the measurement should be done 15 minutes after the medication.

Specific information about how often and when to use a particular inhaler is also emphasized. The child needs to be seen regularly by the physician to evaluate progress and adjust medications. Review signs of respiratory infection: where, when, and whom to call for help. The child and family should be aware of early signs of an asthma attack and methods of limiting such an attack.

Regular exercise is stressed. Swimming is an excellent sport for children with asthma, although they can

Skill 11-2   Use and Interpretation of Peak Flow Meter

Use

1. Move slide marker to zero.
2. Standing upright with no gum or food in mouth, hold meter horizontal.
3. Relax, taking a few slow deep breaths.
4. Close mouth around mouthpiece and keep tongue away from mouthpiece.
5. Blow out hard and as fast as possible.
6. Note the marker number and repeat the previous steps for a total of three times, waiting at least 30 seconds between each time.
7. Record the highest of the three tries.
8. The peak flow meter reading should be done close to the same time each day. Readings should be done at least once a day, preferably in the morning.
9. A chart or record should be maintained.

Interpretation

1. Green zone (80% to 100% of personal best): No symptoms are present and routine treatment plan can be followed.
2. Yellow zone (50% to 79% of personal best): Indicates caution. An acute episode may be present. Medication may need to be increased.
3. Red zone (<50% of personal best): Indicates airway narrowing. Short-acting bronchodilator should be administered. If peak flow meter does not return immediately and stay in yellow or green zone, medical attention should be sought.

participate in many other sports as well. If the child with asthma also has exercise-induced bronchospasm, use of an inhaler before exercising is important.

Listen to and provide support for the child, parents, and siblings. Review stress reduction strategies with the child. These often can avert an impending attack. Parents should be encouraged to allow the child to live a normal life within the limits of a chronic condition. Refer the family to social services for additional support and to the Asthma and Allergy Foundation of America or the American Lung Association. Be certain that all children discharged from the hospital have appropriate inhalation equipment for the home management of their condition (Nursing Care Plan 11-2).

EPIGLOTTITIS

Epiglottitis is a swelling of the tissues **above** the vocal cords—that is, **supraglottic** (Figure 11-9). This results in narrowing of the airway inlet with the possibility of total airway obstruction. It is most frequently caused by *H. influenzae* type b infection and occurs most often in children between 2 and 6 years of age. It can occur in any season. Unlike croup, which progresses over a period of days, the course is rapid and progressive (airway obstruction can occur in a period of hours). Epiglottitis is a life-threatening medical emergency.

Signs and Symptoms

The child with epiglottitis appears acutely ill with a sudden sore throat, high fever, drooling, muffled voice, and rapid respirations with difficulty breathing.

Stridor is a late, *ominous* sign with epiglottitis. Nearly complete airway obstruction is most likely occurring if stridor is heard. The child with epiglottitis prefers to sit upright, leaning forward with the chin up and mouth open while leaning on the arms (tripod position or **sniffing position**). Blood gases fluctuate, and there is leukocytosis. Bacteremia is often present.

 Nursing Brief

If epiglottitis is suspected, do not examine the pharynx (back of the throat) because laryngospasm may occur and resulting in obstruction, which can cause respiratory arrest.

Treatment and Nursing Care

It is important for the nurse to display a calm, soothing, and reassuring attitude toward the child while being alert for respiratory complications. Endotracheal intubation equipment must be readily available. Epiglottitis may require endotracheal intubation to maintain the airway. Occasionally, a tracheostomy may be necessary. Children who have been intubated are cared for in an intensive care unit. The child generally receives oxygen, IV therapy, and antimicrobials. The incidence of epiglottitis has decreased since *H. influenzae* type b vaccine has been administered routinely beginning at 2 months of age.

BRONCHITIS

Bronchitis refers to *bronchial* inflammation. The bronchi are the two lower divisions of the trachea that branch

⭐ Nursing Care Plan 11-2 | The Child with Asthma

NURSING DIAGNOSIS *Gas exchange, impaired, related to increasing airway obstruction from inflammation and mucus*

Goals/Outcome Criteria	Nursing Interventions	Rationales
Child shows adequate gas exchange, as evidenced by: • Pink skin color • Age-appropriate respiratory rate and rhythm • Ability to talk and sleep comfortably • Absence of wheezing, cough	Provide short-acting β2-agonist (SABA) bronchodilators and other medications as ordered; monitor for effects and side effects.	Relax bronchial tissue and open up the airway. Cromolyn prevents late allergic response; steroids reduce inflammation.
	Monitor vital signs and oxygen saturation closely (at least every 2 to 4 hours) for signs of increased respiratory distress. Maintain oxygen saturation between 92% and 95%.	Close monitoring allows rapid recognition of respiratory distress.
	Place child on a cardiac monitor according to hospital protocol.	Side effects of some of the medication include tachycardia.
	Provide humidified oxygen as ordered via least stressful route.	Facilitates adequate oxygenation in the lung.
	Place child in upright position.	Facilitates lung expansion.
	Organize care to provide maximum rest periods.	Decreased energy expenditure decreases need for oxygen.
	Encourage relaxation strategies such as slow, deep, breathing; listening to quiet music or stories. Rock the infant or young child.	Relaxation decreases stress and respiratory effort.

NURSING DIAGNOSIS *Fluid volume, risk for deficient, related to fluid loss from increased expirations and diaphoresis*

Goals/Outcome Criteria	Nursing Interventions	Rationales
Child maintains adequate hydration, as evidenced by: • Supple skin turgor • Adequate urination • Absence of thirst • Moist mucous membranes	Provide intravenous fluids as ordered.	Maintains fluid balance while the child may be unable to take oral fluids.
	Give clear oral fluids when respiratory effort decreases; give fluids child likes.	Providing fluids child likes increases child's interest in taking them.
	Avoid cold fluids.	Can cause bronchospasm.
	Give small, frequent sips rather than larger amounts; use straws, "sippy" cups, or other devices that interest the child.	Giving large volumes of fluid can result in vomiting when the child coughs; large volumes also cause distention, which limits diaphragm movement.
	Monitor intake and output.	Provides data on hydration status.

NURSING DIAGNOSIS *Coping, ineffective, related to stress of acute and chronic illness*

Goals/Outcome Criteria	Nursing Interventions	Rationales
Child has decreased stress: • Appears calm and in control • Demonstrates stress-reducing measures	Encourage regular participation in exercise.	Exercise releases hormones that facilitate a feeling of well-being.
	Advise child to participate in exercise or sports that require short periods of energy (sprints, baseball, gymnastics) or in swimming.	Short bursts of energy allow the child to recover in between; swimming provides external source of moisture for airways.
	Advise child to find enjoyable activities that reduce stress (e.g., bike riding, talking to friends, playing games).	Reducing stress helps the child cope with daily living.
	Advise parents to encourage child to participate in normal developmental activities.	Overprotection increases stress by decreasing the child's self-esteem.

⭐ Nursing Care Plan 11-2   The Child with Asthma—cont'd

NURSING DIAGNOSIS *Deficient knowledge about home management, related to inexperience with equipment, medications, and principles of disease management*

Goals/Outcome Criteria	Nursing Interventions	Rationales
Parent and older child appropriately manage condition at home: • Demonstrate equipment • Describe signs indicating condition is worse • Intervene appropriately • Describe principles of infection prevention	Review teaching about MDI, nebulizer equipment, and PEFR measurements.	Review reinforces teaching.
	Have child and parent demonstrate use of equipment.	Return demonstration allows for evaluation of learning.
	Review medications and when to use them. Provide list of criteria for when it is necessary to adjust medications or call the doctor.	Reinforces teaching.
	Help parents with environmental control measures (e.g., allergy-proofing the home, installing air purification systems or dehumidifiers to reduce mites and molds).	Reducing home allergens can reduce episodes in children with allergic asthma.
	Teach prevention of respiratory infections, avoiding exposure to colds, meticulous cleaning of inhalation equipment, yearly influenza vaccine.	Preventing respiratory infection reduces exacerbations of asthma.

NURSING DIAGNOSIS *Interrupted family processes, related to chronic condition and frequent exacerbations*

Goals/Outcome Criteria	Nursing Interventions	Rationales
Family adjusts to child's chronic illness, as evidenced by: • Appropriate intervention during acute episodes • Child's normal development • Absence of inappropriate anxiety	Encourage parent to participate in child's care during exacerbations.	Involving the parent decreases parental and child stress.
	Keep parent informed about changes in condition.	Parents know more about how their child reacts to situations than the health care personnel.
	Maintain child's usual routine and usual treatment regimen if possible.	Decreases stress associated with hospitalization and increases coping.
	Encourage close communication between family and the school nurse.	Appropriate communication increases consistency in care.
	Listen to family concerns.	Listening provides a basis for planning.
	Refer for financial or psychological help if indicated.	Stress adversely affects family relationships and coping.

Critical Thinking Snapshot

A 12-year-old comes to the community health clinic with his mother. He is wheezing and short of breath; his chest is tight, and he is coughing. He is lethargic and sitting in a tripod position. His color is pale, and his skin is cool and clammy. As the nurse, what is your initial assessment of this child? What are your initial interventions? What changes in his breath sounds would concern you?

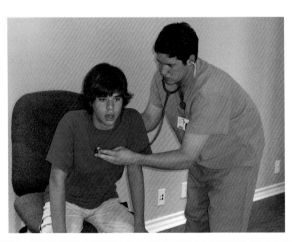

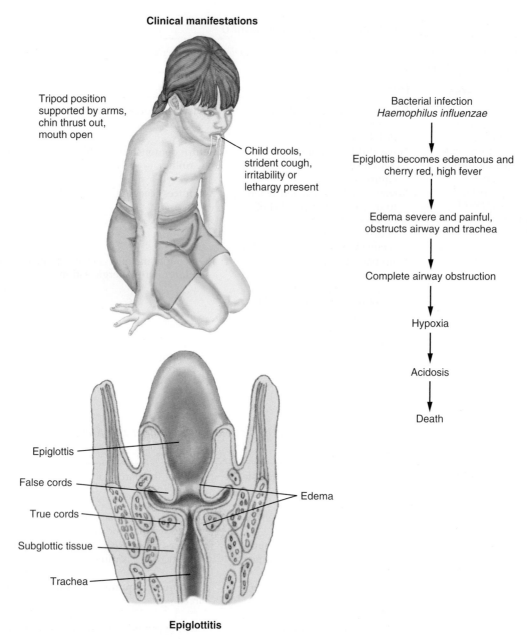

Clinical manifestations

Tripod position supported by arms, chin thrust out, mouth open

Child drools, strident cough, irritability or lethargy present

Bacterial infection
Haemophilus influenzae

↓

Epiglottis becomes edematous and cherry red, high fever

↓

Edema severe and painful, obstructs airway and trachea

↓

Complete airway obstruction

↓

Hypoxia

↓

Acidosis

↓

Death

Epiglottis
False cords
True cords
Subglottic tissue
Trachea
Edema

Epiglottitis

FIGURE 11-9 Pathophysiology of epiglottitis.

off to the lungs. This condition is usually preceded by a viral upper respiratory tract infection. It is more common in winter.

The child may initially have a cold followed by a cough that may or may not be productive. Low-grade fever may be present. Crackles and wheezes may be detected on auscultation. As with all respiratory disorders, fluids are important. Bronchitis is generally self-limiting and resolves in 2 to 3 weeks. Antimicrobials, cough suppressants, antihistamines, and expectorants are not indicated (Kliegman et al., 2007).

PNEUMONIA

Pneumonia is an infection of the lower respiratory tract in which the *alveoli* (air sacs) become filled with

exudate. As the infection progresses, the exudate becomes solidified (consolidation). The affected portion of the lung does not receive enough air. Breathing is shallow. As a result, the bloodstream is denied sufficient oxygen. *Pneumonitis* is a general term for lung inflammation and may or may not be associated with consolidation.

About 80% of pneumonia is caused by viruses and 20% by bacteria. Aspiration of foreign substances such as talcum powder, peanuts, or popcorn may result in pneumonia. Aspirated hydrocarbons (kerosene, furniture polish, paint thinner) damage the lung cells by impairing the surface tension. Gastroesophageal reflux may result in the aspiration of gastric contents, resulting in pneumonia.

Respiratory Disorders CHAPTER 11 223

Viral pneumonia can be caused by RSV, influenza, and adenovirus. This occurs more frequently during the winter months. Bacterial pneumonia generally causes a more severe infection. The common bacterial organisms are *S. pneumoniae,* group A streptococcal, *Staphylococcus aureus,* and *H. influenzae.* Additional agents may cause pneumonia such as acute respiratory syndrome (SARS), Avian flu or bird flu (influenza A, H5N1), and the recent outbreak of H1N1 or swine flu.

Pneumonia might occur as the initial or **primary** disease, or it can complicate another illness, in which case it is termed **secondary** pneumonia. Secondary pneumonia may accompany various communicable diseases or may follow surgery. It is more serious than primary pneumonia because the child is in a weakened condition.

Signs and Symptoms

The symptoms of pneumonia vary with the age of the child and the causative organism. They may develop suddenly or be preceded by an upper respiratory tract infection. The cough is dry at first but gradually becomes productive. Fever rises as high as 103° F to 104° F (39.5° C to 40° C) and may fluctuate widely over a 24-hour period. The respiration rate may increase to 40 to 80 breaths per minute in infants, and in older children to 30 to 50 breaths per minute. Rhonchi and faint crackles may be heard with breath sounds. Respirations are shallow as the child attempts to reduce the chest pain. Sternal retractions may be seen as the assisting muscles of respiration are brought into use. Flaring of the nostrils may appear. The child's color may vary from pale to cyanotic. The child is listless and has a poor appetite. The child tends to lie on the affected side.

Treatment and Nursing Care

The child is given a complete physical examination. A tuberculosis skin test is administered if the child is at risk or if the child has not been tested recently. The doctor pays particular attention to the examination of the child's chest. Radiographs confirm the diagnosis and determine whether there are complications. A differential white blood cell count is routinely done. Blood specimens show a marked increase in the number of white blood cells (16,000 to 40,000/mm3). The number of red blood cells and the amount of hemoglobin may be slightly reduced. Obtaining blood specimens can be traumatic to the child, and crying can increase coughing spells. The nurse or parent should hug and calm the child afterward.

Treatment depends on the severity of the disease and the causative organism. Children who are in severe respiratory distress, dehydrated, vomiting, or are immunocompromised are treated in the hospital. Bacterial pneumonia is treated with antimicrobials. Treatment for viral pneumonia is supportive. The nurse

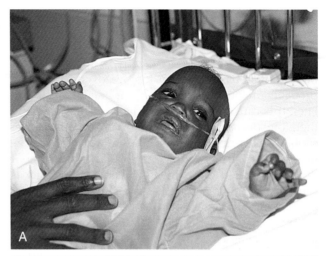

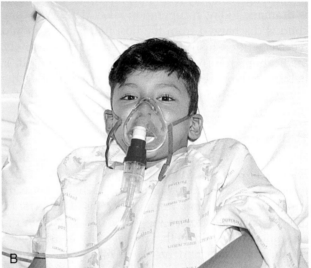

FIGURE 11-10   **A,** Infant receiving oxygen via a nasal cannula. **B,** Child receiving oxygen via face mask.

checks the vital signs at regular intervals. When a child is flushed with fever, remove heavy clothing and blankets and administer antipyretics. The nurse may be asked to give the child tepid sponge baths to help reduce a high fever (see Chapter 3). Oxygen is administered for dyspnea or cyanosis and needs to be monitored with pulse oximetry (Figure 11-10). Rest and conservation of energy are an important part of the treatment of this disease. The nurse needs to organize work so that the child is not disturbed unnecessarily. An increase in fluid intake is important. Encouraging children to increase oral fluid intake is often a goal. Besides water, offer the child Gatorade, juice, or a Popsicle, depending on preference. IV fluids are administered if the child cannot retain fluids because of vomiting or will not take fluids by mouth. They are also given to replace insensible fluid loss from tachypnea and fever. The appetite of the child improves as the condition does. For severe cases that do not resolve, a thoracentesis (surgical removal of fluids using large bore-needle) may be attempted or a chest tube may be placed. Most cases of pneumonia in healthy children can be managed outside of the hospital.

Reposition the child frequently. Although this is painful, it is paramount to total recovery. The child probably prefers the affected side (if pneumonia is unilateral) because it splints the chest on that side and therefore decreases the discomfort. Administer prescribed analgesics to increase the child's comfort. The nurse assists and encourages the child to walk about the room and in the hallways when such activity is prescribed. Small children can exercise their lungs by blowing bubbles through a straw. The respiratory therapist may provide chest percussion and postural drainage exercise.

Although recovery from uncomplicated pneumonia is dramatic today, recuperation takes time. When the child is discharged from the hospital, parents should receive written instructions concerning diet, activity, medication, return appointments, and so on. It is helpful if the parents repeat these instructions to the nurse to determine whether they have interpreted them correctly.

TUBERCULOSIS

Tuberculosis (TB) has been around for a long time. There has been an increase in the incidence of this disease. Several factors contributing to this increase are emigration, HIV, and resistant strains. Pediatric TB directly correlates to the incidence of adult TB in the community. A child with TB is usually considered a primary infection and has been infected by contact with an infectious adult or adolescent (Robinson and El-Sadr, 2006).

Tuberculosis is caused by the acid-fast bacillus, *Mycobacterium tuberculosis.* Transmission of the organism is by inhalation of an infected droplet. It begins to multiply in the lung tissue. If the primary lesion erodes into a blood vessel, dissemination of the organism can occur. When the organism spreads to other tissue, such as bone, kidney, or the brain, the condition is known as **miliary tuberculosis.**

Skin testing is the method of screening for TB. The most accurate form of skin testing is the Mantoux test, which is administered intradermally. The test should be read only by qualified medical personnel. It is recommended that children be screened at 15 months of age. If other risk factors are present, additional screenings may be needed.

Children are most vulnerable to TB when their immune system is the least mature, which is during the first 3 years of life. Another period of vulnerability is just before, during, and after puberty. The risk of becoming infected with TB increases with poverty and crowded living conditions, which can lead to poor hygiene. The highest incidence of TB is among the Hispanic population. Asians represent the second

largest ethnic group. Both of these groups who are foreign-born account for 59% of cases. Children's rates have decreased, but they still continue to be high risk especially if they are from these two groups and are foreign-born (CDC, 2009).

While there is a decrease in the number of cases, another major concern is the developing number of resistant strains. Individuals with HIV are susceptible to TB and should be screened for the exposure. Children with TB should also be tested for HIV.

Signs and Symptoms

Diagnosis is determined with tests including a positive skin test. Chest radiographs can confirm the disease. Gastric washing is done to confirm the presence of the bacillus. Infants and small children may present with a nonproductive cough and mild dyspnea. There also may be a failure to thrive. Symptoms may be variable and can include fever, anorexia, malaise, weight loss, night sweats, and mild dyspnea. As the lungs become more invaded, more respiratory symptoms may develop, such as increased respiratory rate, diminished breath sounds, and rales.

Treatment

Hospitalization is not necessary except for diagnostic procedures. All hospitalized children with active TB must be in respiratory isolation. All health care workers must wear an N-95 respirator when caring for a child with contagious TB (AAP, 2000). All other treatment can be given in a community-based environment and involves nurses in the ambulatory setting, the school, and the public health facilities.

Gastric washing is done to isolate the bacillus. Young children swallow their secretions, and the organism can be obtained from the stomach. The gastric washing is obtained in the early morning after the child has had nothing to eat during the night. A nasogastric (NG) tube is passed, and the stomach is lavaged. The gastric contents are removed and sent to the laboratory for testing.

Currently the first-line medications given for TB are isoniazid (INH), rifampin, pyrazinamide, and ethambutol. These are given daily for 8 weeks (56 doses) as the initial phase of the preferred regimen. A continuation phase continues for either 4 to 7 months depending on chest film and sputum culture results after the first 2 months. The continuation phase medications typically used are isoniazid and rifampin. Modifications of the regimens can be determined by special circumstances such as HIV and pregnancy (CDC, 2010). Because of the difficulty in eradicating this organism and the importance of compliance, most experts recommend that all drug administration be directly observed (DOT) by a health care worker. A fourth drug such as streptomycin or ethambutol may be added in areas where there are resistant strains.

Asymptomatic TB occurs when there is a positive skin test but all other diagnostic findings are negative. The child with asymptomatic TB is treated with INH for 9 months. Even if they have a negative skin test, children younger than 6 years of age who have been exposed to an adult with infectious TB also receive INH therapy. These children are retested after 3 months. If the skin test is again negative, then the INH therapy can be discontinued. If the skin test is positive, the child needs a complete course of treatment. In rare, severe cases, surgery may be needed to remove the involved tissue.

Nursing Care

Emotional support is vital for this family. The treatment of TB takes a long time. This family's life will change, and avenues to support them need to be identified.

Tuberculosis is a communicable disease and therefore is reported to the public health department. A concern for some families may be their status as citizens of the United States. This concern can affect the treatment of the disease because a family may not feel that they can be entirely honest with the health care team.

Parents need to know the side effects of the medication(s) given to their child. They need to understand the importance of the length of treatment. In addition, the source of infection needs to be identified so that the disease can be eradicated in the family and in other families in the community. Older children and adolescents can be involved in their own care and should assist in setting goals. Compliance increases if they are active participants.

Because stress can alter the immune system and make it less proficient, decreasing stress for these children is important. Stress may result from many factors, such as fear of bodily harm, fear of being ostracized, fear of peer rejection, being different, or concern that they can give TB to their friends. A support group can be beneficial for these children so that they can verbalize their fears and concerns.

Proper rest and a balanced diet are important for healing. Families may need assistance in regard to a proper diet. Make sure their needs in regard to culture are addressed.

Most affected children limit their own activities. Participation in competitive sports is usually discouraged during this period of time.

Get Ready for the NCLEX® Examination!

Key Points

- Anatomic differences in the respiratory system predispose infants and children to respiratory distress.
- Respiratory distress should be identified early to prevent respiratory failure.
- When interviewing parents of an infant who died of suspected SIDS, avoid implications of guilt.
- Bronchopulmonary dysplasia occurs primarily in premature and low–birth weight infants who have needed mechanical ventilation for a prolonged period of time.
- Children infected with RSV should be placed in contact isolation.
- Aggressive pulmonary therapy, including antimicrobials and intermittent aerosol therapy, has increased the life expectancy of children with CF.
- Bleeding after a tonsillectomy can be identified by frequent swallowing, restlessness, fast thready pulse, and vomiting of bright red blood.
- Eliminating or minimizing environmental triggers can reduce asthma symptoms, disease severity, and the amount of medications needed to have effective asthma control.
- Suspected epiglottitis requires immediate care.
- Infants and children are at greater risk for TB if they are foreign-born Hispanics or Asians.
- Tuberculosis is a communicable disease and should be reported to the public health department. The public health department oversees the management and treatment of this disease.

Additional Learning Resources

evolve Go to your Evolve website (*http://evolve.elsevier.com/Price/pediatric/*) for the following FREE learning resources:
- 3-D Animations
- Answer Keys
- Appendixes
- Audio Glossary
- Spanish/English Glossary
- Video Clips

Review Questions for the NCLEX® Examination

1. Two clinical features of sudden infant death syndrome (SIDS) that remain constant are: (**Select all that apply.**)
   1. Child is between 2 and 4 months of age.
   2. Death occurs during winter.
   3. Death occurs during sleep.
   4. Infant does not cry or make other sounds of distress.
   5. Autopsy reveals slight respiratory infection or otitis media.

2. A chronic lung disease that occurs in newborns that are premature or have pulmonary disorders that require mechanical ventilator support with high positive pressure and oxygen is:
   1. Asthma
   2. Cystic fibrosis
   3. Infantile apnea
   4. Bronchopulmonary dysplasia

3. All of the following may be used to achieve pain control with a diagnosis of otitis media **except:**

   1. Acetaminophen
   2. Eardrops (Auralgan)
   3. Warm compresses
   4. Antihistamines

4. An infant is diagnosed with bronchiolitis. Which of the following would be an indication for hospitalization?

   1. Oxygen level of 93%
   2. Respiratory rate of 42 breaths per minute
   3. Fever of 102° Fahrenheit
   4. Inability to tolerate oral feeding

5. It is suspected that a child has cystic fibrosis. The study the nurse would expect to be ordered to diagnose this condition is:

   1. Pulmonary function test
   2. Sweat test
   3. Chest x-ray
   4. Magnetic resonance imaging

Cardiac Disorders

Objectives

1. Define the vocabulary terms listed
2. Describe the changes from fetal to neonatal circulation
3. Summarize the symptoms of a congenital heart defect with increased pulmonary blood flow
4. Discuss the corrective interventions for a child with mixed heart defects
5. Develop a teaching plan for an older child who is scheduled for a cardiac catheterization
6. List the symptoms for an infant with CHF
7. List three major and two minor manifestations of acute rheumatic fever as determined by the modified Jones criteria
8. Identify the priority nursing care for a child with rheumatic fever

Key Terms

chemoprophylaxis (KĒ-mō-prō-fe-LAK-ses; p. 241)
ductus arteriosus (p. 227)
ductus venosus (p. 227)
foramen ovale (p. 227)
hemodynamics (HĒ-mō-dī-NĂM-ĭks; p. 229)
infective endocarditis (IE) (p. 238)
Jones criteria (p. 239)

latent (p. 239)
multifactorial (MŬL-tĭ-făk-TŌ-rē-ăl; p. 228)
polycythemia (PA-lē-sī-THĒ-mē-a; p. 230)
shunting (p. 229)
squatting position (p. 230)
subacute bacterial endocarditis (SBE) (p. 233)

CARDIOVASCULAR SYSTEM

The four-chambered heart begins development as a single tube around the third week of gestation and becomes the first fully functioning system by the eighth week of gestation. Some of these defects occur before mothers are aware of their pregnancy. Cardiac defects can be evident at birth or may not be identified until a later age. The heart is a vital organ and when parents are confronted with cardiac problems, fear and anxiety become overwhelming. Families who may not have a basic understanding of the cardiovascular system are being overloaded with new terms and information.

Heart defects are the most common birth defect and are the leading cause of birth defect-related deaths. The incidence rate of infants born with a congenital heart defect is about one per 125 deliveries (March of Dimes, 2006). With the advancement in diagnosis and treatment, about 85% of children live into adulthood. This has created a new subspecialty, the adult with congenital heart disease.

Fetal circulation differs from normal circulation as the organ of oxygenation is the placenta. Oxygenated blood from the placenta flows through the umbilical

vein to the liver and inferior vena cava. A small portion of the blood supports the hepatic tissue, while the rest flows through the ductus venosus into the inferior vena cava. As blood enters the right atrium, most of the flow is directed through the foramen ovale (a septum connection between the right and left atrium) to the left side of the heart and out the aorta. The remaining blood continues to flow to the right ventricle and out the pulmonary arteries to the lungs. Since the lungs are not functioning, only a small amount of the oxygenated blood is needed to provide nutrients to lung tissue. The majority of this oxygenated flow is diverted again through the ductus arteriosus (a connection between the pulmonary artery and the aorta) into the aorta. The oxygenated blood is distributed to the rest of the body and is returned through the umbilical arteries to the placenta (Figure 12-1).

During the birthing process, the dynamics of blood flow changes as the lungs become the organ of oxygenation. Blood flow no longer needs to bypass the lungs, resulting in the closure of the fetal shunts (i.e., the ductus venosus, foramen ovale, and ductus arteriosus). While the ductus venosus and foramen ovale usually close quickly, the ductus arteriosus may take several days to close.

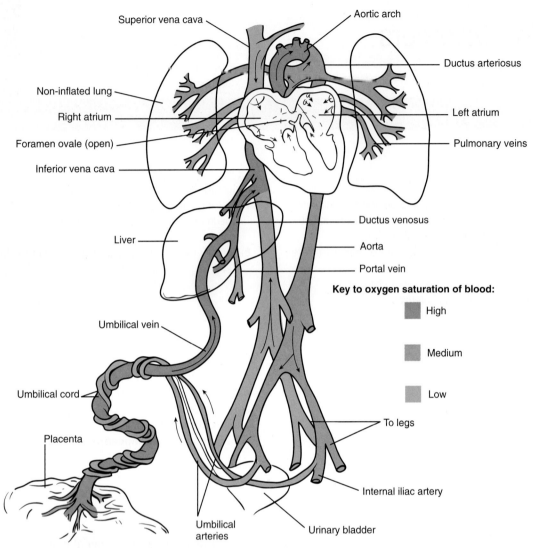

FIGURE 12-1 Diagram of fetal circulation showing the placenta, umbilical vein, and umbilical arteries. The fetal bypasses are also shown. These are ductus venosus, ductus arteriosus, and foramen ovale.

Closures of these shunts impact the pressures in the heart. During fetal circulation, the pressure is higher on the right side of the heart. The closure of the shunts will result in higher left-sided pressures. Direction of blood flow is impacted by the pressures in various parts of the heart. Blood flow will move from an area of higher pressure to an area of lower pressure.

Murmurs are generated by turbulence of blood flow through the heart. They are classified as systolic, diastolic, or continuous. They are graded from 1 to 6 based on increasing loudness. Murmurs may be thought of as functional (innocent) or organic (from improper heart formation). Functional murmurs are caused by the sound of blood passing through a normal heart. Organic murmurs result from blood passing through abnormal openings or normal openings that have not yet closed. Most heart murmurs in the newborn period have been found to be functional, may come and go (transient), and tend not to be serious. However, murmurs should be reported to the physician and the newborn should be checked periodically to rule out other possibilities.

CONGENITAL HEART DISEASE

A baby born with congenital heart disease (CHD) has a defect in the structure of the heart or in one or more of the large blood vessels that lead to and from the heart. The heart or vessels have failed to develop properly during the gestational period.

Research indicates that most congenital defects are a result of genetic-environmental interactions; that is, they are multifactorial. Genetic factors that may increase the risks include a history of CHD in other family members and chromosomal abnormalities such as

Down syndrome. Environmental risk factors include alcoholism, cocaine use, rubella, exposure to *Coxsackie* virus, diabetes mellitus, ingestion of lithium salts, use of Accutane, and advanced maternal age.

Therefore, the nurse must stress the need for good prenatal care and impress on the parents the value of regular checkups at baby clinics. Many organic heart murmurs have been detected early in infancy at a periodic checkup. A careful health history is particularly useful.

Classification

In the past, congenital heart defects were divided into two groups: cyanotic and acyanotic. This categorization has proved inaccurate because children with acyanotic defects may develop cyanosis and those with cyanotic disease may be pink in color. Presently, defects are classified according to the effect the defect has on the movement of circulating blood. The study of blood circulation is termed hemodynamics (*hemo*, blood; *dynamis*, power). Defects can be classified as (1) defects with increased pulmonary blood flow, (2) obstructive defects, (3) defects with decreased pulmonary blood flow, and (4) mixed defects. A list of the hemodynamics and the heart defect(s) associated with each is given in Box 12-1.

The flow of blood through abnormal openings or vessels is called shunting. The direction of the shunt flow is determined by the pressures in the connecting chambers or vessels. Flow will move from a high to a low pressure area. Normally the right side of the heart has a lower pressure than the left side. Flow from the left side to the right is referred to as "left to right shunt." The flow of oxygenated blood into unoxygenated blood results in no mixed blood gaining access to

the systemic system. Flow from the right to the left side is called "right to left shunt." This flow of unoxygenated blood into oxygenated blood results in mixed blood circulating in the systemic system.

Diagnostic Tools

Several diagnostic tools can be used in evaluation of a child with CHD. Not all testing is necessary for each child. The tools include laboratory tests, electrocardiogram, Holter monitor, event recorder, chest radiography, echocardiogram, MRI, and cardiac catheterization. The diagnostic procedures listed in Box 12-2 can be used in identifying the type of heart defect.

Cardiac catheterization is an invasive procedure that provides information about anatomy, cardiac pressures, oxygen saturations, and cardiac function. Sedation is necessary to ensure that the child does not move. Older children and families should be prepared for the procedure. Discussing the sounds and sights of the cath lab and post op care may help decrease anxiety. Following the procedure, the child will have a cardiac monitor and pulse oximetry. The nurse will need to monitor the following:

- Temperature and color of extremity below (distal) insertion site
- Pulse of extremity below insertion site
- Sensation of affected extremity
- Vital signs every 15 minutes for first hour and then hourly
- Dressing for excessive bleeding
- Hydration status

 Safety Alert

The pressure dressing placed over the insertion site is monitored per hospital policy. The infant's diaper area should also be monitored as any bleeding can flow down the child's groin crease. Any wetness or bleeding should be immediately reported, and pressure should be applied above the insertion site. Dressings should not be removed to view the site until ordered.

Box 12-1 Hemodynamics and Examples of Congenital Heart Disease

INCREASED PULMONARY BLOOD FLOW
Atrial septal defect
Patent ductus arteriosus
Ventricular septal defect

OBSTRUCTIVE BLOOD FLOW
Aortic stenosis
Coarctation of the aorta
Pulmonary stenosis

DECREASED PULMONARY BLOOD FLOW
Tetralogy of Fallot
Tricuspid atresia

MIXED BLOOD FLOW
Hypoplastic left heart syndrome
Total anomalous pulmonary venous return
Transposition of the great vessels
Truncus arteriosus

Box 12-2 Diagnostic Procedures in Congenital Heart Disease

History
Physical examination
Chest radiography
Electrocardiography
Echocardiography
Cardiac catheterization
Cardiac magnetic resonance (CMR)
Computed tomography (CT)
Laboratory studies
- Blood gases
- Hemoglobin
- Hematocrit

Box 12-3	General Signs and Symptoms in Congenital Heart Disease	
INFANTS	**CHILDREN**	
Dyspnea	Dyspnea	
Difficulty feeding	Decreased activity	
Stridor or choking spells	tolerance	
Tachycardia	Squatting	
Recurrent respiratory	Tachycardia	
infections	Recurrent respiratory	
Failure to gain weight	infections	
Heart murmurs	Delayed physical	
Cyanosis	development	
Cerebral thrombosis	Heart murmur and thrills	
Anoxic episodes	Cyanosis	
	Clubbing of fingers	
	Elevated blood pressure	

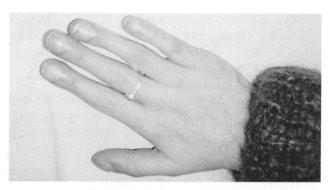

FIGURE 12-2 Clubbing in fingers caused by poor oxygenation.

The child's extremity should be kept straight for 4 to 6 hours depending on hospital policy. Encouraging parents to hold the child may help in decreasing the child's anxiety. Discharge instructions should include signs of infection, fever management, activity restrictions, and bathing guidelines.

Signs and Symptoms

The symptoms, as indicated in Box 12-3, depend on the location and type of heart defect. Some children have mild cases and can lead a fairly normal life with medical management. Others are treated medically until the optimal time for surgery. Heart transplantation is an option in some cases.

The child with CHD may be small for age, and his or her condition may be classified as a physiologic failure to thrive. This is the result of the difficulty the child has feeding and breathing at the same time. In addition, it takes energy to suck and infants may spend more energy eating than gained from their formula. Exercise intolerance may first be identified when the infant experiences dyspnea while feeding or it may not be evident until later, when the child tends to be more active. The older child may assume a squatting position to decrease venous return by occluding the femoral veins and thus lessen the workload of the right side of the heart. The infant can gain this same effect by being placed in the knee-chest position.

Hematocrit and hemoglobin concentration impact the effectiveness of oxygen transportation. Hematocrit (the percent of erythrocytes volume in a given volume of blood) is normally 35% to 49% in infants and children. Hematocrit can range from 44% to 72% in newborns. Hemoglobin (the iron-containing pigment that carries oxygen) can range from 11% to 15% in children. When the body determines there is hypoxemia (decreased oxygen in blood), it compensates by increasing the number of red blood cells to carry oxygen to the tissues. This is known as polycythemia. When there

is an increase in the number of red blood cells, the hematocrit will also be elevated. This results in an increased viscosity of the blood and increased cardiac workload. "Thick" blood causes an increased risk for thromboembolism and cardiovascular accident.

Hypoxia is a result of inadequate oxygenation and can present with cyanosis in children with heart defects. Cyanosis can be generalized or localized such as in the hands, feet, or lips or around the mouth. Cyanosis may be constant or transient and can be influenced by the child's behavior such as crying. Crying can improve or worsen the cyanosis. Overt cyanosis can be difficult to observe in children with dark skin. For these children, cyanosis can be detected in the mucous membranes of the mouth, on the palms of the hands, or on the bottom of the feet. Chronic hypoxia can result in long-lasting pooling of the blood in the capillaries resulting in clubbing of the fingers and/or toes (Figure 12-2). The child may also present with a pale or mottled appearance. Arterial oxygen saturation can differ with each type of defect. Ideally, oxygen saturation is between 95% and 98% in normal children, and saturations below 88% can result in cyanosis. Some of the defects have saturations much lower than 88%. Assessment of the heart rate of a child with hypoxemia is important as hypoxemia can result in bradycardia.

Nursing Brief

Bradycardia can be a warning sign of an impending cardiac arrest. Prolonged hypoxemia and respiratory arrest result in cardiac arrest in children rather than a primary cardiac arrhythmia as seen in adults. Nursing assessment of hypoxemia is a priority for a child with a cardiac defect.

Finally, many CHD children tend to have frequent respiratory infections because of pulmonary vascular congestion. The amount of dyspnea does vary, and in more acute cases, it is accompanied by flaring of the nostrils, mouth breathing, and sternal retractions. The child has more trouble breathing when flat in bed than when being held upright. Signs of air hunger are

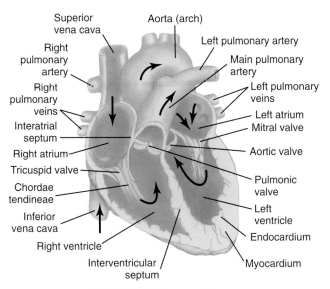

FIGURE 12-3 The normal heart.

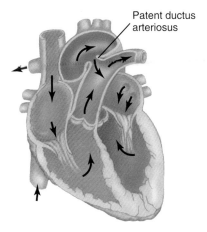

FIGURE 12-4 Patent ductus arteriosus.

edema, vein distention, hepatomegaly, and spleno-megaly can appear. A decrease in perfusion results in decreased urine output, diaphoresis, mottling, cyanosis, and pallor.

Defects with Increased Pulmonary Blood Flow

Patent Ductus Arteriosus. The **ductus arteriosus (PDA)** is the passageway by which the blood crosses from the pulmonary artery to the aorta and avoids the deflated lungs in the fetus. This vessel closes shortly after birth; however, when it does not close, blood continues to pass from the aorta, where the pressure is higher, into the pulmonary artery. This causes oxygenated blood to recycle through the lungs, overburdening the pulmonary circulation and making the heart work harder. A machine-like murmur may be heard. The symptoms of this disorder may go unnoticed during infancy. However, with growth, the child experiences dyspnea, pulses becomes full and bounding on exertion, and there may be failure to thrive. The parents may report frequent respiratory infections, which are a result of pulmonary congestion. Symptoms will depend on the amount of blood flowing through the ductus.

Patent ductus arteriosus is one of the most common cardiac anomalies (Figure 12-4). The word *patent* means open. PDA occurs twice as frequently in females as in males. In the premature infant, indomethacin or ibuprofen may be administered to facilitate closure of the ductus (Sadowski, 2009). If drug treatment is not successful, other nonsurgical intervention may be tried. Recent interventional devices such as coils or the Amplatzer PDA device (Figure 12-5) have provided closure for small ducts during cardiac catheterization. Occluder device risks include leaking and occlusions (Park, 2008). For large ducts, surgical repair includes ligation of the ductus through a left thoracotomy or with video-assisted thoracoscopic surgery (VATS). If this condition is left uncorrected, the child eventually could develop CHF or endocarditis. The prognosis for a corrected PDA is excellent.

irritability, restlessness, and a weak and hoarse cry. Increased respirations over 60 per minute in an infant can indicate distress.

Some common nursing diagnoses associated with CHD are listed in Box 12-4. The normal heart is illustrated in Figure 12-3.

Congestive Heart Failure. A child with a severe heart defect may develop congestive heart failure (CHF). It is not a disease in itself but rather symptoms caused by an underlying heart defect. CHF occurs if the heart is unable to maintain adequate cardiac output to meet body demands. Early symptoms may be subtle. The infant, who requires a longer time period for feeding and has a decrease in intake, may fail to gain weight and be irritable and fatigued. Tachycardia and tachypnea with increased work of breathing (grunting, nasal flaring, wheezing, coughing, retractions) may be observed. As CHF progresses, periorbital and facial

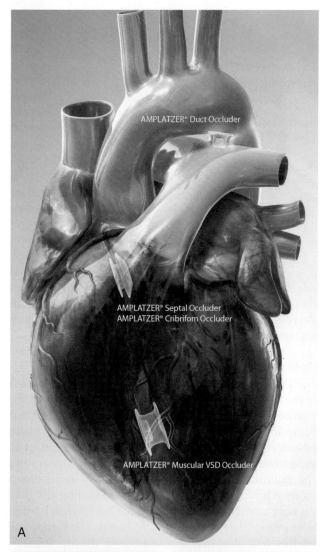

A

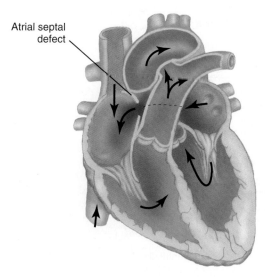

FIGURE 12-6 Atrial septal defect.

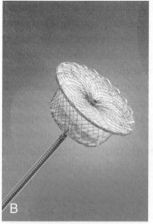

B

AMPLATZER® Duct Occluder
© AGA Medical Corporation

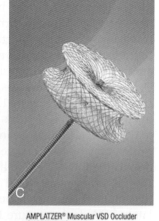

C

AMPLATZER® Muscular VSD Occluder
© AGA Medical Corporation

FIGURE 12-5 Amplatzer devices used with ASD, VSD, and PDA.

Atrial Septal Defect. Atrial septal defect (ASD) is one of the more common congenital heart anomalies (Figure 12-6). The incidence is higher in females than in males. There is an abnormal opening between the right and left atria. Blood that contains oxygen is forced from the left atrium to the right atrium. This type of arteriovenous shunt does not produce cyanosis unless the blood flow is reversed by heart failure. Most children do not have symptoms, but CHF and failure to thrive may be present in those with large openings. Currently, the defect can be repaired either with open heart surgery or percutaneous occluder devices (e.g., the Amplatzer ASD; see Figure 12-5) during cardiac catheterization. Open heart surgery requires the child being placed on the heart-lung machine during the procedure and has all the risks of a surgical procedure. Occluder devices can be used with openings located in certain places along the septum and openings with a small diameter. The occluder devices require shorter hospital stays. The child may require antimicrobial prophylaxis for potential infective endocarditis, and low-dose aspirin or an antiplatelet such as Plavix for clot prevention (Ferri, 2011). Both surgical and nonsurgical procedures have good results.

Ventricular Septal Defect. As the name suggests, in ventricular septal defect (VSD), there is an opening between the right and left ventricles of the heart (Figure 12-7). Increased pressure within the left ventricle forces blood into the right ventricle (left to right shunt). A loud, harsh murmur combined with a systolic tremor is characteristic of this defect. Defects that are moderate to large in size may present with symptoms of CHF. The choice for repair in the past has been surgical intervention, but improvement with percutaneous transcatheter closure has increased usage of this method. Occluder devices (see Figure 12-5) have fewer complications and result in shorter hospital stays. About 75% of small VSDs will close spontaneously by 10 years of age. Routine antimicrobial prophylaxis for dental and surgical procedures is no longer recommended except during the first 6 months postclosure (Ferri, 2011).

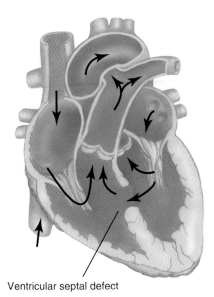

Ventricular septal defect

FIGURE 12-7 Ventricular septal defect.

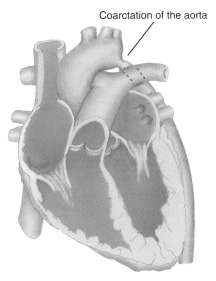

Coarctation of the aorta

FIGURE 12-8 Coarctation of the aorta.

Obstructive Defect

Coarctation of the Aorta. The word *coarctation* means tightening. In this condition, there is a constriction or narrowing of the aortic arch or of the descending aorta (Figure 12-8). Hemodynamic changes consist of increased pressure proximal to the defect with decreased pressure distally. The child may not develop symptoms until later childhood. The child has high blood pressure and bounding pulses in the upper extremities and weak pulses in the cooler lower extremities. Often there are also signs of CHF. Treatment choices for infants and young children can vary from institutions. Balloon angioplasty may be used with infants who are a high surgical risk but has a high rate of recoarctation. Surgical intervention may include resection of the narrowed portion of the aorta and joins its ends. This joining is called an **anastomosis**. If the

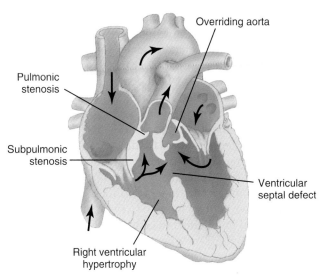

Overriding aorta

Pulmonic stenosis

Subpulmonic stenosis

Ventricular septal defect

Right ventricular hypertrophy

FIGURE 12-9 Tetralogy of Fallot showing the four defects: (1) pulmonary stenosis, (2) VSD, (3) dextroposition of the aorta, and (4) right ventricular hypertrophy.

section removed is large, an end-to-end graft with tubes of Dacron or of similar material may be necessary. Because the graft does not grow and the aorta does, the best time for surgery is between 3 and 6 years of age. There is a high risk for recurrence if the repair is done during infancy. For children who develop a recoarctation, balloon angioplasty (with or without stents) has been used with some success. The prognosis is favorable if there are no other defects. The child will require follow-up every 6 to 12 months to check for recurrence, especially in infants. There can be a risk for developing subacute bacterial endocarditis (SBE) (Parks, 2008).

Defect with Decreased Pulmonary Blood Flow

Tetralogy of Fallot. *Tetra* means four. In tetralogy of Fallot (Figure 12-9), there are four defects: (1) stenosis or narrowing of the pulmonary artery (which decreases blood flow to the lungs), (2) hypertrophy of the right ventricle (enlargement of heart muscle is a result of having to work harder to pump blood through the narrow pulmonary artery), (3) dextroposition (*dextra,* right; position) of the aorta (the aorta is displaced to the right and receives blood from both ventricles), and (4) VSD. This is the most common of the cyanotic heart defects.

When unoxygenated blood enters the aorta, severe heart trouble is evident in the infant. Cyanosis or hypoxemia episodes can present with hyperpnea, irritability, and increasing cyanosis. A "tet spell" (hypoxia) is triggered when there is an acute demand for oxygen such as during a blood draw, defecation, feeding, or crying. Prompt management of these spells include placing the child in a knee-chest position, which will decrease the blood flow to the lower extremities and increase blood flow to the upper body and head. Oxygen may or may not help as the underlying problem is unoxygenated blood being mixed with oxygenated blood and not an oxygenation problem. Morphine is given to stop hyperpnea. Sodium bicarbonate is given for any acidosis. A beta blocker such a propanolol can assist with decreasing the heart rate and oxygen demands.

The older child often rests in a "squatting position" to decrease a hypoxic spell. Squatting reduces the blood flow to the lower extremities and can assist in reducing oxygen demand. Feeding problems, growth retardation, frequent respiratory infections, and severe dyspnea during physical activity are prevalent. There can be clubbing of the fingers and toes. The red blood cells increase (polycythemia [*poly,* many; *cyt,* cells; *hema,* blood]) in an effort to compensate for the lack of oxygen. All children who have cyanosis associated with their heart disease are at risk for neurologic sequelae such as a cerebrovascular accident. Blackouts and convulsions may also occur.

The child or infant is treated medically until corrective surgery can be completed. Open heart surgery is performed for the permanent correction of the defect. Improved surgical procedures allow most defects to be repaired in the first couple of months of life. Palliative procedures may be performed on children who require stabilization before corrective surgery.

Mixed Defect

Transposition of the Great Arteries. In transposition of the great arteries (TGA), the pulmonary artery leaves the left side of the ventricle and the aorta leaves the right ventricle (Figure 12-10). Because the body receives only unoxygenated blood, there must be other defects to maintain life (septal defects, PDA). The condition of the child depends on how much mixing of systemic and pulmonary venous blood is taking place. Infants with large septal defects or a PDA may not be as cyanotic but do develop symptoms of CHF. No murmur

is associated with TGA. If a murmur is present, it is related to the other defects. Prostaglandin E_1 (PGE₁) is given to keep the ductus arteriosus open, and a balloon atrial septostomy may be used as a palliative measure until corrective surgery takes place. Surgery is performed within the first couple of weeks of life and involves switching of the arteries. With the high risk of infective endocarditis, antimicrobial prophylaxis is done for the first 6 months. The mortality rate has greatly improved with corrective surgery. Without surgical intervention, survival is impossible.

Hypoplastic Left Heart Syndrome. With hypoplastic left heart syndrome (HLHS), the left side of the heart is underdeveloped (Figure 12-11). There is hypoplasia of the aorta and left ventricle and mitral valve involvement. Therefore the systemic circulation is provided by the right side of the heart. It is necessary for the ductus arteriosus and the foramen ovale to remain patent to provide oxygenated blood to the body. Prostaglandin E_1 (PGE₁) is administered to maintain a PDA. Without intervention, the infant survives only a few months. Options for treatment include surgical treatment, which is done with a several-staged approach. The Norwood procedure is done in the neonatal period with the Glenn procedure completed at 6 months of age. The Fontan procedure is completed at 18 to 24 months of age. Mortality rates have decreased with improvements in surgical techniques. Transplants have been successful, but there are issues of donor availability, organ rejection, infection, and immunosuppression (Sadowski, 2009).

Treatment and Nursing Care

Nursing goals in the care of children with heart defects include: (1) to reduce the work of the heart, (2) to improve respiration, (3) to maintain proper nutrition, (4) to prevent infection, (5) to reduce the anxiety of the child, (6) to promote normal growth and development, and (7) to support and instruct the parents.

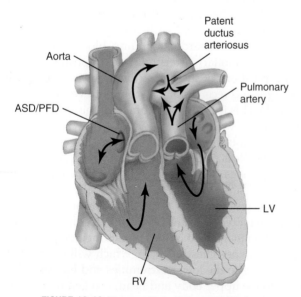

FIGURE 12-10 Transposition of the great arteries.

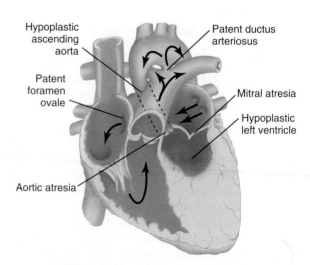

FIGURE 12-11 Hypoplastic left heart syndrome.

Preoperative and postoperative care require an accurate record of intake and output. Signs of dehydration, such as thirst, fever, poor skin turgor, apathy, sunken eyes or fontanel, dry skin, dry tongue, dry mucous membranes, and a decrease in urination, should be brought to the immediate attention of the nurse in charge. Pneumonia can occur rapidly and can present with fever, irritability, and an increase in respiratory distress. The child's position is changed regularly to help prevent respiratory complications. With the increase in numbers of red blood cells circulating within the body (polycythemia), the blood becomes sluggish and prone to clots. When this is accompanied with dehydration, the threat of cerebral thrombosis may become a reality. See Nursing Care Plan 12-1, The Child with Congenital Heart Disease Preoperative, for a general plan of care.

 Nursing Brief

Urine output of 1 to 2 mL/kg/hour is required for adequate output.

Chest tubes may be used after surgery to remove secretions and air from the pleural cavity and to allow reexpansion of the lungs. These are attached to underwater seal drainage bottles or a commercially manufactured disposable system such as Pleur-Evac. Units for infants and older children are available. This system must be *airtight* to prevent collapse of the lung. Drainage containers are always kept below the level of the chest to prevent backflow of secretions. This is especially important during transportation. Emergency equipment should accompany the child with a chest tube at all times. A petrolatum-covered gauze dressing also needs to be available for immediate application over the insertion site when the tubes are removed. This provides an airtight seal over the site.

 Safety Alert

Emergency equipment includes two rubber-shod Kelly clamps for emergency clamping of tubes. Clamps are applied to the tubes as close as possible to the child's chest if a break in the system occurs. Also included is a petrolatum-covered gauze dressing to provide an airtight seal over the site.

 Safety Alert

After cardiac surgery, infants and young children are not picked up under their arms. This can cause damage to the surgical repair sites (e.g., grafts). They should be picked up by placing one hand under their heads and one hand under their hips.

To conserve energy, the nurse must organize care so that the child is not unnecessarily disturbed. A complete bath and linen change should been done after evaluation of the child status. Small frequent feedings are scheduled. The physician may use a higher-calorie formula to maintain adequate intake. An infant is fed in an upright position and burped frequently. The nipple should be soft and the hole large enough for easy sucking. Older children generally tolerate a high-calorie diet with no added salt and a restriction on high-sodium foods. In some cases, nasogastric (NG) tube feedings are advantageous because they are less tiring for the child. Elevating the head may be helpful (Fowler's position) and can facilitate breathing. Oxygen is administered to relieve dyspnea.

Digoxin (Lanoxin) is the most commonly prescribed oral digitalis preparation. Lanoxin is preferred because of its rapid action and shorter half-life. The action of the agent is to slow and strengthen the heartbeat. The nurse counts the apical pulse for **1 full minute** before administering the medication. A resting apical pulse is most accurate. Because the normal pulse ranges vary at different ages, the physician usually indicates at what pulse rate the drug is to be withheld. If this information is not available, it should be clarified with the physician in order to prevent confusion and a possible error. When the drug is withheld, the physician must be notified. A common guideline is to withhold the medication if the pulse is below 90 to 110 beats per minute in infants and below 70 beats per minute in older children. However, the nurse should also be aware of significant changes from the child's previous reading. Tachycardia and irregularities in the rhythm of the pulse are significant and should be reported. Symptoms of toxic effect include nausea, vomiting, anorexia, irregularity in rate and rhythm of the pulse, and a sudden change in pulse.

If the child is discharged while still receiving medication, the parents are taught how to take the pulse and what signs to be alert for when administering the drug (see Home Care Considerations).

 Home Care Considerations

Home Care Administration of Digoxin

Give at regular intervals.

Use an oral syringe to measure medication and not a dropper or spoon.

Check child's pulse and follow physician's directions for when to withhold.

Decrease the risk of hypokalemia by providing adequate potassium in the diet.

Do not repeat dose if child vomits it up.

For missed dose, do not double up on next dose. If missed longer than 4 hours, skip dose and give next scheduled dose.

Report vomiting, poor feeding, and slow heart rate to physician.

⭐ Nursing Care Plan 12-1 | **The Child with Congenital Heart Disease Preoperative**

NURSING DIAGNOSIS *Decreased cardiac output, related to structural defect, myocardial dysfunction, altered hemodynamics*

Goals/Outcome Criteria	Nursing Interventions	Rationales
Child shows adequate cardiac output as evidenced by: • Vital signs within acceptable ranges • Peripheral pulses, strong and equal • Brisk capillary refill within 2 to 3 seconds • Skin warm to touch • Skin color • Adequate urine output • Oxygenation saturation within acceptable range for child • Lack of edema • Activity level within normal limits for defect	Monitor vital signs (heart rate, respiratory rate, blood pressure) every 2 to 4 hours and as needed	Close monitoring allows rapid recognition of altered cardiac output.
	Monitor peripheral pulses including upper and lower extremities.	Monitoring allows recognition of altered cardiac output.
	Place child on a cardiac monitor according to hospital protocol.	Symptoms of impaired cardiac output include tachycardia or bradycardia. Tachycardia is an attempt to maintain adequate cardiac output.
	Monitor capillary refill every 2 to 4 hours and as needed.	Sluggish capillary refill is an indication of impaired tissue perfusion.
	Monitor skin temperature and skin color.	Cool, cold, mottled, or cyanotic skin can be an indicator of poor tissue perfusion.
	Accurate intake and output.	Kidney function is directly related to adequate perfusion. Decrease in urine output indicates inadequate perfusion to the kidneys. 1 to 2 ml/kg/hour indicates adequate urine output.
	Monitor oxygen saturation every 2 to 4 hours or as needed.	Oxygen saturation indicates tissue perfusion.
	Monitor for edema. Daily weight using same scale and approximately at same time.	Assessing for CHF, which can have increased fluid retention resulting in edema, increase in weight, and changes in breathing patterns.
	Assess breath sounds including crackles and rhonchi.	Using same scales at the same time ensures consistency in weight data.
	Offer small, frequent feedings (may use formulas with higher calorie concentration such as 24 to 27 Cal/oz). Infants may require soft, large-hole nipple. Gavage feeding for an infant who tires before consuming recommended amount of feeding or takes longer than 30 minutes to feed.	Feeding requires energy expenditure. Using higher caloric formula decreases amount of formula required and decreases the length of time for feeding. Providing a nipple with a large hole may assist with sucking and decrease energy expenditure. Gavage feeding can decrease energy expenditure and ensure adequate intake.
	Organize nursing interventions to provide maximum rest periods.	Clustering care can decrease fatigue, promote intake, and conserve metabolic demands. Avoid clustering multiple interventions as this can severely fatigue the child.

NURSING DIAGNOSIS *Activity Intolerance, related to fatigue secondary to inadequate cardiac output*

Goals/Outcome Criteria	Nursing Interventions	Rationales
Child will have appropriate activity for age, as evidenced by: • Vital signs within acceptable range. • Ability to perform age-appropriate activities/play appropriate to capabilities	Monitor vital signs every 4 hours or as needed.	Changes in vital signs can indicate inadequate cardiac output resulting in the child's inability to tolerate activity.
	Balance activities and rest.	Promotes balance with energy expenditure.
	Assist with activities of daily living, ambulation, and repositioning as needed.	Prevents fatigue.
	Assist in choosing play activities appropriate for child's energy level.	Provides stimulation for the child while monitoring the child's energy expenditure

⭐ **Nursing Care Plan 12-1** | **The Child with Congenital Heart Disease Preoperative**

NURSING DIAGNOSIS *Ineffective breathing pattern related to pulmonary congestion*

Goals/Outcome Criteria	Nursing Interventions	Rationales
Child will have: • Respiratory rate within normal limits for age and normal respiratory effort • Adequate rest periods • Pink color or maintain baseline cyanosis	Monitor respiratory rate and rhythm. Monitor for presence of retractions, nasal flaring, and/or use of accessory muscles.	Increased pulmonary blood flow to lungs can cause abnormal changes to respiratory rate and effort.
	Position the child with the head of the bed elevated 30 to 45 degrees.	Elevation promotes chest expansion by lowering the diaphragm.
	Administer ordered oxygen as needed	Improves oxygen availability and promotes delivery to tissues. Cautious use is necessary, as oxygen can lower pulmonary vascular resistance, which results in increased pulmonary blood flow and pulmonary congestion.

NURSING DIAGNOSIS *Knowledge deficit about home management, related to inexperience with equipment, medications, and principles of disease management*

Goals/Outcome Criteria	Nursing Interventions	Rationales
Parent and/or child will have adequate knowledge base regarding disease process, treatment, interventions, and home care as evidenced by: • Ability to describe cardiac defect with current and future interventions. • Ability to perform treatments including medication administration. • Asking appropriate questions.	Determine the readiness to learn, anxiety level, and current level of knowledge. Provide factual information in brief sessions, and allow time for parents to develop an understanding of information. Present information at an appropriate level. Encourage family/child to verbalize feelings and concerns in a nonjudgmental environment. Demonstrate skills required for patient care. Observe family/child understanding through return demonstration of skills. Identify community resources for family/child.	Assessment of knowledge level should be considered before development of teaching plan. Effective teaching occurs when information is presented with repetitive explanations. A cardiac defect can be a frightening diagnosis, and providing correct information and allowing the expression of fear and concerns can assist families to cope with the situation. Return demonstrations validate that learning has occurred. Community resources such as support groups can provide additional coping support for the family.

Critical Thinking Snapshot

A 3-week-old is admitted with a diagnosis of tetralogy of Fallot. He is the first child of 20-year-old parents. He is pale with cyanosis, and his skin is cool and clammy. His heart rate is 160 beats per minute, and respirations are 56 breaths per minute. As the nurse, what is your initial assessment of this child? What additional information is essential for your assessment? What are your initial interventions? What should be discussed with the parents?

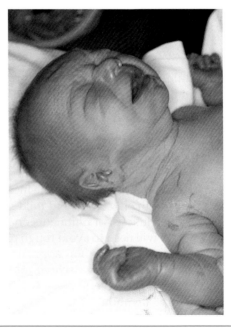

Other mediations that can be prescribed are dopamine, dobutamine, and epinephrine, which increase blood pressure, heart rate, and cardiac output. Amrinone and milrinone help increase cardiac output without increasing heart rate. Common angiotensin-converting enzymes (ACE) inhibitors such as captopril and enalapril assist with vasodilation. Angiotensin II receptor blockers are additional vasodilators that may be used. Blood pressures should be monitored when administering some of these medications.

Diuretics such as furosemide (Lasix) or chlorothiazide (Diuril) are useful in reducing edema. Careful monitoring of serum electrolyte levels can identify electrolyte imbalance, particularly potassium depletion. Hypokalemia can increase digoxin effects, increasing risk for toxicity. The nurse should teach the parents of older children to recognize foods high in potassium, such as bananas, oranges, milk, potatoes, and prune juice. Diapers are weighed to determine urine output. Daily weights of the child also help the physician determine the effectiveness of the diuresis.

Infective endocarditis (IE) is a high risk for children who have a complex cyanotic heart disease or have had surgical intervention to repair heart defects. Organisms attach and grow on the endocardium (inner membrane of the heart) or in areas of turbulent blood flow such as with a VSD. These abnormal growths can break off and attach to other body parts. Symptoms are usually nonspecific but include fever, fatigue, headache, nausea, and vomiting. The effective organism is identified with blood cultures, and this determines the antimicrobial treatment.

Nursing Brief

Nurses working in a cardiac unit should be alert for emergencies such as cardiac and respiratory arrest and should be competent in cardiopulmonary resuscitation techniques and the necessary modifications required for children.

When the child is discharged, the family will need to be comfortable in providing home care. They will need to understand medication administration (see Home Care Considerations) and schedules. If the child has an incision, home care instructions are clarified. In a car seat, a small blanket should be placed over site to prevent straps from rubbing. Cover the incision with a bib or dressing during feeding. The incision site should be cleaned with only water and mild soap. Do not use oils, creams, lotions, or ointments on the incision. An older child will need to avoid rough play, bike riding, or strenuous activities for approximately 6 weeks. The child may return to school after a few weeks. Parents should be able to identify symptoms that require medical attention.

The parents of the child need support and understanding over a long period of time. Parental fears and dependencies come to the surface when an infant is born with a defect. Because the heart is the body's most vital organ, this type of diagnosis causes a great deal of apprehension and anxiety. The physician has to reassure the parents without minimizing the danger involved. If the condition permits, the infant is sent home under medical supervision until the preferred age for surgery. Every effort must be made by the family to provide a normal environment that is within the child's limits. It is easy for parents to become overpermissive because they do not wish the child to become unnecessarily excited. The child senses this and soon gains control of the home. Using limit setting, such as 5 minutes of chair time, if done with consistency, can be beneficial in behavior control.

The patterns formed during infancy can build the framework of a healthy personality for the child. The child with a heart condition who is well integrated into family life has a definite advantage over the child who is made to think he or she is an invalid. Routine naps and early bedtime provide adequate rest for most children. As these children grow, they usually set their own limits on the amount of activity they can handle. Substitutions can be made for strenuous activities, such as bicycle riding, and for rigorous competitive games. The child receives the usual childhood immunizations. Prompt treatment of infections is important. A suitable diet with adequate fluids is necessary, and iron-rich foods are encouraged. Dental care should also be regular. All-day attendance in school may be too tiring for the child, so special provisions in this area may be necessary. The child additionally needs careful evaluation before any type of minor surgery, such as a tonsillectomy.

Some children need hospitalization occasionally for various tests or problems. Simple explanations must be given to children regarding this condition. Whenever possible they should be allowed to handle and to see hospital equipment before its use. Cardiac surgery is generally performed at a medical center with a pediatric cardiac surgery department. Consistent nursing care throughout hospitalization is desirable for both the physical and the psychological welfare of the child. The parents may be referred to a social worker who assists them in seeking needed services and financial assistance. The financial burden on the parents for years of medical and surgical necessities is phenomenal. All avenues for financial aid should be explored by qualified personnel.

ACUTE RHEUMATIC FEVER

Acute rheumatic fever is a systemic disease that involves the joints, heart, central nervous system

(CNS), skin, and subcutaneous tissues. It follows an infection with certain strains of group A β-hemolytic streptococci (GABHS). While the condition is uncommon in the United States, there have been some outbreaks. Its peak incidence rate occurs between 5 and 15 years of age (Steer et al., 2009). Rheumatic fever has a high family incidence and is more common worldwide in lower-income groups and in persons living in overcrowded conditions. It is more prevalent in fall, winter, and spring because carrier rates among schoolchildren are believed to increase during these seasons. Genetic factors also have been implicated. The incidence of rheumatic fever fell dramatically with the widespread use of antimicrobials in the 1960s and 1970s. The disease remains a concern, however, because of its potential to cause permanent cardiac problems.

Rheumatic fever is considered an autoimmune inflammatory response of connective tissue to untreated GABHS. Rheumatic fever typically follows an upper respiratory tract infection (tonsillitis, pharyngitis). Throat cultures done at the time of diagnosis of rheumatic fever are not always positive for streptococci because there is a latent period of 1 to 3 weeks between the streptococcal infection and the onset of rheumatic fever. It is thought that during this period the body becomes sensitized to the organism and develops an immune response to it. This immune response affects the particular body tissues described previously. The disease is self-limiting.

Signs and Symptoms

Symptoms range from mild to severe and may not occur for several weeks after a streptococcal infection. The classic symptoms are outlined in Table 12-1. The diagnosis of rheumatic fever is difficult, and for this reason, the revised Jones criteria have been developed and modified over the years (Figure 12-12). The presence of two major criteria, or of one major and two minor criteria, along with evidence of recent streptococcal infection, indicates a high probability of rheumatic fever. The diagnosis of Sydenham chorea or carditis without any other known cause is sufficient to suggest rheumatic fever (Steer et al., 2009). Abdominal pain, often mistaken for appendicitis, sometimes occurs. Fever varies from slight to very high. Pallor, fatigue, anorexia, and unexplained nosebleeds may be seen.

A careful history and physical examination are done. Certain blood tests are helpful to confirm diagnosis. The erythrocyte sedimentation rate (ESR) is elevated. Abnormal proteins, such as C-reactive protein (CRP), may also be evident in the serum. Leukocytosis may occur but is not regularly present.

Culture demonstration of streptococcal infection may not be possible. Therefore, antibodies against the streptococci (measured with antistreptolysin-O titer) can confirm recent streptococcal infection. Additional studies may include chest radiography.

The electrocardiogram (ECG) is useful. Changes in conductivity, particularly a prolonged P-R interval

Table **12-1**	Symptoms of Acute Rheumatic Fever
SYMPTOMS	**DESCRIPTION**
Carditis	Involves the myocardium (heart muscle), the pericardium, and endocardium, but particularly the *mitral valve*, located between the left atrium and left ventricle. Inflammation causes dysfunction of the valve initially; later, scarring leads to mitral stenosis. Myocardial lesions called *Aschoff bodies* are also characteristic of the disease. Murmurs can be heard, and ECG alterations are present. The burden on the heart is great because it has to pump harder to circulate the blood. As a result, it may become enlarged and fail.
Polyarthritis	Painful, tender, warm, red, and swollen joints, especially the knees, elbows, ankles, wrists, and shoulders. Symptoms in one joint may disappear, only to appear in another joint (migratory arthritis). This pattern may continue for a few weeks without treatment with antiinflammatory medications. There is no permanent joint damage.
Erythema marginatum	Small red circles and wavy lines on the trunk and extremities that appear and disappear rapidly. The rash may come and go for several months.
Sydenham chorea	Characterized by involuntary, purposeless movements of the muscles. Begins as clumsiness, which is often noted by teachers. The child may stumble and spill things and may have difficulty buttoning clothes and writing. When the facial muscles are involved, grimacing occurs. The child may laugh and cry inappropriately. In severe cases, the child may become completely incapacitated and deterioration in speech may be noticeable. Symptoms decrease when the child is at rest. Chorea is self-limiting, and full recovery is expected. It can last as little as 2 weeks or more than a year.
Subcutaneous nodules	Hard, painless swellings that occur most frequently over bony prominences (scalp, spine, joints).

ECG, Electrocardiogram.

MAJOR CRITERIA   MINOR CRITERIA

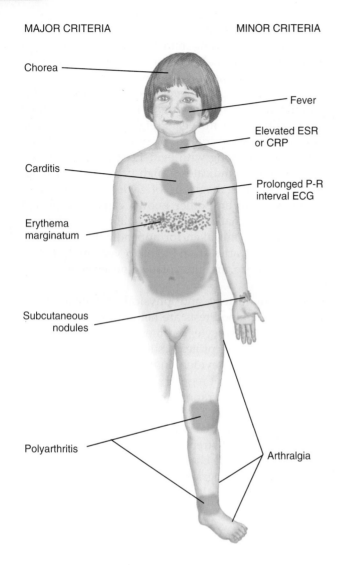

FIGURE 12-12 Major and minor criteria for the diagnosis of acute rheumatic fever.

(first-degree heart block), may indicate carditis. Tests are repeated throughout the course of the disease so that the doctor may determine when the active stage has subsided. Rheumatic fever has a tendency to recur, and each attack carries the threat of further damage to the heart. The recurrences are most frequent during the first 5 years after the initial attack and decline rapidly thereafter.

Treatment and Nursing Care

Treatment is aimed at preventing permanent damage to the heart, relieving uncomfortable symptoms, and preventing recurrence of rheumatic fever. All children should be treated for streptococcal infection at diagnosis. Two methods of control involve primary and secondary prophylaxis.

Primary prophylaxis, a single injection of benzathine penicillin G (Bicillin), is followed by secondary prophylaxis. Intramuscular penicillin benzathine G,

given as an intramuscular injection every 4 weeks, is the drug of choice to prevent recurrence for children with a history of rheumatic fever or evidence of rheumatic heart disease (Steer et al., 2009). Oral penicillin does not have the same reliability but may be considered for children with minimal involvement whose reliability about medications can be ascertained. The duration of therapy varies from 10 years to the lifetime of the child, depending on individual and environmental factors. Sulfadiazine is recommended for long-term therapy for children who cannot tolerate penicillin. A vaccine against group A streptococcal (GAS) infection is being evaluated but is still years away.

🏥 Nursing Brief

Benzathine penicillin G should be given in a large muscle mass. It can be painful and should be warmed to room temperature before administration.

Anti-inflammatory drugs (salicylates or nonsteroidal anti-inflammatory drugs [NSAIDs]) are used to decrease pain and inflammation. Aspirin is the drug of choice for joint disease but should be withheld until the diagnosis has been confirmed because it can mask the migratory nature of the arthritis (Kliegman et al., 2007). The use of steroids is controversial and is reserved for individuals with severe carditis and CHF. Important concerns during therapy include aspirin toxicity and the effect of aspirin therapy on clotting time. More severe reactions such as gastric ulcer, hypertension, overwhelming infection, and psychic disturbances require monitoring.

Chorea is self-limiting, and maintaining a calm environment to decrease overstimulation can be helpful. Medications that may be used are diazepam or haloperidol. Seizure precautions may be necessary. Chorea movements are aggravated by anxiety; therefore the nurse should suggest activities that do not require fine-motor coordination of the hands, thus avoiding frustration. Good communication with school personnel when the child returns to school increases understanding of the child's behavior.

Home Care. Bed rest during the initial attack is not necessary but is recommended if carditis is present. Because most children with rheumatic fever are treated at home, the nurse needs to verify that the parent and child understand any prescribed activity limitations. The child will benefit from access to quiet games and other interesting activities during the acute phase. Suggested passive diversions include an aquarium, growing plants of various types, stories, and quiet music. As the condition improves, part of the time may be taken up with simple self-care tasks. Hobbies such as needlework or stamp collecting are interesting and fun to start. Most children resume moderate activity shortly after the febrile phase.

 Nursing Brief

Nurses need to become skilled at providing quiet activities for the child who is ill. Provisions must be made for the child to carry out school work as the condition permits. If a long period of convalescence is indicated, a tutor is needed unless closed-circuit television or a school-to-home telephone is available.

When painful joints are involved, care should be given to support these joints with the hands when moving the child. Care includes special attention to the skin, especially over bony prominences. The child with anorexia may benefit from being offered small amounts of nutritious food. Providing ethnic food should be considered for a child who is does not normally eat hospital food. Parents should be encouraged to bring favorite foods high in protein for healing.

The child with rheumatic fever is susceptible to sub-acute bacterial endocarditis, which can occur as a complication of dental or other invasive procedures likely to cause bleeding or infection. High-dose antimicrobial prophylaxis is indicated if the child is to undergo dental procedures or surgery, regardless of whether the child is receiving prophylaxis for prevention of recurrent rheumatic fever.

Preparation of the child and family for long-term antimicrobial compliance is extremely important.

Recurrent infections can cause damage to the heart, and nurses should emphasize the importance of infection prevention. Financial assistance is available to children on long-term chemoprophylaxis. Local heart associations and disabled children's services, as well as state and municipal health departments, are among the sources of such aid.

Any disease that has the potential to permanently affect the heart produces anxiety in the child and parents. Keeping the parents informed about the child's condition helps them to cope by relieving anxiety.

Prevention

The nurse is involved in prevention of rheumatic fever in the community by recognizing signs and symptoms of streptococcal infections, doing screening, and referring for treatment. Any child with symptoms who has been exposed to another person with a streptococcal infection needs investigation. Examination of family contacts is also important. Throat cultures are necessary in determining whether the organism is GABHS. The use of rapid antigen detection testing (RADT) has assisted physicians in detecting the organism quickly. There are reports of false-positive results in children, so if a child has a negative RADT, a throat culture is done to confirm the results. Once a diagnosis is established, the nurse stresses the importance of completing antimicrobial therapy; parents sometimes neglect this once the child's symptoms disappear. The absence of acute signs and symptoms may inaccurately be associated with eradication of the organism.

Get Ready for the NCLEX® Examination!

Key Points

- The cardiovascular system is the first system to function in the fetus.
- Cardiac defects are categorized by pathophysiology and hemodynamics: increased pulmonary blood flow, decreased pulmonary blood flow, obstructive blood flow from ventricles, and mixed blood flow.
- Symptoms of decreased cardiac output include diminished pulses, poor color, prolonged capillary refill, and decreased urine output.
- Cardiac catheterization provides information regarding anatomy, hemodynamics, and pressures.
- Congenital heart disease can lead to the development of CHF.
- Signs of CHF include tachypnea, tachycardia, pallor or cyanosis, nasal flaring, grunting, retractions, cough, crackles, periorbital and facial edema, and hepatomegaly.
- Improvements with interventions completed during cardiac catheterization and surgical procedures have improved the life expectancy of children with CHD.
- Endocarditis is an infection that can occur with cardiac disease.
- Rheumatic fever is an autoimmune disease that occurs after a GABHS infection. The primary goal of treatment is to prevent cardiac complications, such as problems with the mitral valve.

Additional Learning Resources

evolve Go to your Evolve website (*http://evolve.elsevier.com/Price/ pediatric/*) for the following FREE learning resources:
- 3-D Animations
- Answer Keys
- Appendixes
- Audio Glossary
- Spanish/English Glossary
- Video Clips

Review Questions for the NCLEX® Examination

1. Environmental factors that can increase the risk of congenital heart disease in children are: (**Select all that apply.**)
   1. Down syndrome
   2. Maternal use of Accutane
   3. Maternal cocaine use
   4. Family history
   5. Advanced maternal age

2. When reviewing the blood test results of a child with congenital heart disease (CHD), the nurse notices an increase in the number of red blood cells (polycythemia). When there is an increase in the number of red blood cells, the:
   1. Hematocrit will also be elevated
   2. Hematocrit will be decreased
   3. White blood cell count will also be increased
   4. Platelet count will be decreased

3. All of the following are true regarding patent ductus arteriosus (PDA) **except:**
   1. A machine-like murmur may be heard
   2. Symptoms are readily apparent at birth
   3. It occurs more frequently in females
   4. Oxygenated blood recycles through the lungs

4. A child is experiencing a "tet spell" secondary to tetralogy of Fallot. What intervention would the nurse expect to implement to stop hyperpnea?
   1. Administer sodium bicarbonate as ordered
   2. Administer oxygen
   3. Assist child into high Fowler's position
   4. Administer morphine as ordered

5. Chest tube drainage containers are always kept:
   1. Below the level of the chest
   2. Above the level of the chest
   3. At the level of the chest
   4. Either below or above the level of the chest

Neurologic and Sensory Disorders

Objectives

1. Define the vocabulary terms listed
2. List the differences found in the neurologic system of a child
3. Describe the signs of increased intracranial pressure in a child with a head injury, including nursing observations necessary to establish a baseline of information
4. Discuss care of the child with intracranial hemorrhage
5. Discuss use of the pediatric coma scale
6. Differentiate between communicating and noncommunicating hydrocephalus
7. Outline the pre- and postoperative nursing care of a neonate with spina bifida cystica
8. Explain how to care for a child with bacterial meningitis or viral encephalitis
9. Differentiate the types of generalized and partial seizures
10. Describe the nursing measures necessary for a child during and after a tonic-clonic seizure
11. Discuss care of the near-drowning victim
12. Differentiate two types of hearing loss
13. Differentiate amblyopia and strabismus

Key Terms

audiometry (ăw-dē-ŎM-ĕ-trē; p. 260)
aura (OR-ĕ; p. 256)
choroid plexus (KŌR-oid PLĔK-sŭs; p. 248)
cover test (p. 262)
habilitation (hă-BĬL-ĭ-TĀ-shŭn; p. 251)
idiopathic (i-dē-e-PA-thik; p. 254)
ketogenic diet (KĒ-tō-JĔN-ĭk; p. 257)
multifactorial (MŬL-tĭ-făk-TŌ-rē-ăl; p. 250)
myelinization (MĪ-e-len-e-zā-shŭn ; p. 243)
neural tube defects (NTDs) (NUR-el; p. 250)
occlusion (e-KLU-zhen; p. 262)
opisthotonic (ō-pĭs-THŎT-ō-nĭc; p. 244)

ototoxic (ō-te-TAK-sik; p. 259)
petechiae (pē-TĒ-kē-ī; p. 252)
postictal (pōst-ĬK-tăl; p. 256)
shunt (p. 248)
syndrome of inappropriate antidiuretic hormone (SIADH) (p. 253)
TORCH (p. 247)
transillumination (TRĂNS-ĭ-LŪ-mĭ-NĀ-shŭn; p. 248)
tympanography (TĬM-păh-nŏ-gră-fē; p. 260)
uncover test (p. 262)
vesicostomy (VES-i-kos-te-mē; p. 251)

THE NERVOUS SYSTEM

The nervous system is made up of the central nervous system (CNS), which is composed of the cerebrum, cerebellum, brainstem, and spinal cord; the peripheral nervous system, which is composed of the cranial nerves and spinal nerves; and the autonomic nervous system, which is composed of the sympathetic and parasympathetic systems. The focus of this chapter is primarily on the CNS and the disorders that occur in childhood.

The cerebellum is the center for consciousness, thought, memory, sensory input, and motor activity. The cerebellum coordinates all muscle movement including walking, talking, and balance. All cranial nerves (except 1) arise from the brainstem and control vital centers.

The nervous system grows rapidly before birth and well into the first year of life. It will slow to a more gradual rate in later childhood. Brain growth is measured with head circumference and plotted during the first 3 years of life. There is an increased cerebral blood flow and oxygen consumption in childhood that is almost twice that of adults (Hockenberry and Wilson, 2007). This is due to the increased metabolic requirement in early childhood. Myelinization of the nerves in the CNS progresses in a head-to-toe (cephalocaudal) and proximodistal sequence. This myelinization and maturation of the nervous system will lead to the development of motor skills in the growth and development process. Brain development will be influenced by environmental stimuli. Box 13-1 reviews additional physical differences.

| Box **13-1** | Pediatric Neurologic Differences |

- Cranium around the brain is not fully fused; this allows for brain growth.
- Anterior and posterior fontanels do not close until 12 to 18 months of age, and 2 months of age, respectively.
- The cranium bones are not fully developed until 12 years of age.
- Head growth is rapid during the first year; by the end of the first year, the brain has increased in weight about 2½ times.
- Myelination is generally completed within the first 2 years.
- Primitive reflexes are present at birth (see Chapter 5).

NEUROLOGIC DISORDERS

INCREASED INTRACRANIAL PRESSURE

The brain, CSF, and blood occupy space within the cranium. A change in volume of any of these components must be compensated for. However, if the capacity increases to the point where compensation cannot occur any longer, there will be a rapid increase in **intracranial pressure (ICP)**. Early signs and symptoms of increased ICP may be subtle; these signs and symptoms become more pronounced as the level of consciousness deteriorates. It is important to remember that as ICP increases, cerebral perfusion decreases or is at least compromised. A decrease in cerebral perfusion causes less oxygen to be delivered to the brain cells. Without oxygen, a cell dies, and brain cells do not replace themselves as other cells may do. Discussion of ICP will continue throughout this chapter.

INTRACRANIAL HEMORRHAGE

Intracranial hemorrhage, a common birth injury, may result from trauma or anoxia. It occurs more frequently in the preterm infant, in whom the blood vessels are fragile. Blood vessels within the skull are broken, and bleeding occurs into the brain. When the diagnosis is made, the specific location of the hemorrhage should be noted: subdural or subarachnoid, epidural or intraventricular (IVH is discussed in Chapter 5). This injury may also occur during precipitated delivery, prolonged labor, or when the newborn's head is large in comparison with the mother's pelvis.

Signs and Symptoms

The symptoms of intracranial hemorrhage may occur suddenly or gradually. Some or all may be present, depending on the severity. They include inability to move normally, lethargy, poor sucking reflex, irregular respirations, cyanosis, twitching, forceful vomiting, a high-pitched shrill cry, and convulsions. Opisthotonic (*opistho*, backward; *tonos*, tension) posturing may be observed. The fontanel may be tense and under pressure, rather than soft and compressible. The pupil of one eye is apt to be small and the other large. If the symptoms are mild, there is a good chance of complete recovery in most cases. Death results if there is a massive hemorrhage. The infant who survives an extensive hemorrhage may have residual defects such as mental retardation or cerebral palsy. The diagnosis is established by the history of the delivery, CT, MRI, evidence of an increase in CSF pressure, and the symptoms and course of the disease.

Treatment and Nursing Care

The newborn is placed in an isolette, which allows proper temperature control, ease in administering oxygen, and continuous observation. The baby is handled gently and as little as possible. The head is elevated. The doctor may prescribe medication to control bleeding and anticonvulsants if convulsions are apparent. The baby is fed carefully because the sucking reflex may be affected. The infant vomits easily. The nurse observes the baby for signs of increased ICP and convulsions. The nurse also assists the physician with such procedures as lumbar punctures and aspiration of subdural hemorrhage.

If a convulsion occurs, the nurse's observation of its character aids the physician in determining the exact location of the bleeding. The following observations are of particular importance: Were the arms, legs, or face involved? Was the right or left side of the body involved? Was the convulsion mild or severe? How long did it last? What was the condition of the infant before and after the seizure? The nurse records observations in the nurses' notes.

HEAD INJURIES

Infants and children suffer from head injuries that may occasionally result in brain damage. Falls, shaken baby syndrome, motor vehicle injuries, and bicycle injuries account for a large number of these statistics. Toddlers especially are famous for the number of blows received to the head. Fortunately, most of these injuries are not serious, but they are alarming to parents. The skulls of infants and young toddlers are more pliable and absorb much of the impact to the head. By 2 years of age, both fontanels have completely closed, and the cranium no longer has the same pliability in response to force. Types of head injuries are discussed in Table 13-1.

Complications

The major complications of head injury are hemorrhage, infections, cerebral edema (swelling of the brain), and compression of the brainstem. The brain and its interrelated compartments are tightly confined by the skull, more so after closure of the fontanels. Enlargement of any intracranial component (brain or subarachnoid, venous, or arterial space) can produce

| Table **13-1** | Types of Head Injuries | | | | |

	SKULL AND SCALP INJURIES	FRACTURES	CONCUSSIONS	CONTUSIONS	HEMATOMAS
Etiology	Falls, blunt trauma, penetrating	Falls, blunt trauma	Blunt trauma	Blunt trauma	Falls, motor vehicle accidents
Manifestations	Lacerations, bleeding, hematoma	Linear: thin, clear line usually with no symptoms; suspect child abuse Depressed: indentation of skull; may have fragments in brain tissue Basilar: fracture at base of skull; symptoms include hemorrhage of nose, nasal pharynx, middle ear, over mastoid bone (Battle sign), and around eyes (raccoon eyes)	Alterations in mental status, with or without loss of consciousness, headache, nausea, vomiting, dizziness, irritability, seizures, retrograde amnesia (of events up to and including the injury)	Bruising or tearing of the brain, usually temporal or frontal sites; focal symptoms depending on area of injury; altered LOC, from confusion and disorientation to obtunded; focal seizures	Lacerations of arteries or veins in the brain; momentary unconsciousness Epidural: usually arterial, may be fatal; sleepiness, headache, bulging fontanel, paresthesias, papilledema, fixed pupils, increased ICP Subdural: usually venous; change in LOC
Treatment	Usually observation at home	Observation, supportive, or surgical intervention	Observation, supportive, and usually at home unless unconscious for more than 5 minutes or if there is amnesia of event	Observation and supportive	Observation or surgical intervention with evacuation of hematoma

ICP, Intracranial pressure; *LOC,* level of consciousness.

increased ICP, which can lead to permanent brain damage or death.

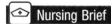

Nursing Brief

Shaken baby syndrome can result in increased ICP. The shearing force that results from brain movement as the baby is vigorously shaken may tear small arteries and cause cerebral edema. Always be alert for signs of ICP in children with the possibility of this diagnosis.

Treatment and Nursing Care

Frequently a child who has had a blow to the head is brought to the hospital for observation to rule out or confirm the diagnosis. Initial care of the child with a head injury includes assessment of the ABCs (airway, breathing, circulation), assessment for spinal cord injury, and documentation of baseline vital signs. The child may have all or some of the following symptoms: headache (manifested by fussiness in the toddler), drowsiness, blurred vision, vomiting, and dyspnea (see Did You Know?). In severe cases, the child may be completely unconscious or having seizures. **Decerebrate** (indicating injury to the midbrain) or **decorticate** (indicating injury to the cerebral cortex) **posturing** may be evident (Figure 13-1). A careful history is obtained to determine any preexisting conditions and to ascertain the exact circumstances of the accident. Of particular importance is the child's state of consciousness immediately after the occurrence. Radiography, CT, and magnetic resonance imaging (MRI) can be used to diagnose the specific head injury. Should the child be alert, without significant symptoms, and the parents reliable, the child can be sent home with instructions for observation.

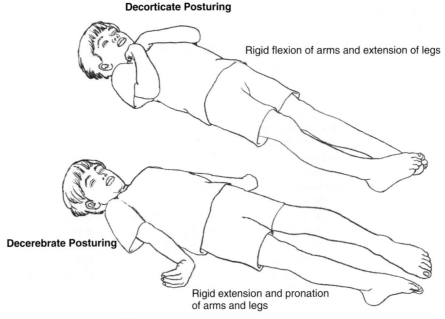

Decorticate Posturing

Rigid flexion of arms and extension of legs

Decerebrate Posturing

Rigid extension and pronation of arms and legs

FIGURE 13-1 Decorticate and decerebrate posturing.

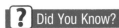 **Did You Know?**

For the Child with Increasing ICP

- Behavior changes; older child may have disorientation
- Restlessness, fussiness; older child may have headache
- Dizziness, ataxia
- Increasing systolic blood pressure; widening pulse pressure
- Changes in respiratory pattern, decreasing pulse
- Several episodes of vomiting
- Pallor
- Listlessness, followed by increasing difficulty in arousing
- Changes in pupil size and reactions to light
- Seizures

 Home Care Considerations

Guidelines for a Child with a Minor Head Injury

Monitor the child, and alert the physician if the child exhibits any of the following:
- Severe headache or vomiting
- Blurred or double vision
- Unequal pupils
- Slurred speech
- Watery fluid from the nose or ears
- Gait problems or unusual weakness in extremities
- Any seizure activity
- Will not awaken from sleep
- Becomes confused or is acting unusual
- Any other symptoms that are worrisome

Further assessment includes the level of consciousness (LOC); changes are particularly meaningful and require immediate medical attention. Changes in behavior can be an *early* sign of increasing ICP.

Response should be correlated with the developmental age of the child. Parents can be helpful in providing information about the child's usual capabilities. In general, the child should be oriented to person, time, and place (may not be accessible in the toddler). Ask "What is your name?" and "Where are you?" Older children may know the day of the week. The child should recognize the parents. Point to the mother and ask "Who is this?" If there is no response to verbal stimuli, note the arousal to tactile stimulation. Determine the presence or absence of crying or speech. It is not unusual for the child to fall asleep, but he or she should be easily aroused. Record changes in sleeping pattern, posture, movements of extremities, and any signs of tremors or restlessness.

The Pediatric Coma Scale (Figure 13-2), based on the adult Glasgow Coma Scale, is valuable in determining various LOCs. It consists of three parts: eye opening, motor response, and verbal response. A numerical value is assigned to each part. The lower the score, the deeper the coma.

Evaluation of pupil and eye movement requires documentation of size, shape, and equality of pupils and their reaction to light and extraocular movements. (Have the child follow your finger from side to side and up and down to detect movement.) Strabismus, nystagmus, "sunset" eyes (eyes deviated downward), and inability to move eyes in all four quadrants indicate abnormality. If ICP is increasing, pupils become sluggish to light stimulus, dilated, and eventually fixed; this is an indication of a medical emergency.

Advanced ICP causes an increase in systolic blood pressure with a widening **pulse pressure** (the diastolic blood pressure usually decreases), a decrease in pulse,

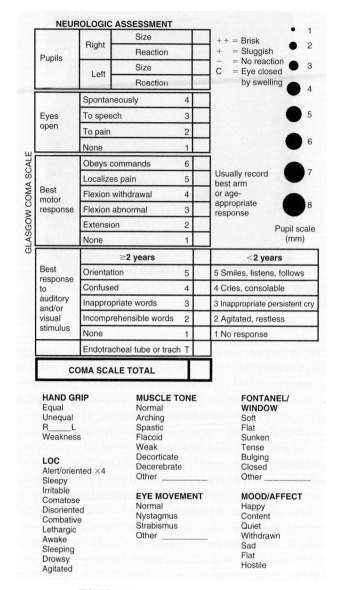

FIGURE 13-2 The Pediatric Coma Scale.

The table within the figure:

NEUROLOGIC ASSESSMENT

Pupils	Right	Size	
		Reaction	
	Left	Size	
		Reaction	

++ = Brisk
+ = Sluggish
− = No reaction
C = Eye closed by swelling

Pupil scale (mm): 1 2 3 4 5 6 7 8

GLASGOW COMA SCALE

Eyes open	Spontaneously	4
	To speech	3
	To pain	2
	None	1

Best motor response	Obeys commands	6
	Localizes pain	5
	Flexion withdrawal	4
	Flexion abnormal	3
	Extension	2
	None	1

Usually record best arm or age-appropriate response

Best response to auditory and/or visual stimulus	≥2 years		<2 years
	Orientation	5	5 Smiles, listens, follows
	Confused	4	4 Cries, consolable
	Inappropriate words	3	3 Inappropriate persistent cry
	Incomprehensible words	2	2 Agitated, restless
	None	1	1 No response
	Endotracheal tube or trach	T	

COMA SCALE TOTAL

HAND GRIP
Equal
Unequal
R____L
Weakness

LOC
Alert/oriented ×4
Sleepy
Irritable
Comatose
Disoriented
Combative
Lethargic
Awake
Sleeping
Drowsy
Agitated

MUSCLE TONE
Normal
Arching
Spastic
Flaccid
Weak
Decorticate
Decerebrate
Other _____

EYE MOVEMENT
Normal
Nystagmus
Strabismus
Other _____

FONTANEL/WINDOW
Soft
Flat
Sunken
Tense
Bulging
Closed
Other _____

MOOD/AFFECT
Happy
Content
Quiet
Withdrawn
Sad
Flat
Hostile

and altered respiratory pattern. This is referred to as the **Cushing triad.** Temperature is routinely monitored. Never take oral temperatures in children prone to seizures. Elevations may result from inflammation, systemic infection, or damage to the hypothalamus, which regulates body temperature. Body temperature may be reduced by administering antipyretics or by using a hypothermia blanket. Mild elevations in temperature are not uncommon in the first 2 days after trauma. Any seizure activity is treated with anticonvulsants.

The quality and strength of muscle tone should be observed in all four extremities. The child should be able to squeeze the nurse's hands. The grip should be equal in both hands. The child should be able to move the legs and push against the examiner's hands with both feet. The face should be symmetrical, and the child should be able to smile and frown. Drooping

of the eyes, ptosis, inability to close the eyes tightly, and drooping of the corner of the mouth are considered adverse signs. The child should be able to raise the arms and turn the palms up and down. Abnormal posturing should be described and recorded.

Record the type and amount of any drainage from the ears and nose. Leakage of cerebrospinal fluid from a fractured skull is seen as clear drainage from the ears or nose. Head circumference (FOC) should be monitored in infants, as should tension of the fontanels and the presence of a high-pitched cry.

Fluids are carefully monitored to control cerebral edema. Overhydration increases the amount of cerebral fluid. Feeding difficulties should be noted as the child's diet is increased. Children should be observed for signs of shock, which can also occur.

Children whose conditions have remained stable are discharged. Parents are instructed about any additional observations and follow-up care.

It is important to teach parents about preventing head injury. Teach parents of infants *never* to leave the child unattended on a changing table or bed. Childproofing the home with stairway gates decreases falls. Teaching the toddler and preschooler not to run out in the street is an important safety measure. As the child becomes older and more active, a helmet should be worn during activities that provide risk, such as biking, rollerblading, and contact sports.

HYDROCEPHALUS

Hydrocephalus (*hydro,* water; *cephalo,* head) is a condition characterized by an increase in cerebrospinal fluid (CSF) in the ventricles of the brain, which causes an increase in the size of the head and pressure changes in the brain. It occurs as a result of an imbalance between production and absorption of CSF. Hydrocephalus may be congenital or acquired. It may occur in conjunction with a meningomyelocele or as a sequela of infections, including congenital TORCH infections (TORCH stands for **t**oxoplasmosis, **o**ther, **r**ubella, **c**ytomegalovirus, and **h**erpes simplex), encephalitis, or meningitis, or because of perinatal hemorrhage. The symptoms depend on the site of obstruction and the age at which it develops. Although there are many causes of hydrocephalus, all result in either an impairment of CSF absorption within the subarachnoid space (communicating hydrocephalus) or an obstruction of CSF flow within the ventricles (noncommunicating hydrocephalus). Hydrocephalus may proceed slowly or rapidly. Two forms of hydrocephalus are the *Arnold-Chiari malformation* and the *Dandy-Walker syndrome.* Because hydrocephalus can cause progressive cerebral damage, early recognition and treatment are important.

It should be recalled that the brain and spinal cord are surrounded by fluid, membranes, and bone. The three membranes, called **meninges,** are the dura mater,

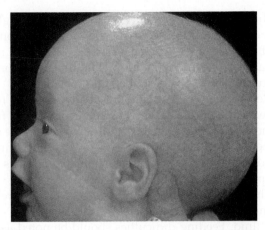

FIGURE 13-3 The head of an infant with hydrocephalus is larger than normal.

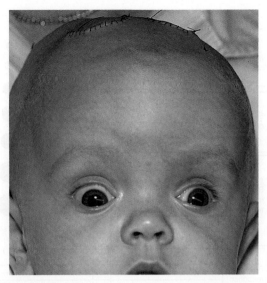

FIGURE 13-4 Marked hydrocephalus with "setting sun" sign and divergence of the eyes.

the arachnoid, and the pia mater. The arachnoid mater (also known as the middle membrane) resembles a cobweb, and its spaces are filled with fluid. CSF is also found in spaces of the brain called **ventricles.** The primary site of formation for CSF is believed to be the choroid plexus.

Signs and Symptoms

Signs and symptoms depend on the time of onset and the severity of the imbalance. The classic sign both in congenital hydrocephalus and in hydrocephalus with onset in infancy is an increase in head size (Figure 13-3). The direction of skull expansion depends on the site of obstruction. Transillumination (*trans,* across; *illuminare,* to enlighten), or the inspection of a cavity or organ by passing a light through its walls, is an older diagnostic procedure used to visualize fluid. (This method uses a flashlight with a sponge rubber collar held tightly against the infant's head in a dark room to indicate areas of increased luminosity.) Another sign is a bulging anterior fontanel and separation of cranial sutures. The scalp is also shiny and the veins dilated. The infant appears helpless and lethargic. The body becomes thin, and the muscle tone of the extremities is often poor. In addition to the infant's shrill and high-pitched cry, irritability, vomiting, and anorexia are present. Convulsions may also occur. In severe infantile hydrocephalus, the eyes may appear deviated downward, which is known as the "setting sun" sign (Figure 13-4). Children with an onset of hydrocephalus later in childhood may have minimal enlargement of the head and display the signs and symptoms of increased ICP.

Diagnosis and Treatment

The child's head is measured daily. Echoencephalography, computed tomography (CT), or magnetic resonance imaging (MRI) is most frequently used to show

the enlarged ventricles and to locate the level of obstruction. Sedation is required. A ventricular tap or puncture may be performed in a special procedures room with sterile technique. The equipment needed is the same as that for a lumbar puncture. The specimen is labeled and sent to the laboratory for analysis.

Treatment is directed toward relief of symptoms, treatment of the underlying problem (such as a tumor), and treatment of complications. If there is an obstruction, such as a tumor, it may be removed surgically. In other conditions, a shunt is placed by inserting special tubing that provides drainage of the CFS from the ventricles to another area of the body, where it is absorbed and eventually excreted. Two types of shunts are used: the ventriculoperitoneal (VP) shunt and the ventriculoatrial (VA) shunt. The VP shunt is the most commonly used (Figure 13-5). New shunt systems now allow for growth and have generally eliminated the necessity for shunt revisions. (Shunts still need to be replaced if a malfunction occurs). Shunts work with a one-way valve that opens at a predetermined intraventricular pressure and closes when the pressure falls below that level. This prevents CSF from flowing back upward. Nurses and parents may be taught how to pump the shunt.

The prognosis for hydrocephalus has improved with modern drugs and surgical techniques. If the brain has not been seriously damaged before the operation, mental function can be preserved. However, motor development may occur at a slower rate, if the child cannot lift the head normally. Complications associated with shunts are usually caused by mechanical flaws (kinking or plugging of tubing) or infection. Shunt malfunction may be identified by headaches, nausea, vomiting, irritability, and lethargy. The shunt is also subject to infection. The symptoms of shunt

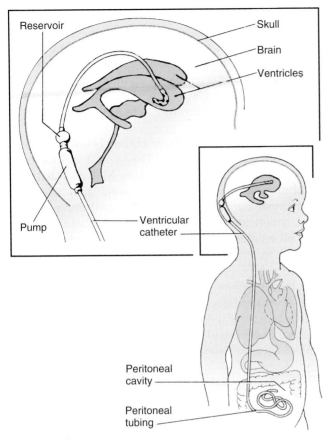

Reservoir

Skull

Brain

Ventricles

Pump

Ventricular
catheter

Peritoneal
cavity

Peritoneal
tubing

FIGURE 13-5 Placement of a ventriculoperitoneal (VP) shunt.

infections may include an unexplained fever and symptoms similar to those of shunt malfunction. If the infections persist, it may become necessary to remove the shunt.

Nursing Care

The general nursing care of an infant with hydrocephalus who has not undergone surgery presents several challenges. The child may be barely able to raise the head. Mental development is also delayed. Lack of appetite, a tendency to vomit easily, and poor resistance to infections pose additional problems.

The position of the infant must be changed frequently to prevent hypostatic pneumonia and pressure sores. Hypostatic pneumonia occurs when there is poor circulation of the blood in the lungs and when the child remains too long in one position. It is particularly prevalent in children who are poorly nourished, weak, or have a debilitating disease. Whenever the nurse turns the child with hydrocephalus, the head must always be supported. To turn the patient in bed, the weight of the head should be borne in the palm of one hand and the head and body should be rotated together to prevent a strain on the neck. When the child is lifted from the crib, the head must be supported by the nurse's arm and chest. The head circumference (FOC) is measured

daily. This measurement is critical, and it is often marked so that daily measurements will be performed in the same location. If there is a deviation in the findings, the charge nurse should be notified. Pressure sores may occur if the child's position is not changed at least every 2 hours. The tissues of the head and ears and the bony prominences have a tendency to break down. A soft fluid-filled pad may be placed under the head to help prevent lesions. In most cases, the nurse may hold the infant for feeding. The nurse sits with the arm supported because the baby's head is heavy. A calm, unhurried manner is necessary. The room should also be as quiet as possible to avoid unnecessary stimulation.

Observations that need to be made include vomiting, condition of skin, motor abilities, restlessness, irritability, lethargy, and changes in vital signs. Fontanels are palpated for size and bulging. Changes in vital signs associated with increased ICP are usually a sign later in infancy. They include elevated blood pressure and a decrease in pulse and respirations. Signs of a cold or other infection should be reported to the charge nurse immediately and recorded.

Many infants and children are treated surgically for hydrocephalus. Postoperative nursing care is complex, and in addition to routine postoperative care and observations, the nurse observes the child for signs of increased ICP and for infection at the operative site or along the shunt line. Pain issues should be included in the care of the postoperative child.

Bacterial infection is a life-threatening complication that sometimes makes it necessary to remove the shunt. Signs of infection include poor feeding, elevated vital signs, decreased level of consciousness, vomiting, and seizure activity. The nurse should also observe for signs of inflammation at the shunt insertion site. If the fontanels are sunken, the infant should be kept flat because too rapid a reduction in fluid may lead to seizures or cortical bleeding. If the fontanels are bulging, the child is usually placed in the semi-Fowler's position to assist in drainage of the ventricles through the shunt. Usually the physician will indicate the position to be maintained and the extent of activity allowed. The child is always positioned so as to avoid pressure on the operative site. Head measurements are recorded. In children with peritoneal shunts, the abdomen should also be measured or observed to detect malabsorption of fluid. Skin care continues to remain a priority. As the child's condition improves, parents are instructed regarding the care of the shunt.

Hydrocephalus, even with a shunt, is a chronic condition, and the child needs to be followed throughout life. Parents are taught how to recognize shunt malfunction and infection. It is also important that family issues and the child's own growth and development be considered.

Community Considerations

The National Hydrocephalus Foundation *(www.nhfonline.org)* provides information and networking opportunities for families.

MYELODYSPLASIA/SPINA BIFIDA

Myelodysplasia refers to a group of CNS disorders characterized by abnormal development of the spinal cord and associated neural tube structures. These defects are categorized as neural tube defects (NTDs). One of these disorders is spina bifida.

Spina bifida (divided spine) is a congenital embryonic NTD in which there is imperfect closure of the spinal vertebrae. There are two forms: **occulta** (hidden) and **cystica** (sac or cyst). Spina bifida occulta is a relatively minor variation of the disorder in which the opening is small and there is no associated protrusion of structures. It is often undetected and occurs most commonly at L5 and S1 levels. There may be a tuft of hair, a dimple, a lipoma, or a port-wine birthmark at the site. Generally, treatment is not necessary unless neuromuscular symptoms appear. These consist of progressive disturbances of gait, footdrop, or disturbances of bowel and bladder sphincter function.

Spina bifida cystica consists of the development of a cystic mass in the midline of the spine (Figure 13-6). **Meningocele** and **meningomyelocele (also called myelomeningocele)** are two types of spina bifida cystica. A meningocele (*meningo,* membrane; *cele,* tumor) contains portions of the membranes and CSF.

The size varies from that of a walnut to that of the head of a newborn infant.

More serious is a protrusion of the **membranes** and **spinal cord** through this opening, or a **meningomyelocele.** Although it resembles a meningocele, there may be associated paralysis of the legs and poor control of bowel and bladder functions. Hydrocephalus is common.

Although the cause of spina bifida is unknown, it is thought to be multifactorial. This would include both genetic and environmental factors. Maternal diabetes, alcohol use, hyperthermia, valproic acid use, and nutritional deficiencies may be contributing factors. The American Academy of Pediatrics recommends that all women of childbearing age take a daily multivitamin that includes 0.4 mg of folic acid. Women with previous NTDs should take 4 mg of folic acid per day one month before planned pregnancy and during the first trimester (Hockenberry and Wilson, 2009). There has been a steady decline of cases of NTDs because of the use of folic acid in pregnancy. It is important that nurses continue to educate women of childbearing age on the use of folic acid during pregnancy.

Treatment

The treatment for spina bifida is surgical closure to prevent meningeal infection. The child is observed for the development of hydrocephalus, and a shunt is placed if this occurs. Urinary retention is managed with catheterization. The prognosis for these children depends on the location of the lesion, the involvement of the spinal cord, and the presence of other anomalies.

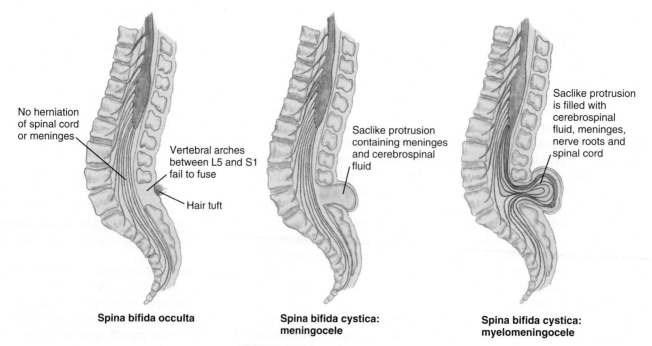

No herniation of spinal cord or meninges

Vertebral arches between L5 and S1 fail to fuse

Hair tuft

Spina bifida occulta

Saclike protrusion containing meninges and cerebrospinal fluid

Spina bifida cystica: meningocele

Saclike protrusion is filled with cerebrospinal fluid, meninges, nerve roots and spinal cord

Spina bifida cystica: myelomeningocele

FIGURE 13-6 Malformation of the spine.

Care of the child involves a multidisciplinary approach that includes neurology, neurosurgery, urology, pediatrics, physical therapy, occupational therapy, and nursing. Depending on the extent of the defect, the child may have problems with hydrocephalus, orthopedic defects, genitourinary abnormalities, and paralysis. Habilitation is necessary after surgery to minimize the child's disability and to put the normally functioning parts of the body to constructive use. Every effort is made to help the child develop a healthy personality so that he or she may live a happy and useful life. Eventually the child may attain some degree of fecal continence and some type of emptying of the bladder (intermittent clean catheterization). Mobility is assisted through bracing, surgery, and the use of a wheelchair.

Nursing Care

The main objectives of the extensive nursing care required include preventing infection of or injury to the sac; correct positioning to prevent pressure on the sac and deformities; good skin care; adequate nutrition; tender, loving care; accurate observations and charting; education of the parents; continued medical supervision; and habilitation.

Immediate care of the sac is essentially the same whether or not the cord is involved. Upon delivery, the neonate is placed in an isolette. Moist sterile dressings of saline solution or an antimicrobial solution may be ordered to prevent drying of the sac. Some method of protecting the mass is necessary if surgery is to be delayed. Pertinent nursing observations include a description of the newborn infant, the size and area of the sac, and any tears or leakage. The extremities are observed for deformities and for movement. There may be spasticity or paralysis of the limbs or they may be normal, depending on the type and location of the cyst. The head is measured to determine the possibility of associated hydrocephalus. Fontanels are observed to provide baseline data. Lack of anal sphincter control and dribbling of urine are significant in the differential diagnosis. In general, the higher the defect is on the spine, the greater is the neurologic deficit. Data are recorded along with the routine observations made for every newborn infant.

Positioning of the child is crucial. The goal is to avoid pressure on the sac and to prevent postural deformities. When positioning children with multiple deformities, the nurse must try to guard against aggravating existing problems. These children may also have hip dysplasia, which can be another factor in positioning the infant. The infant is usually placed prone with a pad between the legs to maintain abduction and counteract hip subluxation, and a small roll is placed under the ankles to maintain a neutral foot position. The position can be maintained with diaper rolls, blankets, or sandbags.

Postoperative nursing care involves neurologic assessment and prevention of infection. The status of the fontanels and any signs of increased ICP, such as irritability or vomiting, are important. Sometimes a shunt is inserted along with the closure of the spine (see the Nursing Care section under Hydrocephalus in this chapter for a discussion of nursing care for the child with a shunt). Complications that can be life-threatening include meningitis, pneumonia, and urinary tract infection.

Skin care is a challenge. Diapering may be contraindicated until the defect is repaired and healing has taken place. Constant dribbling of feces and urine irritates the perineal area and can infect the sac or the incision. Meticulous cleanliness is necessary. Bedding must be dry and wrinkle-free. Frequent cleansing, application of a prescribed ointment or lotion, and light massage help maintain skin integrity. If range-of-motion exercises are ordered, they are performed gently. Because these children have lack of sensation below the spinal lesion, they lack the ability to be aware of skin breakdown or burns. Parents should be instructed to inspect the skin closely.

Nursing Brief

Latex allergy is commonly associated with spina bifida. All equipment used should be latex-free.

Feeding of the child is facilitated by early closure of the defect. In delayed cases, gavage feedings may be used. To bottle-feed the child, one nurse may hold the infant over the shoulder while another administers the formula. Nipple holes should be large enough to prevent exhaustion, which can occur if the infant has to work to get food. A side-lying position in or out of the crib (on the nurse's lap) is effective with some infants.

These children need cuddling and sensory stimulation. If infants cannot be held, the nurse should soothe them by touch. Talk to them, and when possible provide face-to-face (en face position) communication. Mobiles should be placed appropriately. Moving the incubators or cribs periodically provides diversity of view. Soft music is also soothing.

As these children get older, urologic monitoring is essential because many of these children are incontinent of urine. Medication to prevent urinary tract infections may be given routinely. Clean intermittent catheterization is taught. This is a simple procedure that ensures total emptying of the bladder. It can be performed by parents and learned by young children. It is important that this procedure be performed regularly and in a clean manner. A surgical vesicostomy may be necessary. This involves bringing the

Table 13-2	Organisms That Cause Bacterial Meningitis in Various Age Groups
AGE	**ORGANISM**
Birth to 2 mo	Enteric bacilli Group B streptococci
2 mo to 12 yr	H. influenzae b S. pneumoniae Neisseria meningitidis (meningococci)
Over 13 yr	N. meningitidis S. pneumoniae

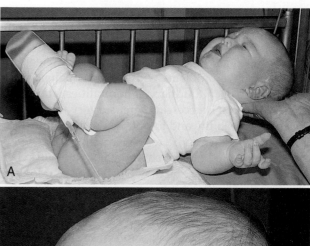
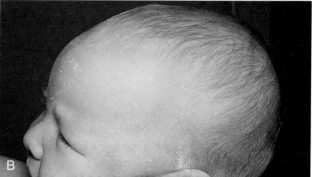

FIGURE 13-7 **A,** An infant shows nuchal rigidity with meningitis. Attempts to flex the neck result in the infant grimacing with pain, neck stiffness, and flexed knees and hips. **B,** A quiet infant shows a bulging fontanel that indicates increased intracranial pressure.

bladder out to the abdominal wall, facilitating continuous urinary drainage.

Special consideration must be given to the establishment of parent-infant relationships. This problem is complicated if the infant is transferred to a large medical center. Understanding and support need to be given to the parents. It is not unusual for them to be overwhelmed by the cyst. Most experience a sense of loss for what was to have been their "perfect baby." Steps of the grieving process may be recognized by the nurse. If the malformation is complex and incompatible with life, a decision must be made about the feasibility of surgical intervention. This is a crisis situation for the most mature of people and an area in which guidelines are not clearly defined. Information and education concerning this disorder can be obtained from the Spina Bifida Association.

BACTERIAL MENINGITIS

Meningitis is an inflammation of the **meninges,** the membranes covering the brain and spinal cord. Different organisms cause bacterial meningitis in different age groups (Table 13-2). Organisms may invade the meninges indirectly by way of the bloodstream from such centers of infection as the teeth, sinuses, tonsils, and lungs or directly through the ear (otitis media), from neurologic procedures, or from a fracture of the skull. Bacterial meningitis is often referred to as **purulent** (pus-forming) because a thick exudate surrounds the meninges and adjacent structures. This can lead to certain sequelae such as subdural effusion and, less frequently, hydrocephalus. The peak incidence for bacterial meningitis is between 6 and 12 months of age. It is less frequently seen in children older than 4 years of age. The nursing care for all types is similar.

Signs and Symptoms
The symptoms of purulent meningitis result mainly from intracranial irritation. The onset of the illness generally follows two courses. Most often the disease is preceded by an upper respiratory infection or gastrointestinal problem. Nonspecific symptoms such as irritability and lethargy may follow. The other course

is sudden rapid onset with shock, **purpura,** changes in level of consciousness, and disseminated intravascular coagulation (DIC). Other nonspecific reactions include headache, drowsiness, delirium, irritability, restlessness, fever, vomiting, photophobia, and stiffness of the neck and spine (Figure 13-7). The infant may have a characteristic high-pitched cry and a bulging tense fontanel. Convulsions may occur. Coma can occur fairly early in the older child. In severe cases, opisthotonis or involuntary arching of the back from muscle contractions is seen. The presence of petechiae, small hemorrhages beneath the skin, is suggestive of meningococcal infection.

Treatment
At the first indication of meningitis, the physician performs a spinal tap for laboratory analysis (see Collection of Spinal Fluid for Culture in Chapter 3). In the early stages of the illness, the fluid may be clear, but it rapidly becomes full of pus. The pressure is increased, and further laboratory analysis indicates many white cells, sometimes too numerous to count. There is an increase in protein and a decrease in glucose.

Isolation is used until the child has received at least 24 hours of antimicrobial therapy. (It is uncommon for others in the family to contract the disease, but the physician orders preventive medicines if necessary. An intravenous line is established. The fluid serves as a vehicle for the administration of antimicrobials, which need to be quickly assimilated, and also aids in the restoration of fluids and electrolytes. Antimicrobials are given in combination and are adjusted on the basis of culture and sensitivity reporting. The initial choice is dictated by the cerebrospinal fluid gram-stained smear and the child's age. Antimicrobials are given according to the child's progress but are always administered for a minimum of 10 days. With increasing antimicrobial-resistant bacteria, medical management has changed to use of third-generation cephalosporins (cefotaxime or ceftriaxone) in combination with vancomycin. Neonates may be treated with ampicillin, gentamicin, and third-generation cephalosporins. Anticonvulsants may also be necessary if the child is having seizures.

Initially, the child may be given nothing by mouth. An accurate record is kept of fluid intake and output, and vital signs and neurologic checks are routinely performed. Fever may be controlled with antipyretics, sponge baths, and the use of a hypothermia blanket. The nurse observes the child for signs of increased ICP, especially a change in alertness, or muscle twitching. New or persistent fever requires reevaluation. Computed tomography (CT) may be helpful in pinpointing secondary sites of infection.

 ## Health Promotion

Decreasing Risks for Meningitis

- The number of cases of meningitis related to *H. influenzae*, *Neisseria meningitidis*, and *Streptococcus pneumoniae* have been decreased with the use of the Hib, pneumococcal, and meningococcal vaccines.
- Immunization should be encouraged for all children.

Nursing Care

The nursing care of the child with meningitis is extensive. The isolation room is prepared in accordance with hospital procedure. Because the child is overly sensitive to stimuli, indirect lighting should be used. **Photophobia** is a common complaint, especially in older children. Shades are drawn on a bright day. The nurse also carefully raises and lowers the crib sides to avoid jarring the bed. Padded side rails ensure that the child is not injured in the event of a convulsion. The nurse avoids startling the child by using a gentle touch when waking the child and by speaking in a low voice. This need is also explained to the parents.

The child is placed on the side to avoid aspiration of vomitus. Because handling must be kept to a minimum during the acute stage, it is important that the nurse organize care so that the child is disturbed as little as possible yet still receives the treatment necessary for survival and recovery. Frequent changes of position are necessary to prevent pneumonia and to avoid breakdown of the skin. However, careful

planning and consolidation of nursing procedures can minimize activity about the child. As the child's condition improves, nursing care should include range-of-motion exercises (easily done during bathtime). In children with long-term conditions, splinting of the extremities may also be necessary to avoid this complication.

Most children with bacterial meningitis develop the syndrome of inappropriate antidiuretic hormone (SIADH). To determine the presence of SIADH, body weight, serum electrolytes, and serum and urine osmolarities should be measured at the time of hospital admission. The intake and output are carefully observed and recorded. If SIADH occurs, there may be fluid restriction. As the child's condition improves, the diet progresses from clear fluids to regular diet. A special formula may be given when NG feedings are necessary. The nurse promptly reports a decrease in output of urine, which could signal **urinary retention.** Bowel movements are recorded each day to detect constipation and avoid fecal impaction (an accumulation of feces in the rectum). Watch for signs of residual effects from the disease, such as weakness of limbs, speech difficulties, mental confusion, behavior problems, and hearing problems.

The diagnosis of meningitis is frightening to parents, as is the prospect of the child undergoing a spinal tap. Early recognition, appropriate antimicrobial therapy, and supportive care have decreased the mortality of the illness. There is also concern for the health of other members of the family. The nurse should direct attention to the parents. Parents should be encouraged to stay.

ENCEPHALITIS

Encephalitis (*encephalo*, brain; *itis*, inflammation) is an inflammation of the brain parenchyma. It is usually more severe than viral meningitis. This disorder can be caused by arboviruses, enteroviruses (RNA viruses), and herpesvirus types 1 and 2; it can be the aftermath of disorders such as upper respiratory tract infections, German measles, or measles or, rarely, an untoward reaction to vaccinations such as DTP (diphtheria, tetanus, pertussis); or it may result from lead poisoning. Other less common etiological agents are bacteria, spirochetes, and fungi.

This disease also affects horses, and during epidemics, newspapers specify the equine variety if this is the case. If the specific virus is determined, it is given the name of the geographic location in which it is found, such as Eastern (United States), Western (United States), St. Louis, or California. The infection is transmitted to horses and humans by mosquitoes and ticks.

Signs and Symptoms

The symptoms of encephalitis result from the response of the CNS to irritation. In general, the viruses invade the lymphatic system and multiply. The bloodstream becomes affected, and consequently various organs are also involved. Characteristically, the history is that of a headache followed by drowsiness, which may proceed to coma. Because coma is sometimes prolonged, encephalitis is sometimes referred to as "sleeping sickness." Convulsions occur, particularly in infants. Fever, cramps, abdominal pain, vomiting, stiff neck, delirium, muscle twitching, and abnormal eye movements are other manifestations of the disease. The child's history is of particular significance. Recent illness, injections, travel, and geographic location are recorded.

Treatment and Nursing Care

At this time, no specific treatment with medication is known, with the exception of the use of corticosteroids and immune globulin; or acyclovir for herpesvirus encephalitis. Parenteral antimicrobials are used until a bacterial cause has been ruled out. A brain scan, electroencephalography (EEG), computed tomography (CT), and cerebrospinal fluid analysis may be useful in determining the diagnosis. Intracranial monitoring may also be used.

Treatment is supportive and aimed at providing relief from specific symptoms. Treatment may include sedatives, fluids given intravenously, seizure control, and monitoring for increased ICP. Catheterization for urinary retention may be necessary. Antipyretics are given as ordered, and seizure precautions are instituted. The nurse provides a quiet dark environment, good oral hygiene, skin care, and frequent change of position. Oxygen is given as needed, and the mouth and nose are kept free of mucus with suctioning. Bowel movements are recorded daily because the child may be constipated from lack of activity. Preventing this and other secondary effects of immobility is paramount. Physical therapy maintains range of motion. The nurse closely observes the child for neurologic changes.

Fatality rates and residual effects are higher among infants than older children. Speech, mental processes, and motor abilities may be slowed, and permanent brain damage and mental retardation can result. Parents are encouraged to help with the care of the child as soon as the condition is stable. They are instructed in the nursing procedures necessary for home care. In long-term cases, rehabilitation services, the services of the home health care nurse, and related agencies are invaluable.

SEIZURE DISORDERS

FEBRILE SEIZURE

Febrile seizures in children occur in association with a fever. They are a common pediatric neurologic disorder and are generally transient in nature.

Approximately 1 in every 25 children will have at least one febrile seizure, and more than one third of these children will have additional febrile seizures before they outgrow the tendency to have them (National Institute of Neurological Disorders and Stroke, 2006). They usually occur between the ages of 6 months and 5 years and are common in toddlerhood. Febrile seizures are associated with an identifiable infection such as otitis media, roseola infantum, gastroenteritis, or pharyngitis. Fever after immunization can also trigger a febrile seizure (Nordi, 2006). Other theories discuss the height of the temperature (39° C or 102.2° F) as a factor; the seizure generally occurs during the rise rather than after a prolonged elevation (Hockenberry and Wilson, 2007).

Simple febrile seizures are often not present when the child reaches the hospital. Causes other than fever are ruled out. Unless the child has neurologic impairments, is younger than 1 year of age, or experiences repetitive or prolonged seizures, epilepsy treatment is not considered. (Epilepsy is discussed in the next section.) Generally, the parents are educated on fever management and seizure precautions, although fever management (such as administering acetaminophen) does not typically reduce the risk for a seizure.

EPILEPSY

The term **epilepsy** (chronic recurrent convulsions) comes from the Greek *epilepsia*, which means seizure. Depending on the type of epilepsy, a child may need treatment for only a specified period of time. Others need lifelong treatment.

Epilepsy is characterized by recurrent paroxysmal attacks of unconsciousness or impaired consciousness that may be followed by alternating contraction and relaxation of the muscles or by disturbed feelings or behavior. It is a disorder of the CNS in which the neurons or nerve cells discharge in an abnormal way. These discharges may be focal or diffuse. The site of general discharge can sometimes be ascertained by observing the child's symptoms during the attack. Types of generalized and partial epileptic seizures are listed in Table 13-3. Treatment is based on accurately diagnosing the type of seizure the child is experiencing. When the cause is unknown, the term idiopathic is used. If a cerebral abnormality is found, the child may be said to have **organic** or **symptomatic** epilepsy.

Idiopathic epilepsy is the most common cause of recurrent convulsions in children older than 3 years of age. It is possible that some specific genetic defect in cerebral metabolism is responsible in many children. It has been pointed out that EEG abnormalities (cerebral dysrhythmias) are more likely to be found in parents and siblings of affected children than in the population at large.

Table 13-3   Generalized and Partial Seizures

SEIZURE TYPE	CHARACTERISTICS
Generalized Seizures	
Tonic-clonic (formerly called *grand mal*)	(Tonic phase) Sudden loss of consciousness with a cry; fall; rigid muscles; (clonic phase) muscle jerking; rolling of eyes; pallor or blue skin color associated with slowing or cessation of breathing; possible loss of bowel or bladder control. Seizure lasts a few minutes, and then breathing resumes. Child is sleepy and confused and often sleeps 30 minutes to 2 hours after the seizure. Postictal state may involve vomiting and intense bifrontal headache. Seizure may be preceded by an aura.
Absence (formerly called *petit mal*)	Simple (typical) absence seizures are characterized by a sudden cessation of motor activity or speech with a blank facial expression and flickering of the eyelids. Usually last about 5 to 10 seconds; are uncommon in children younger than 5 years of age; involve possible eyelid and chewing movements during the seizure. Child resumes full activity when seizure ends, although is unaware of what is going on during the seizure. No aura or postictal state. May experience countless seizures daily. Can cause learning difficulties if not recognized.
Myoclonic	Repetitive seizures consisting of brief muscular contractions with loss of body tone and falling or slumping forward; can cause injuries to face and mouth. May occur with other seizure forms. No postictal state. May or may not lose consciousness.
Infantile spasms	Brief symmetric contractions of the neck, trunk, and extremities. Involve sudden *flexion* of the neck, arms, and legs onto the trunk; *extension* of the trunk and extremities; or a combination. Spasms commonly occur while children are drowsy or immediately on wakening. Onset between 4 and 8 months. May or may not be associated with underlying neurologic disorder or trauma. Poor outlook for normal intelligence.
Atonic	Onset between 2 and 5 years of age; sudden momentary loss of muscle control. Can fall to floor violently and injure face, head, shoulder. Recurs frequently during the day.
Partial Seizures	
Simple partial	Motor activity is the most common symptom. Muscle movements involving face, neck, or extremities; can begin in one location and spread to another. Head turning and eye movements are common. Usually lasts 10 to 20 seconds. Child remains aware and may verbalize during the seizure. There is no postictal period. Often preceded by aura ("feeling funny" or "something crawling inside me"). These should not be confused with tics (e.g., shoulder shrugging, eye blinking).
Complex partial	Begins with simple partial seizure with or without an aura; decreased consciousness—child seems dazed; followed by repetitive movements—lip smacking, chewing, swallowing, and excessive salivation; picking and pulling at clothing, rubbing or caressing objects; child may walk or run around randomly and is fearful. Lasts 1 or 2 minutes. Postictal state with no awareness of the seizure afterward.

Adapted from Kliegman, R., Behrman, R., Jenson, H., et al (2007). *Nelson's textbook of pediatrics* (18th ed.). Philadelphia: Saunders; Hockenberry, M. J., and Wilson, D. (2009) *Wong's essentials of pediatric nursing* (8th ed.). St. Louis: Mosby.

Organic epilepsy may be caused by a number of conditions or injuries that have impaired the brain. Many genetically determined conditions, such as phenylketonuria (PKU), hydrocephalus, and tuberous sclerosis, are associated with seizures. Convulsions may also occur as a result of brain injury during prenatal, perinatal, or postnatal periods. Acute infections may be responsible for epilepsy in infants and toddlers. There are also contributing conditions that can alter the convulsive threshold. If the child becomes overtired or overexcited or is faced with a stressful situation, a seizure may occur. Bright, flashing lights, or flickering images such as those seen in computer games, can trigger seizures in susceptible people. Alterations in serum and brain concentrations of sodium, potassium, and water resulting from fluid retention can be a precipitating factor. Hormonal changes during puberty, excess fluid intake, and photogenic stimulation have also been suggested as triggers.

Signs and Symptoms

Symptoms vary according to the type of seizure (see Table 13-3). Mixed seizures may also occur in people with epilepsy. Seizures may be convulsive or nonconvulsive. Convulsive seizures usually begin with the **tonic** phase, a phase in which the body stiffens and the child may lose consciousness and drop to the floor if sitting or standing. The face becomes pale at first and then cyanotic from arrest of respiratory movements. The eyes roll upward or to one side. The child may utter a brief cry as air is forced out of the lungs across tightly closed vocal cords. The head, back, and legs stiffen. Onset is usually abrupt and may be preceded by an *aura*, which is a particular sensation such as dizziness, visual images, nausea, headache, or an ascending feeling of abdominal discomfort. Children often are unable to describe an aura. The tonic phase lasts about 20 to 40 seconds and is usually followed by the **clonic** phase, which lasts for variable periods. Jerking movements of the trunk and extremities begin. Frothing at the mouth, biting of the tongue, and urinary or fecal incontinence may occur. Muscle contraction and relaxation gradually subside, and the child enters the *postictal* state. The child appears dazed and confused and generally sleeps for a while. On awakening, children may have a headache and may perform more or less automatic acts. This is believed to be caused by malfunctioning of the neurons, which may not be fully recovered. The child has no recollection of the seizure. **Status epilepticus** is a series of convulsions rapidly following one another. The most common cause is abrupt withdrawal of anticonvulsant medication. Families need to be taught to call emergency medical services when this occurs. Status epilepticus is an emergency situation because death can result from respiratory failure and exhaustion. Diazepam (Valium) or lorazepam (Ativan) is given IV.

Nonconvulsive seizures take various forms, including lapses in consciousness, loss of muscle tone, distorted sensations, and **automatisms,** or repetitive movements. Most nonconvulsive seizures are not preceded by an aura.

Treatment and Nursing Care

First aid for a child with a convulsive seizure includes protecting the child from harm, loosening clothing around the neck, turning on the side to maintain an airway, and reassuring the child when consciousness returns. Parents need to be taught first aid as well. During a seizure, the nurse observes and records the following: the child's activity immediately before the seizure; body movements; changes in color, respiration, or muscle tone; incontinence; and the parts of the body involved. When possible, the seizure is timed. The child's appearance, behavior, and level of consciousness after the seizure are also documented. Do not place any hard object in the mouth or try to hold the child down during a seizure. Rescue breathing is not necessary unless the child is not breathing when the seizure is finished. Seizure precautions in the hospital setting include padding side rails and having oropharyngeal suction and oxygen at the bedside. The child's bed should be kept at the lowest position with the rails up at all times.

Initially, treatment of the child with a seizure disorder is aimed at determining the type, site, and cause of the disorder. Diagnostic measures include a complete history and physical and neurologic examinations. Skull radiography and CT are used to establish the presence or absence of tumors, skull abnormalities,

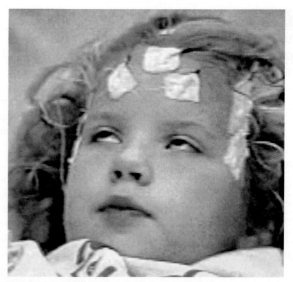

FIGURE 13-8 This absence seizure was recorded during a video electroencephalogram.

hematomas, and intracranial calcifications. Magnetic resonance imaging (MRI) is also used for diagnosis as it is technically superior to CT for this purpose. EEG is also a valuable tool in evaluating seizures. It is especially helpful in differentiating between an absence seizure and a complex partial seizure (Figure 13-8). Video EEG recordings can show more subtle manifestations and provide a permanent record for playback. Prolonged ambulatory EEG monitoring (24 hours) is another advanced technique. Laboratory studies such as a fasting blood sugar, complete blood cell count (CBC), serum calcium, blood urea nitrogen (BUN), and drug screening may detect acute infections, lead poisoning, drug ingestion, or metabolic disorders. A lumbar puncture may be ordered when encephalitis or meningitis is suspected. If the seizure is related to any such underlying cause, appropriate therapy is begun. Anticonvulsive drug therapy is begun only after all such causes have been excluded.

Some common anticonvulsants and their side effects are listed in Table 13-4. The physician determines the child's medication by the type of seizure and other factors. The goal is to achieve the best control with the minimum dosage and the least number of side effects. Serum anticonvulsant levels should be carefully monitored during initial seizure control stages. Doses are altered accordingly. An important aspect of nursing intervention includes reinforcing the need for drug supervision and compliance. The duration of therapy is individual. Initially the physician prescribes the lowest dose likely to control the seizures. A combination of drugs may be necessary. Drowsiness, a common side effect of many anticonvulsants, can interfere with

Table **13-4**   Commonly Used Anticonvulsant Drugs

DRUG	SEIZURE TYPE	SIDE EFFECTS	COMMENTS
Phenobarbital	Generalized tonic-clonic Partial Status epilepticus	Hyperactivity, short attention span, temper tantrums, altered sleep pattern	May cause Stevens-Johnson syndrome and depression of cognitive function. Relatively safe. Routine blood test not indicated.
Primidone (Mysoline)	Generalized tonic-clonic Partial	Aggressive behavior, personality changes	Similar to phenobarbital; routine blood tests not indicated. Relatively safe.
Phenytoin (Dilantin)	Generalized tonic-clonic Partial Status epilepticus	Ataxia, gum hypertrophy, hirsutism (hairiness), rash, nausea, nystagmus, drowsiness, coarsening facial features	Generally effective and safe; regular massaging of gums decreases hyperplasia; is used in combination with phenobarbital or primidone. May be causative agent of Stevens-Johnson syndrome. Many drug interactions. Fosphenytoin for IM or IV use is available.
Valproic acid (Depakene)	Generalized tonic-clonic Absence Myoclonic Partial	Gastrointestinal disturbance, weight gain, alopecia, liver toxicity	Monitor blood counts; take with food or use enteric-coated preparations; potentiates action of phenobarbital and other drugs. Serious side effects include hepatotoxicity (irreversible) and Reye-like syndrome.
Clonazepam (Rivotril)	Absence Myoclonic Infantile spasms Partial	Drowsiness, irritability, agitation, behavioral abnormalities, depression, excessive salivation.	May increase serum phenytoin concentrations when used together.
Carbamazepine (Tegretol)	Generalized tonic-clonic Partial	Diplopia, drowsiness, vertigo	Anemia, neutropenia, hepatotoxic effects.

Adapted from Kliegman, R., Behrman, R., Jenson, H., et al. (2007). *Nelson's textbook of pediatrics* (18th ed.). Philadelphia: Saunders.

the child's activities and requires monitoring. Careful recording of seizure activity and adherence to the drug regimen are of particular importance in determining a suitable program. Medication is given at the same time each day, generally with meals or at bedtime. Parents need to work with the physician to find the medication that works best for their child. Noncompliance can be a problem because of the side effects (hyperactivity, drowsiness). Parents should be told that children often reach a level where they adjust to the medication and side effects may not be as severe. As with all complicated childhood diseases, using a multidisciplinary approach to treatment generally results in increased compliance and improved outcomes.

If it is necessary for the child to take medication during school hours, the parents sign a consent form so that the school nurse may monitor administration. This provides the child and the nurse opportunities to get acquainted and share their knowledge of the disease. Nurse and teacher response, particularly during and after a seizure, has a significant effect on the attitude of classmates toward the disease.

It is important that medication be reduced gradually under a physician's supervision because abrupt withdrawal of medications is the most common cause of status epilepticus. In the hospital, the nurse consults the physician as to whether anticonvulsants are to be withheld if the child is to be NPO. As in any long-term drug therapy, periodic blood and urine tests may be necessary to detect subtle side effects, noncompliance, drug toxicity, and other problems. When children are old enough, they can assume responsibility for their own medications. They should wear a Medic-Alert bracelet. During puberty and adolescence, dosages may have to be adjusted to meet growth needs. Premenstrual fluid retention in girls can sometimes trigger seizures.

The ketogenic diet is sometimes prescribed for children who do not respond well to anticonvulsant therapy. It is high in fats and produces ketoacidosis in the body, which appears to have a calming effect. Some children have a reduction in the number of seizures, whereas others may become seizure-free. The diet is difficult to maintain, however, because food has to be carefully measured and controlled and because it is generally unpalatable to children. Research is ongoing with this diet.

Surgery may be considered for some children with intractable seizures that do not respond to medication. Precisely locating the area of seizure activity is critical for a successful outcome. These children need to be monitored carefully after surgery. Other children may be candidates for a vagal nerve stimulator, which is implanted in the chest wall. A reduction of seizure activity with some children has also been achieved with this device.

Rebellion against medical routine is not uncommon during adolescence. Some states do not allow people with controlled epilepsy to obtain a driver's license, which may be disheartening to the child. Other states have stipulations about the amount of seizure-free time required before licensing is allowed. In terms of diet, excess intake of fluids, particularly alcoholic beverages, can be a source of contention.

 Community Considerations

Parents can obtain valuable information and support from the Epilepsy Foundation of America *(www.epilepsyfoundation. org)*.

The well-controlled child can lead a normal life with a few safety restrictions (e.g., using precautions while swimming). Children can participate in selected athletic and recreational activities. Moderate exercise is encouraged; avoidance of caffeine, alcohol, and trigger factors is recommended. Death or serious injury rarely occurs from a seizure, and a seizure does not cause mental deterioration.

Preventing organic epilepsy includes promoting good prenatal and postnatal care and healthful living for children. Teach parents the importance of providing a safe environment and supervision for small children to prevent injury. Play areas need to be properly supervised, poisonous substances must be stored away from little hands, and proper seat belts should be used in automobiles to prevent head injury. Prevention, early diagnosis, and treatment for such conditions as PKU, meningitis, Reye syndrome, and encephalitis are also crucial in minimizing irreversible brain damage. The abuse of drugs, including alcohol, by teenagers can result in cerebral anoxia and convulsions, and this danger should be stressed in comprehensive health teaching for this age group. It is not possible or desirable to shield children from every stressful situation, but adults can assist growing children by helping them make wise decisions at their level of competency and by being supportive. The response of parents and nurses in stressful situations is also of importance in role modeling. Education of the child and family is

a prime consideration in developing nursing care plans. Children who state that they are subject to seizures indicate that they are aware of their condition, and this encourages others to relate to them in a mature way.

REYE SYNDROME

Reye syndrome is a pediatric disease characterized by a nonspecific encephalopathy with fatty degeneration of the viscera and altered ammonia metabolism. It mainly affects the liver and brain. The disease is triggered by a virus, particularly influenza or varicella. Other controversial causes include genetic makeup, environmental factors, and the use of salicylates. The incidence rate of this disorder has decreased markedly since pediatricians began advising parents not to treat children with aspirin. The younger the child, the higher the morbidity and fatality rates. Early diagnosis is crucial because of the rapid, life-threatening course of the disease.

Signs and Symptoms

The clinical picture is typical in that the child is recovering from an upper respiratory infection or chickenpox (varicella). The recuperation is interrupted by general malaise; then there is the sudden onset of persistent vomiting, which may continue for 24 hours, and lethargy (Table 13-5). Metabolic acidosis and respiratory alkalosis can occur.

The diagnosis is based on the child's history, symptoms, and laboratory data. Examples of the latter include elevated findings on liver function tests (serum glutamate oxaloacetate transaminase [SGOT], serum glutamate pyruvate transaminase [SGPT], lactate dehydrogenase [LDH]) and serum ammonia levels,

Table 13-5	Clinical Staging of Reye Syndrome
GRADE	**SYMPTOMS AT TIME OF ADMISSION**
I	Usually quiet, **lethargic** and sleepy, vomiting, laboratory evidence of liver dysfunction
II	Deep lethargy, **confusion**, delirium, combative, hyperventilation, hyperreflexic
III	Obtunded, **light coma**, with or without seizures, decorticate rigidity, intact pupillary light reaction
IV	Seizures, deepening coma, **decerebrate rigidity**, loss of oculocephalic reflexes, fixed pupils
V	Coma, loss of deep tendon reflexes, respiratory arrest, fixed dilated pupils, **flaccidity/decerebrate** (intermittent); isoelectric EEG

From Kliegman, R., Behrman, R., Jenson, H., et al. (2007). *Nelson's textbook of pediatrics* (18th ed.). Philadelphia: Saunders.

possibly decreased blood glucose levels, and elevated prothrombin times. Liver biopsy may be done if the diagnosis is questionable.

Treatment and Nursing Care

The child is admitted to the ICU. Treatment is supportive. Of particular priority is prevention of brain insult because the disease process in most other organs is reversible. Fluid management in conjunction with treatment of increased ICP is crucial. Medications include osmotic diuretics (such as mannitol), sedatives, and barbiturates. Appropriate therapy for secondary infection is also instituted. The nursing care is similar to any child with increased ICP. In addition, the nurse should evaluate the child's respiratory status frequently. The prognosis depends on the severity of the illness. Most survivors recover completely; however, some have complications of neurologic sequelae.

NEAR-DROWNING

Near-drowning is defined as surviving at least 24 hours after submersion in a fluid medium. Drowning is death from asphyxia. Drowning and near-drowning can occur in any body of water, including a hot tub, toilet, or even mop bucket. Many drownings and near-drownings occur in swimming pools, often because young children are left unsupervised, even if for just a moment. Anticipatory guidance and teaching about water safety is a vital role of the nurse. This is a major cause of accidental death in children older than 1 year of age, but it can be prevented with education.

Signs and Symptoms

Length of submersion time, the victim's physiologic response, and exposure to hypothermia all affect the victim's prognosis (Hockenberry and Wilson, 2009). Hypoxia is the primary problem in near-drownings. Without enough oxygen, brain cells (neurons) will begin to die after 4 to 6 minutes. Cardiac arrest can also occur. Respiratory acidosis results from retained carbon dioxide, and metabolic acidosis results from a buildup of acid metabolites from anaerobic metabolism. Aspiration may result, which leads to airway complications including pulmonary edema and pneumonia. Children are at increased risk for hypothermia (after submersion) because they have a relatively high ratio of body surface area to mass, decreased subcutaneous fat, and limited thermogenic capacity (Kliegman et al., 2007).

Treatment and Nursing Care

On-site CPR, transportation availability to a trauma facility, and intensive pulmonary care affect the prognosis of a near-drowning. Oftentimes victims will be monitored in the hospital because of the potential for pulmonary complications and the risk for cerebral edema. Severe anoxia can result in devastating neurologic deficits or death. The nursing care of these children involves respiratory support with monitoring of vital signs, possible mechanical ventilation, chest physiotherapy, blood gas analysis, IV infusions, treatment of metabolic and respiratory acidosis, treatment of hypothermia, and possibly care for severe neurologic complications. The guilt of the child's caregivers can be overwhelming. Nurses must be supportive of the families in these difficult situations.

SENSORY DISORDERS

EARS

DEAFNESS

Deaf children present special challenges to the nursing team. They may be hospitalized for direct evaluation and treatment of hearing loss, or they may have other medical or surgical problems that are—or are not—related to the deafness. The nurse should have a basic knowledge of the problems that confront deaf children to give them comprehensive nursing care.

The inner ear is fully formed during the first months of prenatal life. If an expectant mother contracts German measles (rubella) or takes medications such as the antimicrobial streptomycin, the child may be born with a hearing loss, which is termed **congenital deafness.** Deafness can also be **acquired.** Infectious diseases such as measles, mumps, chickenpox, or meningitis can result in various degrees of hearing loss. Ototoxic (injurious to the ear) medications or ear infections may also be responsible. Deafness can also be temporary, as a result of wax accumulation that blocks the ear canal.

Hearing loss falls into two major categories. **Sensorineural** hearing loss results from damage to the structures of the inner ear or auditory nerve. This can result from congenital defects of the inner ear or from the effects of certain conditions such as kernicterus (see Chapter 5) or infection. Complications can also arise from ototoxic drugs such as streptomycin, kanamycin, neomycin, and others. In addition, sensorineural hearing loss can be caused by noise pollution, such as loud rock music or target shooting. Symptoms include buzzing in the ears and muffled dull sounds immediately after exposure. Most people with sensorineural deafness benefit to some degree from hearing aids. With an interruption in the transmission of sound waves (from structural problems) from the external or middle ear, **conductive** hearing loss occurs. Common causes of conduction deafness are otitis media (ear infections), injury, foreign bodies, and wax build-up. Many children with this type of deafness can be helped with treatment for infection, surgery, or other measures to remove a blockage. Some children have **mixed** hearing loss, which is a combination of conductive and sensorineural causes.

Signs and Symptoms

It is important that parents know whether their child has hearing problems, especially when the child is young. Early intervention becomes critical for successful childhood development. Parents need to be alert for signs of hearing loss and notify their doctor if their baby:

- Does not startle with sudden loud sounds.
- Does not turn his or her head toward a sound by 3 or 4 months.
- Does not begin babbling by 6 months of age.
- Does not respond by interacting to music by around 8 months of age.
- Does not attempt to speak syllables such as "da" by around 1 year of age.

The various degrees of deafness range from complete hearing loss bilaterally to a loss so mild that the problem is never discovered. **Bilateral** deafness affects both ears. If this is complete, the child misses all the pleasures that sound brings to life and has difficulty communicating because children learn to talk by imitating what they hear. Behavior problems arise because the children do not understand directions. They may become aggressive with other children in their attempts to communicate. If children are ridiculed by playmates, their personality development is affected. Without help, these children become socially isolated and unable to attend school.

Partial bilateral deafness may be responsible for behavior problems and poor progress in school. This may be caused by chronic infections such as otitis media or by blockage of the eustachian tube. It may be a warning signal of more serious defects in later life. Children who are deaf in one ear are less disabled if the hearing in the other ear is normal.

Treatment and Nursing Care

The nurse must stress the importance of proper immunization during childhood to prevent many of the communicable diseases that contribute to acquired deafness. Vaccines against measles (rubeola), mumps, and German measles (rubella) are available, as is the vaccine against *Haemophilus influenzae* type b (a cause of meningitis in childhood). The child should be taken to the doctor for periodic health examinations. Early diagnosis and early intervention are important in the treatment of the deaf child to prevent adverse physical and mental complications.

Complete bilateral deafness is usually discovered during infancy. As discussed in Chapter 5, the Joint Committee on Infant Hearing (JCIH) recommends universal screening of hearing loss in newborns before hospital discharge. Early detection of hearing loss results in a child being able to develop speech and language skills along with peers.

Partial deafness may be unrecognized until the child begins school. Many hearing problems are detected then with standard hearing tests. A machine called an **audiometer** is used. The measurement of hearing as with an audiometer is called audiometry. The child puts on an earphone that is connected to the audiometer. When the audiometer is turned on, it makes various noises and pitches of sound. The child raises a hand on hearing the tones. The results of these tests are interpreted by specialists in this field. A child should be screened two times before a referral is made to avoid unnecessary referrals. Another test used to assess hearing problems in children is tympanography. The tympanogram measures the movement of the eardrum in response to sound waves. Decreased movement of the eardrum causes temporary hearing loss. This happens primarily when children have fluid in the middle ear as a result of an ear infection. Children who fail hearing tests should be referred to an otolaryngologist (specialist in ear, nose, and throat [ENT]) or audiologist for further testing.

Community Considerations

The American Speech-Language-Hearing Association (*www. asha.org*) is committed to ensuring that all people with speech, language, and hearing disorders receive services to help them communicate effectively.

Members of the health team concerned with the child who is hard of hearing include the physician, otolaryngologist, audiologist, speech therapist, specially trained teacher, social worker, psychologist, nurse, and the child's family. Children with a severe loss of hearing may need more extensive help from personnel at special hearing and speech centers. Whether the child should be placed in special classes in a regular school or should attend a school for the deaf is decided on an individual basis. Some children who spend a few years in a school for the deaf can be transferred to a regular school. These children need to begin their education early to help them catch up on what they have missed since infancy.

The deaf child in the hospital needs the same opportunities to develop a healthy personality as the child with normal hearing. The nurse who uses a relaxed manner with the child creates an atmosphere that others will follow. Remember the following points when communicating with a deaf child:

- Smile when approaching a deaf child.
- Face the child when you speak.
- Position yourself so that you are at eye level with the child.
- Use short sentences rather than separate words.

- Speak clearly in a natural tone.
- Use appropriate gestures to accompany your speech.
- Try to talk to the child in an area that is free of background noise (television, radio, loud conversation).

The older child who is able to write can use this as a means of communication. Have the child read aloud what has been written. In this way, you become better accustomed to the child's speech. Regression in speech patterns may occur during hospitalization. Do not assume that because a child is not talking a great deal he or she does not understand what is being said. Repeat or reword certain statements as you would with any child.

Various methods are used to bring the child into the world of sound. Lip reading, sign language, writing, closed captioning (on television), computers, visual aids, music, and amplified sound are but a few examples.

Safety needs have to be addressed also. Flashing lights can be attached to a telephone or doorbell to indicate its ringing. Hearing ear dogs can also be of great assistance for older children and adults. Telecommunications devices for the deaf (TDD or TDY) also help older children and adults. Through these special teletypewriters, deaf persons can communicate with each other over the telephone.

Babies (usually over 3 months of age) can be successfully fitted with hearing aids. Through education, the parent knows that the hearing aid is working correctly. If a hearing aid is indicated in an older child, the child and parent are taught how to use it. A hearing aid is expensive and invaluable to the child. It should be kept in a safe place when it is not in use. Be sure the parents safeguard the hearing aid if their child ever has surgery. Regular checkups ensure that the device is working properly. A malfunctioning hearing aid may cause a child to lose interest in its use. Surgical procedures with cochlear implants are also used. These devices have met with success in profoundly deaf children with sensorineural hearing loss. Amplification technology is critical so that sound can get to the child's developing brain as soon as possible. This enables children to develop at or nearly at a normal rate, enabling them to keep up with peers as much as possible.

Because preventing deafness is so important, the nurse should take advantage of opportunities to demonstrate and teach proper hygiene of the ears to the child and family. No objects should be inserted into the ear canal when cleaning. If a foreign object gets into the ear, the child should be seen by a doctor. Do *not* try to remove any object from the ear yourself. If assisting with an ear examination, have the parent hold the young child in his or her lap with the head pressed against the parent's chest. The parent can hold one hand on the child's forehead and the other securely around the body. The child can also lie on his or her side on the examination table. The parent or nurse may assist in holding the child still. The head is held still so that the delicate ear canal is not injured by the **otoscope.** The doctor may need cotton swabs or other instruments to remove excess secretions from the external ear. The ear **speculum** (a funnel-shaped device that is attached to the otoscope and comes in direct contact with the ear) must be disinfected after each use.

EYES

Preventing and detecting early vision problems in infants and children can improve long-term visual health. Adequate vision is necessary for normal growth and development. Taking a careful history during every well-infant examination with observations on visual tracking and recognition of parent faces is important. Children should have a thorough ophthalmic examination by 3 to 4 years of age. These are crucial years for detecting and treating eye problems that may possibly lead to permanent vision loss.

The nurse should stress the importance of continued proper care of the eyes. Young children who are beginning to read will need books with large type and letters spaced far apart. The lighting provided must be adequate and without glare. Chairs and desks must be of proper height.

Symptoms that may indicate eye strain include inflammation, aching or smarting of the eyes, squinting, a short attention span, frequent headaches, difficulties with schoolwork, or inability to see the blackboard. They may occur suddenly. The child between 6 and 10 years of age often becomes nearsighted and has to hold books close to the eyes to read. If this occurs, an eye examination and, in some cases, a complete physical examination are indicated.

Determining visual acuity for children younger than 3 years of age can only be done indirectly. By 3 years of age, most children can cooperate to obtain a full assessment. The standard Snellen E test is modified and available for nonreaders. A kindergarten eye chart with familiar shapes is also available. Directions for testing are standardized and must be carefully adhered to for proper results.

AMBLYOPIA

Amblyopia is a decrease in or loss of vision, usually in one eye. The vision loss is not caused by structural eye damage but results from the brain "turning off" confusing visual images. This condition occurs when the visual image does not fall on the retina. The prognosis depends on how long the eye has been affected and the age of the child when treatment is begun. Because critical visual development occurs from birth until 6 years of age, treatment should begin as early as possible to prevent permanent vision loss.

Signs and Symptoms

The condition is not usually noticed until the child's first vision screening at approximately 3 to 4 years of age. An observant parent might notice that the child sits closer to the television or appears to have difficulty seeing. Conditions such as congenital cataract or strabismus can alert the ophthalmologist to the possibility of amblyopia.

Treatment and Nursing Care

The goal of treatment is to obtain normal and equal vision in each eye. Treatment consists of glasses for significant refractive errors (hyperopia, myopia) and occlusion (covering) of the unaffected eye. Drops to blur the vision of the unaffected eye (penalization therapy) may be used in place of occlusion therapy (Kliegman et al., 2007). Either treatment works by stimulating proper visual development of the affected eye. With occlusion therapy, an adhesive patch covers the eye for a designated time period throughout the day. This is based on severity. The nurse can help with the treatment methodology by explaining the importance of the procedure and offering support. Listening to children express their feelings is important in promoting healthy self-esteem.

STRABISMUS

Strabismus ("cross-eye") refers to ocular misalignment and is a condition in which the child is not able to direct both eyes toward the same object. If the malalignment is not corrected, the weak eye becomes "lazy" and the brain eventually suppresses the image produced by that eye. Amblyopia can result. There are several kinds of strabismus. Most children with strabismus have **esotropia,** or an inward deviation of one or both eyes (Figure 13-9). Some children have **exotropia,** which is outward turning. Strabismus may be present at birth or may be acquired after a disease.

Signs and Symptoms

Simple tests can be done to detect strabismus. With the **corneal light reflex,** the examiner shines a light into the child's eyes. With the child looking directly into the light, the reflection should be at the same point in each pupil. In the uncover test, the eyes are observed for

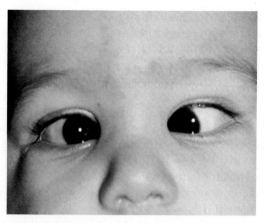

FIGURE 13-9 Infantile esotropia with asymmetrical corneal light reflexes.

compensatory or adjustment movements. The eye is covered and the child looks at a light source; when it is quickly uncovered, the eye should not move. This indicates alignment. If the eye has to shift to focus on the light, malalignment is present. In the cover test, one eye is covered and the movement of the uncovered eye is observed while the child looks at a distant object (preferably 6 m or 20 ft). If the uncovered eye does not move, it is aligned. **Epicanthal folds,** the vertical folds of skin on either side of the nose that are frequently seen in children of Asian descent, can give a false impression of strabismus. Transient strabismus is normal in very young infants (less than 4 months). If present after 4 months of age, infants should be referred to an ophthalmologist.

Treatment and Nursing Care

Depending on the type of strabismus, eye exercises and glasses may be effective ways of treating the condition medically. Surgery is often indicated for strabismus. The child undergoing surgery for strabismus is hospitalized for only a brief period. Parents may visit the child in the recovery room. Eyes will be red after surgery and may be sensitive to light. Eyelids may be swollen. Postoperative care includes the use of eyedrops and ointments, pain relievers, and other comfort measures.

Get Ready for the NCLEX® Examination!

Key Points

- Level of consciousness assessment is the most important evaluation of neurologic status in children.
- Cushing Triad is a late sign associated with ICP.
  - Monitoring FOC is an important nursing assessment when caring for a child with hydrocephalus.
- Shunt infections and malfunction are two complications of shunt surgery.
- Myelodysplasia refers to malformations of the spinal cord.
- The priority with bacterial meningitis is administration of antimicrobials.
- Educating families regarding preventive measures for bacterial meningitis should include Hib.

- Encephalitis is an inflammation of the brain tissue. The child may be at risk for residual neurologic problems such as seizures.
- Education of parents with children having recurrent seizures involves understanding appropriate interventions during a seizure, proper medication administration, and family coping mechanisms.
- Aspirin is not given to children with influenza or chickenpox because of increased risk for Reye syndrome.

Additional Learning Resources

evolve Go to your Evolve website (*http://evolve.elsevier.com/Price/pediatric/*) for the following FREE learning resources:
- 3-D Animations
- Answer Keys
- Appendixes
- Audio Glossary
- Spanish/English Glossary
- Video Clips

Review Questions for the NCLEX® Examination

1. Intracranial hemorrhage in the newborn is associated with all of the following **except**:
   1. Prematurity
   2. Cephalopelvic disproportion
   3. Precipitated delivery
   4. Pre-eclampsia

2. An *early* sign of increased intracranial pressure (ICP) is:
   1. Fixed pupils
   2. Decreased pulse
   3. Changes in behavior
   4. Altered respiratory pattern

3. The **best** nursing intervention to prevent hypostatic pneumonia in the infant with the diagnosis of hydrocephalus is:
   1. Frequent position changes
   2. Assessment of lung sounds every 4 hours
   3. Daily weights
   4. Daily head circumference measurements

4. There has been a steady decline in the cases of neural tube defects because of the use of:
   1. Vitamin D in pregnancy
   2. Folic acid in pregnancy
   3. Ferrous sulfate in pregnancy
   4. Vitamin B-12 in pregnancy

5. Symptoms of encephalitis include: (**Select all that apply.**)
   1. Headache
   2. Drowsiness
   3. Fever
   4. Cramps
   5. Stiff neck

14

Gastrointestinal Disorders

Objectives

1. Define the vocabulary terms listed
2. Describe the changes from infancy with the gastrointestinal system
3. Describe the nursing care of a child with infectious diarrhea
4. Discuss two feeding techniques used for the infant with a cleft lip or cleft palate
5. Summarize the needs of a neonate with tracheoesophageal fistula
6. Identify the nursing care for an infant with biliary atresia
7. Describe the home care of an infant with GER
8. Discuss the different nursing care involved in caring for a child with gastroschisis or omphalocele
9. Discuss the nursing care of a child with celiac disease
10. Identify the difference in symptoms for intussuception and Hirschsprung disorders
11. List the symptoms of appendicitis, and discuss necessary modifications in treatment and postoperative nursing care for a school-age child with a ruptured appendix

Key Terms

acholic (p. 269)
alkalosis (p. 275)
anastomosis (p. 274)
currant jelly stool (p. 273)
fundoplication (p. 277)
gluten (GLŪ-těn; p. 272)
guarding (p. 278)
Guiac stool test (p. 273)
herniate (p. 267)
hypertrophy (p. 269)

incarcerated (p. 271)
Logan bow (bar) (p. 266)
nonbilious vomitus (p. 270)
peristalsis (p. 264)
peritonitis (p. 277)
polyhydramnios (p. 268)
projectile vomiting (p. 270)
pyloromyotomy (p. 270)
regurgitation (p. 264)

GASTROINTESTINAL SYSTEM

The gastrointestinal system includes the mouth; esophagus; stomach; small and large intestine; and accessory organs such as the gall bladder, liver, and pancreas. In the gastrointestinal tract, foods and fluids are ingested, absorbed, and eliminated. The absorption of essential nutrients is necessary for growth and development.

The gastrointestinal system is completely developed at birth but is not fully mature until after the second year of life. The infant's sucking and swallowing are automatic reflexes until about 6 weeks of age when nerve and voluntary muscle control has developed. The stomach capacity of the child increases as the child grows (Table 14-1).

Intestinal motility (peristalsis) is quicker with infants and becomes slower in older children. The emptying time of the stomach is 2 to 3 hours for a newborn and increases to 4 to 6 hours by 2 months of age. These factors explain the necessity for small, frequent feedings with newborns and infants. Infants can have issues with regurgitation of feedings as a result of a relaxed and immature cardiac sphincter.

The infant's small intestine is proportionally greater than an adult's. This allows for more absorption of nutrients to help with meeting the higher caloric demands needed for growth. The infant's large intestine is proportionally shorter than an adult's. With less surface area, less water absorption occurs resulting in the frequent loose stools characteristic of a young infant. With a decreased ability to recapture large amounts of water, the infant and young child are at risk for developing dehydration.

Several digestive enzymes are deficient until about 4 to 6 months of age. Amylase (digests carbohydrates), lipase (fat absorption), and lactase (carbohydrate digestion) are insufficient to aid with digestion. Infants who are given solid foods such as cereal before 4 to 6 months of age may develop gas and diarrhea. Introduction of solid foods should not be started until 6

Table 14-1	Stomach Capacity
Newborn	10-20 mL
1 week	30-90 mL
2-3 weeks	75-100 mL
1 month	90-150 mL
3 months	150-200 mL
1 year	210-360 mL
2 years	500 mL

Modified from James, S., and Ashwill, J. (2007). *Nursing care of children: principles & practice.* (3rd ed.). St. Louis: Saunders.

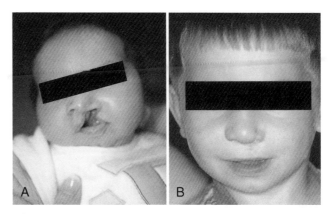

FIGURE 14-1 Child with cleft lip and cleft palate at birth (**A**) and at 3 years of age (**B**).

months of age due to the infant's inability to digest them. It also exposes them to food allergens that may cause food allergies. Despite this recommendation, many parents begin the introduction as early as 2 weeks of age to help the infant sleep better at night or gain weight (Morin, 2004). Iron-fortified infant cereal is usually the first. Rice is suggested as it has low allergy potential. It can be mixed with both breast milk and commercial formula. Fruits and vegetables are next, with meats and eggs by 1 year of age. Either fruits or vegetables can be given first. Whichever, it is highly recommended that only one new food is introduced in a limited amount every 5 to 7 days while monitoring for any reactions. While commercial baby food is very popular, making baby food at home is easy and inexpensive. Steamed fruits and vegetables without seeds can be pureed with water from cooking. Placing small amounts of pureed food in ice cube trays for freezing and storing in freezer bags offers an economical alternative.

Liver function is also immature, but after the first few weeks the infant can conjugate bilirubin and excrete bile. The immaturity of the liver affects the infant's ability to detoxify substances, effectively process medications, and break down vitamins and minerals.

CLEFT LIP

A cleft lip is characterized by a fissure or opening in the upper lip and is a result of the failure of the embryonic structures of the face to unite. In many cases, the condition seems to be caused by hereditary predisposition, coupled with a minor deviation in the intrauterine environment. This disorder appears more frequently in boys than in girls and may occur on one or both sides of the lip. The extent of the defect may vary from slight to severe. Sometimes it is accompanied by a **cleft palate**, a fissure in the midline of the roof of the mouth. Cleft lip and cleft palate are common congenital anomalies, occurring in about 1 in approximately 700 births.

Treatment and Nursing Care

The initial treatment is surgical repair. The cleft lip is usually repaired first because it interferes with the infant's ability to eat. If the infant cannot create a

vacuum in the mouth, there can be difficulty with sucking. Surgery not only improves the infant's sucking, it also greatly improves the appearance. Currently, it is performed any time after birth if the infant's general health is good and there is no infection. Most infants undergo repair at around 10 to 12 weeks of age (Figure 14-1).

Feeding Method for Neonates with Cleft Lip, Cleft Palate, or Both. Babies with cleft lip and/or cleft palate can be fed by bottle or breast. Several specialized feeders (e.g., the Haberman Feeder, Pigeon Bottle, and Mead-Johnson Cleft Palate Feeder) are used to feed the infant before and after surgery. These feeders are designed to provide easy but limited flow of the liquid. Sometimes a soft, cross-cut nipple can be used.

Breastfeeding is possible for these babies but may require the assistance of a lactation specialist. Infants with cleft lip are usually more successful with breastfeeding than the infant with cleft palate or a cleft lip and cleft palate. Mothers who wish to breastfeed to gain all the benefits from breastfeeding should be supported. Skill 14-1 describes mechanical feeding methods that may be used for infants with both cleft lip and cleft palate. After the infant has established a feeding routine, the infant should be able to complete the feeding in 18 to 30 minutes. An infant who requires a longer feeding period could be working too hard and expending too many calories. This would not promote growth, which is a goal for these infants. It is important for the nurse and the caregiver to remain flexible and patient in feeding these infants. It may require trying several different systems and techniques before the best one is found (Figure 14-2).

Postoperative Care

Postoperative nursing goals for a child with cleft lip/palate repair include (1) preventing the child from excessive crying, which could cause tension on the suture line, (2) careful positioning (*never* on the

Skill 14-1 Oral Feeding for Infants with Cleft Lip or Cleft Palate

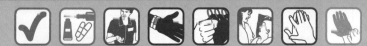

Equipment	Description	Method
✓ Soft, thin-walled nipple (preemie nipple)	• Compresses easily; readily available	1. Use a nipple or feeding system that provides a controllable flow rate and is energy-efficient for the infant.
✓ NUK orthodontic nipple	• Large surface for compression	2. Hold infant in upright position to assist in reducing the amount of nasal regurgitation.
✓ Cross-cut nipple	• Allows easy flow of milk with compression	3. Use a pillow for additional support for infant to assist with longer feeding times.
✓ Ross Cleft Palate Nurser	• For infants with weak suck; has soft tubelike nipple that delivers past the cleft	4. Keep chin tucked because neck extension inhibits swallowing.
✓ Mead Johnson Cleft Palate Nurser	• Soft, long cross-cut nipple; soft bottle for squeezing and monitoring milk flow; can use cross-cut or NUK nipples with this system	5. If regurgitation occurs (milk coming out through the nose), stop feeding and allow infant to cough/sneeze to clear nasal airway.
✓ Haberman Feeder	• Large, squeezable nipple with a slit cut; has one-way valve to reduce amount of air ingested; two nipple lengths available: regular and short	6. Place nipple on top of tongue. Nipple insertion may push tongue to the back of mouth.\n7. Burp the infant frequently because of increased air ingestion.\n8. Monitor for distress and fatigue during feeding.\n9. Limit feeding time to approximately 30 minutes to avoid fatigue.
✓ Pigeon Cleft Palate Nurser	• Larger, more bulbous Y-cut nipple; firm on top with soft bottom; has air valve to prevent collapse and air flow; has flow setting in bottle collar	10. Follow feeding with sterile water to clean any trapped food in the cleft.\n11. Clean mouth and nose.
✓ Asepto syringe, rubber tip	• Readily available; places milk beyond cleft	

Adapted from Cleft Palate Foundation. (2002). *Feeding an infant with a cleft.* Chapel Hill, NC: Author.

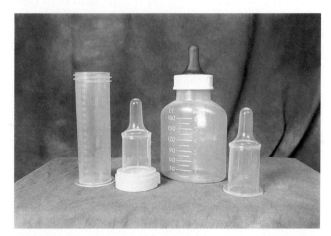

FIGURE 14-2 Devices used to feed an infant with cleft lip and cleft palate. *Right to left,* Haberman Feeder and Mead Johnson Nurser.

abdomen) to avoid injury to the operative site, (3) cleaning the suture line to prevent crusts from forming, which could cause scarring, (4) applying restraints to prevent injury to the operative site and using a butterfly strip or a Logan bow (bar) (to reduce tension on the suture line), and (5) cuddling and other forms of affection to provide for the infant's emotional needs. This last is of particular importance because the infant is unable to obtain the usual satisfactions from sucking.

Suture line care may involve application of an antibacterial ointment, depending on the surgeon's instruction. Cotton-tipped applicators should be avoided to prevent injuring the surgical site. The surgical site may be rinsed with sterile saline solution. The infant receives feedings by special feeder until the wound is completely healed (from 1 to 2 weeks).

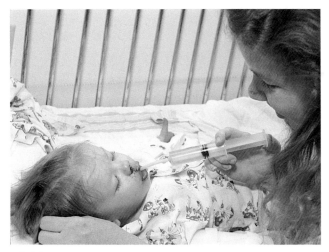

FIGURE 14-3 After a cleft lip repair, a syringe with a rubber tip is used for feeding to prevent trauma to the incision.

CLEFT PALATE

A cleft palate is more serious than a cleft lip. It forms a passageway between the nasopharynx and the nose, which not only complicates feeding but easily leads to infections of the respiratory tract and middle ear and is generally responsible for speech difficulties in later life. Unlike cleft lip, cleft palate is more common in girls than in boys.

Treatment

Most surgeons prefer to operate between 7 to 15 months of age, so that speech patterns are not affected. Even with the advances in surgical techniques, many centers are electing to repair the cleft palate during these times (Campbell et al., 2010). There are several approaches to repair depending on the severity of the defect. While a single surgery may be all that is necessary, future surgical interventions may be required as the child grows.

The management of the child with a cleft lip and cleft palate requires expert teamwork over a long period of time. The emotional problems that sometimes occur with this condition may require more extensive attention than the repair itself. A child born with a facial deformity encounters many problems. It is difficult to be unattractive when society places such importance on good looks. The parent's first reaction to a disfigured newborn infant may be one of shock, hurt, disappointment, and guilt. Some parents may regard the deformity as a result of their inadequacies. It should be strongly stressed that they are not responsible for causing the defect. They may desire to hide the child from relatives and friends. Feedings are difficult. As the child grows, irregular tooth eruptions, drooling, delayed speech, and intermittent hospitalizations and frequent clinic appointments can be frustrating. The developing child senses the feelings of the

parents and acquires either a positive or a negative self-attitude.

In large cities, special cleft palate clinics are available where several specialists can work together in convenient consultation. The parents should be informed of the resources available in the state in which they live. Financial assistance is usually indicated because of the length of treatment required.

Postoperative Management and Nursing Care

Nutrition. Fluids are best taken by a cup, although an Asepto syringe with a rubber tip (gravity feeder) may be used (Figure 14-3). Hot foods and liquids should be avoided to prevent injury to the surgical site. All objects should be kept out of the mouth. This includes straws, tongue blades, spoons, forks, and pacifiers. A wide-bodied spoon may be used if the food is fed from the side of the spoon and does not come in contact with the roof of the mouth. The diet progresses from a clear to a full liquid diet. The older child may go home on a soft diet (nothing harder than mashed potatoes).

Oral Hygiene. The mouth is kept clean at all times. Feedings should be followed by a little water. The doctor may prescribe a mild antiseptic mouthwash.

Restraints. Elbow restraints are generally sufficient for a young child. They should be removed under supervision one at a time periodically to prevent constriction of circulation and to allow normal movement. It is important to prevent the child from placing fingers or objects in the mouth. Discuss with the older child to keep the tongue away from the sore part of the mouth.

Speech. Children who have had extensive repairs or have associated deafness will need the help of a speech therapist. Others simply require a minimum of help from their parents.

Diversion. The goal is for the child to cry as little as possible. Play should be quiet, particularly in the immediate postoperative period. Read to the child or help the child color.

Complications. Otitis media and dental problems may accompany this condition. The parent should seek medical attention at the first signs of earache. Children with cleft palate are at high risk for developing hearing loss and should be closely followed (Kaster et al., 2008). Because of the involvement of the palate, development of teeth may be involved and the orthodontist may be involved until adulthood.

GASTROSCHISIS AND OMPHALOCELE

These two defects allow abdominal contents to herniate outside the abdominal cavity (Figure 14-4). The

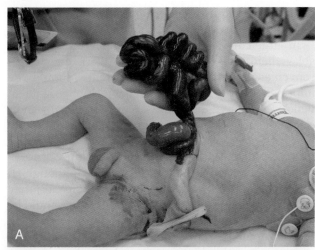

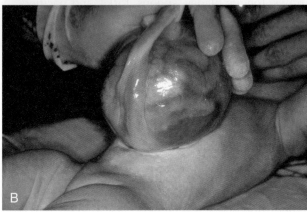

FIGURE 14-4 **A,** Gastroschisis. **B,** Omphalocele.

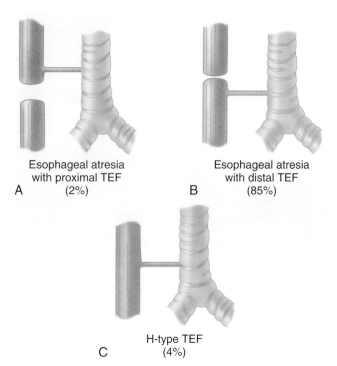

Esophageal atresia
with proximal TEF
A (2%)

Esophageal atresia
with distal TEF
B (85%)

H-type TEF
C (4%)

FIGURE 14-5 **A**, The esophagus ends in a blind pouch with a fistula between the distal esophagus and trachea. **B**, Esophageal atresia with distal fistula. **C**, Tracheoesophageal fistula without esophageal atresia.

gastroschisis usually occurs to the right of the umbilical cord. It is usually a small defect and involves only the bowel. It does not have a sac covering the defect. An omphalocele is a herniation of the gut into the umbilical cord. It is generally a large defect involving the bowel, liver, spleen, bladder, uterus, or ovaries. It is contained in a translucent sac with amniotic fluid. Improvement with survival rates has been helped by prenatal detection and cesarean delivery in a medical facility able to handle the care of this infant.

Treatment and Nursing Care

After delivery, care is given to prevent rupture of the sac with the omphalocele. Any exposed viscera are covered with warm saline-soaked gauze covered with plastic dressing to prevent radiant heat loss. The infant requires monitoring of respirations, temperature, and hydration status. Surgical repair is necessary for both defects. Small defects may be repaired by replacing the exposed viscera back into the abdominal cavity. For large defects, the surgical repair may require a staged repair. A Silastic silo or tubelike material is sutured around the defect. The abdominal contents are within the silo and are slowly pushed into the abdominal cavity. This procedure may take 7 to 10 days, which allows for the abdominal cavity to expand accommodating the bowel.

During the reduction period, the infant is at risk for infection, hypothermia, dehydration and shock, and decreased lower extremity circulation. When the bowel is completely reduced into the abdominal cavity, the infant is ready for complete closure. Postoperative nursing care requires pain control. Nursing priorities include monitoring respiratory and circulatory status and bowel function. Total parenteral nutrition (TPN) provides nutritional needs until bowel function has returned. Feeding is introduced slowly as tolerance is monitored. With the improvement of parenteral nutrition and neonatal care, survival rates are 90% to 95% (Durken and Shaaban, 2009).

ESOPHAGEAL ATRESIA AND TRACHEOESOPHAGEAL FISTULA ATRESIA

Esophageal atresia (EA) is a congenital defect in which the esophagus fails to connect to the stomach. It ends in a blind pouch. Most cases are associated with tracheoesophageal fistula (TEF), which is characterized by an abnormal connection or fistula between the esophagus and the trachea (Figure 14-5). There may be a maternal history of **polyhydramnios** (excess of amniotic fluid in pregnancy).

Treatment and Nursing Care

At birth, the infant presents with excessive oral secretions and accompanying coughing, choking, and cyanosis. These symptoms may worsen when feeding is attempted. Respiratory distress can present when the excessive secretions are aspirated or when the secretions pass into the trachea through a fistula. If an EA is not present, diagnosis may be more difficult. Diagnosis is determined by attempting to pass a small-bore NG tube into the esophagus. If passage is not possible, radiograph is used to diagnosis the defect.

A low-suction catheter is placed in the blind pouch to control secretions. The infant is maintained in an upright position or reverse Trendelenburg position to reduce the risk of aspiration. Priority nursing interventions include monitoring respiratory status, maintaining NPO (nothing by mouth) status, and administering oxygen. Antimicrobials are given for possible infection related to aspiration pneumonia. A gastrostomy tube or button is placed to provide nutrition and gastric decompression.

Surgical intervention is necessary. It involves reattaching the ends of the esophagus and ligation of the fistula. If the distance between the two ends of the esophagus is too far, surgery to connect these may be delayed. The esophagus may need to be lengthened before the ends can be attached.

Postoperative care involves care of a chest tube, a gastrostomy tube, and an NG/orogastric tube connected to low suction. As with any postoperative child, the nurse needs to monitor respiratory status, hydration status, thermoregulation, pain, and infection and assist in providing bonding between parent and infant. The infant may be prescribed peptic acid blockers to help with any reflux. As the infant progresses toward discharge, parents need education regarding home care and feedings. This may be more relevant for infants who require further surgical interventions.

BILIARY ATRESIA

Biliary atresia is a disorder in which an obstruction of the flow of bile results from the destruction or absence of extrahepatic bile ducts. It is more common in girls than in boys. Infants are generally born with a normal birth weight.

Signs and Symptoms

There is persistent jaundice continuing after the period of newborn physiologic hyperbilirubinemia (beyond 14 days of age). The liver becomes enlarged (hepatomegaly), and the abdomen is distended. Lab values for bilirubin are elevated. The body tries to eliminate the excessive bilirubin by excretion through the kidneys, which turns the urine a dark tea color. Bile is deposited in the tissue, causing jaundice and pruritus. Eventually the spleen becomes enlarged (splenomegaly) as the disorder progresses. Early stools may be normal color, but as the disorder progresses, stools become acholic. Lacking bile, the infant is unable to digest fats and absorb A, D, E, and K fat-soluble vitamins. The infant becomes malnourished. The lack of bile flow results in destruction of liver tissue and development of cirrhosis.

Diagnostic tools include liver biopsy, hepatobiliary excretory exam, and ultrasound.

Treatment

Early diagnosis is critical to the course of the disorder. A palliative surgery (hepatoportoenterostomy or Kasai procedure) has the best results when done within 60 days of birth. Untreated biliary atresia has a poor prognosis, with death within 2 years (Feldman, 2006). Most of these children will require a liver transplant. The success rate for transplantation has improved. The availability of small donor livers remains an issue. Advances using partial liver transplantation are promising.

Nursing Care

The diagnosis of biliary atresia is devastating to the family. Parents will need emotional and educational support. Special formulas may be needed to maximize absorption. Monitoring the infant's intake and weight is important. Itching as a result of the deposit of bile salts in the tissue is a frustrating side effect. Medications such as ursodeoxycholic acid (Ursodiol, Actigall) help to increase the bile flow and decrease itching. Diphenhydramine (Benadryl) can be used to help alleviate itching. Skin integrity should be closely monitored. Measures to reduce scratching, such as covering hands and keeping the nails short, are helpful. Tepid baths may also help relieve itching and patting rather than rubbing the skin can help prevent further skin irritation. Children can become irritable with the intense itching. The nurse can assist the family in coping with a child who is extremely irritable.

PYLORIC STENOSIS

Pyloric stenosis (narrowing of the pylorus) is a disorder of the digestive tract. The pylorus, the lower end of the stomach, becomes partially blocked so that food does not empty properly into the duodenum (Figure 14-6). Pyloric stenosis is caused by an overgrowth of the circular muscles of the pylorus. The stomach muscles above the obstructed area also enlarge in their attempt to force material through the narrowed passage. An abnormal increase in the size of an organ or part, such as this, is called hypertrophy. This condition is commonly classified as a congenital anomaly; however, its symptoms do not appear until the infant is 2 or 3 weeks old. Pyloric stenosis is the most common surgical condition of the digestive tract in infancy. Its incidence is higher in boys than in girls, with a tendency for it to be inherited.

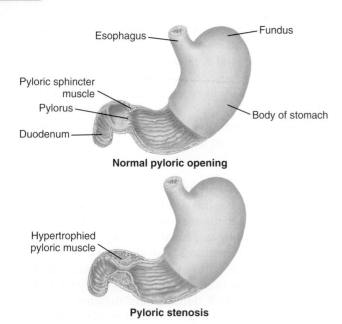

Normal pyloric opening

Pyloric stenosis

FIGURE 14-6 In pyloric stenosis, the pyloric muscle hypertrophies and obstructs the passage of stomach contents into the intestines. Surgically splitting the muscle relieves the obstruction.

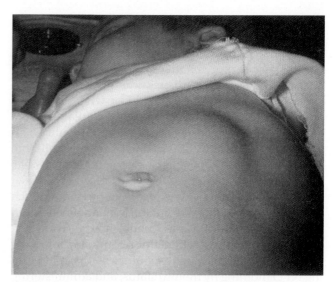

FIGURE 14-7 Visible peristaltic waves associated with pyloric stenosis.

Signs and Symptoms

Vomiting is the outstanding symptom of this disorder. The force of vomiting progresses until most of the food is ejected several inches from the mouth. This is termed projectile vomiting and occurs before and after feedings. The nonbilious vomitus contains mucus and may be blood streaked but does not contain bile. The infant is constantly hungry and eats again immediately after vomiting has occurred. Dehydration, as evidenced by a sunken fontanel, poor turgor, and decreased urination, may occur. An olive-shaped mass may be felt in the right upper quadrant of the abdomen. Ultrasonography is commonly used for diagnostic purposes because it is noninvasive and accurate. In severe cases, the outline of the distended stomach and peristaltic waves are visible during feedings (Figure 14-7). Urine and blood values are alkaline because the fluid being lost from the body is mostly hydrochloric acid from the stomach juices. Bowel movements gradually diminish because little or no food passes into the intestine.

Treatment

The surgery performed for pyloric stenosis is called pyloromyotomy (*pyloro*, gatekeeper; *myo*, muscle; *tomy*, incision of). This procedure can either be laparoscopic or open. The surgeon incises the pyloric muscle in such a way that the opening is enlarged and food may again pass easily through it.

Nursing Care

If the infant is not dehydrated, surgery is usually performed as soon as possible. The dehydrated infant is given intravenous fluids before surgery to restore fluid and electrolyte balance and prevent shock. The infant may be NPO to prevent further losses from vomiting. Monitoring of intravenous fluids intake, accurate urine output, and emesis should be important nursing actions. Comforting the infant and supporting and alleviating parental anxiety are priority actions.

The postoperative care of the infant includes monitoring of vital signs and intravenous administration of fluids. The wound site is inspected frequently for bleeding. Signs of shock are an increase in the pulse rate and respiration rate; pale cool skin; and restlessness. An NG tube may or may not be in place; it is usually removed soon after surgery so that oral feedings can begin. Current views are that the infant may resume full-strength formula or breast milk 4 hours after surgery (Miniati and Albanese, 2004). Vomiting may occur after surgery, but it gradually diminishes. The diaper is placed low over the abdomen to prevent irritation of the surgical sites.

The infant is generally discharged 24 to 48 hours after surgery. Normal feedings are reestablished. Parental instructions should include feeding schedule and wound care. Parents should have instructions regarding symptoms of complications such as wound infection, recurrent vomiting, and dehydration. Follow-up care is stressed.

HERNIA

An inguinal hernia is a protrusion of part of the abdominal contents through the inguinal canal in the groin. The condition is more common in boys than in girls. It is also seen frequently in premature infants. Hernias may be present at birth (congenital) or may be acquired and can vary in size. A hernia is termed **reducible** if the abdominal contents can be put back in place with gentle pressure; if this cannot be done, it is called an **irreducible** or an **incarcerated** (constricted) **hernia**.

Signs and Symptoms

The infant with a hernia may be relatively free of symptoms. Irritability, fretfulness, and constipation are sometimes evident. The diagnosis is made when physical examination shows a mass in the inguinal area that reappears from time to time, particularly when the child cries or strains (Figure 14-8). A **strangulated hernia** occurs when the intestine becomes caught in the passage and the blood supply is diminished. This happens more frequently during the first 6 months of life. Vomiting and severe abdominal pain are present. Emergency surgery is necessary if strangulation occurs, and in some cases a bowel resection is performed.

Treatment and Nursing Care

Inguinal hernias are repaired successfully with the surgical operation called a **herniorrhaphy**. This is a relatively simple procedure that is done in same-day surgery units. Parents remain with the child during the entire time except for the actual procedure. They are encouraged to assist in routine postoperative care if they choose. Often no dressing is applied to the incision or sometimes a waterproof collodion dressing may be used. Postoperative care is directed toward keeping the incision clean. Diapers are left opened and are changed frequently. The child is discharged in about 2 to 3 hours, when fluids are tolerated. Activity is not limited. Parents are provided with written instructions about home management. Follow-up telephone calls may be made by nursing personnel, and return appointments are scheduled.

Children with incarcerated hernias are hospitalized. After surgery, vital signs are carefully monitored.

Nasogastric (NG) suctioning and intravenous fluids are maintained until bowel function returns. The nurse measures and records the child's intake and output. The child is turned frequently to avoid respiratory complications. The nurse observes the child carefully for signs of peritonitis or bowel obstruction.

UMBILICAL HERNIA

An umbilical hernia is a protrusion of a portion of intestine through the umbilical ring, an opening in the muscular area of the abdomen where the umbilical vessels pass through (Figure 14-9). This type of hernia appears as a soft swelling, covered by skin that protrudes when the infant cries or strains. Most small umbilical hernias disappear spontaneously during the first year of life. This type of hernia is not known to become strangulated or to cause other complications.

Treatment

Generally, surgery is not advised unless the hernia causes symptoms, becomes enlarged, or persists until the child is 3 to 5 years of age. The use of tape, coins, or abdominal binding in an attempt to reduce the hernia is ineffective.

CONGENITAL DIAPHRAGMATIC HERNIA

Diaphragmatic hernia can be either congenital or traumatic. Congenital diaphragmatic hernia causes abdominal contents in the fetus to protrude through the

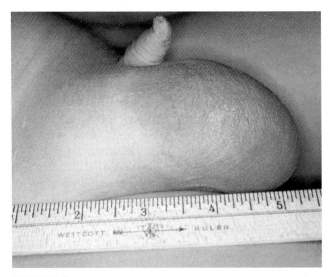

FIGURE 14-8 Inguinal hernia in a male may occur with crying and straining.

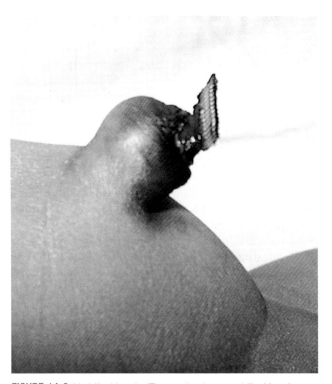

FIGURE 14-9 Umbilical hernia. The predominant umbilical hernia was noted at birth.

diaphragm. The size of the defect can vary from a small to a large opening. Herniation of abdominal contents into the chest cavity impairs lung development, resulting in pulmonary hypoplasia and pulmonary hypertension. In severe cases, the heart can also be impacted. There is an association with other anomalies such as cardiovascular lesions, central nervous system lesions, omphalocele, and esophageal atresia.

Frequently diagnosis is made during a prenatal ultrasound. Postnatal diagnosis may be made with a chest x-ray demonstrating gastric air or bowel loops in the chest. Bowel sounds may be auscultated in the chest. Clinically the newborn may have respiratory distress, which may present at birth or may develop several hours after delivery.

Treatment

In utero fetal surgery has been used in an attempt to remove the abdominal contents from the chest and allow for improved lung development. This procedure is a high risk for both the fetus and mother and has not improved survival (Townsend, 2007). Identification of the defect prenatally provides the opportunity to have the mother followed in a medical center that can handle the infant's postnatal needs.

Postnatal interventions require cardiac and respiratory stabilization before surgery. Intubation is necessary. Surgery to remove abdominal contents is done. These children continue to have long-term neurologic and developmental issues, seizures, and hearing loss.

CELIAC DISEASE

Celiac disease, also known as *celiac sprue* and *gluten-sensitive enteropathy*, is a lifelong, genetic disorder that results in the inability to digest gluten. It is a multi-system disorder with a complex autoimmune response in predisposed individuals, resulting in malabsorption and maldigestion of nutrients, vitamins, and minerals.

Signs and Symptoms

Gluten is a protein found in wheat, barley, and rye. Oats are considered questionable as the harvesting and milling process can allow contamination with gluten. Between the ages of 1 and 5, many foods with gluten (e.g., pasta, bread, cereals) are introduced into the child's diet. Gluten breaks down into *gliadin* in the small intestine. In celiac disease, the gliadin cannot be digested and damage to intestinal mucosal cells occurs. Although symptoms may not be noticed initially, malabsorption results and children begin to manifest symptoms that may include failure to thrive, chronic diarrhea, abdominal distention, muscle wasting, anorexia, and irritability. Stools are described as foul-smelling and fatty in appearance because of the malabsorption. Non-gastrointestinal symptoms include short stature, osteoporosis, iron deficiency anemia,

hepatitis, headache, depression, dermatitis herpetiformis, and diabetes (Kliegman et al., 2007).

Treatment and Nursing Care

Serology tests can assist with diagnosis. Anti-endomysium IgA antibody (EmA) can be used with children as a screening test. A more definitive test is a small bowel (jejunal) biopsy. Once diagnosed, celiac disease is managed through dietary restrictions. All gluten should be removed from the diet. Foods containing wheat, barley, rye, and oats should not be eaten. Rice, corn, and soy are safe to eat if no gluten has been added to them. There are many sources of hidden gluten in prepared foods; therefore it is usually necessary to consult a dietitian to design a gluten-free diet. Symptoms may be relieved in as early as 1 week after introducing a gluten-free diet.

This lifelong diet may be difficult to adhere to. It is important to help the child learn the necessary dietary restrictions to avoid later complications. Parents must read all food labels to identify any gluten. With governmental labeling requirements, wheat has become much easier to identify. Barley and rye may be more difficult to identify. The family and the child will benefit from the assistance of a dietician. Experimentation of new recipes with suitable ingredients, such as Mexican or Chinese dishes that use corn or rice, helps the family adjust. Vitamin supplements may be necessary. Teenagers may also have difficulty maintaining their diet since they do not want to be seen as different. Health care professionals and parents play a vital role in helping children to adapt to the dietary changes necessary to live a fulfilling life.

 Community Considerations

Parents can contact the Celiac Sprue Association/United States of America, Inc, at 877-CSA-4CSA (*www.csaceliacs. org*).

SHORT GUT SYNDROME

Short gut syndrome is a result of the loss of part of the small bowel. There can be a variety of causes for the loss, including gastroschisis, bowel atresias, necrotizing enterocolitis, meconium peritonitis, and trauma. The infant has 200 to 250 cm of small bowel. A bowel length of at least 15 cm with an ileocecal valve or 29 cm without the valve has the potential for survival. In addition to the length of bowel, the sections of bowel that are missing affect survival (Table 14-2).

Treatment and Nursing Care

The goal for treatment is replacement of fluids and nutrition. Total parenteral nutrition (TPN) may be required. A central venous catheter is placed to provide access for TPN and fluids. Enteral nutrition is begun

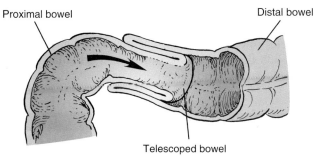

FIGURE 14-10 In intussusception, a portion of the bowel telescopes into itself, causing signs and symptoms of intestinal obstruction.

Table 14-2	Small Bowel Absorption	
SECTION OF SMALL BOWEL	**ABSORPTION ACTION**
Duodenum and jejunum	Calcium, magnesium, phosphorus, iron, folic acid
Proximal small intestine (100-200 cm)	Carbohydrates, protein, water-soluble vitamins
Small intestine	Monoglycerides, fatty acids, triglycerides
Distal ileum	Vitamin B$_{12}$, bile acids
Colon	Water, electrolytes

Adapted from Kliegman, R., Behrman, R., Jenson, H., et al. (2007). *Nelson's textbook of pediatrics* (18th ed.). Philadelphia: Saunders.

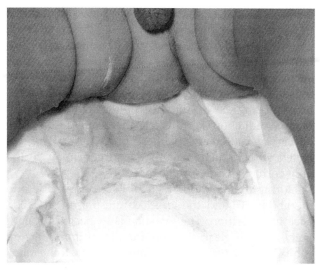

FIGURE 14-11 "Currant jelly" stools are a classic sign of intussusception.

as soon as possible by continuous feeding through an NG or gastrostomy tube. Breast milk is the first choice of feeding as it assists the infant's immune system, contains growth factors, and has a less risk for allergies (Olieman et al., 2010). Feedings are started slowly and advanced based on stool output and abdominal symptoms. It is essential that oral feedings begin as soon as possible to prevent the loss of suck-and-swallow reflexes. A pacifier may help in maintaining sucking.

Infant intestines can continue to grow and adapt, which may help with the prognosis. For children who cannot be weaned from parenteral nutrition and cannot tolerate enteral feeding, bowel transplants may be an option.

INTUSSUSCEPTION

Intussusception (*intus*, within; *suscipere*, to receive) is a slipping of one part of the intestine into another part just below it (Figure 14-10). The condition is frequently seen at the ileocecal valve, where the small intestine opens into the ascending colon. The **mesentery**, a double fan-shaped fold of peritoneum that covers most of the intestine, is filled with blood vessels and nerves and is also pulled along. Edema occurs. Initially, this telescoping of the bowel causes intestinal obstruction, but as peristalsis forces the structures tighter, strangulation takes place. This portion may burst, causing peritonitis.

Intussusception generally occurs in male infants who are otherwise healthy. It can occur at any age but typically affects children under 2 years of age, with the highest incidence rate between 4 and 9 months of age. The exact cause is still in question. Occasionally, the condition corrects itself without treatment. This is termed a **spontaneous reduction**. However, because the child's life is in danger, the physician does not wait for spontaneous reduction. The prognosis is good when the condition is treated within 24 hours.

Signs and Symptoms

In typical cases the onset is sudden. The infant feels severe pain in the abdomen, evidenced by loud cries, straining efforts, and the kicking and drawing of the legs toward the abdomen. Typically, the child is comfortable between pains, but the intervals shorten and the condition worsens. The child vomits; the contents are green or greenish yellow in color because of bile stain, and the contents are described as **bilious**. If the condition is left untreated, fecal vomiting ensues. Bowel movements diminish, and little flatus is passed. Stools with blood and mucus, which contain no feces, are common about 12 hours after the onset of the obstruction; these are termed currant jelly stools (Figure 14-11). Guiac stool testing is used to determine if blood is present. The child's fever may run as high as 106° F (41.1° C), and signs of shock such as sweating, weak pulse, and shallow grunting respirations appear. The abdomen is rigid.

Treatment

Intussusception is an emergency situation, and because of the severity of the symptoms, most parents contact a physician promptly. The diagnosis is determined from the history and physical findings. The physician may feel a sausage-shaped mass in the right upper portion of the abdomen during bimanual rectal and abdominal palpation. An ultrasound may also indicate the mass. Hydrostatic reduction materials such as air, oxygen, saline, and aqueous contrast materials have proven successful to reduce the intussusception (Keating, 2006). Intussusception may recur after manual reduction. For this reason, the child is kept for observation after any of these procedures. If uncorrected with reduction methods, surgery may be the only corrective measure.

During the operation a small incision is made into the abdomen, and the affected intestine is "milked" back into position. The intestine is inspected for gangrene, and, if clear, the abdomen is sutured. Barring complications, recovery is straightforward. If the intestine cannot be reduced or if gangrene has set in, a resection is done and the affected bowel is removed. The cut end of the ileum is joined to the cut end of the colon; this is called an anastomosis.

Nursing Care

Preoperative. Treatment is aimed at combating shock and restoring blood, fluids, and electrolytes. As with any surgery, a written consent for surgery from the parents or guardians of the child is needed. While the surgeon will explain the course of treatment, many times parents need information reinforced.

Gastric suction is necessary to prevent stomach distention. This may be continued for some time after surgery, particularly if a resection is done. Elbow restraints to prevent dislodgment of the nasal tube may be necessary. Preoperative medication is given to relax the child and to prevent the aspiration of secretions. Once the child has been medicated, the surrounding activity should be kept to a minimum. The medical record accompanies the child. Proper safety precautions are taken during transit.

More than likely, this is the first surgery the child has undergone. The parents need to be supported. Explanations concerning the procedures and care of the child are important to them. Most pediatric hospitals allow parents to accompany the child to the surgical preop area. Make sure they know where the family can stay during the surgical procedure. Information provided in a timely manner is consoling and respectful to the family.

Postoperative. After surgery, care is mainly symptomatic. Vital signs are checked frequently, the child's position is changed often, and careful attention is given to the skin. Mouth care is essential because the child receives little or nothing by mouth for a while. The nostrils need cleaning and lubricating because the nasal tube can be irritating. If a urinary catheter is used, drainage is measured and described in the nurse's notes. The incision site is kept clean and dry.

Promptly report any odor from the incision or increased abdominal distention. Clear fluids are begun when bowel sounds are present. The passage of gas, liquids, or solids through the rectum is of particular significance because it indicates peristalsis.

 Safety Alert

The most definitive method for evaluation of abdominal distention is to measure the circumference of the abdomen.

Gastric suction keeps the stomach and upper intestine empty. The gastric tube is attached to suction and is run on low to avoid damage to the lining of the stomach. Small saline irrigations are usually ordered to prevent clogging of the tube. Drainage is measured and recorded every 8 hours or more frequently if necessary. Accurate recording of fluid drainage is essential because this type of drainage removes salts and hydrochloric acid from the stomach, which must be replaced by intravenous fluids.

Pain management is a top priority especially with an infant who cannot verbally express pain. The infant and the family are given supportive help throughout this ordeal. A pacifier may soothe the infant who is deprived of feeding by mouth. Some of these children are at an age when fear of strangers is prevalent; thus their need for the security of parents is paramount.

 Community Considerations

Rotovirus vaccine had been linked to intussusception in the past and resulted in the vaccine being removed from the market. Improved rotovirus vaccines are now available and have no association with an increased risk of intussusceptions. The CDC website provides information for parents regarding this vaccination (Belongia et al., 2010)

HIRSCHSPRUNG'S DISEASE

Hirschsprung's disease, or **aganglionic megacolon**, is characterized by the absence of ganglion nerve cells in the colon (Figure 14-12). This causes abnormal peristalsis and resulting chronic constipation. The affected segment of the colon is in constant contraction and obstructs the flow of stool. The portion of the colon proximal to the affected colon becomes distended (megacolon). The results can be decreased blood flow, ischemia, and breakdown of the intestinal walls. Inflammation (enterocolitis) and infection can result in a life-threatening situation.

Signs and Symptoms

Newborn infants who do not pass meconium stool within 48 hours of birth should be evaluated. Other symptoms include bilious vomiting, abdominal

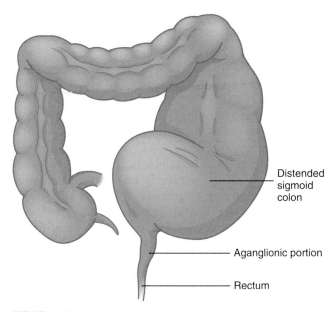

FIGURE 14-12 In Hirschsprung's disease, dilation of the colon occurs proximal to the aganglionic section.

distention, and refusal to eat. Older children have a history of chronic constipation with foul-smelling, pellet-like stools, ribbon-like stools, or liquid stools. They have abdominal distention and may have failure to thrive. Parents may have tried a variety of methods to treat the constipation. Diagnosis is made with a rectal mucosa biopsy and rectal manometry (measures the strength of the internal rectal sphincter).

Treatment and Nursing Care
Nursing interventions include parent education and support during the testing procedures. The disease requires the surgical removal of the affected portion of the colon and anastomosis of the normal bowel to the rectum. The surgical correction of the affected colon can involve a stepped approach with a colostomy in the first few weeks followed by corrective surgery in 3 to 6 months. Another approach is to perform a complete repair without a colostomy on the infant in the first few weeks of life.

Before surgery, the child is NPO and undergoes gastric decompression. Fluids and electrolytes are administered and monitored. Abdominal distention should be monitored with repeated measurements. Antimicrobials may be administered if enterocolitis is suspected. Depending on the age of the child, both child and parents need support and education regarding ostomy care if necessary.

Postoperative care is similar to that of any abdominal surgery. The child is NPO and often has an NG tube to suction for gastric decompression. All fluid output is measured and documented. A Foley catheter may be in place to prevent contamination to the wound site. TPN is used until sufficient enteral intake occurs. Assessment of bowel function is monitored and

indicates the readiness for oral feedings. If a colostomy was performed, the nurse follows routine ostomy care. Rectal irrigations with normal saline help to decrease the risk of postoperative enterocolitis. Special attention to the perineal area is necessary as frequent liquid stools can cause skin breakdown (Verklan and Walden, 2009). Parents should be encouraged to participate in the care of the child in preparing for home discharge. Long-term issues can include constipation and fecal incontinence, which usually improve over time.

ACUTE GASTROENTERITIS

Infections of the gastrointestinal tract are caused by bacteria, viruses, or parasites. Most infections are a result of oral-fecal contamination or ingestion of contaminated food or water. Worldwide infectious diarrhea remains the leading cause for childhood morbidity and mortality. Deaths in developing countries have been drastically reduced with water quality, personal hygiene, sanitation, and food safety. Rotovirus is the most common cause of viral gastroenteritis in children (Kliegman et al., 2007).

Diarrhea, vomiting, and abdominal cramping are the most common symptoms. Quick assessment includes evaluation of the child's hydration status, determination of potential exposure history, and identification of causative agent. Stool examination is used to identify causative agents.

Treatment and Nursing Care
The focus of treatment is to restore hydration. Oral rehydration solutions can be used in the home setting or hospital (see Chapter 15 for discussion on dehydration). If severe dehydration is present, fluids may be replaced through the intravenous route. Once hydration is established, early feeding including breastfeeding is recommended. Complex carbohydrates (rice, potatoes, breads, cereals) are well tolerated. Fatty foods, carbonated drinks, or foods high in simple sugar should be avoided. Most children are able to tolerate milk, so lactose-free formulas are unnecessary (Kliegman et al., 2007). If the causative agent is bacterial, antimicrobials are administered. Prevention of gastroenteritis caused by the rotovirus has been decreased with the use of the rotovirus vaccine (see Chapter 18).

Vomiting is a common problem with gastroenteritis. Persistent vomiting requires monitoring because it results in dehydration and electrolyte imbalance. The continuous loss of hydrochloric acid and sodium chloride from the stomach can cause alkalosis. In this condition, the acid-base balance of the body becomes disturbed because of a loss of chlorides and potassium. This can result in death if left untreated.

Vomiting can result from various other causes. Some of them stem from improper feeding techniques. Sometimes the difficulty lies with the formula. If the fat content is too high, it can slow down the emptying process of the stomach. The introduction of foods of a different consistency may also precipitate this symptom. Infants sometimes instigate vomiting by gagging themselves with fingers or objects of play.

 Communication

When assessing a vomiting infant, the nurse should include the following questions: Was the infant fed too fast or given too much? Was the infant burped frequently and properly positioned after the feeding? Has there been a recent formula increase or change? Were any previous feedings vomited?

Other factors that cause vomiting are ear, nose, and throat infections. Vomiting is seen in the primary stages of many communicable diseases. Specific disorders, such as Reye syndrome, peptic ulcer disease, increased intracranial pressure, strangulated hernia, and various bowel obstructions, are also responsible. In these conditions, the vomiting is not necessarily associated with feedings. When the cause of the illness is discovered and properly treated, the symptom disappears. Aspiration and aspiration pneumonia are serious complications of vomiting. Vomitus becomes drawn into the air passages on inspiration and causes immediate death in extreme cases.

To help prevent vomiting, the nurse must carefully feed and burp the infant, especially an ill child. Treatments are avoided immediately after feedings. The child should be handled as little as possible at this time. To prevent aspiration of vomitus, the nurse places the infant on the right side after feedings. When an older child begins to vomit, the head is turned to one side and an emesis basin and tissues are provided. The child's hands and face are bathed with warm water.

To determine the amount vomited, try weighing the towel, linen, or clothing involved. Factors to be charted include time, amount, color (bloody, bile-stained), consistency, force, frequency, and whether or not vomiting was preceded by nausea or feedings. The diet after vomiting is prescribed by the physician. In the hospital, intravenous fluids may be given. (See Chapter 3 for a discussion on parenteral nutrition.) Oral fluids are withheld for a short time to allow the stomach to rest. Gradually, sips of water are given according to the child's tolerance and condition. The child's intake and output are carefully recorded so that the physician is able to compare the urine output with the total fluid intake.

When vomiting is persistent, drugs such as trimethobenzamide (Tigan) or promethazine (Phenergan) may be prescribed. They are available in rectal suppository form. The nurse lubricates the suppository and inserts it well into the rectum, where it dissolves. Slight pressure is exerted over the anus for a short time to ensure that the suppository is not expelled. Charting includes the time, name of suppository, and whether or not relief from vomiting was obtained.

GASTROESOPHGEAL REFLUX

Gastroesophageal reflux (GER) is one of the most common gastrointestinal disorders in infants. Gastric contents are regurgitated back into the esophagus. GER can be a result of physiologic or pathologic issues. Physiologic GER is common in many healthy infants. An immature lower esophageal sphincter (LES) contributes to the reflux and usually resolves by 1 to 2 years of age. Pathologic GER occurs with other disorders such as cerebral palsy, Down syndrome, or respiratory problems.

Classic symptoms are vomiting and regurgitation especially after feedings accompanied by excessive crying and irritability from the esophagitis. Infants may become difficult to feed, and parents may be reluctant to feed an infant who is constantly spitting up. These factors can lead to failure to thrive. Other complications include apnea, choking, bradycardia, and frequent respiratory infections. Diagnosis includes ruling out other causes. Tests include x-ray, barium swallow, upper GE endoscopy, and pH probe.

Treatment and Nursing Care

Treatment is based on the severity of the symptoms. It will involve dietary and positional changes, medications, and possible surgical interventions. Small, frequent feedings, which may be a predigested formula, are started. This decreases the amount of formula in the stomach and helps decrease reflux episodes. Thickening the formula can help with decreasing the episodes of reflux, decreasing crying, and increasing weight gain for the malnourished infant. Older children should avoid esophageal irritants such as caffeine and spicy or acidic foods.

 Safety Alert

Positioning of the infant with GER after feeding has been controversial. The prone position significantly reduces the number of episodes, but for young infants the supine position is recommended to prevent SIDS. The severity of the reflux will determine if the risk for SIDS outweighs the complications from reflux. Placing the infant in a seated position should be avoided. Either the head elevated prone or flat prone position is recommended for infants with GER.

Medications may be used if feeding interventions and positioning are ineffective. The use of acid suppression drugs includes histamine-2 receptor antagonists (Ranitidine [Zantac]); proton-pump inhibitors (Lansoprazole [Prevacid] or Omeprazole [Prilosec]);

and antacids. Over-the-counter antacids are usually not recommended due to side effects. Prokinetic agents such as metoclopramide (Reglan), which improve gastric emptying, may be used. All medications should be given under the direction of the physician as they all have potentially harmful side effects.

Surgical intervention is done for children with severe GER and respiratory complications. A fundoplication involves wrapping the top of the stomach around the LES. This tightens the sphincter and helps prevent gastric reflux. Many times these children will also have a gastrostomy button to assist with decompression. These children will not be able to be burped or vomit. Review Chapter 3 for care of a child with a gastrostomy button.

PINWORM

Of the several varieties of worms that affect humans, the most common is the pinworm *Enterobius vermicularis* (*enteron*, intestine; *bios*, life; *vermis*, wormlike). Pinworms can affect individuals of all ages but are more common in young children. Crowded living conditions, institutions (schools and daycare centers), and pinworm infestation in the family are factors of high risk. The child infects himself or herself by handling contaminated toys or soiled linen. The route of entry is the mouth. The pinworm looks like a white thread about one third of an inch long. It lives in the lower intestine but comes out of the anus to lay its eggs, generally during the night. Hand-to-mouth activity contributes to reinfection.

Signs and Symptoms

Signs and symptoms include the child scratching the bottom, complaining of itchiness, and becoming irritable and restless. Weight loss, poor appetite, and fretfulness during the night may develop. The rectal area may become irritated from scratching. Worms may be seen on the surface of stools or around the anus. A special pinworm diagnostic tape or paddle or a tongue blade covered with cellophane tape, sticky side out, may be placed against the anal region in an attempt to obtain pinworm eggs. This is done early in the morning or after a period of inactivity. The tape is examined in the physician's office with a microscope.

Treatment and Nursing Care

Several effective **anthelmintics** are available. Mebendazole (Vermox) is a single-dose chewable tablet that is appropriate for children older than 2 years of age. It is generally the drug of choice because it is safe and effective and has few side effects. Pyrantel pamoate (Antiminth) can be used and is taken as a single dose that is repeated in 2 weeks. It is not recommended for children younger than 2 years of age. Potential anthelmintic overdose precautions should be discussed with the family.

Home Care Considerations

- All other family members are treated to prevent reinfection.
- Toilet seat is scrubbed daily.
- Underwear and bed linens are washed in hot water.
- Bed linens are handled carefully to avoid spreading the infection.
- Parents are taught the danger of anthelmintic overdosage.

APPENDICITIS

Appendicitis occurs when the opening of the appendix into the cecum becomes obstructed. This may have a number of causes, among them fecaliths (blockage with fecal matter), infection, and allergy. Diet has also been implicated. Appendicitis is rare before 2 years of age but is the most common cause of abdominal surgery during childhood. The incidence rate is higher in boys.

Signs and Symptoms

Symptoms in older children are similar to those in adults and include nausea, with or without vomiting; abdominal tenderness; fever; constipation or diarrhea; and an elevated white blood cell count. Pain, which is initially about the umbilicus, localizes in the right lower quadrant (RLQ) midway between the umbilicus and the iliac crest (McBurney's point).

The symptoms of appendicitis in the young child are more obscure. The child has to be observed carefully over a period of time to determine the diagnosis. The child cries, is restless, and has a low-grade fever. Pain is more generalized and harder to pinpoint, and nausea and vomiting may occur. Because these symptoms accompany many childhood disorders, the diagnosis is more difficult to establish than in adolescents or adults. Having the child stand on the toes and then drop onto the heels often helps localize the pain in cooperative younger children. Pain, followed by a sudden absence of pain, can indicate rupture of the appendix. If the appendix ruptures, the infected contents spill into the abdominal cavity and a generalized infection called peritonitis results.

Absent or diminished bowel sounds, rigid abdomen, and rebound tenderness are also indicative of appendicitis. **Rebound tenderness** can occur when pressure placed on the RLQ is followed by quick release of pressure, resulting in severe pain. Rebound tenderness in the RLQ, although classic for appendicitis, is not reliable in children. Because it can be falsely negative or positive, eliciting it in the child can cause needless pain. Rectal examination elicits tenderness. Diarrhea may be present in retrocecal appendicitis.

A chest radiograph may be ordered to rule out lower lobe pneumonia, which sometimes mimics appendicitis. A careful history and physical examination are paramount. The presence of vomiting and the degree of change in the child's behavior are considered particularly significant. Children almost always refuse solids and liquids. The child may guard the abdomen or voluntarily lie down. Guarding is characterized by tightening or rigidity of the abdominal muscles when the abdomen is palpated. One position frequently seen in the child with appendicitis pain is lying on the side with the knees flexed toward the abdomen.

Treatment and Nursing Care

Appendicitis is treated with a surgical operation called an **appendectomy**. Surgery is performed immediately after diagnosis unless the child is dehydrated and needs rehydration. Antimicrobial therapy is instituted before surgery in the child with a perforated appendix.

> ⚠ **Safety Alert**
>
> Heat is never applied and cathartics are not given because they might cause a rupture, leading to the possibility of peritonitis.

Uncomplicated Appendicitis. Oral fluids and feedings are withheld pending surgery. As in other emergency situations, emotional support is given by the nurse and the child's family. The prognosis of uncomplicated appendicitis is good.

Temperature, pulse, respirations, and blood pressure are monitored. The dressing is observed for drainage. If an intravenous line is running, the type, amount, and rate are observed. The state of consciousness (e.g., alert, groggy), the presence of nausea or vomiting, the appearance of any drainage, and any other pertinent observations are noted.

The child's position is changed frequently. Teach the child to take deep breaths; an incentive spirometer can be used, as can bubbles for younger children. An accurate record of intake and output is kept. The first void should be noted. If the child has not voided by change of the shift, the nurse should report this. The physician's orders indicate whether or not the child with nausea can have sips of water or ice chips.

As soon as the child is able to take and retain water and other fluids by mouth, intravenous feedings are discontinued. Vital signs and bowel sounds are monitored as ordered or according to institutional policies. The child is encouraged to move about in bed; reluctance to move and anorexia may be early signs of complications. Evidence of pain is reported, and analgesics are administered as ordered.

Children recuperate quickly from uncomplicated surgery. Ambulation is generally not a problem. Children usually can return to school in 1 or 2 weeks, but specific instructions concerning restriction of activity should be reviewed before hospital discharge.

Ruptured Appendix. Early recognition of appendicitis decreases the danger of perforation. Parents may be confused by early symptoms and hesitate to obtain medical attention. With a ruptured appendix, the child is acutely ill and the recovery period prolonged. After the appendix ruptures, the abdomen rapidly becomes rigid.

Medical management to prevent shock, dehydration, and infection is instigated before surgery. This usually includes intravenous administration of fluids and electrolytes, systemic antimicrobials, nasogastric suctioning, and positioning in a low Fowler's position or on the right side to facilitate drainage into the pelvic area. The child is given nothing by mouth. Intermittent suction is maintained at appropriate negative pressure, and irrigations are carried out as ordered to ensure patency of the nasogastric tube.

> **Communication**
>
> The nurse can use nonverbal cues such as restlessness and a pain scale with faces for a younger child to identify the level of pain.

Penrose drains may be placed in the incision to drain exudate or abscess. Some surgeons prefer to leave the incision open and packed with Betadine or saline gauze. The nurse may do a wet-to-dry dressing change several times a day, removing the contaminated dressing, and repacking the wound. Wound precautions are followed according to hospital procedure. The area is kept clean and dry, and medication is applied if ordered. Administer analgesics for pain relief. Monitor intake, output, and bowel sounds. Supply nutritious foods as the diet is increased. Administer nursing care as described for the child with simple appendicitis, including appropriate modifications and interventions in nursing care plans. The child should be placed in a semi-Fowler's position to prevent respiratory complications. The child's hospital stay is increased, and intravenous antimicrobial therapy is given.

OBESITY

Obesity is the accumulation of excess body fat. It is the most common nutritional disorder in Western society today, and its treatment record is dismal. Obesity has become an important issue with children. The Centers for Disease Control and Prevention (CDC) has developed growth charts that use body mass index (BMI) for age to determine percentiles. Obesity in children is defined as having a BMI greater than the 95th percentile for age. Children with a BMI between the 85th and 95th percentile for age are defined as overweight. (See Chapter 4 for a discussion on growth standards.)

Signs and Symptoms

Weight gain can occur at any age but appears most frequently in the first year of life, at 5 to 6 years of age, and during adolescence (Kliegman et al., 2007). Most children stay plump during puberty and then return to their normal size after growth is complete.

Obesity becomes particularly significant during adolescence, when feelings of inadequacy are pronounced. Obese adolescents are concerned about their appearance. They are often the subject of cruel ridicule. For instance, overweight males frequently appear to have developed breasts, white striae may appear on the abdomen, and the penis appears disproportionately small. Obese teenagers date less and may feel rejected, unattractive, and unloved. Accompanying the emotional anxieties are the more obvious physical handicaps. Overweight teenagers may be unable to participate in sports or other school activities and are more accident-prone. Their choice of careers is more limited. Although some obese adolescents experience emotional consequences, many do not and become well-adjusted adults. However, the physical consequences of obesity can adversely affect adult health.

Causes

There are many theories concerning the causes of obesity. In reality, the etiology is complex, and researchers are only beginning to discover some of the underlying genetic and emotional contributing factors. The onset of obesity can be traced to excess food intake, reduced physical activity, or both. Contrary to popular belief, obesity due to abnormal function of the glands is rare. Children born to obese parents are more likely to become obese. However, environmental factors such as ethnic diet, family eating practices, and psychological factors are also operating, making it difficult to isolate these from genetic factors.

 Health Promotion

The only way to obtain a permanent solution to obesity is to decrease intake and increase the amount of energy used through activity.

Treatment and Nursing Care

The optimal treatment of obesity usually includes a combination of diet modification and exercise. Often the goal is not to lose weight but to avoid gaining weight. Teaching the family and the child about good nutrition, proper food choices, and the importance of regular moderate exercise helps develop healthy patterns for the future.

If a diet is necessary, it must be carefully planned with a nutritionist or dietitian to ensure enough calories and nutrients for growth. Dieting is difficult and often unsuccessful. When obesity begins in early childhood, a person is faced with a lifetime of fighting calories. This is complicated by the fact that food is readily available in the United States and that advertisers bombard the public with tempting treats. Parents must be keenly interested in helping control their child's weight if a diet is to be successful. Changing methods of cooking and types of food prepared to create a healthy plan for the entire family is more successful than preparing different food for the dieting child. Many specialized cookbooks and magazines help families prepare meals that are appealing yet not high in fat or calories. Cookies and cakes should be avoided, and fresh fruits should be substituted for between-meal snacks. Older children and adolescents are apt to go on diets that they invent themselves, which can be dangerous to their health.

Behavior modification techniques have shown success. This approach helps a person identify and control poor eating patterns. Such techniques include eating only at the table, using a smaller plate, eating only at specific times, recording food intake (food diary) and feelings at the time of eating, and so on. A point system or system of rewards is established on initiation of this technique. Groups such as Weight Watchers, Overeaters Anonymous, or diet workshops, although helpful, are frequented mostly by adults.

Support groups specifically for children are more acceptable. These are usually found in teenage clinics, schools, and specialized summer camps (Huelsing et al., 2010). Diet pills are not recommended. Their long-term effectiveness is minimal, and the potential for misuse by the adolescent is high. Jejunoileal bypass, or lap banding, can have complications and is seldom advised unless the child is morbidly obese. The long-term consequences of this procedure have yet to be established.

Prevention of obesity in children is important. The earlier in life this begins, the better. Identification of the infant or child at risk is necessary while the child is still under parental control and before eating and activity patterns are firmly established. Breastfeeding is desirable for infants. Solid foods should be delayed until 6 months of age. Inform mothers that an infant's food requirements diminish greatly as growth slows at about the first year. Discourage overfeeding because fat babies are not necessarily healthy babies. Advise parents that a crying infant does not necessarily mean that the infant is hungry.

 Health Promotion

Parents should foster activities that promote freedom of movement and exercise during the first few years of life. If there are any questions concerning weight gain, these should be voiced during well-baby visits.

During the school years, nutritious snacks rather than junk foods should be kept in the home. Television viewing and video games should be restricted to 2 hours per day, and walking and other exercise should be encouraged. Parents need to promote participation in a regular exercise program. Sound nutritional practices are of particular importance during puberty, when there is an increase in fat cells. Teenagers are capable of assuming responsibility for what they eat.

Helping the child's self-esteem through encouragement, praise, and support is essential. The depressed young person may turn to food as an outlet for emotions. Be generous and specific with praise. Sprinkle conversation with such comments as "I knew you could do it," "That's quite an improvement," "You made it look easy," "I couldn't have done better myself." This type of positive approach may help the child or young person feel better and decrease the need to overeat.

Get Ready for the NCLEX® Examination!

Key Points

- Cleft lip and cleft palate cause feeding difficulties that can lead to nutritional issues.
- Omphalocele has a protective covering of the internal organs, whereas gastroschisis does not.
- Jaundice, itching, and irritability are common problems in a child with biliary atresia.
- Tracheoesophageal fistula can be identified during feedings with choking, cyanosis, and coughing.
- Pyloric stenosis is characterized with projectile vomiting.
- Celiac disease is managed through dietary restrictions. All gluten should be removed or reduced from the diet.
- Rotovirus is an organism that causes diarrhea and dehydration in infants and small children.
- GER is managed through dietary and positional changes, medications, and possible surgical interventions.
- The typical hand-to-mouth behavior of young children makes them prone to pinworm infestation.
- Appendicitis is difficult to diagnose in the young child because the child's vague symptoms may resemble other gastrointestinal problems.
- Obesity is an epidemic in children and adolescents and can lead to serious health problems.
- Childhood is a critical period for beginning obesity that has implications for future coronary heart disease.

Additional Learning Resources

evolve Go to your Evolve website (*http://evolve.elsevier.com/Price/pediatric/*) for the following FREE learning resources:
- 3-D Animations
- Answer Keys
- Appendixes
- Audio Glossary
- Spanish/English Glossary
- Video Clips

Review Questions for the NCLEX® Examination

1. All of the following are interventions for the postoperative care of a child with cleft lip **except**:
    1. Application of antibacterial ointment with cotton-tipped swabs
    2. Rinsing of surgical site with sterile saline solution
    3. Application of restraints
    4. Prevention of excessive crying

2. An omphalocele is a herniation of the gut into the umbilical cord that generally involves the: (**Select all that apply.**)
    1. Ovaries
    2. Liver
    3. Spleen
    4. Pancreas
    5. Gallbladder
    6. Urinary bladder

3. Diagnosis of esophageal atresia (EA) is determined by:
    1. Presentation of symptoms
    2. Barium swallow
    3. Attempting to pass a small-bore nasogastric tube into the esophagus
    4. Placing a low-suction catheter in the blind pouch

4. When caring for the child with biliary atresia, the nurse would expect the color of the urine to be:
    1. Light yellow
    2. Dark tea
    3. Bloody
    4. Amber

5. Postoperative care of the child following a herniorrhaphy is directed toward:
    1. Activity limitation
    2. Strict measurement of intake and output
    3. Careful monitoring of nasogastric tube drainage
    4. Keeping the incision clean

Fluid Balance, Renal, and Reproductive Disorders

Objectives

1. Define the vocabulary terms listed
2. Explain why infants and young children are more easily dehydrated than adults
3. Discuss the nursing care of the child with a urinary tract infection
4. Compare and contrast acute glomerulonephritis and nephrotic syndrome
5. Differentiate hydrocele and cryptorchidism
6. Discuss the impact STDs have on a teenager's life
7. Discuss the nursing care of a child with acquired immunodeficiency syndrome

Key Terms

anuria (ăn-ŪR-ē-ă; p. 287)
dysmenorrhea (dĭs-měn-ō-RĒ-ă; p. 292)
glomerulus (glō-MĔR-ū-lŭs; p. 286)
homeostasis (hō-mē-ō-STĀ-sĭs; p. 281)
hypertonic (hī-per-TŎN-ĭk; p. 283)

hypotonic (hī-pō-TŎN-ĭk; p. 283)
isotonic (ī-sō-TŎN-ĭk; p. 283)
mittelschmerz (MĬT-ĕl-shmärts; p. 292)
oliguria (Ō-lig-Ū-rē-ă; p. 286)
premenstrual syndrome (PMS) (prē-MĔN-strū-ăl; p. 292)

PRINCIPLES OF FLUID BALANCE IN CHILDREN

Infants and small children have different proportions of body water and body fat than do adults (Figure 15-1), and the water needs and water losses of the infant, per unit of body weight, are greater. In children younger than 2 years of age, the surface area is particularly important in fluid and electrolyte balance because more water is lost through the skin than through the kidneys. The surface area of the infant is two to three times greater than that of the adult in proportion to body volume or body weight. Metabolic rate and heat production are also two to three times greater in infants per kilogram of body weight. This produces more waste products, which must be diluted to be excreted. It also stimulates respiration, which causes greater evaporation through the lungs. Compared with adults, children younger than 2 years of age have a greater percentage of body water contained in the extracellular compartment.

Fluid turnover is rapid, and dehydration occurs more quickly in infants than in adults. The infant cannot survive as long as the adult can in the presence of continued water depletion. A sick infant does not adapt as rapidly to shifts in intake and output because the kidneys lack maturity. Their kidneys are less able to concentrate urine and require more water than an adult's kidneys to excrete a given amount of solute. Disturbances of the gastrointestinal tract frequently lead to vomiting and diarrhea (discussed in Chapter 14). Electrolyte balance depends on fluid balance and cardiovascular, renal, adrenal, pituitary, parathyroid, and pulmonary regulatory mechanisms. Many of these mechanisms are maturing in the developing child and are unable to react to full capacity under the stress of illness.

In order to understand fluid balance and imbalance in children, it is important to understand fluid volume requirements. Box 15-1 refers to the daily maintenance fluid requirements for children.

FLUID IMBALANCE

Dehydration

When a person is in good health, fluid intake and output balance and homeostasis (a uniform state) exist. This is accomplished by appropriate shifts of fluids and electrolytes across cellular membranes and by elimination of those products of metabolism that are no longer needed or that are in excess. The volume of blood plasma and interstitial and intracellular fluid (ICF) remains relatively constant. Dehydration occurs whenever fluid output exceeds fluid intake, regardless of the cause. The degree of dehydration and the symptoms are discussed in Box 15-2.

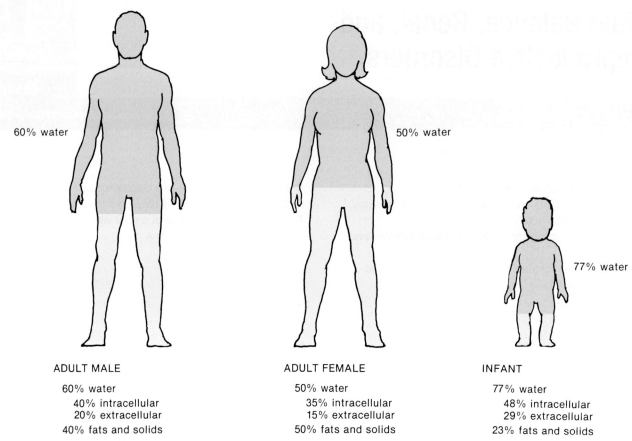

60% water

50% water

77% water

ADULT MALE

60% water
40% intracellular
20% extracellular
40% fats and solids

ADULT FEMALE

50% water
35% intracellular
15% extracellular
50% fats and solids

INFANT

77% water
48% intracellular
29% extracellular
23% fats and solids

FIGURE 15-1 Average body weight composition. Water (particularly extracellular water) makes up a larger percentage of an infant's total body weight than an adult's. Because extracellular water is lost first when water loss occurs in illness, trauma, or environmental stress, the infant is extremely susceptible to fluid and electrolyte imbalances.

Box 15-1 | Daily Maintenance Fluid Requirements

1. Calculate weight of child in kilograms:

$$\frac{\text{Weight of child (in pounds)}}{\text{Divided by 2.2 lb/kg}} = \text{Weight in kilograms}$$

2. Allow 100 ml/kg for first 10 kg.
3. Allow 50 ml/kg for second 10 kg.
4. Allow 20 ml/kg for remainder of weight in kilograms.
5. Divide total amount by 24 hours to obtain rate in milliliters per hour.

Nursing Brief

Output in infants is determined by weighing the wet diaper (urine or liquid stool), subtracting the weight of a comparable dry diaper, and recording the difference. It is important to monitor both intake and output when a child is dehydrated or can potentially become dehydrated.

Disorders of fluids and electrolytes (sodium [Na], potassium [K], calcium [Ca], and magnesium [Mg]) are more complex in children who are growing. A newborn infant's total weight is approximately 78% water, compared with 60% in adults. This varies with the amount

of fat. Also, the daily turnover of water in an infant is equal to almost 24% of total body water, compared with about 6% in adults. An infant's body surface in comparison with weight is three times that of the older child; therefore the infant is subject to greater evaporation of water from the skin. The younger the child, the higher the metabolic rate and the more unstable the heat-regulating mechanisms. (Elevations in temperature are also higher, increasing the rate of water loss.) Rapid respirations speed up this process, and when diarrhea is present (see Chapter 14), additional fluid is lost in the stools. Immaturity of the kidneys impairs the infant's ability to conserve water. Preterm and newborn infants are also more susceptible to dehydration from variations in room temperature and humidity. Cessation of intake alone can result in significant depletion. When this is coupled with higher fluid losses, life-threatening deficits can occur in a few hours.

Problems of fluid and electrolyte disturbance require evaluation of the type and severity of dehydration, clinical observation of the child, and chemical analysis of the blood. Types of dehydration are classified as follows according to the amount of **serum sodium:**

isotonic (the child has lost equal amounts of fluids and electrolytes), hypotonic (the child has lost more electrolytes than fluids), and hypertonic (the child has lost more fluids than electrolytes). These classifications are important because each form of dehydration is associated with different relative losses from intracellular fluid (ICF) and extracellular fluid (ECF) compartments, and each requires certain modifications in treatment. **Maintenance therapy** replaces normal water and electrolyte losses, and **deficit therapy** restores preexisting body fluid and electrolyte deficiencies. The replacement of a deficit may take several days, and the deficit continues unless adequate maintenance therapy is also provided. The physician calculates the volume of fluids to be administered through the use of various formulas on the basis of caloric expenditures because daily physiologic water losses are directly proportional to caloric expenditure. The child's temperature and activity (coma, restlessness) must also be considered. **Basal calories** are determined by the weight of the child. Volume is calculated on a 24-hour basis. Isotonic dehydration is the most common form in children. Signs of isotonic, hypertonic, and hypotonic dehydration are discussed in Table 15-1.

Adjustments in fluid therapy are made constantly, according to the condition of the child. The higher daily exchange of water that occurs in child leaves less volume reserve with dehydration. Shock (hypovolemia) is the greatest threat to life in isotonic dehydration. The electrolyte content of oral fluids is particularly significant in the care of infants and small children with disorders of fluid balance and those receiving infusions. Commercially prepared electrolyte solutions are available by bottle; however, the nurse should ascertain whether they are to be given freely or by physician's order only. Children with hypotonic dehydration—that is, excess water with sodium electrolyte depletion—are at risk for water intoxication. This can also occur if tap water enemas are given to small children. Loss of potassium occurs in almost all states of dehydration. Replacement potassium is administered only after normal urinary excretion is established.

Box 15-2 Clinical Signs of Dehydration in an Infant

MILD DEHYDRATION (UP TO 5% WEIGHT LOSS)
Vital signs are normal
Alert and thirsty
Turgor is normal
Capillary refill time is normal
Anterior fontanel is normal
Tears are present
Slight oliguria

MODERATE DEHYDRATION (6% TO 9% WEIGHT LOSS)
Heart rate and respiratory rate are increased
Blood pressure is normal or slightly decreased
Behavior: restless or irritable
Marked thirst
Turgor shows tenting
Capillary refill time is 2 to 3 seconds
Lips and mucous membranes of the mouth are dry
Anterior fontanel is sunken
Tears are absent
Oliguria

SEVERE DEHYDRATION (10% AND GREATER WEIGHT LOSS)
Heart rate and respiratory rate are increased
Blood pressure is normal or slightly decreased
Behavior: lethargic or comatose
Turgor shows severe tenting
Capillary refill time is greater than 3 seconds
Skin is cold and clammy
Cyanosis may be present
Mucous membranes are extremely dry
Anterior fontanel is severely sunken
Tears are absent
Severe oliguria

Table 15-1 Signs of Isotonic, Hypertonic, and Hypotonic Dehydration

| BODY RESPONSES | SIGNS OF DEHYDRATION | | |
	ISOTONIC	HYPOTONIC	HYPERTONIC
Level of consciousness	Irritable to lethargic	Lethargic to coma	Lethargic, hyperirritable with stimulation
Skin turgor	Diminished turgor, feels dry	Diminished to absent turgor; "tenting"	Fair turgor, feels thickened, "doughy"
Skin temperature	Cold	Cold	Cold to hot
Eyes	Sunken	Sunken	Sunken
Tearing and salivation	Absent or decreased	Absent or decreased	Absent or decreased
Mucous membranes	Dry	Dry to slightly moist	Parched
Fontanel	Sunken	Sunken	Sunken
Body temperature	Afebrile to febrile	Afebrile to febrile	Afebrile to febrile
Respiration and pulse	Rapid	Rapid	Rapid
Blood pressure	Normal to low	Normal to low	Very low

Oral Fluids. Whenever possible, fluids are given by mouth to the child with dehydration. It is the most natural and satisfactory method. The nurse must use ingenuity to encourage the sick child to take enough fluids because he or she may refuse food and water and cannot understand their relation to recovery. The infant and small child become dehydrated faster than the adult does. The busy nurse must find time to offer fluids and must be patient and gently persistent. Liquids are offered frequently and in small amounts. Some common clear liquid fluids used to replace lost fluid are popsicles, lemon-lime drinks, and the oral replacement solutions such as Pedialyte. Brightly colored containers and drinking straws may help. The nurse keeps an accurate record of the child's intake and output. The physician cannot determine whether a child needs IV fluids with a partially completed chart. **The importance of this particular responsibility on the pediatric unit cannot be overemphasized.**

Parenteral Fluids. Parenteral (*para,* beside or apart; *enteron,* intestine) fluids are those given by some route other than the digestive tract. This is necessary when sickness is accompanied by vomiting or loss of consciousness or when the gastrointestinal system requires rest. Use of parenteral fluids is important in severe cases of vomiting and diarrhea in which the excessive loss of water and electrolytes leads to death if untreated.

The infant or child receiving parenteral fluids needs the nurse's warmth and affection. Babies still need to be held and derive the pleasures they receive from sucking a pacifier if it is not contraindicated. Intake and output should be charted on all children receiving parenteral fluids.

Overhydration

Overhydration results when the body receives more fluid than it can excrete. This can occur in children with normal kidneys who receive intravenous fluids too rapidly. It can also occur in a child receiving acceptable rates of fluid, especially when the child's illness is related to disorders of fluid mechanism. These disorders include kidney disease, burns, cardiovascular disease, protein deficiencies, and certain allergies. Hormonal therapy also may disrupt fluid mechanisms.

Edema is the presence of excess fluid in the interstitial spaces. Trauma to or infections of the head can cause cerebral edema, which can be life-threatening. A constrictive dressing may obstruct venous return, causing swelling, particularly in dependent areas. Early detection and management of edema are essential. Taking accurate daily weights is indispensable, as is close attention to body weight changes. Vital signs, physical appearance, and changes in urine character or output are noted. Edema in infants may first be seen about the eyes and in the presacral, occipital, or genital areas. In **pitting edema,** after exerting gentle pressure with the finger, the nurse should notice an impression in the skin that lasts for several seconds.

RENAL SYSTEM

The renal system includes the kidneys, ureters, bladder, urethra, and the renal arteries and veins. The primary functions of the urinary system includes waste excretion; maintaining homeostasis with fluid, electrolyte, and acid-base balance; and hormonal function (production of renin for blood pressure regulation, production of erythropoietin, and metabolism of vitamin D). The kidneys function normally at birth but are not fully developed. There is also a decrease in the ability to concentrate urine and to cope with fluid imbalances. As discussed in Chapter 5, the infant should void within the first 24 to 48 hours after birth. Urine output increases as the child ages and is monitored closely in children with renal conditions.

 Nursing Brief

The rule of thumb for urine output is 2 mL/kg/hr for an infant and 0.5 to 1 mL/kg/hr for a child.

URINARY TRACT INFECTION

Urinary tract infections (UTIs) are caused by bacterial invasion of the upper urinary tract (kidney and ureters) or lower urinary tract (bladder and urethra). Genitourinary anatomy is reviewed in Figure 15-2. They generally occur in children between 2 and 6 years of age, unless a structural anomaly is the cause. Urinary tract infections are more commonly found in girls because the distance infectious organisms need to travel to enter the bladder is considerably shorter than in boys. Boys have a much longer urethra.

Several factors contribute to the incidence of UTIs in children. These include congenital malformations of the urinary tract and conditions resulting in urinary stasis (such as ignoring the urge to urinate or neurogenic bladder in children with conditions such as myelomeningocele). In affected infant boys, the incidence is higher in uncircumcised infants. Mechanical factors such as tight diapers or underwear, chemical irritation from bubble bath, inflammatory conditions of the external perineal area, and pinworms all contribute to UTIs. Although UTI in young girls is not uncommon, repeated UTIs can suggest possible sexual abuse.

Vesicoureteral Reflux

Vesicoureteral reflux (VUR) is a primary contributing factor to UTIs. As urine fills the bladder or as the bladder contracts during voiding, the opening to the ureter is normally occluded. With VUR, a malfunctioning valve at the junction of the ureter and bladder

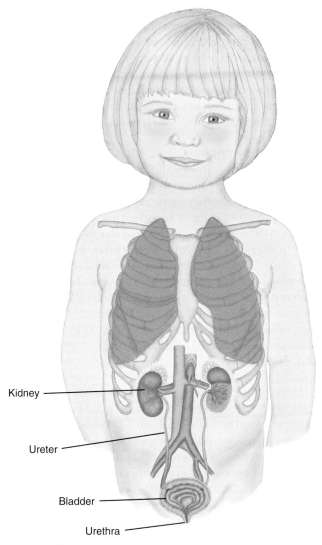

FIGURE 15-2 Anatomy of the genitourinary system.

Kidney

Ureter

Bladder

Urethra

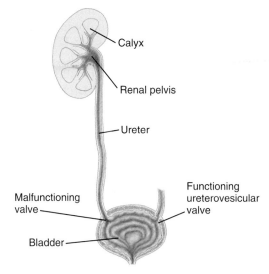

Calyx

Renal pelvis

Ureter

Functioning ureterovesicular valve

Malfunctioning valve

Bladder

FIGURE 15-3 Mechanics of vesicoureteral reflux.

allows urine to reflux upward into the ureters toward the kidney (Figure 15-3). This allows bacteria in the urine to be carried upward, possibly all the way into the kidney. This can cause pyelonephritis and renal damage. In addition, the urine can return to the bladder, creating a residual that becomes a medium for bacterial growth or infection. VUR is graded I to V (1 to 5), with grade V involving a gross dilation of the ureter and pelvis and calyces of the kidney. Diagnosis is generally made after ultrasound and a voiding cystourethrography (VCUG). During a VCUG, contrast medium is injected into the bladder through a urethral catheter; radiographs are taken before, during, and after voiding. This procedure visualizes the bladder outline and urethra, and it identifies reflux and other structural complications. All children (1 to 10 years of age) are treated initially with antimicrobial prophylaxis. At the end of 1 year, if VUR is not resolved, endoscopy therapy is recommended for children with lower grades of reflux. Open surgery is used if

endoscopy is unsuccessful; it may also be used from the outset if children have higher grades of reflux (Greenbaum and Mesrobian, 2006).

Signs and Symptoms

Signs of UTIs in infants and young children are easily missed. The child exhibits poor feeding, fussiness, delayed growth, foul-smelling urine, and incontinence (in a child who has been previously trained). Unexplained fever in infants may be caused by a UTI, and this should be considered when no other source for the fever is found. Many adolescent girls exhibit classic signs of UTI (frequency, urgency, pain on urination, blood in the urine) after the first episode of sexual intercourse. High fever, chills, flank pain, and abdominal pain can indicate kidney infection (pyelonephritis).

Urinary tract infection is diagnosed with urine culture. The specimen is obtained with a clean midstream urine collection in potty-trained children or with catheterization or suprapubic aspiration in infants and untrained children. The culture shows organism growth; usually colony growth exceeding 100,000 of a single organism is diagnostic from a midstream specimen. *Escherichia coli* and other gram-negative organisms are frequently the cause. Antimicrobial sensitivities determine the treatment. Blood, protein, and white blood cell casts might be found in the urine. A complete renal workup to detect urinary tract abnormalities includes ultrasonography, VCUG and radionuclide cystography, renal nucleotide scans, and CT or MRI.

Treatment and Nursing Care

Treatment of a UTI with older children is a 7- to 14-day course of an appropriate antimicrobial, generally sulfamethoxazole/trimethoprim (Bactrim, Septra).

Penicillins, cephalosporins, and nitrofurantoin may also be ordered. Children who do not improve within 2 days of starting antimicrobials for UTI should be reevaluated with ultrasound and VCUG. Nurses need to teach proper hygiene (no bubble baths or irritating diaper wipes; wiping from front to back).

It is important to explain procedures using terms with which the child is familiar. If a catheterized urine sample is necessary, the nurse needs to reassure the child that the tube does not harm the body but helps find out what is wrong. Practice relaxation breathing exercises with the child before inserting the catheter, and encourage the child to sing or breathe slowly as the tube is being inserted. Sphincter relaxation decreases the amount of discomfort the child might experience.

Other preventive measures include wearing cotton underwear, adequate fluid intake, encouraging children to not put off going to the bathroom when needed, investigating and treating signs of intestinal parasites (pinworms), and avoiding bubble baths. Acidification of the urine with cranberry juice may be helpful. Some clinicians may recommend drinking cranberry juice to help prevent urinary tract infections. Sexually active girls should urinate after sexual intercourse. If urine specimens are obtained at home, teach the parent to bring the specimen immediately to the laboratory. If the parent is unable to get to the laboratory within 30 minutes, the specimen should be refrigerated.

ACUTE (POSTSTREPTOCOCCAL) GLOMERULONEPHRITIS

Acute glomerulonephritis (AGN) occurs as an immune reaction (antigen-antibody) to an infection in the body. The most common of the noninfectious renal diseases in childhood is acute poststreptococcal glomerulonephritis. The infection is generally caused by a Group A beta-hemolytic streptococci infecting the throat or the skin. It may appear after the child has had scarlet fever or skin infections (impetigo). The body's immune mechanisms appear to be important in its development. Antibodies produced to fight the invading organisms react against the glomerular tissue. Glomerulonephritis is the most common form of nephritis in children and occurs most frequently in boys between 3 and 7 years of age. It has a seasonal incidence, with peaks in winter and spring. Both kidneys are affected.

The nephron is the working unit of the kidneys. Nephrons number in the millions. Within the bulb of each nephron lies a cluster of capillaries known as the glomerulus. It is these structures that are affected, as the name of the disease implies. They become inflamed and sometimes blocked, permitting red blood cells and protein, which are normally retained, to enter the urine. Sodium and fluid are retained, leading to edema and oliguria (decreased urine output). The kidneys become pale and slightly enlarged.

The prognosis is excellent. Children with mild cases of the disease may recover within 10 to 14 days. Children with protracted cases may show urinary changes for as long as a year but have complete recovery. Chronic nephritis is seen in a small number of children; renal failure can result from this. These severe complications, plus hypertensive changes, necessitate careful observation and care of each child.

Signs and Symptoms

Symptoms range from mild to severe. From 1 to 2 weeks after a streptococcal infection has occurred in the child, the mother may notice that the urine is smoky brown in color or bloody. This is frightening to the mother and child; medical advice is immediately sought by most parents. **Periorbital edema** (mild swelling about the eyes) may also be present in the morning, and the edema spreads to the abdomen and extremities as the day progresses. The child may have fatigue, headache, abdominal discomfort, and vomiting. After an initial acute phase, the child spontaneously diureses and the symptoms begin to abate. Blood and protein can be found in the urine for several weeks.

Urinary output is decreased. Protein, red blood cells, white blood cells, and casts may be found on examination. The BUN level can be elevated, as can the serum creatinine and erythrocyte sedimentation rates. The serum complement level is usually reduced. For a definitive diagnosis, it may be necessary to have positive confirmation of a streptococcal infection, either with culture or with antibody titer. Mild-to-severe hypertension may be seen. Complications such as renal and cardiac failure and encephalopathy may also occur.

Treatment and Nursing Care

Although the child may feel well, activity should be limited until gross hematuria subsides. The urine should be examined regularly. Every effort should be made to prevent the child from becoming overtired, chilled, or exposed to infection. Because renal function is impaired, there is a danger of accumulation of nitrogenous wastes and sodium in the body. A low-sodium diet may be ordered. Parents need to be educated by the dietitian on this diet. Protein restriction is not usually necessary. Fluid restriction may be necessary for some children. Furosemide (Lasix) may be given if significant edema and fluid overload are present and renal failure is not severe (Hockenberry and Wilson, 2007). Penicillin is given if the streptococcal infection persists, but it usually does not alter the course of the disease. Recurrent glomerulonephritis is rare.

The nurse should try to make the period of bed rest as pleasant as possible by providing quiet diversions. When the child is allowed up, the nurse observes him or her frequently for signs of fatigue. The child should be protected from contact with persons with infections.

The child's vital signs are taken regularly, preferably with the same apparatus. A rise in blood pressure is reported immediately. Between readings, the nurse should be alert for symptoms such as headache, drowsiness, vomiting, and blurring of vision. If any of these are noticed, the child is returned to bed and the crib sides or rails are raised. Because seizures can occur, someone should remain with the child until medication is given. Hypotensive drugs, including short-acting calcium channel blockers such as *nifedipine,* may be ordered by the physician. Parameters for administration are specific. These reduce the blood pressure rapidly, and the cerebral symptoms subside. If cardiac failure is evidenced with an ECG or chest radiograph, sedation, oxygen, and digitalis may be necessary.

The nurse accurately records the child's daily weight, fluid intake, and urine output. Fluids may be restricted, especially if the urinary output is scant. In this circumstance, the physician orders the oral intake allowed; for example, 650 mL daily. This must be distributed throughout the 24-hour period. Each shift should know the specific amount of fluids the child is to receive for that shift so that an excess amount is not given. The greater amounts of fluid are allotted to the day shift, when thirst is more pronounced and when the child is awake. The individual needs of the child should be observed and incorporated into the day's events. Persistent anuria (suppression of urine formation) may necessitate dialysis.

Although glomerulonephritis is generally benign, it can be a source of anguish for parents and child. If the child is treated at home, the parents must be creative if he or she has restricted activity orders. They must understand the importance of continued medical supervision because follow-up urine and blood tests are necessary to ensure that the disease has been eradicated.

NEPHROTIC SYNDROME (NEPHROSIS)

Nephrotic syndrome refers to a number of different types of kidney conditions that are distinguished by the presence of marked amounts of protein in the urine. Minimal change nephrotic syndrome, idiopathic nephrosis, in which the cause is seldom determined, is discussed here because it is the most common type seen in early childhood. Table 15-2 compares poststreptococcal glomerulonephritis and nephrotic syndrome.

The **glomeruli,** the working units of the kidneys that filter the blood, become damaged and allow albumin and other proteins to enter the urine. Proteinuria is massive. There is a fall in the level of protein in the blood, termed **hypoproteinemia,** and a rise in cholesterol content, termed **hyperlipidemia.**

Table 15-2	Comparison of (Poststreptococcal) Glomerulonephritis and (Minimal Change) Nephrotic Syndrome	
MANIFESTATIONS	**APSGN**	**MINIMAL CHANGE NEPHROTIC SYNDROME**
Streptococcal antibody titers	Elevated	Normal
BP	Elevated	Normal or decreased
Edema	Periorbital and peripheral	Generalized, severe
Circulatory congestion	Common	Absent
Proteinuria	Mild to moderate	Massive
Hematuria	Gross to microscopic	Microscopic or none
BUN and serum creatinine	Elevated	Normal
Serum potassium levels	Normal or increased	Normal
Serum protein levels	Minimal reduction	Markedly decreased
Serum lipid levels	Normal	Elevated
Peak age at onset	3-7 yr	2-7 yr
Recurrence	Uncommon	Common

Data modified from Hockenberry, M., Wilson, D., Winkelstein, M., et al. (2007). *Wong's nursing care of infants and children* (8th ed.). St. Louis: Mosby.

Nephrosis is more frequently seen in boys than in girls and is seen most often in toddlers and preschoolers. The prognosis for children with nephrosis is usually positive. Most children have repeated relapses until the disease resolves itself. Children with types other than minimal change nephrotic syndrome do not have as good a prognosis. They may have renal failure develop and need dialysis or transplantation.

Signs and Symptoms

The characteristic symptom of nephrosis is **edema.** This occurs slowly; the child does not appear to be sick. It is noticed at first about the eyes and ankles but later becomes generalized. The edema shifts with the position of the child during sleep. The child gains weight because of the accumulation of this fluid. The abdomen may become so distended that striae, or stretch marks similar to those that appear on the skin of a pregnant woman, may occur. The child is pale, irritable, and listless and has a poor appetite. The child becomes more susceptible to infection.

The urine appears dark and frothy. Urine output can be decreased. Urine examination reveals albumin. Vomiting and diarrhea may also be present. Renal biopsy may be done.

Treatment and Nursing Care

Control of Edema. Steroid therapy is initiated, and diuresis occurs as the urinary protein excretion diminishes in 7 to 21 days. Prednisone, which comes in liquid form for young children, is the drug of choice. The drug is continued until the urine is free of protein and remains normal for a prescribed period. The dosage is tapered to discontinuation. Immunosuppressive therapy (e.g., cytoxan, chlorambucil) has shown promise for some steroid-resistant children.

Diuretics are given as ordered to aid in the elimination of excessive fluid. The child is weighed daily to determine changes in the degree of edema. The child is weighed on the same scale each time and at about the same time of day. Abdominal girth (circumference) should also be measured every day.

Albumin may be administered intravenously to help restore normal fluid volume and reduce the amount of edema present. IV furosemide (Lasix) is given following administration of albumin to decrease the chance for fluid volume overload.

Because of the amount of edema in the lower extremities and fluid stasis, cellulitis can occur. Peritonitis can also develop; therefore oral penicillin is frequently given to reduce the risk for such infections.

Diet. The child's appetite is generally poor. A well-balanced diet high in protein is desirable because protein is constantly being lost in the urine. Salt is restricted during periods of massive edema, and a diet with no added salt may be recommended after remission to assist in decreasing the salt appetite. Normal amounts of water are given unless otherwise ordered.

Fluid Balance. The child's urine must be carefully measured. This is difficult with the child who is not toilet-trained or who has had a regression in urinary habits. Diapers are weighed on a gram scale. The character, odor, and color of the urine are also important.

Care of the Skin. Good skin care is especially important during periods of marked edema. Special attention is given to the neck, underarms, groin, and other moist areas of the body. The male genitals may become edematous; supportive clothing may be necessary. Cotton or clothing may be used to separate the skin surfaces to prevent a rash from forming.

Positioning. The child is repositioned frequently to prevent respiratory infection. A pressure-equalizing mattress reduces the risk for skin breakdown. A pillow placed between the knees when the child is lying on the side prevents pressure on edematous organs. The child's head is elevated during the day to reduce edema of the eyelids and to make him or her more comfortable. Children with mild edema can participate in usual activities with frequent periods of rest.

Infection Prevention. Because steroids mask the signs of infection, the child must be watched closely for more subtle symptoms of illness. Examine the child's skin for redness at sites of punctures, wounds, catheters, and so on. Watch for temperature variations, increased blood pressure, and changes in behavior. Report suspicions promptly because septicemia is life threatening. Prompt antimicrobial therapy is begun when an acute infection is recognized.

Nurses make every effort to protect the children from exposure to upper respiratory tract infections. Proper hand hygiene is crucial. Children should be separated from other infectious patients. **No live immunizations should be administered during therapy with steroids.**

Emotional Support. The nursing care of the child with nephrosis is of the greatest significance because this disease requires long-term therapy. The child might be hospitalized periodically and becomes a familiar personality to hospital personnel. Parental guidance and support should be given by all members of the nursing team. Family education about weighing, measuring abdominal girth, and determining urine specific gravity and urinary albumin is necessary. The parents should be encouraged to remain with the child as much as possible.

Whenever possible, the child is treated at home and brought to the hospital for therapy only. Parents are instructed to keep a daily record of the child's weight, urinary protein, and medications. Signs of infection, such as abnormal weight gain, and increased protein in the urine must be reported promptly. The child is allowed to be up and about after the acute stage of the illness subsides to participate in normal childhood activities.

The child with nephrosis is kept under close medical supervision over an extended period. The prognosis is considered favorable but depends on the child's response to drug therapy (Nursing Care Plan 15-1).

ENURESIS

Enuresis, or bedwetting, is a common disorder among children that generally occurs at night (nocturnal). According to Hockenberry and Wilson (2009), the inappropriate voiding of urine occurs at least twice a week for at least 3 months, and the age of the child (chronologically or developmentally) is at least 5 years. While it is bothersome to the child and family, the important thing to remember is that the child should never be punished. Positive reinforcement and reassurance are important for the child's self esteem. While this occurs more often in boys, it can also interfere with girls' lives. Enuresis is considered *primary* if the child has never been dry for an extended period of time. *Secondary* enuresis is the onset of bedwetting after the child has been dry for a period of time.

Nursing Care Plan 15-1 | The Child with Nephrotic Syndrome

NURSING DIAGNOSIS *Excess fluid volume, related to fluid shift from intravascular to interstitial spaces, as a result of glomerular damage*

Goals/Outcome Criteria	Nursing Interventions	Rationales
Child begins to lose accumulated interstitial fluid as evidenced by: • Increased urinary output • Decreased edema • Weight loss	Administer medications as prescribed; liquid medication is more appropriate for children. Test urine daily for protein. Weigh daily with the same scale and at the same time of day. Measure abdominal girth.	Steroids act on the glomeruli by suppressing the immune response; diuretics may be indicated. Trace amounts or absence of urine protein indicates the disease is in remission. Monitors fluid gain or loss. Monitors fluid accumulation in abdominal area.
Child maintains normal intravascular fluid volume as evidenced by: • Moist mucous membranes • Good skin turgor • Stable vital signs	Strictly measure intake and output: • Place input and output sign on bedside. • Instruct all visitors to keep track. • Weigh wet diapers (1 g weight = 1 mL of fluid). • Use toilet "hat" for urine output measurement. • Measure intake amount in "sippy cup" if used. • Provide sufficient amounts of the child's favorite fluids—fluids should neither be restricted nor encouraged. Monitor vital signs. Allow child to participate in usual activities as tolerated, but provide sufficient rest.	Provides data about fluid balance. Caretakers need to have understanding of importance of keeping accurate record. Decreasing BP, increasing pulse can indicate hypovolemic shock. Excess fluid volume can deplete energy.

NURSING DIAGNOSIS *Imbalanced nutrition, less than body requirements, related to decreased appetite*

Goals/Outcome Criteria	Nursing Interventions	Rationales
Child eats sufficient amounts to maintain usual growth	Provide a well-balanced diet; adequate protein and no added salt is recommended during acute phase. Serve small quantities of favorite nutritious foods on brightly colored dishes; use colored straws. Encourage the child to eat with others. Allow the child to choose foods with parent's help.	A well-balanced diet is essential for growth and energy. Small quantities are not too overwhelming to a preschool child; interesting plates can often entice a reluctant child to eat. Eating is a social process. Encourages child's autonomy.

NURSING DIAGNOSIS *Risk for infection, related to altered immunity*

Goals/Outcome Criteria	Nursing Interventions	Rationales
Child remains free of infection as evidenced by: • Normal body temperature • Intact skin with no redness or exudate • Normal respiratory function	Use meticulous hand hygiene. Reduce contact with others who are ill. Monitor vital signs. Examine the skin at sites of punctures: wounds, IV, catheters. Teach parent how to recognize and report signs of infection. Administer antimicrobials as directed and for the entire period prescribed.	Prevents spread of infectious organisms. Reduces opportunities to acquire an infection. Fever can indicate an underlying infectious process in the absence of other signs. Local redness, swelling can suggest infectious process. Many children with nephrosis are treated at home; parents need knowledge. Used to treat infections.

Continued

✦ Nursing Care Plan 15-1   The Child with Nephrotic Syndrome—cont'd

NURSING DIAGNOSIS *Risk for impaired skin integrity, related to pressure from edema*

Goals/Outcome Criteria	Nursing Interventions	Rationales
Child's skin remains intact with no areas of redness or evidence of abnormal pressure	Bathe daily and clean diaper area as needed.	Reduces surface microorganisms, reduces action of acidic urine or feces on skin.
	Dry meticulously, particularly in skin folds; separate skin surfaces with cotton or clothing.	Moist areas are prime mediums for organism growth.
	Support edematous scrotal area with pad and t-binder.	Helps reduce pressure in the area.
	Turn and reposition frequently if child is on bed rest; use a pressure-equalizing mattress.	Prevents undue pressure in the same areas.
	Advise parent to avoid dressing the child in tight clothing.	Prevents chafing and skin irritation.

NURSING DIAGNOSIS *Ineffective coping, related to stress of long-term remissions and relapses*

Goals/Outcome Criteria	Nursing Interventions	Rationales
Child and family describe adaptation to usual lifestyle.	Teach parents what to expect about the course of the illness.	Knowing what to expect increases control and decreases stress.
Child and family show stress-reducing strategies.	Teach management strategies, such as urine testing, monitoring for infection, skin care, daily weights, medication administration.	Participation in management increases coping.
Family promptly reports changes in the child's condition and complies with illness regimen.	Refer to Social Services or appropriate agency for financial help if needed.	Coping with illness is facilitated if financial worries are decreased.
	Allow family members to express concerns.	Listening and providing emotional support reduces stress.

Critical Thinking Question

1. The mother of a 6-year-old child with nephrotic syndrome is asking why her child is "so puffy." She also wants to know why her child is on prednisone and how long this needs to continue. How do you explain all of this to her? What discharge instructions need to be given to this mother?

Organic causes of bedwetting must be ruled out. Some children sleep very soundly and do not awaken to void. Oftentimes there is a familial component. Therapy includes medications (antidiuretics, anticholinergics, and tricyclic antidepressants), restricting fluids after the evening meal, waking a child to void, bladder training, and devices such as alarms that attempt to awaken a child upon the initiation of voiding (Hockenberry and Wilson, 2009). Usually it is time that is needed for the child to simply outgrow this disorder. Most children will outgrow this by 8 years of age.

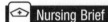 **Nursing Brief**

Normal bladder capacity (in ounces) is the child's age plus 2.

REPRODUCTIVE SYSTEM

HYDROCELE

A hydrocele (*hydro*, water; *cele*, tumor), an excessive amount of fluid in the sac that surrounds the testicle, causes the scrotum to swell. Its appearance in the neonate is not uncommon, and in many cases the condition corrects itself as the baby grows.

If a chronic hydrocele persists in the older child, it is corrected with surgery. Routine postoperative nursing care is given. Same-day or outpatient surgery may be arranged.

UNDESCENDED TESTES (CRYPTORCHIDISM)

The **testes** are the male sex glands. These two oval bodies begin their development in the abdominal cavity below the kidneys of the embryo. Their function is to produce spermatozoa (male sex cells) and male hormones, particularly testosterone. Toward the end of the fetal period, they begin to descend along a pathway into the scrotum. If, for reasons that are still unclear, this descent does not take place normally, the testes may remain in the abdomen or inguinal canal. This condition is common in about 30% of low–birth weight infants. When one or both testes fail to descend into the scrotum, the condition is termed **cryptorchidism** (*kryptos,* hidden; *orchi,* testis). The unilateral form is seen more frequently. Because the testes are warmer in the abdomen than in the scrotum, the sperm cells begin to deteriorate. If both testes are affected, sterility can result. Other complications include increased exposure to injury, an increase in tumor formation, and emotional problems, particularly in the school-age boy, who may be ridiculed by his peers. An **inguinal hernia** often accompanies this condition. Secondary sex characteristics such as voice change, growth of facial hair, and so on are not affected because the testes continue to secrete hormones directly into the bloodstream.

Treatment and Nursing Care

Occasionally, spontaneous descent of the testis or testes occurs during the first 6 months of life. If this does not happen, treatment is recommended at 9 to 15 months. The testes can be brought down to the scrotum with a surgical intervention called **orchiopexy** (*orchio,* testicle; *pexy,* fixation). Although orchiopexy improves the condition, the fertility rate among these patients, even when only one testis is undescended, may be reduced. For boys with congenital absence of a testis, a testicular prosthetic may be psychologically important. In addition, although testicular tumors are rare, their incidence is increased in these patients during adulthood. Parents are told to teach the growing child the importance of self-examination of the testes.

The psychological approach of the nurse to the child and family is of importance because of the embarrassment involved in cases of this nature. People may ask the child why he is having surgery when there is no visible evidence of trauma. This problem is frequently compounded by the fact that the older child has been told not to discuss his condition. In addition, his understanding of his problem and just what is going to happen in surgery really may be vague. Therefore it is important that the nurse caring for the child knows just what he has been told and how he feels about his operation to give emotional support during his care. Terminology needs to be clarified. The nurse should assure the child that his penis will not be involved in the surgery.

The parents also may have anxieties that they cannot verbalize. It is difficult for many parents to communicate with their child in matters such as these. They may also fear that the child will become homosexual or less virile. A thoughtful, sensitive nurse who tries to anticipate these and other related feelings and fears is a definite asset to the child's adjustment.

HYPOSPADIAS AND EPISPADIAS

Hypospadias is the most common congenital anomaly of the penis. In **hypospadias**, the opening of the urinary meatus is on the ventral or underside of the shaft of the penis. In **epispadias**, the urethral opening is on the dorsal or upper surface of the shaft (Figure 15-4).

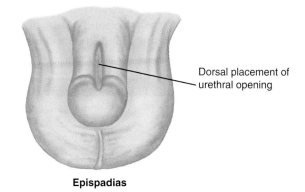

Epispadias

Dorsal placement of urethral opening

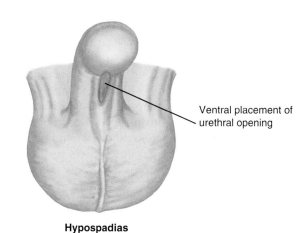

Hypospadias

Ventral placement of urethral opening

FIGURE 15-4 Possible locations of the urethral meatus in the child with hypospadias and epispadias.

Chordee, a downward curvature of the penis, is the result of a tight fibrous band and may be seen with hypospadias. The displacement of the urinary meatus opening should not interfere with continence.

Treatment and Nursing Care

The nurse may discover the defect while the infant is in the nursery. Treatment is determined by the location of the defect. The ultimate goals are for the child to be able to void standing up, to prevent any possible psychological problems, and to avoid potential difficulties with sexual function. Surgical repair is usually performed between 6 and 12 months of age. New microsurgery techniques may allow for an earlier repair. Repair may be done in stages. Circumcision is avoided because the foreskin may be needed in reconstruction. After surgery, a urinary catheter or **urethral stent** may be placed to allow for healing of the meatus. A pressure dressing may be on the penis and is removed by the physician. Parents need instruction for home care of such devices. Fluid intake is important, and increased amounts are necessary to decrease the risk for infection. Antimicrobials and medications for bladder spasms may be administered. Before discharge, parents should be instructed to observe for signs of urinary infections such as cloudy urine or foul smell. The child's temperature should be monitored.

 Nursing Brief

Surgical correction may occur at a developmental stage that involves fear of separation and anxiety of mutilation. These concerns should be included in providing care for the child. Parents should be instructed on the possible fears that the child may experience.

DYSMENORRHEA (PRIMARY)

Primary dysmenorrhea, or painful menstruation, denotes pain associated with the menstrual cycle in the absence of organic pelvic disease. It is distinguished from **secondary dysmenorrhea**, in which the child may have an underlying condition such as endometriosis, pelvic inflammatory disease, ovarian cysts, adhesions, or congenital abnormalities. Mittelschmerz refers to midcycle pain during ovulation. For many years, dysmenorrhea was thought to be psychological. It is now recognized that painful menses result from myometrial stimulation by prostaglandins E_2 and F_{2a}, produced in the endometrium (Kliegman et al., 2007). The concentration of these prostaglandins is higher in women with dysmenorrhea than in control subjects.

About two thirds of postpubescent teenagers in the United States have some degree of dysmenorrhea. Approximately 10% are incapacitated from 1 to 3 days per month. Dysmenorrhea is the greatest single cause of lost school and work days in women. Its onset is usually before age 20 years.

Signs and Symptoms

Symptoms include cramping, abdominal discomfort, and leg aches, all of which begin at the onset of menses. Systemic symptoms such as nausea, vomiting, dizziness, diarrhea, backache, and headache can occur. Dysmenorrhea is graded from mild to severe. Primary dysmenorrhea occurs in the absence of organic disease. Secondary dysmenorrhea occurs as a result of organic disease.

Premenstrual syndrome (PMS) is more common in adults than in teenagers. Although the symptoms may overlap with those of dysmenorrhea, weight gain, breast tenderness, irritability, and insomnia before menstruation are also seen. The symptoms of PMS resolve with the onset of menses. PMS does not generally occur before ovulatory cycles begin.

Treatment and Nursing Care

Painful menses should be evaluated to rule out any structural problem such as pelvic inflammatory disease, tumors, or endometriosis. Primary dysmenorrhea should be treated with NSAIDs, which are prostaglandin inhibitors and assist in decreasing myometrial contractions. Ibuprofen or naproxen should be taken every 4 hours and usually requires 2 to 3 days of medications. These drugs should not be taken on an empty stomach and can cause fluid retention. Applying a warm heating pad to the lower abdomen may also decrease discomfort. When these measures fail, a thorough history and pelvic examination by a gynecologist should be performed to rule out organic disorders. Children with dysmenorrhea who are also in need of contraception may be candidates for combination (estrogen-progesterone) oral contraceptives.

SEXUALLY TRANSMITTED DISEASES

Sexually transmitted disease (STD) is the general name given to an infection that is spread through direct sexual activity. This replaces the term *venereal disease*, which was used in the past. The two most common types of STDs are chlamydial infection and gonorrhea; however, more than 20 other diseases are now considered to be prevalent. Some of these are syphilis, genital warts, herpes progenitalis, cytomegalovirus infection, hepatitis B, and AIDS (acquired immunodeficiency syndrome). Other conditions, such as scabies and pediculosis pubis, can also be transmitted sexually. The effects of some untreated STDs can be debilitating and irreversible. More than one STD can be contracted at the same time. Many can be transmitted by a pregnant woman to her unborn child, causing serious problems in the fetus, such as blindness, birth defects, and death.

 Global Perspective

The incidence of AIDS continues to increase, and public awareness of spread through sexual contact is a priority in prevention. Because persons with HIV infection may remain asymptomatic for many years, they may unknowingly spread the disease to others.

It was thought that with the advent of penicillin, STDs would be eradicated, but there has been a widespread resurgence. The reasons for this resurgence are many and include intertwining cultural, economic, social, and moral factors. Specific reasons include changing values and lifestyles in society; an increase in sexual contact, particularly in the middle and upper classes; an increase in the mobility of society and surges in the population; the reluctance of many persons to seek medical help (particularly adolescents); inadequate education about the diseases; increasing intravenous drug use; organism resistance to antimicrobials; widespread apathy among professionals; social equality of the genders; and a change in common methods of contraception. The occurrence of an STD in a prepubertal child should always prompt investigation into the possibility of sexual abuse.

The incidence of STDs among teenagers is high. The reasons are physical and psychosocial. Today's adolescents are maturing earlier than previous generations, marrying later, engaging in sexual intercourse at younger ages, and having multiple sexual partners. Despite intense efforts to provide comprehensive sex education, adolescents continue to engage in risky behaviors. Alcohol and drug use contribute in large part to an increase in sexual activity among today's youth. Media images in popular music videos, commercials, and teen magazines are becoming an important source of inaccurate sex information for adolescents. Although misinformation contributes to the problem, adolescents are surprisingly well-informed about how to avoid risky behaviors. However, a discrepancy appears between what they know and what they actually do. Although the causes for this discrepancy are not fully understood, contributing factors include lack of appropriate adult role modeling; reacting in an emotional rather than intellectual manner in pressure situations (the heart ruling the head); lack of concrete practice with prevention techniques (putting on a condom, using a diaphragm or foam, and so forth); and low self-esteem.

Signs and Symptoms

Table 15-3 describes the clinical manifestations of the major STDs in the United States. Some additional information follows.

CHLAMYDIA INFECTION

Chlamydia trachomatis infection has become the most common STD in the United States. The condition can persist for months or years and remain undiagnosed because it is often asymptomatic. The incubation period is approximately 1 week. Should an infected woman give birth vaginally, the infant is at risk for development of neonatal conjunctivitis and pneumonia. Infants should be treated with erythromycin.

A positive culture for *Chlamydia trachomatis* from conjunctival, nasopharyngeal, vaginal, or rectal areas is diagnostic. Nonculture tests, such as immunoassays and fluorescent antibody tests, are available but should not be used if sexual abuse is suspected because of false-positive results.

GONORRHEA

The infectious agent that causes this highly communicable disease is *Neisseria gonorrhoeae,* an anaerobic bacterium that penetrates the mucous membrane surfaces lining the genital tract, rectum, and mouth. The bacteria thrive in warm, moist areas of the body and can also survive in the tissues around the eyes of the newborn infant and in the immature vulvar tissues of prepubescent girls. They quickly die outside the human body. The common names for this disease include *GC, clap, dose, strain,* or *drip.*

Symptoms in males appear within 2 to 7 days after sexual contact with an infected person (although some males are asymptomatic). The germs invade the urethral canal, causing a painful burning sensation during urination. Pus that gradually becomes thin and watery is discharged from the penis. Increased burning, urinary frequency, and urgency are signs of bladder infection. The disease may spread to the prostate gland, seminal vesicles, and testes. The scrotum, when inflamed, is hard, swollen, painful, and heavy.

Some 80% to 90% of females with gonorrhea are asymptomatic; therefore they may spread the infection without knowing it. Those who have symptoms experience mild burning or smarting in the genital area, with or without a light yellow discharge. There may be slight inflammation and swelling of the Bartholin glands, which makes sitting or walking painful. The patient may also have a feeling of pelvic heaviness and discomfort in the abdomen. Anal itching and urinary symptoms may prevail. After one or more menstrual periods, untreated disease may invade the reproductive organs, including the fallopian tubes and ovaries, or may spread to the pelvis, causing pelvic inflammatory disease. Scar tissue may cause sterility. The disease can be transmitted by homosexual practices in both male and female patients. Anal gonorrhea is increasing in prevalence and causes no symptoms. In both genders, arthritis, endocarditis, and death may occur if gonorrhea is untreated.

The diagnosis of gonorrhea is based on medical history, symptoms, and laboratory test results. In men, a smear of the discharge from the penis is taken with a cotton swab and transferred to a special culture plate or bottle, where the organisms are grown for identification. The physician may want to take separate cultures a week or two apart. In women, the doctor usually takes a specimen for culture from within the vagina. Fluorescent-tagged antibody methods are the most accurate laboratory tests in women but should not be used in young children because of the risk of false-positive results. Procedures are simple and painless, and the results are confidential. If the patient is a minor, he or she can still receive free, confidential treatment without parental consent from the city or state health department or most physicians. If the test results are positive, sexual contacts are traced so that they may be treated before complications arise.

SYPHILIS

Syphilis, also known as *lues,* causes destruction throughout the body. The disease is caused by the spirochete *Treponema pallidum,* a spiral organism that reproduces rapidly in warm, moist areas of the body and quickly invades other tissues and organs. The organisms enter the body during coitus or through cuts or other breaks in the skin and mucous

Text continued on page 300

Table 15-3 Sexually Transmitted Disease Summary

DISEASE	CLINICAL PRESENTATION	THERAPY	COMPLICATIONS AND SEQUELAE	TEACHING
Chlamydia trachomatis Chlamydia	Asymptomatic infection to acute inflammatory symptoms. Males have urethritis and epididymitis. Females have urethritis, vaginitis, and cervicitis. Can be passed from mother to infant during delivery. Infants can develop conjunctivitis and pneumonia.	Specific antimicrobials are prescribed, including doxycycline, azithromycin, ofloxacin, levofloxacin, and erythromycin.	In females, Inflammation can progress to chronic pelvic inflammatory disease, which can cause infertility or ectopic pregnancy. Lymphogranuloma venereum (LVG) with genital lesions and regional lymphadenitis is a chronic consequence. Pneumonia in infected infants can be severe.	Identification and treatment during pregnancy can prevent infection in the neonate. Routine screening for Chlamydia during yearly pelvic examinations in sexually active adolescents aids in identification and treatment. Evaluate sexual contacts, and treat if the last sexual contact was within 30 days of the first appearance of symptoms or within 60 days of diagnosis in an asymptomatic patient.
Neisseria gonorrhoea Gonorrhea	Asymptomatic. Men usually have dysuria, frequency, and purulent urethral discharge. Women may have abnormal vaginal discharge, abnormal menses, dysuria, or abdominal pain. Anorectal and pharyngeal infections may be symptomatic or asymptomatic	Specific antimicrobials are prescribed, including ceftriaxone, cefixime, and azithromycin.	Women with untreated gonorrhea may have pelvic inflammatory disease develop and are at risk for its sequelae. Men are at risk for urethral stricture, epididymitis, and infertility. Newborns born to women with untreated infection are at risk for scalp abscess at the site of fetal monitors, ophthalmia neonatorum, rhinitis, disseminated infection, or anorectal infections. Untreated persons are at risk for disseminated gonococcal infection (e.g., septicemia, arthritis, dermatitis, disseminated gonococcal infection [DG], meningitis, and endocarditis).	Understand how to take any prescribed oral medications. Return for evaluation if symptoms persist or recur after treatment. Refer sexual partner(s) for examination and treatment. Avoid sex until patient and partner(s) are cured. Use condoms to prevent future infections.

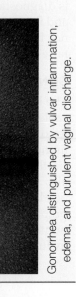

Gonorrhea distinguished by vulvar inflammation, edema, and purulent vaginal discharge.

Genital warts (human papillomavirus [HPV])

Present as single or multiple soft, fleshy, papillary or flat, painless growths around the anus, vulvovaginal area, penis, urethra, or perineum. Subclinical infection, particularly of the cervix, may occur and is best recognized with culdoscopy with application of 3% to 5% acetic acid (vinegar), which turns lesions white.

Most anogenital warts are thought to be caused by HPV type 6 or 11. Other types (principally 16, 18, and 31) have been associated with genital dysplasia and carcinoma. The presence of genital warts in children suggests sexual abuse and requires follow-up. All women with anogenital warts should have an annual Pap smear, and atypical, pigmented, or persistent warts should be biopsied. Lesions may enlarge and produce tissue destruction. Giant condylomata may simulate carcinoma yet be histologically benign.

In pregnancy, warts enlarge and are extremely vascular. Rarely, they may obstruct the birth canal, necessitating cesarean section. HPV can cause laryngeal papillomatosis in infants.

The goal of treatment is removal of warts and the amelioration of signs and symptoms, not the eradication of HPV. Treatment with podofilox 0.5% solution or gel or imiquimod 5% cream if patient applied; trichloroacetic acid may be administered by the provider. Other approaches include cryotherapy, electrocautery, laser surgery, or surgical removal.

Note: For women with cervical warts, dysplasia must be excluded before treatment is begun. Management should therefore be carried out in consultation with an expert.

... ... follow-up until lesions have resolved. Women should have annual Pap smears. Partners should be examined for warts. Abstain from sex or use condoms during therapy. Using condoms may help prevent future infections.

Two HPV vaccines are licensed: a quadrivalent vaccine (HPV4) for the prevention of cervical, vaginal, and vulvar cancers (in females) and genital warts (in females and males) and a bivalent vaccine (HPV2) for the prevention of cervical cancers in females.

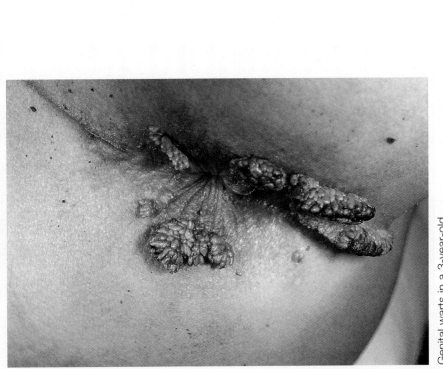

Genital warts in a 3-year-old.

Continued

Table 15-3 Sexually Transmitted Disease Summary—cont'd

DISEASE	CLINICAL PRESENTATION	THERAPY	COMPLICATIONS AND SEQUELAE	TEACHING
Herpes simplex virus type 2	Single or multiple vesicles on the genitalia. Vesicles spontaneously rupture to form shallow ulcers that may be very painful. Because the vesicular phase may be missed, especially in women, genital ulcers may be the initial presentation. Lesions resolve spontaneously without scarring. The first occurrence is termed *initial infection* or *first clinical episode* (mean duration 14-21 days). Subsequent, usually milder, occurrences are termed *recurrent infections* (mean duration of lesions 8-12 days). The interval between clinical episodes is termed *latency*. Viral shedding may occur intermittently during latency.	No known cure exists. Systemic acyclovir treatment of acute disease may reduce symptoms and signs of herpes episodes and may accelerate healing but does not eradicate the infection or affect subsequent recurrences. First clinical episode (genital) as well as episodic therapy: acyclovir, famcyclovir, or valacyclovir. Suppression of recurrent genital herpes infection: Continuous treatment reduces the frequency or severity of active disease in at least 70%-80% of patients with frequent (at least 6 per yr) recurrences. Acyclovir, twice a day. Famciclovir and valacyclovir can also be used for suppressive therapy.	Aseptic meningitis may occur during the first clinical episode. Initial acquisition of HSV infection during pregnancy increases the likelihood of maternal-to-infant transmission; women with recurrent infection infrequently transmit the virus to the neonate during vaginal delivery. Neonatal herpes ranges in severity from clinically inapparent infection to local infections of the eyes, skin, or mucous membranes to severe disseminated infection that may involve the central nervous system.	Keep involved area clean and dry. Because both initial and recurrent lesions shed virus, patients should abstain from sex while symptomatic. An undetermined but presumably small risk for transmission also exists during asymptomatic intervals. Condoms may offer some protection. The risk for fetal infection should be explained to all patients. Nonpregnant women should be reassured that genital herpes does not affect their ability to have children and that, in the great majority of cases, delivery can be performed vaginally. Pregnant women should make their clinicians/obstetricians aware of any history of herpes. Genital herpes (and other diseases-causing genital ulcers) has been associated with increased risk for acquiring HIV infection. Latex condoms can reduce risks.

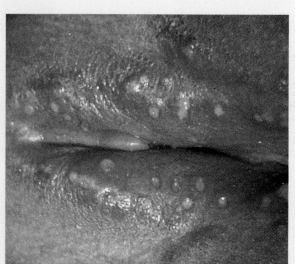

Herpes simplex with thick-walled vesicles and perineal pain.

Treponema pallidum
Syphilis

Primary: The classic chancre is painless, indurated, and located at the site of exposure.

Secondary: A highly variable skin rash, mucous patches, condylomata lata, lymphadenopathy, or other signs.

Latent: Patients are without clinical signs, although they may intermittently have signs of secondary stage.

Neurosyphilis: Neurosyphilis may be asymptomatic. If symptomatic, a variety of neurologic symptoms and signs occur, including lightning pains, ataxia, bladder disturbances, confusion, and obtundation.

Primary, secondary, or early latent syphilis: benzathine penicillin G; 2-week course of oral tetracycline or doxycycline for patients with penicillin allergy.

Late latent syphilis (or unknown duration): benzathine penicillin G.

Tertiary syphilis without neurologic involvement: benzathine penicillin G.

Neurosyphilis (inpatient therapy recommended): Aqueous crystalline penicillin G.

Both late syphilis and congenital syphilis are preventable complications on prompt diagnosis and treatment of early syphilis. Sequelae of late syphilis include neurosyphilis (although neurosyphilis may occur at any stage), cardiovascular syphilis (thoracic aortic aneurysm, aortic valve disease), and localized gumma formation. Congenital syphilis affects multiple organ systems. In addition to stillbirth and intrauterine growth retardation, sequelae of congenital syphilis may include mucocutaneous, skeletal, hematologic, central nervous system, and ocular involvement.

Return for follow-up blood studies as indicated (usually 6 and 12 mo after therapy). Follow-up may be of longer duration or at more frequent intervals. Understand the importance of returning for follow-up treatment or taking oral medications correctly, if prescribed for evaluation and treatment. Avoid sexual activity until patient and partner(s) are cured.

Use condoms to prevent future infections. Understand the risks associated with syphilis during pregnancy. Pregnant women should be screened early in pregnancy. Syphilis (and other diseases causing genital ulcers) has been associated with an increased risk for acquiring HIV infection. HIV-infected patients treated for syphilis should be followed clinically and serologically at 1, 2, 3, 6, 9, and 12 mo after treatment.

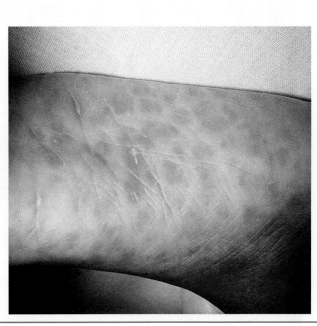

Skin rash of a child with secondary syphilis. Appears on palms of the hands and soles of the feet.

Continued

Table 15-3 Sexually Transmitted Disease Summary—cont'd

DISEASE	CLINICAL PRESENTATION	THERAPY	COMPLICATIONS AND SEQUELAE	TEACHING
Hepatitis B	Clinical symptoms and signs are indistinguishable from other forms of hepatitis and may include various combinations of anorexia, malaise, nausea, vomiting, abdominal pain, dark urine, and jaundice. Skin rashes, arthralgias, and arthritis may also occur. Only 33% to 50% of acute infections are symptomatic. Acute infections may resolve, resulting in permanent immunity. In approximately 90% of infants who acquire the infection perinatally and 5% to 10% of acute cases in the older child, infection is persistent, resulting in a chronic carrier state, which can be asymptomatic.	No specific therapy is available for acute hepatitis B or for the chronic carrier state. Universal hepatitis B vaccine administration is recommended for all infants and for unimmunized children before they reach adolescence. Hepatitis B vaccine is also recommended for persons at risk for acquiring hepatitis B virus (HBV) infection. HIV coinfection reduces the humoral response to the hepatitis B vaccine. Infants born to infected (HBsAg-positive) mothers should receive both hepatitis B immune globulin (HBIG) at birth and hepatitis B vaccine at birth, at 1 mo, and at 6 mo. Sexual partners of persons with acute hepatitis B should receive the hepatitis B vaccine and should receive HBIG if seen within 14 days of the last exposure. Sexual partners of persons who are found to be chronic carriers of HBV should receive the hepatitis B vaccine. Before treatment, testing of sexual partners for susceptibility to HBV infection is recommended if it does not delay treatment beyond 14 days.	Long-term sequelae include chronic persistent and chronic active hepatitis, cirrhosis, hepatocellular carcinoma, hepatic failure, and death. Rarely, acute infection may be fulminant with hepatic failure, resulting in death. Infectious chronic carriers may be asymptomatic but are at increased risk for developing chronic liver disease or liver cancer later.	Long-term sequelae include chronic persistent and chronic active hepatitis, cirrhosis, hepatocellular carcinoma, hepatic failure, and death. Rarely, acute infection may be fulminant with hepatic failure, resulting in death. Infectious chronic carriers may be asymptomatic but are at increased risk for developing chronic liver disease or liver cancer later. Although often asymptomatic, hepatitis B can be life-threatening and can cause serious complications. Hepatitis B is prevented by hepatitis B vaccine, which is both safe and highly effective. Persons at risk for exposure should be immunized with hepatitis B vaccine. Persons whose sexual partners have acute HBV infection should receive postexposure prophylaxis with hepatitis B vaccine and HBIG if seen within 14 days of the last exposure. Persons whose sexual partners are found to be chronic carriers of HBV should receive the hepatitis B vaccine. All pregnant women should be screened for HBsAg during pregnancy to ensure optimal management of the infant. Homosexually active men and parenteral drug users are at increased risk for both HBV and HIV infections. The frequency of clinical follow-up of persons with acute HBV infection is determined by symptomatology and the results of liver function tests. Use condoms to prevent sexual transmission to susceptible persons.

| HIV infection and AIDS | Initial symptoms in young children are failure to thrive and frequent episodes of oral Monilia infection. Other signs and symptoms include those specific to opportunistic diseases: shortness of breath and nonproductive cough resulting from *Pneumocystis carinii* pneumonia (PCP) and glossitis, dysphagia, and retrosternal pain associated with oral and esophageal candidiasis. | Although no vaccine or cure is available for HIV infection or AIDS, the development of treatment therapies, including antiretroviral agents, immunomodulators, and others, is progressing rapidly. For persons with HIV infection, zidovudine (ZDV, formerly called AZT), ddl, Epivir, d4T, and ddC may be effective in delaying the clinical conditions of HIV disease. ZDV, 3TC, and lopinavir/ritonavir or nelfinavir have been shown to produce prolonged viral suppression (Kliegman et al., 2007). Aerosol pentamidine and sulfamethoxazole/trimethoprim has been shown to be effective in preventing *Pneumocystis carinii* pneumonia. These drugs have serious side effects and require careful monitoring by knowledgeable clinicians. For persons diagnosed with AIDS, standard therapy consists of antiretroviral therapy, infection prophylaxis, and aggressive treatment of opportunistic diseases as they occur. Early treatment with ZDV (during pregnancy, at labor and delivery, and administration to newborns at birth) to HIV-positive pregnant women has decreased transmission to newborns to about 8%. Newborns of HIV-infected mothers are treated with ZDV for several weeks after birth. | Although most persons with HIV infection eventually have some symptoms develop related to their infection, some remain asymptomatic for 10 yr or more. About 30% of infants born to HIV-infected women are infected with HIV. The prognosis for these infants is poor, but therapeutic advances are being made. | Individuals initiating a sexual relationship should be counseled about sexual practices that reduce the risk for HIV transmission. Sexual partners should be informed of HIV seropositivity. Sexual practices should be limited to those that do not permit any exchange of blood, semen, or vaginal secretions. Condoms should be used consistently. Persons should not inject illicit drugs. Drug users should enroll or continue in a drug treatment program. If drug use practices continue, needles and syringes should never be shared. If sharing does occur, cleaning the "works" with bleach may decrease the risk for HIV transmission. Alcohol and other drugs that are not injected may result in carelessness in practicing safer sex. Women of childbearing age who may be at risk for HIV infection should be counseled about the risks for perinatal transmission and about contraception options. Pregnant women with known or suspected HIV infection should promptly notify their physicians to ensure optimal management of the pregnancy. STDs causing genital ulcers have been associated with an increased risk for acquiring or transmitting HIV infection. Persons with HIV infection should be skin-tested for tuberculosis. |

Therapy data modified from Centers for Disease Control and Prevention: Sexually transmitted disease curriculum for clinical educators. Retrieved October 5, 2010, from *www.cdc.gov/stdtraining/readytouse*.

membranes. The incubation period is usually 3 weeks but may be anywhere from 10 to 90 days.

The symptoms of syphilis occur in three stages: primary, secondary, and tertiary (third). The primary stage consists of the appearance of a painless sore called a **chancre** (pronounced "shanker"), which appears where the spirochete enters the body on genital, anal, or oral membranes. In females, the chancre may go unnoticed if it is located around the cervix or in the vagina. It disappears without treatment in about 6 weeks. During this time, the serologic blood test results are negative, but the organism can be identified with examination of the scrapings from the sore under the dark-field microscope. Although the chancre disappears, the destructive work of the spirochete continues as it invades various body systems.

Secondary syphilis can begin from 4 weeks to 6 months after the infection. Symptoms subside and reappear intermittently. If left untreated, the disease enters a latent period in which there are no symptoms. The latent period may last for many years. The disease remains contagious during the first 2 years, after which it is generally not communicable. Serologic test results are positive.

The tertiary stage occurs after the fourth year. The disease is noninfectious at this time but is very serious. The spirochetes attack the heart, blood vessels, brain, and spinal cord, in any of which the infection can cause death. Insanity and blindness can result. Bone tissue is destroyed, and there is severe crippling or paralysis.

Because a mother who has syphilis can infect her unborn child, obstetricians perform a serologic test (VDRL, for Venereal Disease Research Laboratories, or RPR, for rapid plasma reagin) at the first prenatal visit and just before delivery. This has been successful in preventing **congenital syphilis**. When the result is positive, the mother is treated with penicillin G, which effectively permeates the placenta regardless of the stage of pregnancy and protects the fetus. If the syphilitic mother is untreated, abortion, stillbirth, or congenital syphilis may result. Young unwed mothers and their babies are in jeopardy, particularly when early prenatal care is neglected. Case finding in adults is furthered by means of preemployment physicals, required by many companies, and by preinduction physicals by the uniformed services. The adolescent who has been raped and is at risk may need prophylactic treatment.

GENITAL HERPES

Herpes simplex virus (HSV) type II causes an STD of the genitalia. Its frequency among teenagers appears to be increasing. Genital herpes usually is caused by type II, but there is an increase of type I. The type I virus is isolated most frequently from lesions above the umbilicus, whereas the type II virus is generally isolated from genital lesions (American Academy of Pediatrics, 2006). The virus becomes latent after the initial infection, only to recur later. The incubation period is from 5 to 10 days, and the lesions may persist from 3 to 6 weeks. The infection can be extremely painful, especially if the urethra and bladder are involved. Sitz baths, heat lamps, and local compresses of Burow's solution can bring relief. Systemic symptoms include fever, headache, malaise, and anorexia. Tissue culture isolates and identifies the virus. There is no known cure, although acyclovir administration can hasten healing and the course of the episode.

HSV type II, which can be fatal to the newborn infant, is acquired from the mother during passage through the birth canal. Overwhelming infection involving many of the body systems occurs. A cesarean section is generally performed on mothers known to have this virus.

Herpes is thought to be a predisposing factor in cancer of the cervix. Regular follow-up Pap smears detect early carcinoma.

Treatment and Nursing Care

Table 15-4 describes the treatment methods and public health approaches for the most frequently seen STDs. Regardless of how health care professionals may feel about the changes in society and sexual permissiveness, they must recognize that STDs exist and deal with them appropriately. For nurses to be of help to teenagers with an STD, they must create an environment in which the teenagers feel at ease. To support adolescents' self-esteem, nurses should listen carefully to concerns with a nonjudgmental attitude.

The nurse approaches the patient with sensitivity, recognizing that the teenager is embarrassed and in need of privacy, especially during examinations. Girls are often afraid of and always nervous about a pelvic examination. This is true even when their outward manner may seem otherwise. The nurse provides careful explanations of the procedure, indicates what the patient can do to relax, drapes the patient appropriately, and remains during the examination to provide reassurance. The findings are discussed with the patient, and questions are encouraged. Most teenagers need help in being drawn out and do not readily ask questions even when they do not understand.

The reporting of sexual contacts, required by law, is an emotionally charged topic that often prevents patients from seeking help. The person who is assured of confidentiality and who has been treated in a dignified manner is more apt to cooperate. Sexually active girls must take responsibility for their own health and should be encouraged to request a chlamydial and gonorrheal culture as a routine part of their physical examination.

The nurse needs to explain to adolescents of both genders that it is particularly important to seek immediate medical attention if they suspect that their partner

Table 15-4 Interventions for the Child or Adolescent with a Sexually Transmitted Disease

ISSUE	GOALS	INTERVENTIONS
Anticipatory guidance for children under 12 yr	To provide anticipatory guidance concerning sexuality at a level that the young person can comprehend throughout the developmental cycle	Encourage educational programs that explore sexuality issues according to developmental level Provide age-appropriate instruction concerning sexuality during well-child visits Teach children strategies to deal with inappropriate touching by others Emphasize the importance of telling an adult if anything inappropriate should occur
Anticipatory guidance for adolescents	To prevent infection through anticipatory guidance	Discuss sexuality risk factors at each well checkup; include information about the relationship between sexual activity and drug and alcohol use Review structure and function of the reproductive system and personal hygiene Discuss values and decision making, possible sexual behavior and consequences, prevention of pregnancy, and STDs Advocate for a comprehensive health education program in the schools
Suspicion of infection	To identify early symptoms and facilitate prompt treatment if infection occurs	Create a nonjudgmental atmosphere, listen, assess level of knowledge, observe nonverbal behavior, establish confidentiality Provide privacy when assisting with pelvic or genital examination; ensure proper draping of patient Inquire about sexual partners and direct them to treatment, if warranted; persons with multiple sexual partners, homosexuals, persons with new partners, and those with history of prior STD are at particular risk for infection Realize anger is often a mask for depression or grief; do not take it personally Suspect sexual abuse if the child is under age 12 yr; report to Department of Social Services if disease is confirmed or sexual abuse is suspected
Compliance with treatment	To ensure that treatment plan is followed and to prevent infection of others	Advise to abstain during treatment and to use condoms if sexual activity continues Advise to take all of the prescribed medication; if the patient is taking tetracycline or doxycycline, advise to take it 1 hr before or 2 hr after meals (on an empty stomach) and to avoid dairy products, antacids, iron, and sunlight. Tell patients taking tetracycline or doxycycline that these medications decrease the effectiveness of oral contraceptives, so they should use other methods of birth control during the treatment course
Preventing complications	To prevent reinfection and sequelae	Emphasize the importance of follow-up and routine Pap smears Discuss the possible complications of specific disorders, such as birth defects and infertility

has an STD. Menstruation should not interfere with gaining medical help. Advise young people that sex with only one partner does not eliminate the risk because this person may have had contact with others; the partner needs only one sexual experience with one infected person to transmit the disease.

Sexual experimentation, lack of education, and lack of caution make adolescents highly susceptible to STDs. The goals of care should include reducing the patient's fear, obtaining a thorough history, and developing a trusting relationship. If a therapeutic relationship develops between the adolescent and the nurse, then preventive teaching can take place. See the Health Promotion box.

 Health Promotion

ABCs for STD Prevention

- Abstinence
- Be faithful (selective in choosing partner) for those who are sexually active
- Condoms
- Diagnosis (obtain screening and treatment)
- Education

Adapted from Polizzotto, M.J. (2005). Prevention of sexually transmitted diseases. *Clin Fam Pract, 7*(1), 127-137.

The percentage of patients hospitalized with STDs is small because of adequate outpatient treatment measures. Diagnosed cases are isolated. Nevertheless, because of the insidious nature of these disorders, nurses must practice scrupulous hand hygiene techniques when assisting with vaginal and rectal examinations on new admissions and when handling equipment such as rectal thermometers and douche nozzles. Hands should be kept away from the face to prevent gonorrheal conjunctivitis.

An STD that affects the reproductive organs is a serious threat to self-image and creates a great deal of anxiety. The nurse needs to assess the person's level of knowledge and provide information at that level. Many young people have little knowledge of their bodies and their developing sexuality. Others have mild to deep-seated emotional problems that need to be addressed. They may be using sex as an escape from reality, to express hostility or rebellion, or to call attention to themselves. They may be involved in relationships they no longer desire, so they need help in formulating positive attitudes toward themselves. They also need help understanding their behavior and that of others. In particular, adolescents need to learn that they are responsible for their own actions if they choose to be sexually active.

The prevention of STDs is everyone's concern and demands individual initiative and responsibility. Nurses must keep themselves informed about the latest techniques in diagnosis and treatment. Education of the public, particularly young people, is paramount. Nurses who work in settings frequented by teenagers can distribute some of the many excellent health pamphlets available. Structured courses in sex education should include presentations on STDs (there are also excellent audiovisual aids) and discussions on how to establish healthy sexual behavior patterns. The community health or school nurse is involved in case finding and referral. Delays because of fear of disclosure are tragic. Legislation has now been enacted in all 50 states that permit physicians to treat infected minors without first obtaining parental consent.

ACQUIRED IMMUNODEFICIENCY SYNDROME

Acquired immunodeficiency syndrome (AIDS) is caused by a retrovirus identified as the human immunodeficiency virus (HIV). This virus attacks T-helper cells that support immune functioning. T-suppressor cells that shut down the immune system are not altered by the virus. This causes an imbalance between these two cells, and the child is at great risk for infections.

The majority of the children affected contract the virus by mother-to-child transmission in utero, during birth, or through breastfeeding. With the early identification of pregnant HIV mothers and the use of antiretroviral therapy, the number of transmissions to the infant has been reduced from approximately 25% to

less than 8% (Kliegman et al., 2007). Drug use and sexual transmission have been the major sources of HIV infection in the adolescent.

Because the risk for HIV transmission through blood products has diminished significantly, the main focus is preventing perinatal transmission. Pregnant women at greatest risk for carrying this disease are intravenous drug users and those with multiple sexual partners. The disease can be transferred even if the mother is asymptomatic. Many women do not know they are positive for HIV when they become pregnant, and the CDC guidelines recommend that HIV screening be included in prenatal care. A portion of children born to HIV-positive mothers remain positive. With advances in prenatal treatment with zidovudine (ZDV, also known as AZT) and the aggressive use of this treatment, the overall risk for perinatal transmission has been reduced.

Signs and Symptoms

With perinatal-acquired HIV, most infants develop symptoms by 18 to 24 months. The most common signs and symptoms in infants include failure to thrive, chronic diarrhea, repeated respiratory infections, oral candidiasis, and enlargement of the liver and spleen. Developmental delays have also been noted. Kaposi's sarcoma, which is common in adults, is rare in children. The ELISA (enzyme-linked immunosorbent assay) can be used for children 18 months and older. The PCR (polymerase chain reaction) blood test is the most commonly used test for infants. Two positive PCR tests are needed to confirm HIV. Two negative PCR tests after 1 month of age can indicate negative HIV in an exposed infant.

Box 15-3 Antiretroviral Medications

NUCLEOSIDE REVERSE TRANSCRIPTASE INHIBITORS
Abacavir
Didanosine (ddI)
Lamivudine (3TC)
Stavudine (d4T)
Zalcitabine (ddC)
Zidovudine (ZDV, AZT)
Zidovudine plus lamivudine

NONNUCLEOSIDE REVERSE TRANSCRIPTASE INHIBITORS
Delavirdine (DLV)
Efavirenz
Nevirapine (NVP)

PROTEASE INHIBITORS
Amprenavir
Indinavir
Nelfinavir (NFV)
Ritonavir (RTV)
Saquinavir (SQV)

Treatment and Nursing Care

Therapy is discussed in Table 15-3. The child should receive a high-protein, high-calorie diet. Frequent, small meals should be served. The child is on intake and output checks, and daily weights are taken. The child should be immunized against the common childhood diseases but generally should not receive live vaccines. Those caring for the child should observe good hand hygiene and avoid contact with anyone who is infectious. Parents should be educated in these two areas. Box 15-3 lists antiretroviral medications.

Get Ready for the NCLEX® Examination!

Key Points

- Infants and children are at greater risk for dehydration than are adults.
- Monitoring of hydration status includes intake and output, vital signs, and level of consciousness.
- Several factors contribute to the incidence of UTIs in children; one of the most common is VUR.
- Acute poststreptococcal glomerulonephritis is caused by an untreated strep infection.
- Management of nephrotic syndrome includes reducing loss of proteins in the urine, decreasing edema, and preventing infection.
- STDs can be prevented through education from health care professionals

Additional Learning Resources

evolve Go to your Evolve website (*http://evolve.elsevier.com/Price/pediatric/*) for the following FREE learning resources:
- 3-D Animations
- Answer Keys
- Appendixes
- Audio Glossary
- Spanish/English Glossary
- Video Clips

Review Questions for the NCLEX® Examination

1. It is determined that a child has lost more electrolytes than fluids and requires intravenous treatment. This type of dehydration is considered:
   1. Isotonic
   2. Hypotonic
   3. Hypertonic
   4. Infectious

2. All of the following are potential treatments for the child with vesicoureteral reflux (VUR) **except**:
   1. Endoscopy therapy
   2. Open surgery
   3. Antimicrobial prophylaxis
   4. Voiding cystourethrography

3. Glomerulonephritis: (**Select all that apply.**)
   1. Occurs most frequently in girls
   2. Peaks in winter and spring
   3. Affects both kidneys
   4. Has a poor prognosis
   5. Is generally caused by Group A beta-hemolytic streptococci

4. An excessive amount of fluid in the sac that surrounds the testicle is called:
   1. Hydrocele
   2. Cryptorchidism
   3. Hypospadias
   4. Chordee

5. Genital warts result from infection from:
   1. Gonorrhea
   2. Syphilis
   3. Human immunodeficiency virus
   4. Human papillomavirus

16

Integumentary Disorders

Objectives

1. Define the vocabulary terms listed
2. Differentiate diaper dermatitis from candidiasis
3. Summarize the nursing care for an infant who has atopic dermatitis, and give the rationale for each nursing measure
4. Discuss care of the child with impetigo
5. Identify complications associated with Staphylococcus
6. Discuss care of the child with cellulitis
7. Define two sources of pediculosis transmission
8. Identify two methods of evaluating burn injury
9. Discuss wound management precautions associated with burn injury
10. Discuss precautions taken with accutane use

Key Terms

allergens (A-lər-gənz; p. 305)
allograft (A-lə-graft; p. 315)
autograft (O-tō-graft; p. 315)

comedo (KŎM-ĕ-dō; p. 316)
eschar (ES-kär; p. 315)
sebum (SĒ-bŭm; p. 315)

INTEGUMENTARY SYSTEM

The integumentary system consists of the skin and associated structure (hair, nails), as well as the subcutaneous tissue. The skin is the largest organ in the body. The epidermis is the thinner, outer layer of the skin and the dermis is the inner, thicker layer of skin. The dermis contains the hair, nails, sebaceous and sweat glands, blood vessels, nerve endings, and sensory organs. Below the dermis is the subcutaneous layer, which literally means "under the skin."

The skin functions to protect the body from pathogens; provides sensory receptors regarding pain, touch, pressure, and temperature; aids in production of Vitamin D; provides cosmetic covering; and regulates temperature as blood vessels dilate and perspiration occurs.

There are many disorders related to this system. Skin disorders range from those caused by infection to those associated with injury. It is important to remember that the *immune system* is affected by a weakened integumentary system. Skin disorders such as acne can lead to concerns about appearance and have a psychological impact on children, especially adolescents. The disfigurement from burns can have a lifelong effect on children.

Discussion of the skin disorders will begin with those occurring in infants. The mucosal (mucous membrane) disorder "thrush" will be included in the discussion as diaper dermatitis oftentimes accompanies this disorder.

THRUSH (ORAL CANDIDIASIS)

Thrush is an infection of the mucous membranes of the mouth caused by the fungus *Candida*. This organism is normally present in the mother's vagina and is nonpathogenic. However, the altered conditions in the vagina produced by pregnancy may lead to the development of **monilial vaginitis**. The mucous membranes of the baby's mouth may become infected by direct contact with this infection during delivery or by contact with the mother's or nurse's contaminated hands. Cross-infection of other newborn infants may then result. Breastfed infants may transfer the infection to the mother's nipples if good hygiene is not followed. Thrush can also occur when oral flora is altered as a result of antimicrobial therapy.

Signs and Symptoms

White patches that resemble milk curds are visible on the tongue, inner lips, gums, and oral mucosa. Initially, these are painless but do not wipe away. The patches may bleed if attempts are made to scrape them away. Because of the discomfort, anorexia may be present. The systemic symptoms are mild if the infection remains in the mouth; however, it can pass along the mucous membranes into the gastrointestinal tract, causing inflammation of the esophagus and stomach.

The infant may develop a beefy red, weeping diaper rash in the genitalia area (see Diaper Dermatitis).

Treatment and Nursing Care
This infection responds well to local application of antimicrobial *suspensions*. Nystatin, for example, may be applied with a swab or a gloved finger. The mouth is swabbed three or four times a day, after feedings, with a sterile applicator moistened with the prescribed solution. The remainder of the dose is deposited in the infant's mouth to be swallowed, treating any other lesions of the gastrointestinal tract. With treatment, the disease is usually self-limiting in an otherwise healthy infant. Topical antifungal ointment such as Nystatin may be administered to skin areas that have been affected.

 Nursing Brief

In the home, parents are taught to place nystatin or other medication slowly into each cheek pocket of the baby's mouth. Medication needs to remain in contact with "patches" as long as possible. The baby should not be fed after medication administration. Instruct parents to watch for dehydration (decrease in number of wet diapers and so on, caused by the baby's refusal to take fluids because of mouth discomfort).

Prevention of this infection begins in the prenatal period. Mothers suspected of having *Candida* infection can be properly treated. Effective hand hygiene to prevent reinfection from the mother is necessary. This is particularly true if she is breastfeeding her infant. If bottles are used, nipples require scrupulous cleaning because they come in direct contact with the lesions. Nurses and other personnel must maintain a high quality of nursing care to prevent cross-infection.

DIAPER DERMATITIS (DIAPER RASH)
Diaper dermatitis is an inflammatory disorder caused by prolonged contact with an irritant such as urine or feces. Irritants in diapers or diaper wipes can also cause diaper rash. Washing cloth diapers in harsh laundry detergent can also be a contributing factor.

Signs and Symptoms
Reddened, irritated skin occurs in the diaper area and may be accompanied by blistering. The skin folds often are not affected. A beefy red rash is generally indicative of Candidiasis (Figure 16-1).

Treatment and Nursing Care
Diaper dermatitis responds well to zinc oxide ointments (Balmex, Desitin). See previous discussion for Candidiasis treatment. Frequent diaper changes, liberal application of a zinc oxide–based barrier cream, and using a moist, damp cloth for cleansing are generally all that is needed for diaper dermatitis control.

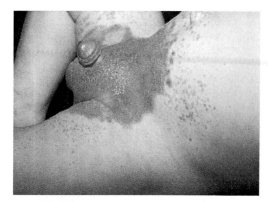
FIGURE 16-1 Candidiasis of the diaper area.

Only mild soap and water should be used to remove stool from the skin, particularly if commercial wipes are irritating. Petroleum jelly can be an inexpensive barrier that helps prevent diaper dermatitis. Powder is not recommended because it can be aspirated into the lungs. Powder can also become a skin irritant, especially if it becomes "caked" on. If it *must* be used (parental preference), parents need to be taught to first apply it to their hand, then to the dry diaper area. Always keep powder containers closed and out of the infant's reach as they can be a choking and aspiration hazard.

 Nursing Brief

If cloth diapers are used, use overwraps that allow air to circulate; do not use "plastic" pants.

ATOPIC DERMATITIS (INFANTILE ECZEMA)
Atopic dermatitis is an inflammation of genetically hypersensitive skin. The pathophysiology is characterized by local vasodilation in affected areas. This progresses to **spongiosis**, or the breakdown of dermal cells and the formation of intradermal vesicles. Chronic scratching produces weeping and results in **lichenification**, or coarsening of the skin folds. The exact cause of this condition is unclear, but several factors may contribute to the condition. Factors can include a family history and/or triggers such as household aeroallergens (dust mites, cat dander, mold), environmental irritants (soaps, detergent, clothing, smoke), extreme temperatures, chemical vapors and gases, food sensitivities, and infections. Atopic dermatitis is seen less frequently in breastfed babies, and delaying introduction of solid food can decrease atopic dermatitis in the first 4 years of life. It seems to have a familial tendency, and emotional factors are often involved.

Development of symptoms indicates that the infant is oversensitive to certain substances called allergens, which enter the body via the digestive tract (food), inhalation (dust, pollen), direct contact (wool, soap,

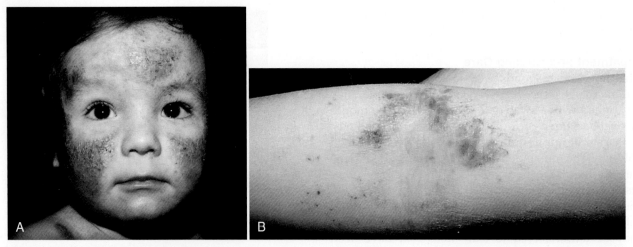

FIGURE 16-2 **A,** Infantile atopic dermatitis or eczema is shown with acute weeping lesions on the cheeks and forehead. **B,** In childhood, eczema can involve the flexor surfaces of extremities.

strong sunlight), or injections (insect bites, vaccines). Of children who have atopic dermatitis, 50% to 60% present with symptoms in the first year of life and 80% to 85% present by 5 years of age. Overall, 10% to 20% of children are affected by the disease (Cardona et al., 2006). Many children (80%) develop the triad of atopic dermatitis, asthma, and allergic rhinitis.

Signs and Symptoms

The lesions form vesicles that weep and develop a dry crust. They are more severe on the face (Figure 16-2) but may occur on the entire body, particularly in the skin folds. Eczema is worse in winter than in summer and has periods of temporary remission.

The infant scratches because the itching is constant and he or she becomes irritable and unable to sleep. The lesions are easily infected by bacterial or viral agents. Herpes simplex is the viral agent of particular concern. Infants and children with eczema should not be exposed to adults with "cold sores." Streptococcal and staphylococcal infection can also complicate the disease process. Eczema may flare up after immunization. Laboratory studies may show an increase in immunoglobulin E (IgE) and eosinophil levels.

Treatment

Treatment is aimed at maintaining the skin integrity, skin hydration, decreasing pruritus, and identification and avoidance of triggers. Treatment includes topical corticosteroids, topical immunosuppressants, and antihistamines. Corticosteroids vary from low potency to strong potency. They are used for different severities and areas of the body. Topical immunosuppressants (tacrolimus or pimecrolimus) are effective on all body areas, and because they cause fewer side effects, they are appropriate for long-term usage. Antihistamines (Atarax, Benadryl) given at bedtime can help control nighttime itching and enhance sleep. Sleep deprivation is a major problem for children with atopic dermatitis. If pharmacologic therapy is not effective, food allergies should be explored. Foods to which these infants may be sensitive include eggs, wheat, cow's milk, peanuts, and citrus fruits. If food allergies are identified, a restrictive diet may be required.

An emollient bath may provide a soothing effect on the infant's skin. Oatmeal and a mixture of cornstarch and baking soda are examples of substances prescribed. Tepid baths (15 to 20 minutes of soaking) and immediate application of emollient moisturizer afterward are key to skin hydration. Occlusive ointments such as Aquaphor, Eucerin, and Cetaphil are effective. Lotions are less effective and not recommended. Application of moisturizer while the skin is damp assists in hydration of the skin. Any lotions with alcohol should be avoided.

Nursing Care

The nurse plays a vital role in the treatment of children with skin problems. Shortening fingernails and putting cotton mittens on hands and feet can be effective. Medicated or oatmeal baths may be part of the treatment. The child should be patted or air-dried, not rubbed. Children with eczema should not be overdressed because undue warmth adds to their discomfort. One-piece soft clothing to prevent binding and irritation is recommended. Wool should be avoided.

Wet dressings are applied to the areas to reduce itching and in some cases to remove crusts. A gauze bandage is dipped into the prescribed solution (such as Burow's solution), squeezed gently to remove excess fluid, and applied to the involved area. The bandage must cover the entire rash. Soaks are usually ordered to be done continuously, and their effectiveness depends on their being *wet*. When they are left on too long and become dried out, itching increases. This type of bandage is **not** covered with towels or rubber sheeting in an effort to protect the bed linens because the itching is relieved by the cooling effect of the medication, and covering the bandage prevents evaporation. Observations for the nurse to chart regarding the application of wet soaks include time of application, name of solution, strength of solution, area to which it was applied, length of time applied, general condition of the involved area (changes in the appearance or area of the rash), and comfort and tolerance of the patient during and after the procedure.

The physician may prescribe an elimination diet. A basic diet consisting of only hypoallergenic foods is given to the child initially. One new food at a time is added to determine the infant's reaction. When the baby is allergic to cow's milk, a substitute such as soybean milk can be used. Vitamin supplements are needed, particularly if the infant is not consuming enough of the prescribed fruits and vegetables. The nurse charts the kind and amount of food taken at each meal and any allergic reactions that may have occurred.

Home Care Considerations

The Child with Atopic Dermatitis (Eczema)

- Use tepid water for bathing.
- Avoid irritating soaps.
- Avoid washcloths or scrubs.
- Air-dry skin and pat with a soft towel.
- Apply topical corticosteroid before emollient.
- Apply emollient within 3 minutes of bath.
- Keep fingernails short and clean.
- Use cotton "mitts" at night.
- Use cotton sheets and pajamas.
- Moisturize skin often until skin is soft and pliable.
- Use mild laundry detergent.
- Discontinue topical corticosteroid when skin clears.

Nursing Brief

An effective moisturizer that is also inexpensive is Crisco shortening (Cardona et al., 2006). Parents need to be taught that it should not be used around the eyes or nasal passages.

The nurse should establish a good working relationship with the parents. Families report high stress and feelings of helplessness in caring for children with atopic dermatitis. Parents express issues with the child's sleeplessness due to itching and the child's decreased self-esteem due to his or her physical appearance. The nurse should listen to ensure that parents understand the physician's instructions and should clarify matters as needed (Nursing Care Plan 16-1).

IMPETIGO

Impetigo is an infectious disease of the skin caused by staphylococci or by group A beta-hemolytic streptococci. There are two classifications: **bullous** (impetigo bullosa) and **nonbullous** (impetigo contagiosa). Both forms are generally seen in children ages 2 to 5 years. The bullous form, seen primarily in infants, is usually caused by *Staphylococcus aureus*, whereas the nonbullous type can been seen in children of all ages and is caused by either staphylococci or streptococci. Impetigo tends to spread from one area of skin to another and is quite contagious.

Signs and Symptoms

The first symptoms of a nonbullous lesion are red papules (Figure 16-3). These eventually became small vesicles or pustules surrounded by a reddened area. When the blister breaks, the surface beneath is raw and weeping and appears like a partial thickness burn. The

Nursing Care Plan 16-1 The Child with Atopic Dermatitis (Eczema)

NURSING DIAGNOSIS *Imbalanced nutrition, less than body requirements, related to irritability, sensitivity to certain foods, and increased metabolic needs*

Goals/Outcome Criteria	Nursing Interventions	Rationales
The child has an adequate diet, as evidenced by: • Maintenance of weight or an increase in weight	Assess diet according to age.	As the child grows, the nutritional needs change.
	Determine with history whether the child is sensitive to any specific foods.	Food sensitivity can trigger a stronger response to the condition.
	Administer hypoallergenic diet.	Hypoallergenic foods have been found to be less offensive to many people.
	Observe child for any food sensitivity.	Any food item can be a potential substance to which the body is sensitive.
	Administer vitamins and minerals as prescribed.	May be given in supplemental form to aid the body in healing and growth.
	Provide adequate fluids.	Fluids are important to the child because the child's body is made up of a higher percentage of fluids than the adult's. If fluid is lost through the skin, the child can easily become dehydrated.

Continued

Nursing Care Plan 16-1 The Child with Atopic Dermatitis (Eczema)—cont'd

NURSING DIAGNOSIS *Deficient knowledge related to the nature of the disorder*

Goals/Outcome Criteria	Nursing Interventions	Rationales
The parents understand the nature of the disorder, as evidenced by: • Ability to verbalize the information given to them • Asking questions • Describing routine care of the skin	Assess the knowledge of the parents.	Allows the nurse to teach the parents.
	Instruct the parents in the care of the child's skin	These are all areas that decrease the irritation to the skin or aid in healing of the skin.
	• Remove clothing that might irritate the skin (e.g., wool).	Wool is an irritant to the skin.
	• Provide loose cotton clothing.	Cotton absorbs if it is loose, does not constrict.
	• Use a mild detergent to launder clothing.	Decreases the irritation of soap in the clothing.
	• Thoroughly rinse clothing.	Ensures that most of the soap is removed from the clothing.
	• Bathe the child in tepid water.	Tepid water decreases the amount of vasodilation, thus causing a decrease in stimulation to the skin and resulting in a decrease in itching.
	Expose infant to sunlight but monitor closely.	Sunlight can be healing to the skin, but because of the skin's condition, too much sunlight can cause more irritation.
	Help parents identify products that contain wheat, milk, eggs, and peanuts.	These foods have been found to cause allergic reactions in children.
	Advise parents to expect exacerbations and remissions.	Eczema can recur. If the parents know this, treatment can be sought earlier and the intensity of the condition can be lessened.

NURSING DIAGNOSIS *Risk for impaired skin integrity, related to scratching and irritation of the skin*

Goals/Outcome Criteria	Nursing Interventions	Rationales
The child is free of skin infection, as evidenced by: • Intact skin • Skin warm, dry, and pink • Skin free of discharge	Assess the skin.	Reveals any breaks in the skin, discharge, or lesions.
	Describe any type of lesion.	Allows the lesions to be monitored to see whether the condition improves or worsens.
	Provide elbow restraints.	Helps the child refrain from scratching. A proper fit is important. Restraints should never be used in place of supervision.
	Hold and comfort the child as needed.	The child may be irritable and restless because of the condition of the skin. Holding and consoling may help the child rest.
	Keep the child's fingernails short, and cover the hands with a sock or mitten.	Decreases the child's ability to scratch.
	Administer medicated baths as ordered.	Soothing to the skin.
	Apply dressings, and teach parents proper application.	Soothing and healing for the skin.
	Administer antimicrobials as ordered.	Used to prevent or resolve a skin infection.
	Teach parents the importance of proper hand hygiene.	Proper hand hygiene decreases the transfer of organisms.

Critical Thinking Question

1. A mother of an 8-month-old child comes to the clinic for a follow-up appointment. She tells the nurse that the doctor told her the baby had eczema. She says that she has been giving her baby a bath in hot, soapy water twice a day. She is putting hand lotion on the lesions, but they seem to be getting worse. She cannot seem to stop the baby from scratching. What teaching interventions by the nurse would be appropriate?

⭐ **Nursing Care Plan 16-1**   **The Child with Atopic Dermatitis (Eczema)—cont'd**

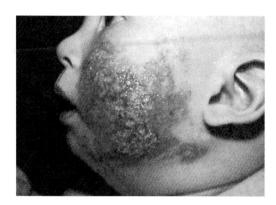

Critical Thinking Snapshot

In evaluating this child with eczema, what are important areas that need to be documented? How should the description of the lesions be noted? What would be expected if the lesions worsen? What symptoms would warrant the parent to seek immediate medical treatment?

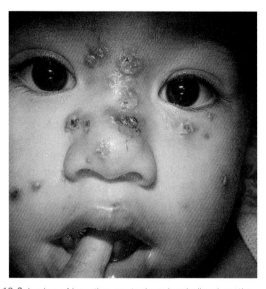

FIGURE 16-3 Lesion of impetigo contagiosa (nonbullous) on the child's face, showing the honey-colored crust.

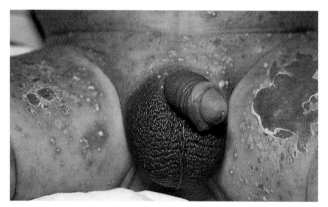

FIGURE 16-4 Infant with Staphylococcus diaper dermatitis has multiple small, thin-walled pustules that rupture rapidly, leaving a shallow base and superficial peeling rims.

lesions may occur anywhere but are most often found on the face, neck, and extremities. A honey-colored crust forms.

Bullous lesions present as vesicles that become fluid-filled. The fluid-filled sac can be tense or flaccid. It eventually ruptures, collapses, and leaves a base with a peeling rim (Figure 16-4). Both forms can cause itching, and the resulting scratching can spread the lesions.

Treatment and Nursing Care

The lesions may be cleaned three or four times a day with soap and water to remove crusts. This cleansing is followed by the application of topical antimicrobial ointment (Bactroban). Oral antimicrobials may also be given (dicloxacillin or cephalexin [Keflex]). The prognosis with proper treatment is good. Nursing care consists primarily of preventing this disease with proper aseptic methods. Once the diagnosis is made, preventing spread to other infants and children becomes an issue. Parents need instructions regarding mode of transmission, which is person-to-person, and preventive measures. Acute glomerulonephritis may occur as a complication of beta-hemolytic streptococcal infections (see Chapter 15 for discussion on glomerulonephritis).

STAPHYLOCOCCUS AUREUS INFECTION

The bacterial genus *Staphylococcus* comprises common bacteria that are found in dust and on the skin. In normal conditions, they do not present a problem to healthy body defenses. If the number of organisms increases in infants whose general resistance is low, skin infections may occur. Neonates have fragile skin that can be traumatized with the use of electrodes or lancets. For the critically ill newborn, technological advances such as indwelling catheters or hyperalimentation can provide routes for infection. An infection or abscess may form, and in some cases of delayed treatment, infection may enter the bloodstream. This condition is called **septicemia** or **bacteremia**. Pneumonia, osteomyelitis, or meningitis may result. Infection may spread easily from one infant to another in the newborn nursery. Pustules must be reported and appropriate isolation precautions taken to prevent further exposure.

Treatment and Nursing Care

Antimicrobials effective against the particular strain are administered. Ointments may be applied locally. Some of the staphylococci have developed resistance to current drugs. Methicillin-resistant *S. aureus* (MRSA) infections have developed. When MRSA is diagnosed, vancomycin is often prescribed. Some of these strains have become vancomycin-resistant (VRSA). Linezolid (Zyvox) is currently used for vancomycin-resistant enterococcus infections. There is ongoing research with both the MRSA and VRSA infections. This resistance makes treatment difficult and has prompted the careful use of antimicrobials. Three distinctive disorders have been identified: staphylococcal scalded skin syndrome, staphylococcal scarlet fever, and toxic shock syndrome (Table 16-1 and Figure 16-5).

Control of the spread of this infection is sometimes difficult because health care providers can act as carriers. The chief reservoir in the carrier for harboring this organism is the nose. To prevent staphylococcal infections, strict standards must be upheld in all facilities. The number and quality of personnel and their health status are also important factors. Washing hands before and after touching each patient and before and after handling equipment is **essential** and supported by the CDC. Medical follow-up remains important for these patients.

CELLULITIS

Cellulitis is a bacterial infection of the skin and subcutaneous tissue, caused by Streptococcus, Staphylococcus, or *Haemophilus influenzae*. It can occur from injuries such as bug bites or trauma and can be associated with other conditions such as otitis media.

Signs and Symptoms

Clinical manifestations include edematous, reddened skin that is tender and warm to the touch. There may be red streaks and involvement of regional lymph nodes. It can progress to abscess formation. The child often presents with fever and malaise and if untreated, cellulitis can result in septicemia.

Treatment and Nursing Care

Children with cellulitis that involves only an extremity or the trunk are often managed at home with oral antimicrobials. Application of warm, moist compresses will increase circulation and promote healing. Children who have cellulitis of the face or those with more extensive cellulitis are hospitalized and receive parenteral antimicrobials with continued treatment at discharge. The family is taught the importance of good hand hygiene, completing all prescribed antimicrobials, and applying warm, moist compresses.

PEDICULOSIS

The infestation of humans by lice is known as *pediculosis*. The three types of pediculosis are pediculosis capitis, or head lice; pediculosis corporis, or body lice; and pediculosis pubis, or crab or pubic lice. The various types usually remain in the part of the body designated by their name. They are transmitted from person to person or from contaminated articles. Their survival depends on the blood they extract from the infected person. Severe itching in the affected area is the main symptom. Treatment in all cases is aimed at ridding the patient of the parasite, treating the excoriated skin, and preventing the infestation of others. The most common form seen in children is head lice. The child or parents may be embarrassed by the presence of lice, but infestations spread quickly in schools and do not reflect on the hygiene of the families.

Head lice affect the scalp and hair. The adult louse attaches numerous eggs, known as *nits*, to the hair shafts approximately $\frac{1}{8}$ inch from the scalp (Figure 16-6). Nits hatch within 3 or 4 days. Head lice are more common in girls than in boys because of hair length.

Table **16-1** *Staphylococcus Aureus* Infections

TYPE	SIGNS AND SYMPTOMS	SKIN MANIFESTATIONS	TREATMENT
Scalded skin syndrome	Sudden onset of fever and irritability; vomiting	Generalized erythema, tender to touch, bullous lesions; skin sloughs	Antimicrobials (e.g., vancomycin); fluids
Staphylococcus scarlet fever	Fever; irritability; malaise	Erythematous rash (sandpaper) in skin creases; skin cracks, weeps, and sheds	Oral antimicrobials
Toxic shock syndrome	Life threatening; abrupt fever with vomiting and abdominal pain; multiorgan involvement and dysfunction; hypotension	General exanthema with macular rash; strawberry tongue; sloughing of skin	Antimicrobials; fluids; cardiovascular and respiratory monitoring

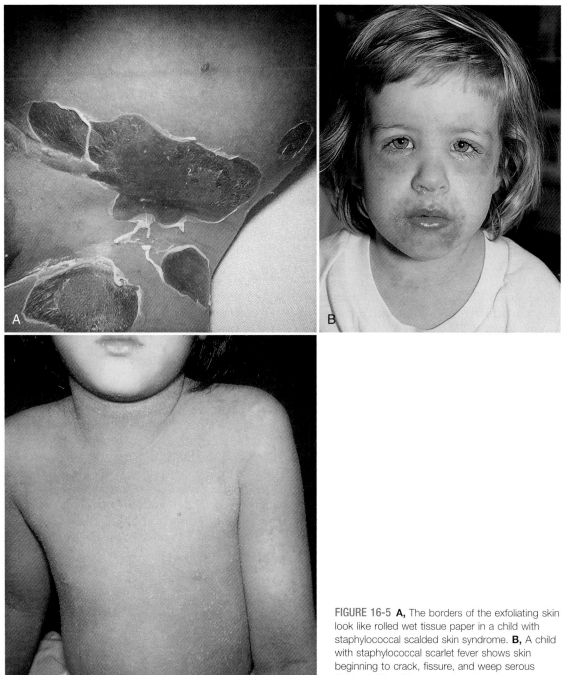

FIGURE 16-5 **A,** The borders of the exfoliating skin look like rolled wet tissue paper in a child with staphylococcal scalded skin syndrome. **B,** A child with staphylococcal scarlet fever shows skin beginning to crack, fissure, and weep serous fluids. **C,** The diffuse macular skin eruption in a child with staphylococcal toxic shock syndrome.

The parasite may be acquired from hats, combs, or hairbrushes. It is easily transferred from one child to another and is seen most frequently in the school-age child and in preschool children who attend daycare centers.

Signs and Symptoms
The child has severe itching of the scalp. Scratching of the head can cause further irritation. The hair may become matted. Occasionally pustules and excoriations are seen about the face. Nurses who admit patients to pediatric units should be on the alert for

head lice. In particular, inspect the hairline at the back of the neck and about the ears. Crusts, nits, and dirt may cause matting of the hair and a foul odor.

Treatment and Nursing Care
Management is directed toward killing the adult lice, getting rid of the nits, and treating any infections of the face and scalp. Family members and playmates of the child should be examined and treated as necessary. The drug of choice is 1% permethrin (Nix) or pyrethrin A-200 (RID) products, which must be applied at least twice, as they are not completely

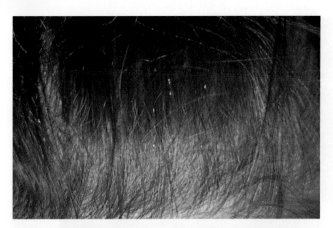

FIGURE 16-6 Head lice nits appear as tiny white dots along the hair shaft. Typically they are firmly attached to the hair around and behind the ears.

ovicidal. Both are nonprescription. Watch for an allergic response, particularly in children with a history of skin problems. Lindane (Kwell) has also been used; however, it has more reported side effects and should not be used to treat head lice in children. In 2009, the FDA approved the use of Ulesfia lotion (benzyl alcohol) for children 6 months and older. A second treatment is needed to kill the nits. Side effects include irritation of the skin, scalp, and eyes; numbness of the scalp has also been reported. If the eyebrows and eyelashes are involved, a thick coating of petrolatum (Vaseline) is applied, followed by removal of remaining nits. Nits on the head are removed by combing the hair with a fine-tooth comb.

Charting includes date and time, condition of scalp and hair before treatment, odor (if noticeable), type of shampoo used, how the procedure was tolerated, and the amount of relief obtained. Any signs of systemic infection should also be documented.

Clothing or bedding should be laundered in hot water. Mattresses may be sprayed with a disinfectant. Wool clothing requires dry cleaning or can be placed dry into a clothes dryer set on hot cycle for at least 20 minutes. Clothing and items that are nonwashable can be sealed in a plastic bag and stored for 2 weeks. Children should be cautioned against swapping caps, headphones, helmets, bandanas, hair ties, brushes, and combs. Combs and brushes are disinfested by soaking them in hot water for at least 5 to 10 minutes. Parents are instructed to inspect the child's head regularly. Encourage parents to report infestations to the school nurse because widespread outbreaks are encountered periodically.

Cutting the child's hair is discouraged because it can be a source of stress to the child, who is already being singled out as "the child with lice." Oral Benadryl may be given for pruritus. Parents should be cautioned to watch for symptoms of secondary infection caused by breaks in the skin from scratching.

BURNS

Burns are a leading cause of accidental death in children. Most burns are minor and can be treated on an outpatient basis. However, some burns are quite severe and require hospitalization either locally or at a burn center. Toddlers may pull hot liquids down on themselves. Older children sometimes misuse matches and flammable materials. One common preventable burn is caused by a curling iron. Burns are categorized as thermal, radiation, electrical, or chemical. Severe burns cause fluid and electrolyte imbalances and can affect every body system. Infection, scarring, and functional disabilities are major complications of severe burns.

Signs and Symptoms

The burn wound is classified according to percentage of body surface involved, depth, location of the injury, and association with other injuries. The age of the child and the presence of respiratory involvement are also important factors.

A method for determining the percentage of skin surface area in children at various ages is presented in Figure 16-7. The "rule of nines," which is used with the older adolescent and the adult, is not applicable in the infant and small child because of the difference in body proportions.

Depth of burn injury is described in Table 16-2. Burns are described as superficial, partial-thickness (superficial and deep), and full-thickness. Some references differentiate full-thickness and deep full-thickness; deep full-thickness would include fascia and muscle with potential for bone and tendon damage. Superficial burns heal in 3 to 7 days, whereas partial-thickness burns can take weeks to months, provided there is no infection. This is because partial-thickness burns involve the epidermis and the dermis. Full-thickness burns generally do not heal without skin grafting. Scarring is present in deep partial-thickness and full-thickness burns. Full-thickness burns (Figure 16-8) involve total destruction of the epidermis and dermis and underlying tissues. The wound is leathery, tan, dark red or brown, and not as painful as the partial thickness burn. Although the patient may not have pain at the actual wound site, there is pain along the edges of the wound where nerve endings are intact. Full-thickness burns require debridement, topical antimicrobials, and grafting; they are managed at a burn center. The child with first- and second-degree (superficial and partial-thickness) burns covering less than 10% of total body surface area may be treated on an outpatient basis if there is adequate family support and there are no issues of child neglect or abuse (Kliegman et al., 2007). Inhalation burns, chemical burns, burns that involve the joints or face, burns that involve the genitalia or perineum, and electrical burns should be treated in a specialized setting such as a burn unit. Patients who have preexisting medical conditions or

Table 16-2 Depth of Burn Injury

| | NORMAL SKIN | SUPERFICIAL (FIRST-DEGREE) | PARTIAL-THICKNESS (SECOND-DEGREE) | | FULL-THICKNESS (THIRD-DEGREE) |
			SUPERFICIAL	DEEP	
	Normal skin				
Morphology		Destruction of epidermis; physiology functions remain intact	Destruction of epidermis and some dermis	Destruction of epidermis and dermis	Destruction of epidermis, dermis, underlying tissue; may include fascia, muscle, tendon, bone
Blister formation		After 24 hr (e.g., from sunburn)	Within minutes; thin-walled, fluid-filled	May or may not appear as fluid-filled blisters; often they are flat, dehydrated, and like tissue paper; body fluids lost through burn tissue must be replaced	Rare; may appear as a tissue paper-like layer that is flat and dehydrated
Appearance		Peels after 24-48 hr	Red to pale ivory, moist surface	Mottled, waxy white, dry surface	White, cherry red, or black
Healing time		3-7 days	7-21 days if no infection develops	30 days to several months if no infection; if infected, this type of burn may convert to full-thickness	Will not heal; skin grafting required; very small areas may heal from edges after a period of weeks
Patient reaction		Moderate discomfort, pain; chills; nausea; vomiting	May cause considerable pain	Severe pain on exposure to air or water because nerve endings are intact	No pain in area of full-thickness burn because nerve endings are destroyed; surrounding areas of lesser depth are painful
Scarring		None	Minimal; influenced by genetic predisposition	Greatest because the slow healing of these burns increases scar tissue; scar formation influenced by genetic predisposition	Autograft scarring minimized by early excision and grafting; scar formation influenced by genetic predisposition

Modified from McKinney E., James S., Murray, S., et al. (2009). *Maternal child nursing* (3rd ed.). Philadelphia: Saunders.

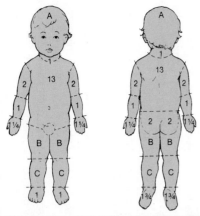

RELATIVE PERCENTAGES OF AREAS AFFECTED BY GROWTH

AREA	BIRTH	AGE 1 YR	AGE 5 YR
A = ½ of head	9½	8½	6½
B = ½ of one thigh	2¾	3¼	4
C = ½ of one leg	2½	2½	2¾

A

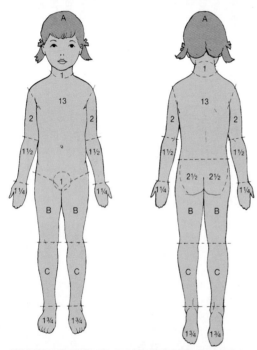

RELATIVE PERCENTAGES OF AREAS AFFECTED BY GROWTH

AREA	AGE 10 YR	AGE 15 YR	ADULT
A = ½ of head	5½	4½	3½
B = ½ of one thigh	4½	4½	4¾
C = ½ of one leg	3	3¼	3½

B

FIGURE 16-7 Burn chart for children.

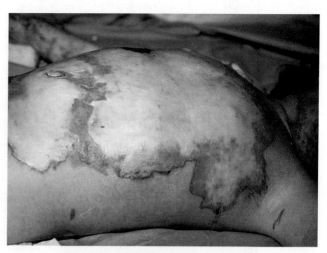

FIGURE 16-8 Full-thickness thermal injury.

trauma associated with the burn injury should also be treated in a specialized setting.

Treatment and Nursing Care

The primary goal in the initial treatment of major burns is the maintenance of an airway and the prevention of shock (*airway, breathing, circulation*). Airway obstruction should be suspected if the child has inhaled smoke or the burn involves the face. Oxygen is administered, and oxygenation is monitored closely. An endotracheal tube is inserted if the child is in respiratory distress. After assessment of the airway and respiratory status, fluid resuscitation is the next priority. *Burn shock* occurs with major burns as a result of massive capillary leakage of circulating fluid into the surrounding tissues. The fluid loss resulting from major burns must be replaced to prevent shock. An intravenous (IV) infusion is started, and fluid volume restoration is initiated. Ringer's lactate in 5% dextrose solution is often used for initial resuscitation (Kliegman et al., 2007). Various formulas for fluid replacement are used, based on practitioner's preference. Blood pressure, capillary refill, heart rate, and urine output must be monitored. A Foley catheter is placed; 1 to 2 mL/kg/hr of urine output serves as the guideline for ensuring successful fluid volume restoration (Duffy et al., 2006). After initial stabilization, the child with a major burn is transferred to a burn treatment facility.

Wound Management. A superficial burn does not require topical antimicrobial medication. Cool compresses and soothing lotions may be used for superficial burns. An antimicrobial agent such as Bacitracin or Neosporin is best used for a superficial partial-thickness burn that is expected to heal within 2 to 3 weeks. Bacitracin may also be used on the face. Silvadene is an antimicrobial cream that has bactericidal activity and is commonly used on partial- and full-thickness burns to prevent wound sepsis. It should not be used on children with known sulfa sensitivity. Sulfamylon is similar, yet effective against *Pseudomonas aeruginosa*; it is used as a topical antimicrobial for a partial- or full-thickness burn (Duffy et al., 2006). Burn wounds may be treated as open (wound uncovered) or covered with a range of thin gauze to bulky gauze. Dressings are changed one to three times daily.

Hydrotherapy can be used to remove the old dressing and to clean the wound and the child. Range-of-motion exercises can be done during this time. Hydrotherapy can be done in a tub or shower. Debridement is done to remove dead tissue. Burned tissue called eschar must be removed to prevent infection. Breaking blisters is controversial. Pain management during dressing change is essential. The goal of care is to prevent infection in the wound. Tetanus prophylaxis should be given if the child is not current in this immunization.

In full-thickness burns where reepithelialization does not take place, grafting (skin transplant) is necessary. Temporary grafts, such as biological or synthetic skin coverings, may be needed until permanent grafting can take place. Cultured skin can actually be grown under special conditions from a postage stamp-sized piece of skin from the patient and then grafted back to the patient. Allograft skin is obtained from human cadavers that have been screened for communicable disease and serves as a temporary graft. Permanent grafts are obtained from an undamaged area of the patient's body (autografts).

Nursing Brief

Biobrane (Smith and Nephew) is a biosynthetic skin dressing that can be used on superficial and partial-thickness wounds and donor sites. It is composed of a silicone-nylon mesh (porcine) and increases healing time while decreasing pain. Integra Artificial Skin (Integra Life-Sciences) is a two-layered dressing that serves as a temporary synthetic epidermis and as a foundation for regrowth of dermal tissue.

Wound care is extremely painful and causes emotional consequences in children if the pain is not addressed. Adequate use of pharmacologic and non-pharmacologic pain relief approaches is essential. Maintenance of strict sterile technique reduces the chance of infection.

Scarring can be minimized through application of continuous pressure to the scar during the rehabilitative phase. Wearing pressure garments prevents scarring by applying a counter pressure to the wounded area. These garments should be worn at all times, except for bathing or cleaning the garment. They may be necessary for up to 18 months. If scarring is extensive, especially around joints, joint limitation and contractures can result. Physical therapy and surgery to release contractures may be necessary.

Infection Prevention. According to Kliegman and colleagues (2007), penicillin may be ordered prophylactically to prevent infection in the burn patient (erythromycin is used with penicillin allergies). There is also the belief that antimicrobials are only ordered if infection occurs. Careful monitoring of central venous catheters as well as monitoring for other signs of infection is critical in the burn patient.

Pain Control. Morphine sulfate is the drug of choice for severely burned patients. It should be given intravenously. Special attention should be given to respiratory rates when morphine is given. Acetaminophen with codeine may be given for less severe pain.

Nutritional Management. The child may be on nothing by mouth (NPO) restriction for the first 24 to 48 hours if the burn is severe and bowel sounds are absent. A nasogastric tube may be inserted.

Metabolism increases and severe protein and fat wasting occurs in response to severe burns. The child requires a high-protein, high-calorie diet. Oral feedings are preferred, although it may be necessary to supplement with nasogastric feedings. Many of these children have poor appetites, and facilitating adequate intake is a challenge. Small, frequent feedings of favorite foods should be provided. Supplements may be added to foods to meet the high protein and calorie needs. Parents may be able to bring favorite foods from home. Daily weights and intake and output are recorded.

Social and Emotional Issues. The nurse must always be aware of the psychological needs of the family and the child at this time. Families may be dealing with guilt, anger, grief, denial, and fear. Body image concerns become paramount for the older child as recovery progresses. Encourage parents to spend as much time as possible with the child. Because this may be a long-term admission, parents may not be able to be with the child at all times. Provide activities appropriate for the child's age and condition. Schooling needs should be met when the child is of school age. Encourage the child to help with bath, dressing change, feeding, and other self-care activities. Provide opportunities for the family and child to talk about feelings and changes in body appearance. Provide for visits by siblings and friends. Accept negative behaviors expressed by the child. Assist in ventilating negative feelings through play therapy and the use of a play therapist, social worker, child life specialist, or psychologist.

ACNE VULGARIS

Acne is an inflammation of the sebaceous glands and hair follicles in the skin. At puberty, because of hormonal influence, the sebaceous follicles enlarge and secrete increased amounts of a fatty substance called sebum. Genetic factors and stress are also thought to play a part. The course of acne may be brief or prolonged (lasting 10 or more years). Premenstrual acne in girls is not uncommon. The principal lesions include comedones, papules, and nodulocystic growths.

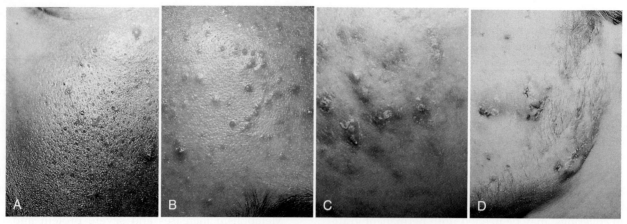

FIGURE 16-9 Acne. **A,** Comedonal acne with blackheads. **B,** Comedonal acne with whiteheads. **C,** Papulopustular acne with inflamed papules and pustules. **D,** Cystic acne with deep cysts and marked erythema that can cause future scarring.

Signs and Symptoms

A comedo (plural, *comedones*) is a plug of keratin, sebum, and bacteria. Keratin is a protein substance that is the main constituent of epidermis and hair. There are two types of comedones, open and closed. In the open comedo, or blackhead, the surface is darkened by melanin. Closed comedones, or whiteheads, are responsible for the inflammatory process of acne. With continued buildup, the walls of the follicle rupture, releasing their irritating content into the surrounding skin. A pustule may appear when this develops near the exterior (Figure 16-9). This process occurs no matter how carefully the teenager washes because surface bacteria are not involved in the pathogenesis. Acne is usually seen on the chin, cheeks, and forehead. It can also develop on the chest, upper back, and shoulders. It is usually more severe in winter.

Treatment and Nursing Care

The basic treatment of acne has changed considerably over the past few years. It is no longer thought that certain foods trigger the condition; therefore chocolate, peanuts, and cola drinks are not restricted unless the patient is convinced of a correlation between a specific item and the condition. A regular well-balanced diet is encouraged. Patients who are not taking tetracycline or vitamin A benefit from sunshine. General hygienic measures of cleanliness, rest, and avoidance of emotional stress may help prevent exacerbations.

Cleansing with mild soap and water removes surface oil, although excessive cleansing should be avoided because it leaves the skin dry and irritated. Lipid-free cleansers, synthetic detergent bars, astringents, and exfoliants can be used to clean the skin. Squeezing pimples increases local inflammation. Use of a flesh-colored topical preparation over active lesions can improve appearance while lesions are resolving.

If topical preparations are needed, over-the-counter benzoyl peroxide lotions or prescription-strength gels act to dry and peel the skin and suppress fatty acid growth. Topical retinoic acid derivative (Retin-A) aids in the elimination of keratinous plugs. It is applied daily, beginning with the lowest strength and increasing the strength until acne is controlled without excessive peeling or irritation. Vitamin A acid can increase sensitivity to the sun, so precautions should be taken when it is used. Antimicrobial topical preparations, such as erythromycin solution in easy-to-use pads, minimize surface bacteria. They can be used in conjunction with benzoyl peroxide.

For adolescents with severe acne that does not respond to topical treatment, systemic medications may be indicated. Tetracycline, doxycycline, or erythromycin may be given in conjunction with topical medications in more serious cases. Monilial vaginitis is a secondary complication sometimes seen with the use of these drugs and should be explained to the unsuspecting female teenager. Tetracycline can interfere with the action of certain birth control pills, so the adolescent girl needs to be sure to tell the dermatologist if she is using oral contraceptives.

Accutane (13-*cis*-retinoic acid) is used for patients with severe pustulocystic acne who have not benefited from other types of treatment. It has many side effects, including conjunctivitis, hypertriglyceridemia, elevated blood cholesterol serum, blood dyscrasia, elevated liver enzymes, dry mucous membranes, photosensitivity, and pruritus. The patient requires careful monitoring. The physician now has to be registered in the manufacturer's System to Manage Accutane-Related Teratogenicity (SMART) program to prescribe the medication. **Because of its highly teratogenic effects, Accutane is not prescribed during pregnancy or to those at any risk for pregnancy because of the possibilities of fetal deformity.** Due to this effect, physicians will prescribe oral contraceptives in conjunction with Accutane. The long-term effects of this medication have not been established. There have been concerns regarding depression and suicide with the use of Accutane; however, at present there is no established correlation. **Dermabrasion** (planing of the skin to minimize scarring) is done selectively because it is not always successful.

Acne is very distressing to the adolescent, particularly when the face is extensively involved. Sometimes even a minimal problem is seen as disastrous when it happens before an important event. The self-conscious young person feels different and embarrassed. The nurse who is attuned to the feelings of individuals can provide understanding support. Although the teenager is educated to assume responsibility for his or her regimen, inclusion of the parents helps prevent conflict surrounding it.

Get Ready for the NCLEX® Examination!

Key Points

- Diaper dermatitis is best prevented by keeping the baby clean and dry; use of a zinc oxide cream may be helpful.
- Nursing care of a child with atopic dermatitis includes frequent moisturizing of the skin.
- Head lice do not jump from individual to individual but are transferred by direct contact.
- Minor burns can usually be handled at home. Major burns need to be handled by a hospital burn unit.
- Risk for infection is a major concern with burn injuries.
- Acne is a common problem that can have serious psychological effects on the adolescent; severe acne can be successfully treated with Accutane.

Additional Learning Resources

evolve Go to your Evolve website (*http://evolve.elsevier.com/Price/pediatric/*) for the following FREE learning resources:
- 3-D Animations
- Answer Keys
- Appendixes
- Audio Glossary
- Spanish/English Glossary
- Video Clips

Review Questions for the NCLEX® Examination

1. The nurse notices white patches that resemble milk curds on the tongue and oral mucosa of an infant. The physician is made aware and makes the diagnosis of thrush. The nurse is aware that thrush is an infection of the mucous membranes of the mouth caused by:
    1. Hepatitis B
    2. Candida
    3. Staphylococci
    4. Streptococci

2. Parents of a child diagnosed with infantile eczema have been educated on various treatments. Which of the following statements would indicate the need for further education?
    1. "An emollient bath may provide a soothing effect on the infant's skin."
    2. "Lotions can be very effective when applied generously after a cool bath."
    3. "If food allergies are identified, a restrictive diet may be required."
    4. "Antihistamines given at bedtime can help control nighttime itching and enhance sleep."

3. All of the following are true regarding nonbullous impetigo (impetigo contagiosa) **except:**
    1. It is primarily seen in infants.
    2. The first symptoms are red papules.
    3. Lesions are most often found on the face, neck, and extremities.
    4. It can be caused by either staphylococci or streptococci.

4. The drug(s) of choice to treat head lice in infants younger than 6 months of age is/are: (**Select all that apply.**)
    1. Lindane (Kwell)
    2. Vaseline
    3. Ulesfia lotion (benzyl alcohol)
    4. 1% Permethrin (Nix)
    5. Pyrethrin A-200 (RID)

5. A burn where there is destruction of the epidermis and **some** of the dermis is considered a:
    1. Superficial (first-degree) burn
    2. Partial-thickness (second-degree) superficial burn
    3. Partial-thickness (second-degree) deep burn
    4. Full-thickness (third-degree) burn

chapter
17

Musculoskeletal Disorders

℮volve

http://evolve.elsevier.com/Price/pediatric/

Objectives

1. Define the vocabulary terms listed
2. Describe the musculoskeletal changes that occur from infancy
3. Identify two ways in which the bones of a toddler differ from those of an adult
4. List the home instruction needed for a infant in a Pavik harness
5. Describe the nursing care of a child with Duchenne muscular dystrophy
6. Discuss the nursing measures for a child in a body cast
7. List various types of pediatric fractures
8. Identify the pathophysiology of Legg-Calvé-Perthes disease and the management approach
9. Formulate a nursing care plan for the adolescent confined in a brace for the treatment of scoliosis
10. Describe several measures designed to prevent sports injury

Key Terms

arthroscopy (p. 337)
asymmetry (ā-SĬM-ĕ-trē; p. 332)
ataxia (ă-TĂK-sē-ă; p. 323)
compartment syndrome (p. 326)
contractures (p. 323)
dysarthria (dĭs-ĂR-thrē-ă; p. 323)
epiphyseal plate (i-pi-fə-SĒ-al; p. 325)
fat embolism (p. 325)
Gower maneuver (p. 324)
intention tremor (p. 323)

open reduction (p. 325)
Ortolani's sign (p. 320)
ossification (ä-sə-fə-KĀ-shen; p. 318)
osteomyelitis (äs-tē-ō-mī-ə-LĪ-təs; p. 336)
Pavlik harness (p. 320)
Ponseti method (p. 319)
pseudohypertrophy (sü-dō-hī-PER-trō-fē; p. 324)
subluxation (sə-blək-SĀ-shən; p. 319)
Trendelenburg gait (p. 320)

MUSCULOSKELETAL SYSTEM

Bones, joints, muscle, and cartilaginous tissue make up the musculoskeletal system. Beginning in the fetus, embryonic connective tissue develops into cartilage, which converts into bone. This process, called ossification, continues until the child is about 20 years of age. The bone marrow in the skeletal system also produces erythrocytes, lymphocytes, and platelets.

Musculoskeletal disorders can be either acquired or congenital. The impact of these disorders on the child's movement can influence the child's development.

At birth infants have all their muscle tissue, and growth affects the size of the muscle but not the number. Bones are largely cartilage in the infant, which makes them more flexible and requires more force to produce a fracture. It is unusual for children younger than 1 year of age to have fractures. As the child grows, secondary ossification of the long bones occurs causing them to be less dense and more porous. This explains why older children have a higher risk of fractures.

The infant's skull is not rigid, has flexible suture lines, and has two openings (anterior and posterior fontanels). The posterior fontanel closes at 6 to 8 weeks, and the anterior fontanel closes at 16 to 18 months to allow for growth of the brain.

The periosteum is the covering of the bone. It contains blood vessels, nerve fibers, and lymphatic vessels. In the young child, this covering is stronger and tougher to allow the child to absorb more force trauma before the bone breaks. The rich periosteum also assists in the fast healing process seen in children. The growth of long bones occurs in the epiphyseal plates. Any injury or fracture of these plates can result in disturbed bone growth.

CLUBFOOT

Clubfoot, one of the most common congenital deformities of the skeletal system, is characterized by a foot that has been twisted inward or outward or toes higher or lower than the heel (Figure 17-1). These deformities can vary from mild and flexible to severe and rigid.

318

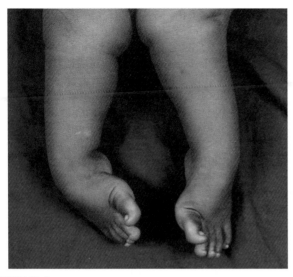

FIGURE 17-1 The child with clubfoot has a flexed ankle, a turned heel, and an adducted forefoot.

The incidence rate is about 1 in 1000 births, with boys affected twice as often as girls. Several variations are recognized. Talipes (*talus,* heel; *pes,* foot) equinovarus (*equinus,* extension; *varus,* bent inward) is seen in 95% of cases. The feet are turned inward, and the untreated child walks on the balls of the foot and the outer borders of the feet. Bilateral clubfeet occur in 50% of cases.

While the exact cause is unknown, recent investigations suggest a genetic influence (Horn and Davidson, 2010). Clubfoot may occur in children with congenital and chromosomal syndromes such as cerebral palsy, spina bifida, and myelomeningocele. Idiopathic clubfoot is thought to result from an unrecognized neuromuscular disorder.

Treatment and Nursing Care

The treatment of clubfoot is typically started shortly after birth; otherwise, the bones and muscles continue to develop abnormally. During infancy, conservative treatment consisting of manipulation and casting to hold the foot in the right position is carried out. Manipulation, known as the Ponseti method, and casting are repeated weekly for the first 6 weeks and then at 1- to 2-week intervals. This is done to allow for rapid growth and to help the foot obtain and retain a more anatomically correct position. If the deformity is corrected, the infant is placed in a brace that maintains the correct position. The brace may be worn for 23 hours a day for an extended length of time, and then only while the child is sleeping. If manipulation or casting does not work, surgery is performed. Although surgery is tailored to the type of deformity, in most cases it involves releasing tight tendons and repositioning and pinning the foot bones. The goal is to complete the treatment by 1 year of age so that the child can use normal shoes when he or she starts walking.

Cast Care. Most casts are made of synthetic materials (fiberglass, polyurethane, or a combination). Synthetic casts dry quickly (in less than 30 minutes) and are lighter, which allows for greater mobility.

A plaster cast takes approximately 24 to 72 hours to dry. The cast should be left uncovered until it dries. The cast dries from the inside out. The child should be turned every 2 hours. When lifting the cast, the nurse should use the palms, not the fingers, to prevent indentations that could press on the underlying skin and cause damage.

> **Nursing Brief**
>
> Important in the long-term care of orthopedic patients is educating parents about orthopedic devices, cast care, exercise and hygiene, and treatment goals. The nurse explains the importance of frequent clinic visits, reinforces physician information, and clarifies directions as necessary.

The toes are left exposed for observation. **The nurse checks them for signs of poor circulation, which would be indicated by pallor, cyanosis, swelling, coldness, numbness, pain, or burning.** If the child's circulation is impaired, the cast may be slit to relieve the pressure or it may need to be removed and reapplied. The nurse should also report any irritation of the skin around the edges of the cast and/or lack of movement of the toes. Adhesive petals may be placed around the edges of the cast to prevent skin irritation.

It is difficult to keep a child's cast free of food particles or small objects, which cause skin irritation. The child needs supervision so that he or she does not place bits of food or small objects under the edges of the cast. Powder and oil should not be used after the bath because they can build up beneath the cast and cause skin irritation.

If surgery on tendons and bones has been performed, the nurse should also observe the cast for evidence of bleeding. If a discolored area appears on the cast, the nurse should circle it, record the time, and notify the physician.

DEVELOPMENTAL DYSPLASIA OF THE HIP

Developmental dysplasia of the hip (DDH) is a common orthopedic deformity. The term **hip dysplasia** is a broad description applied to various degrees of deformity that may involve subluxation or dislocation and may be either partial or complete. The head of the femur is partially or completely displaced from a shallow hip socket (acetabulum). Both hereditary and environmental factors appear to be involved in the cause (Box 17-1). Hip malformation, joint laxity, breech position, and race may all contribute. DDH is seven times more common in girls than in boys. Newborn infants seldom have complete dislocation. When the infant begins to walk, the pressure exerted on the hip can cause a complete dislocation. Accordingly, early detection and treatment are of particular importance in this condition.

Signs and Symptoms

Subluxation of the hip is commonly discovered at the time of the newborn examination. Ongoing screening for DDH should be done during routine health examinations during the first year of life. One of the most reliable signs is a limitation of abduction of the leg on the affected side. When the infant is placed on the back with knees and hips flexed, the physician can press the femur related to the normal hip back until it almost touches the examining table. On the affected side, however, this can be accomplished only partially. Also, the knee on the side of the dislocation appears to be shorter and the skin folds of the thigh are often asymmetrical. When the infant is prone, one hip is higher than the other (Figure 17-2). In some infants younger

than 4 weeks of age, the physician can actually feel and hear the femoral head slip into the acetabulum under gentle pressure. This is called **Ortolani's sign** or Ortolani's click and is considered diagnostic. If the child has begun walking and has had no treatment, he or she will display the characteristic waddling gait and will test positive for the **Trendelenburg gait** test (pelvic drops on the side of the affected hip joint when standing on one leg). Bilateral dislocation may occur; however, unilateral dislocation is more common. Radiographs and ultrasound scans confirm the diagnosis.

Treatment

Treatment is begun as soon as the dislocation is detected and varies with the age of the child. The goal of treatment is to form a normal joint by keeping the head of the femur within the hip socket. This constant pressure enlarges and deepens the acetabulum, thus correcting the dislocation. The bones of small children are fairly pliable because they contain more cartilage than bones of adults.

From birth to approximately 6 months of age, abduction of the hips is maintained with the use of the **Pavlik harness** (Figure 17-3). The harness is worn full time until stability is attained plus 2 months, then a decrease in wearing time begins. Weaning time from the harness is gradual until normal hip function is established by ultrasound or x-ray. The Pavlik harness allows the infant to move the legs. If the dislocation is severe or has not been detected until the child has begun to walk, it may be necessary to use traction. This pulls the head of the femur down to the correct position opposite the acetabulum. After the traction has

Box 17-1	High Risk Factors for Developmental Dysplasia of the Hip

- Family history
- Female
- First born
- Breech delivery
- Neuromuscular disorders
- Congenital deformities (clubfoot)
- Ethnicity (White Caucasian and Navajo Indians)
- Cultural practices (swaddling with hip extension)

Adapted from Canale, S., and Beaty, J. (2008). *Campbell's operative orthopaedics* (11th ed). Philadelphia: Mosby.

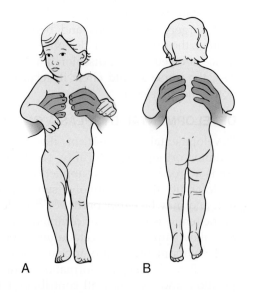 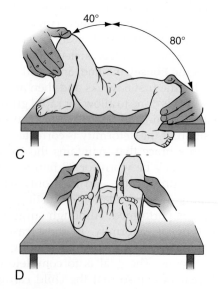

FIGURE 17-2 Three classic signs of DDH. **A** and **B,** Unequal skin folds; **C,** limitation of abduction; and **D,** unequal knee height.

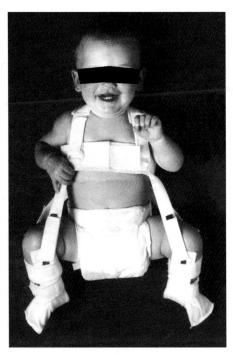

FIGURE 17-3 The Wheaton™ Pavlik Harness is used to maintain the hips in a position of flexion and abduction.

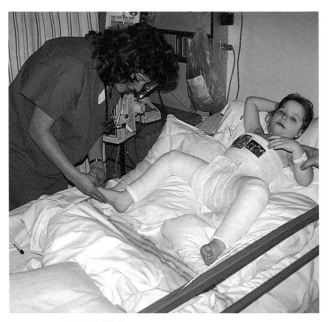

FIGURE 17-4 A spica cast after hip surgery.

stretched the muscles enough to allow the hip to be placed in the acetabulum, the dislocation is reduced with general anesthesia and a spica cast is applied to hold the abduction. This type of cast is shown in Figure 17-4. The length of time that the child remains in the cast varies according to progress, growth, and the condition of the cast; however, it is usually from 3 to 4 months. During this time, the cast may be changed

about every 6 weeks. Sometimes surgery is necessary. In this case, open reduction of the dislocation or repair of the shelf of the hip bone is done. A cast is applied after surgery to keep the femur in the correct position. After removal of the spica cast, some children may require an abduction brace. The brace is worn for 4 to 8 weeks, and then only at nighttime for 1 to 2 years (Canale and Beaty, 2008). For children 6 to 18 months of age, the Pavik harness is less effective and traction is required.

Nursing Care

Parents require instruction regarding skin care while the infant wears the Pavik harness. A T-shirt and long socks can protect the infant's skin from rubbing as the harness allows the infant to move his or her legs. Parents need assurance that they may hold the infant and provide normal activity experiences.

The **body spica cast** encircles the waist and extends to the ankles or toes. General cast care should be reviewed (see Cast Care section under Clubfoot in this chapter). Skill 17-1 describes how to turn and position a child in a body cast.

Firm, plastic-covered pillows are placed beneath the curvatures of the cast for support. Older children may benefit from an overhead bar and trapeze. Do not elevate the head or shoulders of a child in a body cast with pillows because this thrusts the child's lower chest against the cast and can cause discomfort or respiratory difficulty. The head of the child's bed should be slightly elevated so that urine or feces drains away from the body of the cast. A fracture bedpan should be available for appropriate children. To prevent soiling of the cast from urine and feces, plastic wrap or wide cloth tape can be tucked around the edges of the cast at the openings between the legs. A disposable diaper can be tucked under the edges around the buttocks for the same purpose. As these coverings become soiled, they must be changed immediately. Frequent changing of position is important; immobilized children need to be turned often. A covering or bib should be used during feedings to prevent food particles from getting under the cast.

Itching is a particular problem with a child in a body cast. Use of a fan facing toward the opening of the cast or a hair dryer on cool setting may relieve the discomfort. An antihistamine can sometimes help alleviate itching. Any methods that might cause injury to the skin beneath the cast are discouraged because any break in the skin under a cast is difficult to treat. Avoid giving children small objects that could be inserted inside the cast. Be aware of any foul odor from the cast, as this can indicate an infection or skin breakdown. These findings should be reported immediately to the physician.

The child with a long-term disability such as this requires help in meeting the activities of daily living

Skill 17-1   Turning and Positioning a Child in a Body Cast

Method

1. Use two people to turn a child in a body cast.
2. Lift the child and place in the prone position.
3. Do not use crossbars between the legs as handles.

4. With the child in the prone position, place a pillow under the chest and under each leg to prevent pressure on the toes.
5. With a bedpan, support the upper back and legs with pillows so that body alignment is maintained.

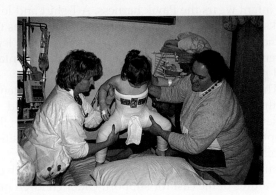

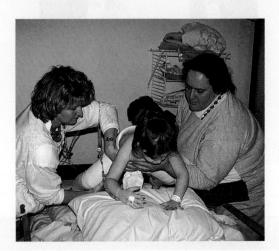

(ADLs). The child is growing and developing rapidly. Dressing and clothing can be a problem. The child also may not be able to use regular furniture or play equipment enjoyed by other children. Transporting children in spica casts can be challenging. Specific equipment is available for a child with a spica cast. Wagons with pillow support, car seats that accommodate a spica cast, and reclining wheelchairs for older children are helpful. A referral to home health agencies can assist parents in obtaining equipment.

CEREBRAL PALSY

Cerebral palsy (CP) refers to a group of nonprogressive disorders that affect the motor centers of the brain, causing problems with movement and coordination. Often children with CP have associated language, perceptual, and intellectual deficits. It is one of the most common disabling conditions seen in children, occurring in approximately 2.5 per 1000 live births (Dodge, 2008).

This condition can be caused by one or more of several factors, which most frequently include the following:

- Congenital problems involving the central nervous system (e.g., hydrocephalus, hemorrhage)
- Postnatal trauma (head injuries) or infections (meningitis, encephalitis)
- Conditions of pregnancy or labor that interfere with oxygen reaching the fetal brain (e.g., premature separation of the placenta, prolonged labor)
- Exposure during pregnancy to infections (e.g., German measles or rubella, cytomegalovirus, toxoplasmosis) or toxins

Signs and Symptoms

The symptoms of CP vary with each child and may range from mild to severe (see Did You Know?). About two thirds of children who have CP are intellectually impaired (National Institute of Neurological Disorders and Stroke, Cerebral Palsy: Hope Through Research, 2010). CP is suspected during infancy when developmental milestones are not met. Diagnostic tests include MRI, electroencephalography, computed tomography (CT), and screening for metabolic disorders. Brain tumors must also be ruled out. **Early recognition is important so that early intervention can begin.**

For the Child with Cerebral Palsy

- Apgar score of less than 5
- Seizures, usually within 48 hours of birth
- Delay in reaching developmental milestones such as sitting, crawling, creeping, standing, and reaching for objects
- Difficulty with fine-motor skills such as holding feeding utensils, writing, and using scissors
- Feeding difficulties such as poor sucking and swallowing, drooling, and persistent tongue thrust
- Involuntary movements such as uncontrolled writhing motions of the hands
- Increased muscle tone: Infant may be rigid when pulled to a sitting position; infant reflexes do not disappear at the normal time

Children may have symptoms of more than one type of CP. **Spastic** CP is characterized by tension in certain muscle groups. When the child tries to move the voluntary muscles, jerky motions result, and eating, walking, and other coordinated movements are difficult to accomplish. The lower extremities are usually involved. The legs cross and the toes point inward **(scissoring).** Toe walking can occur from muscle tightness (Figure 17-5). Upper extremities, or upper and lower extremities on only one side of the body, can be affected. With **athetoid** or **dyskinetic** CP, the child has uncontrolled, slow, writhing movements that can increase during periods of emotional stress and disappear during sleep. These abnormal movements usually affect the hands, feet, arms, or legs and, in some cases, the muscles of the face and tongue, causing grimacing or drooling. Problems can also occur with the coordination of muscle movements needed for speech (dysarthria). Ataxia, or lack of muscle coordination, can be shown by disturbances of balance and depth

perception. A wide-based gait accompanied by unsteadiness is generally present. Intention tremor may also be observed. As the child begins a voluntary movement, such as reaching for a book, there is a resultant trembling that affects the body part being used and worsens as the individual gets nearer to the desired object. **Mixed** CP is usually a combination of spastic and athetoid movements; however, other combinations of symptoms are possible.

Treatment and Nursing Care

The goal of treatment is to help children make the most of their assets and guide them into becoming happy, well-adjusted adults who perform at their maximum ability. Both short- and long-term goals must be realistic and attainable. Parents work with a multidisciplinary team including a physician, such as a pediatrician or orthopedist; a physical therapist; an occupational therapist; a speech and language pathologist; and a social worker. The long course of this disability is financial burden, and contact with social service agencies can assist families in this regard. Parents need to be informed of community resources available to them.

The specific treatment of CP is highly individualized, depending on the severity of the disease. Treatment often includes physical and occupational therapy to assist with ADLs, special education and communication devices, and recreational activities designed for the child's developmental level and adapted to functional limitations. Sometimes surgery is necessary to correct deformities, improve function, or reduce spasticity. The speech therapist helps with communication. Many children with CP cannot produce intelligible speech.

Medications may improve overall function in children with CP. Dantrolene reduces calcium release, thereby decreasing excitation-contraction in skeletal muscle. Skeletal muscle relaxants such as baclofen may decrease spasticity. Intrathecal baclofen delivered via a pump reservoir can help with spastic quadriparesis. Botulinum toxin type A (Botox) has also been successfully used to reduce spasticity (Burg et al., 2006). Antianxiety agents may relieve excessive motion and tension, especially in the athetoid child. Anticonvulsants are prescribed for children with seizures.

All precautions are taken to prevent the formation of contractures (degeneration or shortening of the muscles because of lack of use). The damage may be permanent, resulting in loss of function of the part involved, such as a leg, arm, or finger. Children should be encouraged to do as much as they can for themselves. Other measures used to prevent deformities include frequent changes of position, passive range-of-motion (ROM) exercises, stretching exercises, and use of braces or splints. Assessment of the skin is essential for these children.

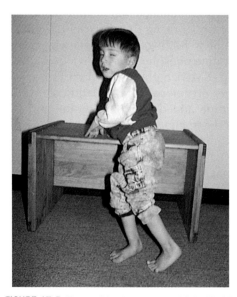

FIGURE 17-5 Toe walking in a young child with CP.

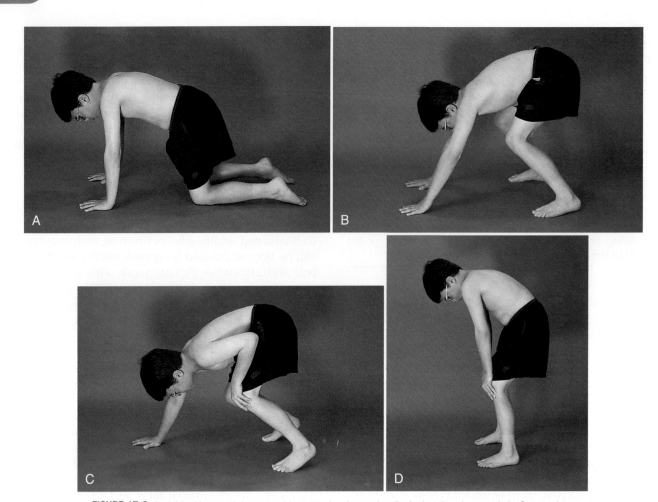

FIGURE 17-6 A child with pseudohypertrophic muscular dystrophy displaying the characteristic Gower sign.

Feeding problems may occur because of swallowing and sucking difficulties. Aspiration is often a risk that requires monitoring. Feeding time should be adequate to facilitate chewing and swallowing. Older children require improved seating and adaptive eating utensils to enhance their nutritional intake. High-caloric diets are necessary to replace calories used by the constant muscle tension. Gastrostomy feeding devices may be essential to provide adequate calories.

DUCHENNE MUSCULAR DYSTROPHY

The muscular dystrophies are a group of disorders in which progressive muscle degeneration occurs. The childhood form, Duchenne muscular dystrophy (DMD), is the most common type. It is an X-linked recessive trait and affects males. Mothers are likely carriers for the disease; however, spontaneous mutations also occur. The gene locus for the disease has been identified, and women at risk may choose to be evaluated and counseled about the carrier state.

Signs and Symptoms

The onset is generally between 2 and 6 years of age; however, a history of delayed motor development during infancy may be evidenced. A waddling gait, slowness in running or climbing, and enlarged rubbery muscles are indicative of this disorder. The calf muscles, in particular, develop pseudohypertrophy from the accumulation of fat and connective tissue. Other signs include frequent falling, clumsiness, contractures of the ankles and hips, and the Gower maneuver, a characteristic way of rising from the floor (Figure 17-6).

Laboratory findings show marked increases in blood creatine phosphokinase (CK) levels. An **electromyogram (EMG),** a graphic record of muscle contraction as a result of electrical stimulation, shows decreases in amplitude and duration of motor unit potentials from the destruction of muscle and not nerves. Electrocardiographic (ECG) abnormalities are also common because of progressive cardiomyopathy. A muscle biopsy may be considered. It reveals degeneration of muscle fibers and replacement of these fibers by fat and connective tissue.

The disease becomes progressively worse. With orthopedic bracing, physical therapy, and sometimes surgery, the child may be able to maintain ambulation until 12 years of age. About one third of boys with DMD have some degree of learning disability, although few are seriously mentally impaired. Life expectancy averages between the late teens and mid-thirties.

Death usually results from cardiac failure or respiratory infection.

Treatment and Nursing Care

Treatment at this time is mainly supportive. It consists of passive exercises to prevent joint contractures, bracing, weight control, surgery for joint contractures, and referrals to appropriate social service agencies. Corticosteroid treatment has been explored with these children. The steroids improve muscle strength, but weight gain from steroid use may prove to be more of a problem. Infections are treated with antimicrobials. Although cardiac manifestations are usually late events, digoxin and diuretics may be beneficial in the early stages of the disease. Keeping weight down is essential; a low-calorie diet may be encouraged. The psychological impact related to the chronic and progressive nature of the disease and its fatal outcome should be addressed. Family denial of the diagnosis is common early in the disease, when symptoms are fairly benign.

Compared with other children with disabilities, children with muscular dystrophy may appear passive and withdrawn. Early on, they may become depressed because they are unable to compete with their peers. Social and emotional pressures on the child and family are great. Financial pressures become magnified as medical and surgical costs escalate. In addition, expensive alterations to the family lifestyle, home, and vehicles are sometimes necessary.

Nurses function as team members along with personnel from many other disciplines in the care of the child with muscular dystrophy. The child should be encouraged to be as active as possible to delay muscle atrophy. Swimming and other activities that promote ROM and mobility for as long as possible are helpful. Nurses provide support for the many daily issues that occur by referring parents to other parents, camp programs, respite care, the Muscular Dystrophy Association *(www.mdausa.org),* public health nurses, home health agencies, family therapists, and eventually hospice care. Although there is no cure at present, different drug therapies, genetic engineering, and stem cell research are beginning to show promise and continue to be investigated (Quintero et al., 2009).

FRACTURES

Description

A **fracture** is a break in a bone and is caused mainly by accidents. With children, falls are responsible for a large number of fractures. A fracture is characterized by pain, tenderness on movement, and swelling. Discoloration, limited movement, and numbness may also occur. In a **simple fracture,** the bone is broken but the skin over the area is not. In a **compound fracture,** a wound in the skin accompanies the broken bone and there is the added danger of infection. Figure 17-7 depicts the various types of pediatric fractures.

Fractures heal faster in children than in adults. The child's periosteum is stronger and thicker, and there is less stiffness with mobilization. Injury to the cartilaginous epiphyseal plate, found at the ends of long bones, is serious if it happens during childhood because it may interfere with the longitudinal growth plate.

Treatment and Nursing Care

Common fracture sites in children include the ulna, tibia, femur, and clavicle. Children typically have pain, and swelling may be obvious with a fracture. If a fracture is suspected, immobilize the extremity. An ice pack, covered with a cloth to prevent skin damage and applied over the fracture site, may minimize swelling. If the fracture is compound, cover the injury lightly with a sterile dressing.

For nurses in the community setting, such as the school nurse, moving the child requires application of a splint. The joints above and below the break are immobilized with a rolled newspaper or bath towels and tied beyond the injury. Commercially made splints are available; for example, a padded board that is bandaged to the extremity or air splints that can be inflated. If the arm is injured, keep it elevated with a sling to reduce swelling and hemorrhage. If a back or neck injury is evident, the child should not be moved unless the injury is life threatening. The EMS system should be activated for these injuries.

X-ray is the most effective method of determining the type of fracture that has occurred. Fractures are treated with closed or open reduction. Closed reduction involves manually aligning the break followed by immobilization. Figure 17-8 shows a child in a long arm cast. Open reduction involves surgical insertion of fixation devices, such as pins, to maintain alignment while healing occurs. In some cases, the child is hospitalized and monitored for possible complications, including infection, neurovascular complications, and fat embolism. Fat embolism can occur as a result of orthopedic trauma. Particles of fat escape from the fracture sites and are carried through the circulatory system; they can lodge in the lung capillaries, causing respiratory distress. The child exhibits signs of altered respiratory status and possible altered level of consciousness (LOC). Such condition changes must be reported immediately.

Any change in general condition or any signs or symptoms of infection, including elevated temperature, pinsite redness, drainage, or odor, need to be reported. Signs of neurovascular compromise also need to be reported. The nurse checks the child's affected extremity frequently to see that toes or fingers are warm and that their color is good. Cyanosis, numbness or irritation from attachments, tight bandages, severe pain, or absence of pulse in the extremities must be reported immediately to the nurse in charge. Refer to Did You Know? on p. 326 for specifics on lower extremity neurovascular checks.

Pediatric fractures are seldom complete breaks. Rather, children's bones tend to bend or buckle because of increased flexibility. This flexibility is due to a thicker periosteum and increased amounts of immature bone.

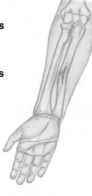

Greenstick

Break occurs through the periosteum on one side of the bone while only bowing or buckling on the other side. Seen most frequently in forearm.

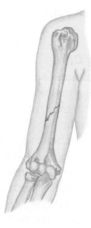

Spiral

Twisted or circular break that affects the length rather than the width. Seen frequently in child abuse.

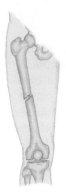

Oblique

Diagonal or slanting break that occurs between the horizontal and perpendicular planes of the bone.

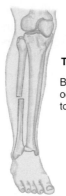

Transverse

Break or fracture line occurs at right angles to the long axis of the bone.

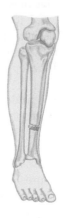

Comminuted

Bone is splintered into pieces. This is a rare occurrence in children.

FIGURE 17-7 Pediatric fractures.

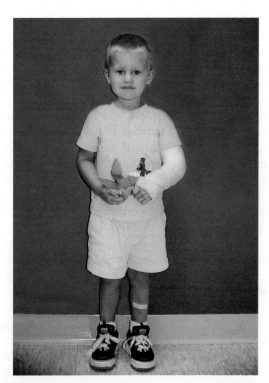

FIGURE 17-8 Most children adapt well to their casts, although they may fear the removal.

? Did You Know?

Signs Suggesting Lower Extremity Neurovascular Impairment

Circulation: Decreased pedal pulse, pallor, toes feel cool to the touch, slowed capillary refill (pink color slow to return after toe is pressed and released)

Sensation: Child complains of numbness or "pins and needles" sensation, pain

Motion: Toes swollen, not moving well

Compartment syndrome can occur as a result of pressure on tissues resulting from edema or swelling. Circulation is compromised. Paralysis and necrosis can occur. Neurovascular checks alert the nurse to possible compartment syndrome.

Nursing Brief

Remember the 5 Ps when performing neurovascular checks: pain, pallor, pulselessness, paresthesia, and paralysis.

Traction. Skin or skeletal traction may be used to reduce the fracture, to keep the bones in proper place, and to immobilize the leg. The type of traction depends on the age of the child and extent of the injury. **Bryant** traction is no longer recommended. This skin traction positioned the child's legs at a 90-degree angle to the body. This type of traction could cause circulatory problems that result from constant elevation of the legs (Hockenberry and Wilson, 2007). For children older than 6 years of age, 90-90 femoral traction with a boot cast on the lower leg and a skeletal Steinmann pin or Kirschner wire through the distal femur is commonly used. Other types of traction that are frequently used in children with lower extremity fractures are Russell traction and balanced suspension traction with a Thomas ring and Pearson attachment. Various types of traction are shown in Tables 17-1 and 17-2.

Table 17-1   Types of Skin Traction

TYPE	ILLUSTRATION	USES	NURSING CONSIDERATIONS
Cervical		Neck sprains or strains Torticollis Cervical nerve trauma Nerve root compression	Limit of weights of 5 to 7 pounds. Avoid compressing the throat or ears with the chin strap. Elevating the head of the bed 20 to 30 degrees helps maintain alignment.
Dunlop (Side-arm 90-90) Can be either skin or skeletal		Fractures and dislocations of the upper arm or shoulder Supracondylar elbow fracture of the humerus	Hand may feel cool because of its elevation. Hand can be covered with sock or mitten if desired. Avoid pressure over bony prominences or nerves.
Buck extension traction		Hip and knee contracture Legg-Calvé-Perthes disease	Remove boot every 8 hours and assess skin. Leg may be slightly abducted.
Russell traction		Supracondylar femur fracture Stabilizes fractured femur until callus forms Legg-Calvé-Perthes disease	Sling may need to be repositioned often; mark leg to ensure proper placement. Avoid pressure over bony prominences or nerves. Weights are not added or removed without physician's order.

Table 17-2   **Types of Skeletal Traction**

TYPE	ILLUSTRATION	USES	NURSING CONSIDERATIONS
Cervical (Crutchfield) skeletal tongs		Preoperative spine distraction Fractures or dislocations of cervical or high thoracic vertebrae	A special bed may be used to assist with turning the child. Logroll the child while maintaining straight body alignment.
Halo cast or vest		Postoperative immobilization after cervical fusion Fracture or dislocation of cervical or high thoracic vertebrae	Balance is altered with a halo cast; child's ambulating need close supervision. Cast may need to be sawed in case of emergency; front panel of brace may need to be removed in case of emergency.
90-90 femoral traction		Femur fractures	Encourage child to dorsiflex foot often to prevent foot drop, or lower leg may be casted. Ensure that weights do not catch on bottom of the bed.
Balanced suspension with Thomas ring and a Pearson attachment		Femur fracture Hip fracture Tibial fracture	Avoid pressure to the area behind the knee, which could cause popliteal nerve injury. If the system is truly balanced, the splint can be placed at any height and will remain there.

The nurse monitors the traction cables to be sure that they are intact and in the wheel grooves of the pulleys and that the child's body is in proper alignment. Elastic bandages stabilizing skin traction should be neither too loose nor too tight. The child should avoid turning from side to side. Do not remove the weights once they have been applied. Continuous traction is necessary. The weights must hang free, and the pull of the weights must not be obstructed by furnishings such as a chair or table.

Initially, the child might have pain, both from the fracture itself and from the muscle spasms associated with the traction and fracture. The pain is spasmodic and can be severe. Pain assessment with age-appropriate pain scales and treatment are essential. Pain assessment and management are discussed in Chapter 3.

Skin care is a priority. Skin should be kept clean, dry, and free from pressure. Keeping sheets free from wrinkles is necessary. Pin care is done to keep crusting around the pins to a minimum, to minimize unnecessary pulling of the skin at the pin sites, and to prevent infection. *Osteomyelitis* is the most serious complication associated with skeletal traction (discussed later). This bone infection manifests itself with localized pain, warmth, swelling, tenderness, or unusual odor. Antimicrobials are prescribed if this complication occurs.

The child is encouraged to drink lots of fluids and to eat foods that are high in fiber content to prevent constipation caused by lack of exercise. Stool softeners may be necessary. A fracture pan is used for bowel movements, and a careful record is kept of eliminations. Deep breathing is encouraged through the use of breathing exercises, blowing bubbles, or moving a windmill toy. Diversional therapy is important because hospitalization can last for a month or longer. ROM exercises for unaffected extremities are important. Try to encourage ROM exercises by making it a game whenever possible. Toys may be suspended over the child's head within reach. The older child can use an overhead trapeze to assist with movement in the bed. DVD movies, computer games, stories, and other forms of entertainment are essential to the total nursing care plan. Parents are encouraged to stay with the child when possible. Children's bones heal faster than those of adults. The prognosis for children with this condition is good with proper treatment. The care of a child in leg traction is illustrated in Nursing Care Plan 17-1.

DISLOCATIONS

Dislocations of the elbow (often referred to as "nurse-maid's elbow") are typically seen in young children between 1 and 4 years of age who have tried to twist their hand out of a parent's hand. The pulling and twisting motion most often dislocates the radial head. Symptoms of a dislocated elbow are immediate and marked. The child splints the affected arm with the unaffected hand and refuses to move it. Often the child cries and appears anxious or in pain. Even when distracted with a toy, the child does not move the affected arm. Treatment of a dislocated elbow is simple and provides immediate relief in most cases. The physician turns the hand and forearm in an upward direction while placing pressure at the elbow until a click is heard or felt. The child is able to move the arm shortly after treatment. Because repeated incidents of elbow dislocation are common, the nurse should advise the parent to avoid placing any pulling motion on the child's arm.

Elbow dislocations may occur in older children as the result of a fall on a hyperextended elbow. There may also be an associated elbow fracture. Reduction is performed under conscious sedation. If stable, it is then immobilized until ROM exercises are ordered (Burg et al., 2006).

LEGG-CALVÉ-PERTHES DISEASE (COXA PLANA)

This disease is one of a group of disorders called the **osteochondroses,** in which the blood supply to the **epiphysis,** or end of the bone, is disrupted. The tissue death that results from the inadequate blood supply is termed **avascular necrosis.** Legg-Calvé-Perthes disease affects the development of the head of the femur. Its cause and incidence are unknown. The disease is age related and is seen most commonly in boys between 4 and 8 years of age. Healing occurs spontaneously over a period of 2 to 3 years; however, marked distortion of the head of the femur may lead to an imperfect joint or degenerative arthritis of the hip in later life.

Signs and Symptoms

The classic symptom is "painless" limping. Other symptoms include intermittent thigh pain that might be referred to the knee and limitation of motion. A number of cases are diagnosed in sports clinics. Legg-Calvé-Perthes disease may or may not be preceded by trauma or infection. Radiographs confirm the diagnosis and show the extent of femoral head involvement.

Treatment and Nursing Care

The prognosis is more favorable with a young age of onset. Children who are older than 8 years of age may have degenerative arthritis develop. Treatment goals are to prevent femoral head deformity, obtain pain relief, and preserve joint motion. This is accomplished through the use of ambulation-abduction casts or braces that prevent dislocation of the femoral head and enable the acetabulum to mold the healing head in such a way that it does not become deformed. This treatment may be preceded by bed rest and traction to relieve muscle irritation. Newer surgical reconstruction and containment methods show promise in shortening the length of treatment. The prognosis in

Nursing Care Plan 17-1 | The Child in Leg Traction

NURSING DIAGNOSIS *Impaired physical mobility, related to restrictions of the traction apparatus and the child's injury*

Goals/Outcome Criteria	Nursing Interventions	Rationales
Child is free of hazards related to immobility, as evidenced by: • Intact skin • Normal elimination patterns for age • Normal respiratory function • Maintenance of muscle tone	Place child on sheepskin or pressure-equalizing mattress.	Equalizing pressure on the back reduces pressure areas and skin breakdown.
	Change child's position in bed every 2 hr. Observe for and gently massage reddened areas.	Promotes circulation to the area and prevents skin breakdown.
	Keep crumbs and small toys off the sheets.	Can get underneath the child and cause skin irritation.
	Keep back clean and dry. Use flat fracture bedpan.	Perspiration can cause skin irritation.
	Encourage increased fluids and high-fiber foods. Use stool softeners if ordered.	Promotes adequate elimination.
	Encourage deep breathing and muscle movement through play such as singing, blowing bubbles or a pinwheel, bean bag toss, Nerf basketball, and simple games.	Deep breathing inflates the lungs, decreasing respiratory compromise.
	Allow child to use overhead trapeze if appropriate, and encourage frequent changes of position.	Muscle movement enhances muscle tone in unaffected extremities. Improves tone of upper extremities; keeps child in alignment.
	Encourage child to feed, bathe, and dress within traction limitations; provide foods high in calcium.	Enhances self-care and muscle movement; calcium promotes adequate bone healing.

NURSING DIAGNOSIS *Acute pain related to tissue injury and muscle spasm*

Goals/Outcome Criteria	Interventions	Rationales
Child exhibits relief from pain, as evidenced by: • Minimal to no pain on the pain rating scale • Sleeping comfortably • Able to play with others • No crying or expressions of pain	Provide pharmacologic pain relief as ordered around the clock for the first 24 to 48 hr.	Giving medication around the clock provides more effective pain control than waiting until the child has pain.
	Monitor the effects of the medication. Note and report any adverse effects.	Proper effectiveness of pain relief depends on achieving the maximum possible relief with the minimum amount of sedation.
	Use age-appropriate rating scale to monitor pain levels.	Rating scales are the most effective way to monitor pain in children.
	Use nonpharmacologic methods of pain relief such as distraction, storytelling, music, play, and gentle touch.	Effective use of nonpharmacologic methods decreases the number of pharmacologic agents necessary.
	Encourage relaxation and deep breathing during muscle spasms.	Conscious muscle relaxation decreases muscle spasms.

NURSING DIAGNOSIS *Fear, related to injury, traction apparatus, hospitalization*

Goals/Outcome Criteria	Nursing Interventions	Rationales
Child adjusts to being in traction, as evidenced by: • Cooperating with plan of care • Sleeping well, no nightmares • Playing appropriately with others • Exhibiting behavior that is consistent with usual temperament	Use imaginary play frequently in care.	Helps toddler deal with fear and loss of control.
	Bring child to the playroom if hospital policy permits.	Seeing other children decreases fears.
	Continue regular routine.	Following routines and rituals helps adjustment.
	Review with parents and child the purpose of the traction, keeping alignment, and what they can do to help.	Knowledge increases cooperation with care.

⭐ Nursing Care Plan 17-1   The Child in Leg Traction—cont'd

NURSING DIAGNOSIS *Risk for infection, related to skin irritation at pin sites*

Goals/Outcome Criteria	Nursing Interventions	Rationales
Child remains free of infection, as evidenced by: • Intact skin • No redness, tenting, swelling, or purulent drainage at site	Monitor vital signs. Monitor pin sites at least once a shift; document condition of skin around pin entry sites. Provide pin care according to hospital protocol.	Elevated temperature can signify infection; elevated pulse and respiration can indicate subtle pain. Frequent monitoring allows for more rapid recognition of infection. Keeping the site clean can prevent infection.

NURSING DIAGNOSIS *Risk for peripheral neurovascular dysfunction, related to edema and traction apparatus*

Goals/Outcome Criteria	Nursing Interventions	Rationales
Child maintains adequate peripheral perfusion, as evidenced by: • Strong pedal pulse • Good movement of toes • No numbness or tingling • Toes warm and pink, good capillary refill	Monitor peripheral circulation, sensation, and motion every 4 hr when stable. Note edema of toes or feet. Encourage child to move the toes of the affected foot frequently. Remove and reapply elastic bandages of skin traction as ordered (use another person to stabilize traction adhesive tapes).	Frequent monitoring detects problems for early intervention. Edema contributes to decreased peripheral circulation. Movement increases circulation locally. Periodic removal of tight bandages promotes circulation to the extremity.

NURSING DIAGNOSIS *Risk for injury related to traction apparatus and confinement to bed*

Goals/Outcome Criteria	Nursing Interventions	Rationales
Child remains free from injury: • Remains quietly in bed • Cooperates with plan of care	Check traction apparatus frequently: • Weights swing freely • Ropes on pulleys • Child in straight alignment • Affected leg supported properly in sling, if used. Cover sharp pin sites with foam or tape. Keep side rails up. Keep snacks, toys, and TV or call buttons within child's reach.	Frequent monitoring of traction apparatus and alignment ensures appropriate traction on the affected extremity. Sharp pin edges can lacerate the unaffected extremity. Prevents falls. Reduces the chance that the child will lean too far and fall.

Critical Thinking Question

1. How would the nurse design a routine for the toddler or young child in traction to avoid boredom, overcome fear, and maintain mobility of nonimpaired extremities? Consider pain control, risk for injury, and prevention of complications.

Critical Thinking Snapshot

In evaluating this child in traction, what would be documented regarding the traction setup? What precautions need to be taken for the child in traction? What would the nurse evaluate and document regarding the child? What are the signs and symptoms if this child has complications from infection? What information would be reported to the physician?

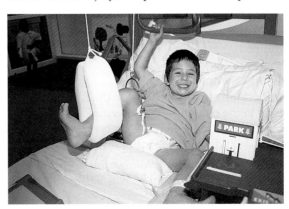

Legg-Calvé-Perthes disease depends on the age at onset, the stage of the disease at diagnosis, and the type of treatment initiated.

Nursing considerations depend on the age of the child and the type of treatment. When immobilization of the child is necessary, the general principles of traction, cast, and brace care are used. Total or partial immobility is particularly trying for children and their families. Braces and casts hinder the child's move toward independence and deprive him or her of many natural outlets for relieving stress. It is important to emphasize safety principles when school-age children are in mobility braces.

Review brace care with the parent and child. Braces must be applied appropriately and preferably over light clothing. Observe the skin underneath the brace for signs of skin breakdown. Keep the skin clean and dry. Check the brace regularly to be sure all parts are working properly.

If the child is admitted to the hospital for surgery, routine preoperative teaching is done. Postoperative care includes monitoring circulation, sensation, pain, and motion, and other routine observations.

SCOLIOSIS

Scoliosis refers to an *S*-shaped curvature of the spine. It is the most common nontraumatic skeletal condition in children. Not all scoliotic curves are progressive, and some may require only periodic evaluation. Untreated progressive scoliosis can lead to back pain, fatigue, disability, and thoracic insufficiency syndrome (TIS). TIS is the impairment and restriction of lung growth and function as a result of the deformity of the thoracic cavity (Cruz and Smith, 2010).

Scoliosis is categorized by age of onset and cause. The cause for **idiopathic scoliosis** is unknown. This category is subdivided into three subcategories based on age of onset: infantile (before 3 years of age), juvenile (4 to 9 years of age), and adolescent (10+ years of age). **Neuromuscular scoliosis** is a result of diseases such as cerebral palsy, spina bifida, or muscular dystrophy. **Congenital scoliosis** defects occur in utero resulting from abnormal fetal vertebral development. The most common occurrence of scoliosis is idiopathic. Most commonly affected is the adolescent. In many cases, scoliosis affects multiple family members, although the exact inheritance pattern has not been determined.

Signs and Symptoms

An important nursing action for the identification of scoliosis in the community is screening. This is usually done in school, preferably at the beginning of fourth grade. It should also be a part of every yearly physical given to prepubescent youngsters. Early recognition is of utmost importance in detecting mild cases amenable to nonsurgical treatment.

Often the first sign the child notices is an uneven hemline and difficulty fitting clothes. During an exam, the examiner looks initially for general body alignment and asymmetry (one side of the body looks different from the other). When viewed from the front, the child with scoliosis can have uneven shoulder levels, unequal arm-to-body spaces, or a protruding hip. One arm may appear longer than the other when the child bends forward. Sometimes the child complains of a "crooked back." When viewed from the back, bent at the waist, the child might have a protruding scapula, with one side of the back appearing higher than the other (Figures 17-9 and 17-10). A definitive diagnosis can be made from spinal radiographs, which show the severity and location of the curve.

Treatment and Nursing Care

Treatment is aimed at correcting the curvature and/or preventing further curvature progression. The course of treatment is determined by the child's age, the skeletal maturity, the degree and location of the curvature, and any underlying disease processes. Curves up to 20 degrees do not require treatment but are carefully followed, particularly if the adolescent is prepubertal. Follow-up examinations every 4 to 6 months can detect any progression of the curve.

Progressive curves between 20 and 40 degrees most often require bracing until the child's skeletal system is mature (Figure 17-11). Braces used are the Boston brace, which uses plastic shells, the thoracolumbosacral orthosis (TLSO), a custom-molded jacket, and the Milwaukee brace. For lower back curves, a plastic molded brace is used. Such a brace contributes to better compliance with the treatment program because it can be worn under clothing and is barely distinguishable (Nursing Care Plan 17-2). In addition to bracing, the child might also be involved in an active exercise program.

The intention for bracing is usually wearing the brace for 23 hours a day, although some experts believe that the same effect can be obtained from wearing the brace for fewer hours (16 hours). This allows the child to avoid wearing a brace to school. It is worn over a T-shirt. Because appearance is such a concern for adolescents, a brace is used only for curves whose apex is higher than the eighth thoracic vertebra.

Curvatures greater than 50 degrees or an increasing curve most likely require surgical intervention in the form of a spinal fusion, with stabilization through the use of instrumentation (rods, wires, screws). There are many instrumentation systems available, such as Dwyer instruments, the Cotrel-Dubousset procedure (rods and wires), Zielke, and TSRH (Texas Scottish Rite Hospital). Depending on the procedure chosen, the surgical approach can be posterior or anterior. The anterior approach requires insertion of a chest tube.

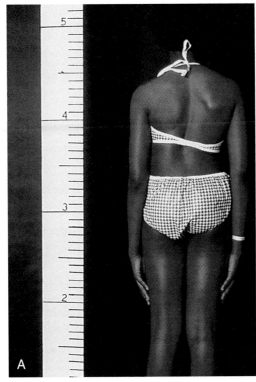
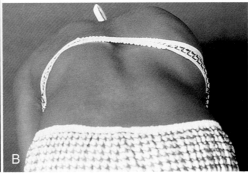

FIGURE 17-9 Idiopathic scoliosis. **A,** Scapular asymmetry is easily seen. Back bra strap can also assist in detecting asymmetry. **B,** Forward bending reveals a mild rib hump deformity.

What is Scoliosis?

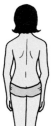

Normal
• head centered over mid-buttocks
• shoulders level
• shoulder blades level, with equal prominence
• hips level and symmetrical
• equal distance between arms and body

1a

Possible Scoliosis
• head alignment to one side of mid-buttocks
• one shoulder higher
• one shoulder blade higher with possible prominence
• one hip more prominent than the other
• unequal distance between arms and body

1b

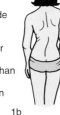

Normal
• both sides of upper and lower back symmetrical
• hips level and symmetrical

2a

Possible Scoliosis
• one side of rib cage and/or the lower back showing uneven symmetry.

2b

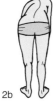

• Scoliosis is a sideways (lateral) curving of the spine.

• One in 10 persons will have scoliosis. Two to three persons in every 1000 will need active treatment for a progressive condition. In one out of every 1000 cases surgery may be necessary.

• Frequent signs are a prominent shoulder blade, uneven hip and shoulder levels, unequal distance between arms and body, and clothes that do not "hang right."

• Eighty percent of scoliosis cases are idiopathic (cause unknown). Scoliosis tends to run in families and affects more girls than boys.

• Spinal curvature is best dealt with when a young person's body is still growing and can respond to treatments such as a body brace. Mild cases may not need treatment, but must be monitored.

• Kyphosis (round back) may occur in developing adolescents. It should be screened for and may need to be treated.

• You, your physician and/or your school screening program (now required in many schools) can perform a 30-second annual screen during these growing years (See diagrams.) An annual 30-second screening for scoliosis and kyphosis during the bone-growing years can make the difference between a preventable condition and a disability in adult years.

Normal
• even and symmetrical on both sides of the upper and lower back

3a

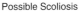

Possible Scoliosis
• unequal symmetry of the upper back, lower back, or both

3b

Also Screen for Kyphosis:

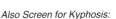

Normal
• smooth symmetrical even arc of the back

4a

Possible Kyphosis ("round back")
• lack of smooth arc with prominence of shoulders and round back.

4b

Screen Out Scoliosis!
If one or more physical features suggest scoliosis or kyphosis, professional diagnosis must be sought.

FIGURE 17-10 Scoliosis screening.

⭐ Nursing Care Plan 17-2 | **The Adolescent with Scoliosis in a Brace**

NURSING DIAGNOSIS *Risk for impaired skin integrity, related to uneven pressure from the brace*

Goals/Outcome Criteria	Nursing Interventions	Rationales
The skin remains smooth without areas of redness or irritation or signs of skin breakdown.	Advise the child to wear a soft cotton T-shirt under the brace; be sure that the shirt is free from wrinkles.	Placing a thin layer of fabric between the brace and the skin reduces friction rubbing.
	Inspect areas under the brace daily after the adolescent showers.	Routine inspection allows for rapid identification of problem areas.
	Report persistent reddened areas to the brace fitter.	Brace modification can reduce friction areas.

NURSING DIAGNOSIS *Risk for injury, related to altered body weight and function from bracing*

Goals/Outcome Criteria	Nursing Interventions	Rationales
The adolescent remains free from injury.	Demonstrate and have the adolescent demonstrate alternative body movements used to accomplish activities of daily living. • Bending from the knees to pick something up • How to get out of bed by rolling to a side-lying position before pushing upright • Putting clothing on lower part of the body while sitting on the edge of a bed or chair	Demonstration helps the adolescent visualize changes that need to be made.
The adolescent adapts appropriately to altered body movements caused by the brace.	Encourage parents to be aware of and remove any potential hazards in the environment (e.g., slippery rugs, toys, other objects on the floor).	Alerting parents to environmental hazards prevents injury.
	Advise the adolescent to be aware of hazards at school; make special arrangements for walking in corridors between classes if necessary.	Because schools are crowded, the injury potential is high and special arrangements may be necessary.
	Advise the adolescent to try activities slowly at first.	Helps adolescent adjust to altered body weight before resuming activity.

NURSING DIAGNOSIS *Disturbed body image, related to the appearance of the brace*

Goals/Outcome Criteria	Nursing Interventions	Rationales
The adolescent adapts appropriately to any changes in appearance or function resulting from the brace, as evidenced by • Ability to verbally express concerns • Participation in activities of interest • Continued contact with peers	Encourage the adolescent to discuss feelings about the appearance or limitations of the brace	Facilitating expression of feelings helps the nurse identify and assist with concerns.
	Help the adolescent and family choose loose, stylish, colorful clothing to minimize the appearance of the brace and boost the adolescent's confidence. Describe any activity restrictions (e.g., competitive sports), and help the adolescent explore alternate activities of interest (e.g., walking, slow jogging, moderate dancing); encourage the adolescent to be physically active.	Attractive clothing helps boost an adolescent's self-image and decreases feelings of being different from peers. Helps the adolescent identify areas of interest and activities that maintain physical fitness and promote socialization with peers.

Nursing Care Plan 17-2   The Adolescent with Scoliosis in a Brace—cont'd

NURSING DIAGNOSIS *Ineffective therapeutic regimen management, related to length of treatment time*

Goals/Outcome Criteria	Nursing Interventions	Rationales
The adolescent complies fully with the treatment, as evidenced by • Wearing the brace the required amount of time • Stating the long-term benefits of the treatment	Reinforce the long-term positive outcome from the bracing	Continued reinforcement helps validate the rationale for treatment and encourages compliance
	Be sure that the brace fits well and that the adolescent is comfortable; refer to the brace fitter if adjustments are needed	Comfort increases compliance
	Allow the adolescent to express anger and frustration if needed.	Allowing expression of feelings prevents them from building up

Critical Thinking Question

1. An 11-year-old girl is admitted to the ICU after surgery for correction of scoliosis. She has an IV, a nasogastric tube to low suction, a HemoVac, and a Foley catheter. She is NPO and on strict intake and output. She is repositioned by log-rolling every 2 hours. Her vital signs are as follows: temperature, 99.8° F; pulse, 96 beats per minute; respiration, 32 breaths per minute; and blood pressure, 135/78 mm Hg. She is moaning. What are the nurse's initial actions? What actions should be done first, and what needs continual evaluation?

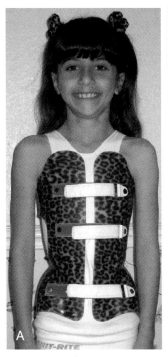 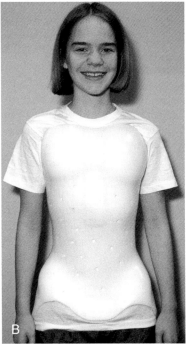 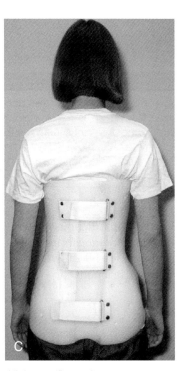

FIGURE 17-11 A brace can be custom designed to meet the child's specific needs.

Some procedures are followed by bracing for several months.

Preoperative Care. The usual preoperative preparation of the child is necessary for spinal fusion. It is important that the nurse evaluate and document the child's neuromuscular status at this time so that it may be used as a basis for comparison after the procedure. All four extremities are observed for color, temperature, capillary filling, edema, sensation, and motion. The nurse explains to the child that breathing exercises and frequent changes of position are necessary to prevent heart and lung complications. If postoperative log-rolling is anticipated, it can be practiced before surgery.

Postoperative Care. After surgery, the child can spend some time in the intensive care unit. When they return to the unit, they usually have a fairly extensive dressing, intravenous fluids, round-the-clock pain medications (often patient-controlled anesthesia), nasogastric tube, urinary catheter, wound drains, and a chest tube (if the anterior approach was used). Early ambulation is encouraged as soon as pain allows. A physical therapist assists with ambulation.

In addition to routine postoperative management, the nurse carefully assesses the child's vital signs and neurologic, cardiovascular, and respiratory status frequently. Any changes in motion or sensation of the extremities, fever, or abnormal wound drainage, which can indicate infection, should be reported immediately because the danger of osteomyelitis (bone infection) is great.

Children often are reluctant to assume self-care after spinal surgery. In addition to being in pain, they are concerned about their safety. They express reluctance to move because of fear that they will dislodge or break the fusion. They should be reassured that careful movement does not harm the surgical site. The sooner the child can participate in self-care, the faster he or she will progress. Encourage the child to shower as soon as is permitted. Some may need to use a shower chair initially.

Nursing Brief

Insertion of a metal device should not affect an airport security scanner because titanium does not activate the alarm. If the alarm is activated, other forms of scanning such as "wanding" can be done. Some airport securities will accept a note from the physician or a card from the manufacturer of the instrument as a clearance for air travel.

Begin home care instructions early in treatment. If bracing is needed, demonstrate application of the brace to the parent and child. Give written instructions for any activity restrictions or necessary follow-up care.

OSTEOMYELITIS

Osteomyelitis is an infection of the bone. The long bones of the lower extremities are the most common location. It can be an acute or chronic infection that spreads to surrounding tissue. While the causative organism can be bacterial, viral, or fungal, *Staphylococcus aureus* is the most common. Trauma, surgical interventions, or infections in other parts of the body can be the initial causes. The microorganism enters at an injury site or spreads through the bloodstream, and then becomes established in the bone. Inflammation results in pus, edema, vascular congestion, and abscesses, which can interrupt the blood supply to the bone and surrounding tissue. If left untreated, necrosis of the bone can result.

Signs and Symptoms

One of the first signs may be the child's refusal to walk or use the affected extremity. Pain, edema, redness, decreased mobility of a joint, and fever may also be present. Many times the onset is rapid and in older children may be thought to be a sports injury.

Treatment and Nursing Care

Laboratory tests that demonstrate infection, elevated white blood cells, elevated erythrocyte sedimentation rate (ESR), C-reactive protein, and blood culture are drawn. X-ray, CT scan, MRI scan, and bone scan can identify the location of the infection. A biopsy or incision and drainage (I&D) may be done to identify the causative organism and determine which antimicrobial will be effective.

Since *Staphylococcus aureus* is the most common organism, broad-spectrum antimicrobials may be started before culture results. With the increased incidence of methicillin-resistant *S. aureus* (MRSA), the physician may begin with antimicrobials that are effective against MRSA. When culture results are available, medications may be altered. These infections can be difficult to eliminate and may require extended intravenous therapy. After several days of therapy, if there is no change in the status of the infection, a surgical incision and drainage (I&D) is done. The child may be discharged with home intravenous therapy. For long-term home intravenous infusion, a device such as a port-a-cath or PICC line will be placed. Antimicrobial therapy can require 3 to 6 weeks or longer.

Home care instructions should begin early in the hospitalization. Parents need to be comfortable if they are administering the antimicrobials. Dressing changes for the IV access is taught. If a home health agency is involved, families should have all contact numbers. Some children have limited ambulation, and parents need suggestions on how to keep the child active. For some older children, parents may need assistance for scheduling schooling options. While some children may be able to attend school, others may require homebound tutoring.

SPORTS INJURIES

There has been an increase in the number of children of both genders participating in team and solo sports. Even children with chronic conditions such as asthma, diabetes mellitus, and seizures can participate in sports. Athletic participation teaches valuable lessons about cooperation, achieving goals, persistence, and confidence building. Many states and school facilities require a pre-participation physical before the participation in the sport. The American Academy of Pediatrics (AAP) has devised a sport classification system to identify the level of potential contact (Box 17-2). Children should be evaluated for suitability for a particular sport. For example, a child with seizures should not

Box 17-2 Sport Contact Classification System

CONTACT
Basketball
Cheerleading
Football-tackle
Gymnastics
Soccer
Skiing

LIMITED-CONTACT
Baseball
Bicycling
Football-flag
Softball
Volleyball

NON-CONTACT
Bowling
Dance
Golf
Running
Swimming

Adapted from Rice, S. (2008). Policy revision: medical conditions affecting sports participation. *Pediatr,* 121(4), 841-848.

participate in contact sports. In addition, the AAP provides an extensive list matching medical conditions with acceptable sports participation (Rice, 2008). The sport classification can assist parents in selecting activities that are most appropriate for their child.

Many sports, however, have the potential for causing both minor injuries, such as strains and soft tissue injury, and catastrophic permanently disabling injuries. The injury potential of an individual sport depends on several factors, among them the amount and type of protective equipment required, rule enforcement, correct assignment of athletes to teams based on developmental level and maturity, and adequate training of the coaching staff. Parents should be aware of the potential injuries. Overuse syndrome has increased in the pediatric population as the demand for excelling in sports is expected.

Sport-related concussion has become a primary focus when caring for adolescents participating in contact sports. Concussions can have significant acute and long-term effects. Many times the athlete, athletic personnel, and the family do not recognize the signs and symptoms of a concussion. The athlete may not understand the implications of a head injury or may be fearful of being excluded from participation. These issues can cause a delay in seeking medical treatment.

Signs and Symptoms

The symptoms of the most common sports injuries are presented in the Did You Know? on Frequently Seen Sport Injuries. In addition to those injuries described, athletes can sustain fractures and dislocations. Altered

tissue blood flow, electrolyte deficiencies, or minor tissue injury can cause muscle cramps, which are experienced at one time or another by all athletes. Nurses need to be aware that some injuries can damage a skeletally immature child's growth plate, interfering with growth potential. Other injuries, such as anterior cruciate ligament tears, can be particularly severe, resulting in several months' loss of participation time and requiring extensive rehabilitation.

? Did You Know?

Frequently Seen Sports Injuries

INJURY	DESCRIPTION
Strain	Caused by stretch injury to soft tissue structures (muscle, tendon), often associated with overuse. Pain on movement, swelling (extent depends on severity of the injury).
Sprain	Ligament tear, most frequently seen in ankle, knee, shoulder, or elbow. Pain, "popping" feeling at time of injury, extensive swelling, bruising, joint instability, movement limitation.
Stress fracture	Fracture occurring at a bony insertion site, usually caused by overuse or from physical exercise without adequate training or preparation. Commonly seen in the lower extremities, depending on the sport involved (e.g., running, ballet, gymnastics). Intermittent pain or limp that worsens with activity; local tenderness or swelling. Fracture is shown with radiography or more sensitive imaging studies.
Shin splints	Pain and discomfort in anterior lower leg from repeatedly running on a hard surface such as concrete.
"Stinger" or "burner"	Described as an "electric jolt" resulting from contact of an athlete's head with another athlete's body. Usually mild and disappears suddenly.
Concussion	Altered mental status caused by a blow to the head. Possible loss of consciousness, headache, vomiting.

Sports injuries are diagnosed using radiography or other bone-imaging procedures. Arthroscopy, a surgical procedure designed to assess joint damage, is used to diagnose knee and shoulder injuries. Some tissue repair can be done with arthroscopy.

Treatment and Nursing Care

First aid treatment for most extremity injuries includes **RICE** (**r**est, **i**ce, **c**ompression, and **e**levation) during the first 48 hours. Immobilizing and elevating the injured limb at the scene prevents further injury until the child can be evaluated. Crutches may be necessary for several days to keep the injured area rested. Compression of the injury with an elastic bandage helps minimize tissue bleeding and swelling.

For soft tissue injuries, such as strains and sprains, apply ice for 20 minutes three to four times a day for the first 48 hours. If using ice in a pack, protect the skin with a thin cloth before applying the pack.

Usually the physician prescribes a rehabilitative physical therapy program for athletes with severe tissue injury. Muscle-strengthening exercises and weight work are usually necessary to stabilize the injured area before an athlete can return to the sport. Some severe injuries may require casting or surgical intervention. In these instances, nursing care is similar to that for any child undergoing surgery or casting.

Initially, for children with concussions, complete physical and cognitive rest is implemented. A step approach is used to return the child to full unrestricted activities. The steps include advancement to light aerobics (walking) to sport-specific training (running for football) to non-contact drills (passing for football) to full contact with medical clearance (Patel and Reddy, 2010).

Prevention

Several factors help prevent sports injuries (Box 17-3). The nurse plays an important role in educating and directing parents to sources of accurate information to ensure that the physical, emotional, and maturational levels of the child are appropriate for the activity.

An often overlooked factor that contributes to sports injuries is emotional pressure. Many parents and coaches place undue pressure on the athlete to be the best or to win at all costs. Parents and coaches often argue with referees and umpires; they criticize their athletes if mistakes are made or if times are not good enough. Many athletes leave their sport because of intolerable pressure to succeed. This can cause decreased self-esteem at a time when positive self-esteem is developmentally important. Nurses need to

Box 17-3 Factors That Decrease Sport Injuries
• Adequate warm-up and cool-down periods • Year-round conditioning • Careful selection of sport according to physical maturity, size, and skill • Proper adult supervision • Safe, well-fitting equipment • No physical participation when in pain • Proper diet and fluids

Adapted from NIAMS. (2009). Handout on health: childhood sports injuries and their prevention: a guide for parents with ideas for kids. Retrieved November 1, 2010, from *www.niams.nih.gov/Health_Info/Sports_Injuries/child_sports_injuries.asp*.

reinforce to parents the value that participating on a team has for a child and the dangers involved with too much pressure.

Pre-Participation Examinations

Authorities disagree about what constitutes a good sports physical examination; however, they are unanimous about the need for regular and pre-participation medical examinations. Most athletes are required to have a yearly sports physical for continued participation. Such examinations are updated with a questionnaire asking about any injury acquired between sports during a given year. The family history and an orthopedic screening are important in identifying risk factors. The problem with this approach is that children who have yearly sports physicals often do not have regular comprehensive examinations. Because the physicals are specific for sports participation, other areas of health promotion (e.g., assessment of risk behaviors, diet, other illnesses that affect sports participation, and emotional health) can be neglected. Sports physicals should include a more thorough assessment of adolescents, or sports-specific assessments should be included as part of the comprehensive physical examination.

Get Ready for the NCLEX® Examination!

Key Points

- Neurovascular assessments should be performed on children in casts and in traction.
- Children with CP should be involved in stimulation programs that assist them in achieving their highest level of functioning.
- Maintaining activity and mobility for as long as possible is an essential nursing goal for children with Duchenne muscular dystrophy.
- Children wearing body braces need to receive instruction in proper wearing techniques. Home

instructions should be carefully discussed as should compliance issues.
- Immobilization from casts or traction can impact other systems such as respiratory and gastrointestinal.
- Children in skeletal traction require diversional therapy and physical outlets for their lack of physical activity.
- A child with a cast should have a neurovascular assessment, and parents should be taught signs and symptoms for home assessment.
- A child with osteomyelitis may require long-term IV antimicrobial therapy.

- Overuse injuries are common in the adolescent. Rest, ice, compression, and elevation are primary treatments.
- Sports-related concussions require medical attention as there can be long-term effects.
- Sports-related concussions can have long-term effects and should be medically evaluated.

Additional Learning Resources

evolve Go to your Evolve website (*http://evolve.elsevier.com/Price/pediatric/*) for the following FREE learning resources:

- 3-D Animations
- Answer Keys
- Appendixes
- Audio Glossary
- Spanish/English Glossary
- Video Clips

Review Questions for the NCLEX® Examination

1. The nurse is caring for a child following a synthetic cast application. When assessing circulatory status, the nurse is aware that signs of poor circulation include: **(Select all that apply.)**
   1. Swelling
   2. Numbness
   3. Sweating
   4. Pain
   5. Pallor

2. The most likely treatment to be implemented for a 2-month-old with developmental dysplasia of the hip (DDH) would be:
   1. Traction
   2. The Pavlik harness
   3. Spica cast application
   4. Surgery

3. All of the following factors can cause cerebral palsy **except**:
   1. Infections
   2. Prolonged labor
   3. Postnatal trauma
   4. Advanced maternal age

4. A disease in which the blood supply to the epiphysis, or end of the bone, is disrupted is:
   1. Duchenne muscular dystrophy
   2. Legg-Calvé-Perthes disease
   3. Scoliosis
   4. Avascular necrosis

5. The most common location for osteomyelitis to occur is the:
   1. Long bones of the lower extremities
   2. Thoracic spine
   3. Facial bones
   4. Long bones of the upper extremities

Objectives

1. Define the vocabulary terms listed
2. Identify the components of chain of infections and specific interventions to break the chain
3. Discuss transmission modes for communicable diseases in children
4. Identify interventions to decrease transmission of a communicable disease
5. Identify the appropriate isolation precaution for each communicable disease
6. Develop a plan for home care for a child with a communicable disease
7. List the immunizations given during the first year, and include the approximate age for each
8. Discuss ways to educate parents about the importance of immunizations
9. Discuss precautions/contraindications of immunizations

Key Terms

acquired immunity (p. 341)
active immunity (p. 341)
antibody (p. 341)
antigen (p. 341)
communicable (p. 340)
encephalopathy (p. 352)
endemic (p. 352)
epidemic (p. 342)
exanthema (p. 341)
immunity (p. 342)
immunizations (p. 342)

incubation period (p. 341)
pandemic (p. 341)
passive immunity (p. 341)
period of communicability (p. 341)
portal of entry (p. 340)
portal of exit (p. 340)
prodromal symptoms (prō-DRŌ-măl; p. 341)
reservoir (p. 340)
vector (p. 340)
virulence (p. 341)

A communicable disease is an infection that has been transmitted by direct or indirect contact, vehicle or vector, or airborne route. Communicable diseases are also known as infectious diseases. Infectious and communicable diseases account for the major cause of illness for infants and children. There are several factors that make infants and children susceptible to these diseases. Their immune system is not fully developed until 6 years of age (see Chapter 19), and they have not developed antibodies against many of the organisms. Many children attend day care during the first year of life, which increases their risk of exposure. Developmentally, infants have hand-to-mouth behavior, which is a source of infection. While many toddlers are still in diapers and are learning to be toilet trained, they may not always wash their hands, and this increases the risk of transmission. They are also exploring their environment and coming in contact with animals. School-age children are exposed to many

potential infections through their school. Many are lax with hand hygiene, and they share items among their peers.

Prevention and control are key factors in limiting the spread of communicable diseases. Nurses can play an important role in prevention. The chain of infection must be disrupted to prevent disease. The chain components are as follows:

- Infectious microorganism
- Reservoir (environment in which the organism exists and multiplies)
- Portal of exit (route by which the organism leaves the reservoir)
- Transmission mode (airborne, contact, droplet)
- Portal of entry to host (route by which the organism enters the host)
- Host susceptibility

The chain can be broken at any point along the process by using preventive measures. The nurse can

Table 18-1	Common Terms Used with Communicable Diseases		
Active immunity	Antibody production is stimulated without causing disease (e.g., a vaccine)	Endemic	Diseases that occur in expected cycles or continuously.
Acquired immunity	Antibody production resulting from exposure to antigen (e.g., having a communicable disease)	Epidemic	Disease that attacks many people at the same time in the same geographic location.
Passive immunity	Antibodies produced by a person and given to another (e.g., when maternal antibodies transfer across the placenta to the fetus)	Pandemic	Disease that is epidemic in different parts of the world.
Antibody	Protein that combines with antigens to assist with body's destruction of the antigen.	Vaccine	Suspension containing live attenuated or killed inactivated microorganisms given to prevent a specific infection.
Antigen	A cell marker that identifies the cell as foreign.	Virulence	Strength of effect produced by pathogen
Chain of infection	Factors and conditions that must be present for an infection to begin.	Incubation period	Period of time between exposure to infection and appearance of first symptoms.
Vector	A carrier that transfers an infectious agent from one host to another.	Prodromal period	Period of time between first symptoms and appearance of rash and fever.
Live attenuated vaccine	Vaccine produced with diminished potency (virulence) so it will not cause full-blown disease.	Period of communicability	Period of time in which infected individual can pass the infectious agent to another person.
Killed inactivated vaccine	Vaccine that contains inactivated pathogens and causes limited immune response.	Exanthema	An eruption or rash that appears on the skin.
Toxoids	Bacterial toxins that are inactive (e.g., diphtheria or tetanus)		

promote these preventive measures during family teaching. Discussions with the families regarding the specifics of infections can help them understand the infectious process. Included in the discussion is the way infections are spread; measures for preventing spread (hand hygiene and cleanliness); care of the ill child; and monitoring sanitation in their child's day care. Immunizations are a major component for prevention (discussed later in chapter), and nurses should be advocates for the immunization of infants and children.

COMMUNICABLE DISEASES

When a communicable disease is suspected, a thorough history must be obtained. The nurse asks whether the child has recently been exposed to a communicable disease, has been immunized, or has already had the disease. The nurse may inquire whether the child has experienced any of the prodromal symptoms (symptoms indicating the onset of a disease). Table 18-1 lists common terms used with communicable diseases.

Most communicable diseases can be treated at home unless the child is immunosuppressed or complications occur. Many of these diseases have identical symptoms and require the same supportive care and comfort. Parents may not be aware of appropriate measures that may be used to help alleviate the discomforts that accompany these diseases. Others may not be aware that some home remedies are no longer considered safe for children. The use of alcohol to reduce a fever has been a method used in the past, but it can be dangerous for infants and small children and is no longer recommended. Parental understanding of the transmission modes and measures to decrease transmission can help decrease the spread of the infection to others.

Home Care Considerations

Home Care Considerations for a Child with a Communicable Disease

- Tepid baths using oatmeal, baking soda, or colloid products such as Aveeno can relieve pruritus and discomfort.
- Drying lotions such as calamine can assist in healing lesions. Care should be taken as certain over-the-counter lotions also contain diphenhydramine (Benadryl).
- Nails should be kept short, and mittens may be worn by younger children who persist in scratching.
- Clothing should be lightweight to decrease skin irritation and decrease body temperature.
- Diphenhydramine (Benadryl) or hydroxyzine (Atarax) may be given to assist with pruritus and discomfort. Avoid overdosing if using lotions containing the same ingredient.
- Acetaminophen or ibuprofen is given for an elevated temperature and mild discomfort. Aspirin should be avoided because of its connection with Reye syndrome.
- Older children may gargle with saline rinses or use lozenges for sore throat relief.
- Adequate hydration is important, and children can be provided with cool, favorite fluids.
- Anorexia is common, and children should be encouraged to eat favorite nutritious foods.
- Quiet activities should be provided to allow for rest and diversion.

Table 18-2 summarizes the nursing care of several common communicable diseases. Smallpox is included to familiarize the student with information on a disease that might be used in an event of bioterrorism.

Global Perspective

Smallpox was determined to be globally eradicated in 1986, and all routine vaccinations have been discontinued. There is no known treatment for the disease, and the only preventive measure available is vaccination. As a result of concerns about the use of smallpox as a bioterrorism agent, the CDC and public health departments have stockpiled enough vaccine to vaccinate every person in the United States (CDC, 2009).

Community Considerations

The Centers for Disease Control and Prevention (CDC) play an active role in researching diseases, including those that could result from bioterrorism. All health care providers should be aware of their educational resources: CDC *(www.cdc.gov/)* and WHO *(www.who.int/en/)*. Information is also available in Spanish and other languages.

IMMUNIZATIONS

Immunizations have dramatically affected the course of many childhood infectious diseases. Immunizations work by stimulating the body to produce antibodies to defend against the weakened or killed microorganism found in the vaccine. These antibodies assist in providing immunity to the child. Immunizations assist in preventing communitywide disease and illness and possible adverse sequelae.

Health personnel must educate parents regarding the importance of immunizations. A delay in immunizations can lead to undue risks for serious illness, with potential fatal complications. Measles, pertussis, and other preventable diseases continue to strike children today. Health experts warn that unless more young children are immunized, epidemics could possibly occur. Current immunization policies and recommendations are updated annually by the American Academy of Pediatrics (AAP), the Advisory Committee on Immunization Practices (ACIP) of the CDC, and the American Academy of Family Physicians (AAFP) in response to the changing needs of the community and the child The nurse can emphasize to employed parents that unimmunized children may become sick, resulting in a loss of valuable working hours. Immunizations can prevent numerous doctor and hospital expenses. In addition, many states require immunization before a child enters school. Accurate record keeping can be difficult and confusing, so parents are encouraged to keep a copy of their child's immunization record.

 Nursing Brief

A delay or interruption in a vaccination series does not interfere with final immunity. Restarting any series is not necessary, regardless of the length of delay.

Contraindications to routine immunizations include acute febrile conditions, some chronic diseases, a recent blood transfusion or an injection of immune serum globulin, severe allergy to a vaccine component, severe reaction after previous administration of an immunization, malignant disease, chemotherapy, and steroid therapy. Those individuals with an altered immune system generally do not receive live virus vaccines because multiplication of the virus could be enhanced, causing a severe vaccine-induced illness (Hockenberry and Wilson, 2007). Other stipulations are described in drug inserts. The common cold is not considered sufficient reason for delaying immunization. Any questions regarding these or other conditions should be brought to the attention of the physician or the health care provider *before* immunization.

Changes have been made in the recommendations for immunizations because of increases in the outbreak of disease and the development of new vaccines. The American Academy of Pediatrics (AP), in collaboration with the Advisory Committee on Immunization Practices (ACIP) of the Centers for Disease Control and

Text continued on page 351.

Table 18-2   Communicable Diseases

DISEASE	COMMUNICABILITY PERIOD AND ROUTE	CLINICAL MANIFESTATIONS	TREATMENT AND NURSING CARE	COMPLICATIONS
Chickenpox (Varicella) Incubation period: 10-21 days Causative agent: Varicella-zoster virus	5 days after onset of rash and until all lesions are crusted Route: Airborne, droplet infection; direct or indirect contact Dry scabs are not infectious	General malaise, slight fever, anorexia, headache. Successive crops of macules, papules, vesicles, crusts. These may all be present at the same time. Itching of the skin. Generalized lymphadenopathy.	Oral acyclovir should be considered for otherwise healthy people at increased risk (e.g., people older than 12 yr of age, individuals with pulmonary disorders). IV antiviral therapy is recommended for immunocompromised children. Symptomatic. Prevent child from scratching. Keep fingernails short and clean. Sedation may be necessary. Use soothing lotions to allay itching. If secondary infections occur, antimicrobials may be given. Do not give aspirin because of high risk for Reye syndrome. Salicylate therapy should be stopped in a child who is exposed to varicella.	Bacterial superinfection; thrombocytopenia, arthritis, encephalitis, nephritis, Reye syndrome (with aspirin use).
Diphtheria Incubation period: 2-7 days or longer Causative agent: *Corynebacterium diphtheriae*	In untreated persons, organisms can be present in discharges from the nose and throat and from eye and skin lesions for 2-6 wk after infection Route: Droplets from respiratory tract of infected person or carrier; contact with discharges from skin lesions	Local and systemic manifestations. Membrane over tissue in nose or throat at site of bacterial invasion. Hoarse, brassy cough with stridor. Toxin from organism produces malaise and fever. Toxin has affinity for renal, nervous, and cardiac tissue.	A single dose (IV preferred) of equine antitoxin should be administered on the basis of clinical diagnosis, even before culture results are available (test for sensitivity to horse serum). Antimicrobial therapy with erythromycin or penicillin G procaine is given for 14 days in addition to antitoxin. Strict bed rest. Prevent exertion. Cleansing throat gargles may be ordered. Liquid or soft diet. Gavage or parenteral administration of fluids may become necessary. Observe for respiratory obstruction. Equipment for suctioning should be available. Oxygen and emergency tracheostomy may be necessary. Isolate.	Local infections: low-grade fever with gradual onset. Serious complications include severe neck swelling (bull neck), upper airway obstruction, myocarditis, and peripheral neuropathies.

Continued

Table 18-2 Communicable Diseases—cont'd

DISEASE	COMMUNICABILITY PERIOD AND ROUTE	CLINICAL MANIFESTATIONS	TREATMENT AND NURSING CARE	COMPLICATIONS
Epidemic Influenza Incubation period: 1-4 days Causative agent: Influenza virus types A, B, and C	Route: Airborne, droplet infection; direct contact	Manifestations in respiratory tract. Sudden onset with chills, fever, muscle pains, cough. If infection is severe and spreads to lower respiratory tract, air hunger may develop.	Symptomatic. Provide bed rest and increased fluid intake. Antimicrobials and sulfonamides may prevent secondary infection. Acetaminophen (antipyretic), drugs to control cough, and analgesics for pain may be given. Do not give aspirin because of high risk for Reye syndrome. Amantadine, rimantadine, Zanamivir, and oseltamivir (antiviral medication) are approved for treatment in children 1 yr of age and older, but different strains have developed some resistance.	In severe cases, pulmonary edema and cardiac failure. Secondary invaders may produce bacterial infections of respiratory tract.
Erythema Infectiosum (fifth disease) Incubation period: 4-14 days or longer Causative agent: Parvovirus B19	Uncertain Route: Droplet; infected persons	Three-stage rash: Erythema on face, mostly on cheeks (disappears in 1-4 days). One day after face rash, maculopapular red spots appear on upper and lower extremities, progressing proximal to distal; lacy appearance. Rash subsides but reappears if skin is irritated (sun, heat, cold); may last 1-3 wk. Child not contagious after rash appears.	Reinforce benign nature of the condition to parents. No treatment indicated. Exposed pregnant women should notify their obstetrician. Avoid exposing immunosuppressed children and children with sickle cell disease.	Aplastic crisis in children with sickle cell anemia.
Exanthema Subitum (Roseola) Incubation period: 9-10 days Causative agent: Human herpesvirus type 6	Unknown Route: Droplet; primarily affects children younger than 2 yr of age	Persistent high fever for 3-4 days in child who appears well. Precipitous drop in fever to normal with appearance of rash. Rash: discrete rose-pink macules appearing first on trunk, then spreading to neck, face, and extremities. Nonpruritic, fades on pressure, lasts 1-2 days.	Antipyretics to control fever. Anticonvulsants for child who has history of febrile seizures. Teach parents measures for combating high temperature. Reinforce benign nature of illness.	Febrile seizures during febrile period. Bulging fontanel.

Continued

Hepatitis Type A	Manifestations occur rapidly and vary from mild to severe, from mild fever, anorexia, generalized malaise, nausea, vomiting, unpleasant taste in mouth, abdominal discomfort, and nonexistent or mild jaundice to severe jaundice, coma, and death. Early leukopenia is seen. Bile may be detected in urine; bowel movements are clay-colored. Liver function tests are useful for diagnosis.	Symptomatic. No specific therapy for uncomplicated HAV infection. Enteric precautions are necessary for 1 wk after onset of jaundice. Persons caring for those who are not toilet-trained, have diarrhea, or are incontinent should use disposable gloves when carrying fecal waste. Prevention: In daycare centers, practice thorough hand hygiene after changing diapers and before preparing and serving food. Because HAV may survive on objects in the environment for weeks (e.g., infant changing tables), adequate environmental hygiene is essential. Children should be immunized at 1 yr of age (12-23 mos). Administer immunoglobulin to contacts of affected child younger than 1 yr of age in a daycare setting.	Usually benign in children. Liver damage, recurrence of symptoms. May be a source of chromosomal damage.
Incubation period: 15-50 days (average 28 days) Causative agent: Hepatitis A virus (HAV)	1-2 weeks before onset of jaundice or elevation of liver enzymes Route: Oral contamination by intestinal excretions; contaminated food, milk, or water Hepatitis A is a major potential health problem in daycare centers		
Hepatitis Type B	Manifestations occur slowly. See hepatitis A for clinical manifestations.	Symptomatic. Children should be allowed to regulate own activity. Diet should be high-protein, high-calorie, high-carbohydrate, and low-fat. Food should be served in small, attractive, frequent feedings. Chief reasons for hospitalization are persistent vomiting and toxicity. Fluids may be given parenterally. Prevention: Universal immunization of infants and preteen children not immunized during infancy. Careful handling of blood and secretions; universal precautions. No specific therapy for acute HBV vaccine is available. HBIG and corticosteroids are not effective.	Acute fulminating hepatitis characterized by rapidly rising bilirubin, encephalopathy, edema, ascites, and hepatic coma. Chronic HBV-infected persons are at risk for serious liver disease including primary hepatocellular carcinoma (HCC) with advancing age.
Incubation period: 45-160 days (average 90 days) Causative agent: Hepatitis B virus (HBV)	Few days before to 1 mo or more after onset Route: Person-to-person by percutaneous introduction of blood; direct contact with secretions or blood contaminated with HBV. Routine preexposure immunization recommended for all infants; appropriate immunoprophylaxis of infants born to HBsAg-positive women and of infants born to women with unknown HBsAg status; some risk in children on hemodialysis, children receiving blood or blood products (including those with hemophilia), and IV drug users		

Table 18-2 Communicable Diseases—cont'd

DISEASE	COMMUNICABILITY PERIOD AND ROUTE	CLINICAL MANIFESTATIONS	TREATMENT AND NURSING CARE	COMPLICATIONS
Lyme Disease Incubation period: 1-32 days but up to months or years Causative agent: *Borrelia burgdorferi*	Not communicable from person to person; persons with active disease should not donate blood Route: Spread by ticks; most common hosts are white-tailed deer and white-footed mice	Begins with a skin lesion at the site of a recent tick bite. The painless red macule expands to form a large papule with a raised border and a clear center. Systemic manifestations include malaise, lethargy, fever, headache, arthralgias, stiff neck, myalgias, and lymphadenopathy. Late manifestations involve the joints and the cardiac and neurologic systems. Often first appears as single joint redness, swelling, and limitation.	Early treatment is doxycycline for children 8 yr of age and older. All ages: amoxicillin or cefuroxime. Later-stage disease is treated with high-dose IV ceftriaxone or penicillin. Prevention by teaching parents to observe for signs of disease during tick season. Protective clothing should be worn in areas where tick exposure is likely. Ticks should be removed.	Neurologic complications, carditis, and chronic arthritis may develop. Transplacental infection has resulted in fetal death, prematurity, and congenital anomalies.
Measles (Rubeola) Incubation period: 8-12 days Causative agent: RNA virus	From 4 days before to 5 days after rash appears Route: Direct contact; airborne by droplets and contaminated dust	Coryza, conjunctivitis, and photophobia are present before rash. Koplik spots in mouth, hacking cough, high fever, rash, and enlarged lymph nodes. Rash consists of small reddish brown or pink macules changing to papules; fades on pressure. Rash begins behind ears, on forehead or cheeks, progresses to extremities, and lasts about 5 days.	Symptomatic. Keep child in bed until fever and cough subside. Light in room should be dimmed. Keep hands from eyes. Irrigate eyes with physiologic saline solution to relieve itching. Tepid baths and soothing lotion relieve itching of skin. Encourage fluids during fever. Humidify the child's room. Antimicrobial therapy given for complications. Vitamin A supplementation is recommended once daily for 2 days to reduce mortality. Immunoglobulin (IG) can help prevent or modify measles within 6 days of exposure.	Vary with severity of disease: otitis media, pneumonia, tracheobronchitis, nephritis. Encephalitis with permanent brain damage may occur. Death from respiratory and neurologic complications. Subacute sclerosing panencephalitis (SSPE), a rare degenerative central nervous system (CNS) disease, may occur. The mean incubation period is 7 yr after measles illness.

Disease	Communicability/Route	Signs and Symptoms	Treatment/Nursing Care	Complications
Measles, German (Rubella) Incubation period: 14-23 days Causative agent: Virus	During prodromal period and for 5 days after appearance of rash Route: Direct contact with secretions of nose and throat of infected person; airborne by contaminated dust particles	Fetus may contract rubella in utero if mother has the disease; slight fever, mild coryza. Rash consists of small pink or pale red macules closely grouped to appear as scarlet blush that fades on pressure. Rash fades in 3 days. Swelling of posterior cervical and occipital lymph nodes. No Koplik spots or photophobia as in measles.	Symptomatic. Bed rest until fever subsides. Children should be excluded from school or daycare for 7 days after onset of rash. Infants with congenital rubella should be considered contagious until 1 yr of age unless cultures are repeatedly negative.	Chief danger of disease is damage to fetus if mother contracts infection during first trimester of pregnancy. Neonate may have congenital rubella syndrome with permanent defects (e.g., cataracts, cardiovascular anomalies, deafness, microcephaly, mental retardation). Virus can be isolated from blood, urine, throat, cerebrospinal fluid, lens, and other involved organs. Infants may shed virus for 12-18 mc. Severe complications are rare. Encephalitis may occur.
Mumps (Infectious Parotitis) Incubation period: 16-18 days Causative agent: Rubulavirus in the Paramyxoviridae family	1-2 days before swelling to 5 days after onset of swelling Route: Direct or indirect contact with salivary secretions of infected person. Droplet	Salivary glands are chiefly affected. Parotid, sublingual, and submaxillary glands may be involved. Swelling and pain occur in these glands either unilaterally or bilaterally. Child may have difficulty swallowing, headache, fever, and malaise.	Local application of heat or cold to salivary glands to reduce discomfort. Liquids or soft foods are given. Foods containing acid may increase pain. Bed rest until swelling subsides. Children are excluded from school or daycare for 9 days from onset of parotid gland swelling. Mumps vaccine should be given at least 2 wk before or 3 mos after administration of IG or blood transfusion.	Complications are less frequent in children than in adults. Meningoencephalitis, inflammation of ovaries or testes, or deafness may occur.

Continued

Table 18-2 Communicable Diseases—cont'd

DISEASE	COMMUNICABILITY PERIOD AND ROUTE	CLINICAL MANIFESTATIONS	TREATMENT AND NURSING CARE	COMPLICATIONS
Pertussis (Whooping Cough) Incubation period: 7-10 days Causative agent: Bordetella pertussis	4-6 wk from onset Route: Direct contact; airborne by droplet spread from infected person	Begins with symptoms of upper respiratory tract infection. Coryza, dry cough, which is worse at night. Cough occurs in paroxysms of several sharp coughs in one expiration, then a rapid deep inspiration, followed by a whoop. Dyspnea and fever may be present. Vomiting may occur after coughing. Lymphocytosis occurs. Duration of illness is 6-10 wk.	Symptomatic. Azithromycin is the drug of choice for treatment or prophylaxis of pertussis in infants younger than 1 mo of age. Erythromycin may limit communicability. Protect child from secondary infection. Erythromycin for household and daycare contacts. Primary or booster vaccination of exposed children younger than 7 yr of age. Provide mental and physical rest to prevent paroxysms of coughing. Provide warm, humid air. Oxygen may be necessary. Avoid chilling. Offer small, frequent feedings to maintain nutritional status. Refeed if child vomits. Small amounts of sedatives may be given to quiet the child. Most infants younger than 6 mos of age are hospitalized; intensive care may be required.	Very serious disease during infancy because of complication of bronchopneumonia. Otitis media, marasmus, bronchiectasis, and atelectasis may occur. Hemorrhage may occur during paroxysms of coughing. Encephalitis may occur.
Poliovirus Infection (Poliomyelitis) Incubation period: 3-6 days Causative agent: Enteroviruses	During period of infection, latter part of incubation period, and first week of acute illness Route: Oral contamination by pharyngeal and intestinal excretions, respiratory route	Acute illness. Initial symptoms of upper respiratory tract infection, headache, fever, vomiting. Nonparalytic: Previous symptoms plus sore or stiff muscles of neck, trunk, and extremities. Nuchal rigidity. Paralytic: Includes muscular paralysis. Clinical manifestations may vary from mild to very severe following symptomless period after initial symptoms.	Both parents and child need support and reassurance, for they are fearful of the term *polio*. Treatment and nursing care are symptomatic. Because oral polio vaccine is no longer available in the United States, the chance for exposure to vaccine-type polio is remote.	Emotional disturbances, gastric dilation, melena, hypertension, or transitory paralysis of bladder may occur. Severe complications of paralytic polio include respiratory failure and permanent muscle deficits.

Rotavirus
 	
Incubation period:
  1-3 days
 	
Causative agent:
  Rotovirus
	Route: Fecal-oral	Acute onset of fever and vomiting followed 24-48 hr later by watery diarrhea.	Oral or parenteral fluids and electrolytes are given to prevent and correct dehydration.
			
			No antiviral therapy is available.
			
			Contact precautions are used when diapering or cleaning incontinent children during illness.
				Dehydration, electrolyte abnormalities, and acidosis.

Smallpox (Variola)
 	
Incubation period:
  7-17 days
 	
Causative agent:
  Virus (variola)
 	
Note: A smallpox vaccination plan has been implemented in the United States; however, the plan does not currently include immunization of children.
	Persons are not infectious during the incubation period or febrile prodrome but become infectious with the onset of mucosal lesions, which occur within hours of the rash; the first week of rash illness is the most infectious period, although individuals remain infectious until all scabs have separated
	
	Route: Droplets (from the oropharynx of infected individuals); may be transmitted from aerosol and direct contact with infected lesions, clothing, or bedding
		Severe prodromal illness with high fever (generally 102° F-104° F [38.9° C-40° C]), malaise, severe headache, backache, abdominal pain, and prostration (exhaustion), lasting for 2-5 days. May include vomiting and seizures. Prodromal period is followed by lesions on the mucosa of the mouth or pharynx that last less than 24 hr before the onset of rash. The child is considered infectious once the lesions appear. The rash begins on the face and spreads rapidly to the forearms, trunk, and legs in a centrifugal distribution. Many have lesions on the palms and soles After 8-10 days, lesions begin to crust. Once all lesions have separated (3-4 wk), the child is no longer infectious.	Treatment is supportive. Vaccinia immune globulin (VIG) is used for certain complications of immunizations and has no role in treatment of smallpox. The vaccination may provide some protection against the disease if administered within 3-4 days of exposure. Children are isolated in a private, airborne infection isolation room with negative pressure ventilation. Anyone entering the room must wear an N95 or higher-quality respirator, gloves, and gown even if there is a history of recent successful immunization. If thechild leaves the room, he or she should wear a mask and be covered with sheets or gowns to decrease the risk for possible transmission.
			
			Cidofovir has been suggested as having a role in smallpox therapy, but no data are available.
				Fatality rates reached 30% in the past; death occurred during the second week of illness from overwhelming viremia. The potential for modern supportive therapy in improving outcome is not known.

Continued

Table 18-2 Communicable Diseases—cont'd

DISEASE	COMMUNICABILITY PERIOD AND ROUTE	CLINICAL MANIFESTATIONS	TREATMENT AND NURSING CARE	COMPLICATIONS
Streptococcal Infection, Group A Beta Hemolytic (Streptococcal Sore Throat, Scarlet Fever, Scarlatina) Incubation period: 2-5 days Causative agent: Betahemolytic streptococci, Group A strains	Onset to recovery Route: Droplet infection; direct and indirect transmission may occur	Initial symptoms of streptococcal sore throat are seen in the pharynx. The source of this organism may also be in a burn or wound. Toxin from site of infection is absorbed into bloodstream. Typical symptoms of scarlet fever are headache, fever, rapid pulse, thirst, vomiting, lymphadenitis, and delirium. Throat is injected, and cellulitis of throat occurs. White tongue coating desquamates, and red strawberry tongue results. Other manifestations may include otitis media, mastoiditis, and meningitis.	Penicillin G is the drug of choice. Erythromycin is used for penicillin-sensitive individuals. Adequate fluid intake, bed rest, pain-relieving drugs, and mouth care are important. Diet should be given as the child wishes: liquid, soft, or regular. Warm saline throat irrigations may be given to the older child. Increased humidity for severe infection of upper respiratory tract. Cold or hot applications to painful cervical lymph nodes.	Complications are caused by toxins, the streptococci, or secondary infection. Complications of pneumonia, glomerulonephritis, or rheumatic fever may occur.
Tetanus Incubation period: 3-21 days (average 8 days) Causative agent: *Clostridium tetani*	Route: Wound contaminant; umbilical stump contamination in neonates	Early signs are headache, restlessness, followed by spasm of masticatory muscles (chewing), difficulty opening the mouth, dysphagia. Progresses to opisthotonos (severe arching of back and head bending to back), seizures.	Human tetanus immune globulin is given to neutralize neurotoxins to stop the infectious process. Surgical wound debridement Quiet environment as muscle spasms are aggravated by external stimuli. Metronidazole is the drug of choice for 10-14 days; an alternative is Penicillin G, IV. Diazepam (Valium) to alleviate muscle spasms	Respiratory failure requiring support. Seizures.

Modified from the American Academy of Pediatrics. (2009) In Pickering, L., Baker, C., Kimberlin, D., et al. (Eds). *Red book: 2009 Report of the Committee on Infectious Diseases* (28th ed.). Elk Grove Village, L: American Academy of Pediatrics. Retrieved November 5, 2010, from *http://aapredbook.aappublications.org*.

Prevention and the American Academy of Family Physicians (AAFP), has approved a Recommended Childhood Immunization Schedule for the United States. **The Immunization Schedule,** found on the Evolve site, shows the recommendations for immunizations. The schedule is dated to ensure that health care providers are following the most recent schedule. The most up-to-date schedule can be obtained from the Centers for Disease Control and Prevention (*www.cdc.gov*).

In the United States, by the time a child is 2 years old, he or she should be immunized against the following diseases: polio, diphtheria, tetanus, pertussis (whooping cough), hepatitis A, hepatitis B, *Haemophilus influenzae* type b, mumps, measles, rubella, varicella (chickenpox), rotavirus, and *Streptococcus pneumoniae* (pneumococcus). The influenza vaccine is now recommended for all children 6 months to 18 years of age. Varicella vaccination recommendations have been updated. The first dose should be administered at 12 to 15 months of age, and a newly recommended second dose should be administered at 4 to 6 years of age. The human papillomavirus (HPV) vaccine is recommended in a 3-dose schedule for girls 11 to 12 years of age. The human papillomavirus (HPV4) is recommended in a 3-dose schedule for boys 9 to 18 years of age to reduce the risk of acquiring genital warts. In February 2006, the U.S. Food and Drug Administration licensed an oral rotavirus vaccine; the three doses are administered at 2, 4, and 6 months of age. The meningococcal conjugate vaccine should be given to all children at the 11- or 12-year-old visit as well as to children 2 to 10 years of age with persistent complement component deficiencies, anatomic or functional **asplenia,** or otherwise considered high risk. Table 18-3 shows the vaccines, the number of doses needed, and the recommended age when the vaccination should be administered.

Nursing Brief

Immunizations must be stored/refrigerated correctly to ensure potency. Always check dose and the route of administration for any vaccine because this varies with the age and in some cases the weight of the child.

Precautions/Side Effects

Precautions need to be taken when dealing with vaccines. Parents should be made aware of the possible side effects of various vaccines. These side effects are usually mild, and **the benefits of protection greatly outweigh the risks.** Other than the health care provider recommendation of the prophylactic use of acetaminophen or ibuprofen for fever or discomfort, no specific treatment is necessary. However, a persistent high fever, continued crying (longer than 3 hours), a

Table 18-3	Immunization Doses Related to A
DOSE	**AGE RECEIVED**
Hep B IM	
First dose	Birth
Second dose	1-2 mo
Third dose	6-18 months
DTaP IM	
First dose	2 mo
Second dose	4 mo
Third dose	6 mo
Fourth dose	15-18 mo
Fifth dose	4-6 yr
Td, Tdap	11-12 yr
HIB IM	
First dose	2 mo
Second dose	4 mo
Third dose	6 mo
Fourth dose	12-15 mo
IPV subq or IM (Polio)	
First dose	2 mo
Second dose	4 mo
Third dose	6-18 mo
Fourth dose	4-6 yr
MMR subq	
First dose	12-15 mo
Second dose	4-6 yr
Varicella subq (chickenpox)	
First dose	12-15 mo
Second dose	4-6 yr
PCV IM	
First dose	2 mo
Second dose	4 mo
Third dose	6 mo
Fourth dose	12-15 mo
Hepatitis A IM	
First dose	12-23 mo
Second dose	6 mo after first dose
Influenza IM	Yearly, starting at 6 mo
Rotavirus oral	
First dose	2 mo
Second dose	4 mo
Third dose	6 mo
Meningococcal IM	11-12 yr (MCV)
Booster	16 yr
Human Papillomavirus (HPV) lay flat rt syncope*	
First dose	11-12 yr
Second dose	2 mo after first dose
Third dose	6 mo after first dose

decrease in responsiveness, and/or possible seizure activity are **not** routine, and the health care provider should be notified in any of these cases.

 Community Considerations

For vaccine information, the Immunization Action Coalition (*www.immunize.org*) provides extensive free provider and patient information, including translations of Vaccine Information Statements into multiple languages. The Vaccine Adverse Events Reporting System (VAERS) sponsored by the CDC, provides a mechanism for reporting suspected adverse effects of vaccinations (*http://vaers.hhs.gov/index*).

Hepatitis B (Hep B) Vaccine. Hepatitis B vaccine is given to the newborn before dismissal from the hospital. Some tenderness at the injection site and a mild fever may be seen. Three doses are needed to ensure proper immunization. If the newborn's mother has a positive surface antigen for hepatitis B, the newborn will receive the hepatitis B vaccine as well as hepatitis B immune globulin (HBIG). Anaphylactic reaction to common baker's yeast is a contraindication to receiving the hepatitis B vaccine. This vaccine is given intramuscularly.

Rotavirus Vaccine. This oral vaccine's precautions include altered immunocompetence, moderate to severe illness (including gastroenteritis), preexisting chronic gastrointestinal disease, previous history of intussusception, or administration of antibody-containing blood products within the past 42 days. Side effects may include irritability or mild, temporary diarrhea or vomiting.

Diphtheria-Tetanus-Pertussis Vaccine (DTP) and Diphtheria-Tetanus-Acellular Pertussis Vaccine (DTaP). DTaP contains acellular pertussis and is recommended for all doses in the series. Contraindications include encephalopathy within 7 days after administration of a previous dose of DTP/DTaP. Precautions include persistent, inconsolable crying that lasts for more than 3 hours and occurs within 48 hours of receiving a previous dose; seizures within 3 days after immunization; fever of 40° C (105° F) or above within 48 hours after the previous dose; or hypotonic-hyporesponsive episode within 48 hours of the previous dose (Guide to Vaccine Contraindications and Precautions, 2009). Possible side effects of DTaP include a mild fever and redness and swelling at the injection site. The infant/child may be fussy, and a slight decrease in appetite may be seen. These effects are temporary and should resolve in approximately 24 to 48 hours. DTaP requires excellent intramuscular injection technique to prevent complications. Tdap was licensed in 2005. It contains a full concentration of

tetanus and lower concentrations of both diphtheria and pertussis. It is the first pertussis-containing vaccine licensed in the United States for older children, adolescents, and adults. It is currently recommended as a once-only booster for children 11 to 18 years of age (CDC, 2011).

Haemophilus Influenzae Type B (Hib) Vaccine. The side effects from Hib vaccine are usually mild. There may be some redness at the injection site and a slight fever, which resolves itself within 2 to 3 days. Hib vaccine is administered as an intramuscular injection.

Pneumococcal Vaccine (PCV). This vaccine can cause fever, fussiness, or local erythema. It is given intramuscularly.

Polio Vaccine (OPV and IPV). Contraindications include anaphylactic reaction to neomycin, streptomycin, or polymyxin B. Vaccination is avoided with pregnancy. In the past, the polio vaccine was given orally. However, because several cases of active polio were related to the administration of oral polio vaccine (OPV), the Advisory Committee for Immunization Practices of the Centers for Disease Control and Prevention recommended the use of the inactivated polio vaccine (IPV) as of January 1, 2000. The IPV is given as a subcutaneous or intramuscular injection. Side effects from polio vaccine are rare and consist of mild soreness at the site.

 Global Perspective

OPV continues to be used in the remaining countries where polio is endemic. OPV is recommended for global polio eradication activities in polio-endemic countries due to its advantages over IPV in providing intestinal immunity and providing secondary spread of the vaccine to unprotected contacts. Department of Health and Human Services, Centers for Disease Control and Prevention, 2010.

Influenza Vaccine. This intramuscular injection is recommended for children 6 months of age and older. For healthy persons 5 to 49 years of age, the intranasal live attenuated influenza vaccine (LAIV) may be used as an alternative. The influenza vaccine is contraindicated in children who have anaphylactic hypersensitivity to eggs. LAIV is contraindicated during pregnancy, with chronic illnesses of the pulmonary or cardiovascular system, with metabolic disorders, and with hemoglobinopathies including sickle cell disease. It is also contraindicated with immunodeficiency disorders and with children and adolescents on aspirin or salicylate therapy.

Mumps, Measles, and Rubella Vaccine (MMR). Contraindications include pregnancy, known altered immunodeficiency, or anaphylactoid reaction to neomycin or gelatin. The MMR vaccine is contraindicated with immunodeficiency, and precautions include recent administration of antibody-containing blood products or thrombocytopenia. The health care provider should be consulted regarding children who are sensitive to eggs. Measles vaccine may produce a fever and a rash, which occur about 7 to 12 days after vaccination and last only a few days. Encephalitis rarely occurs. The mumps vaccine has essentially no side effects other than an occasional mild fever. The rubella vaccine may produce a rash within a few days that may last 1 or 2 days. Joint pain and swelling can occasionally be seen about 2 weeks after vaccination. Be aware of the time delay. This is more common in older children. With the combination MMR, side effects may include a mild fever, possibly a rash, and only occasional mild swelling of the glands in the cheeks or the neck. MMR is administered subcutaneously.

Varicella Vaccine. This vaccine is contraindicated in immunocompromised individuals, in pregnancy, in children receiving steroids, and in those who had a previous anaphylactic reaction to neomycin or gelatin. Precautions include recent administration of antibody-containing blood products. Most individuals who receive the vaccine have a mild reaction. A mild vaccine-associated maculopapular or varicella rash can occur. Soreness and edema at the site and a mild fever may be the only reaction. The vaccine remains safer than the disease itself. Varicella vaccine is administered subcutaneously. Note: If the varicella and MMR vaccines are not given on the same day, the interval between the administrations should be at least 1 month.

 Community Considerations

The MMR and varicella vaccines can be safely administered to household members and caregivers of immunocompromised children.

Hepatitis A (Hep A) Vaccine. Sensitivity to alum or 2-phenoxyethanol is a contraindication. In some cases, local erythema (redness) may occur. This vaccine is administered with an intramuscular injection.

Meningococcal Vaccine (MCV). The most frequent adverse reactions are pain and redness at the injection site. This intramuscular injection is contraindicated with known hypersensitivity to any component of the vaccine.

Human Papillomavirus (HPV). This vaccine prevents infection from HPV but will not treat existing diseases or conditions caused by prior HPV infection. It is now available for males. The most common side effect is pain, redness, and swelling at the site of injection. Syncope can occur after administration, so it is recommended to observe the child for 15 to 20 minutes after administration (Knudtson et al., 2009; CDC, 2010). See Table 15-3 in Chapter 15 for further discussion of HPV.

Health Problems and Immunizations

Children who have asthma, lung disease, heart disease, kidney disease, metabolic disorders such as diabetes, or blood disorders should not receive the LAIV vaccine (live attenuated influenza vaccine, known as FluMist). They should only receive inactivated influenza vaccine. In addition, if children have cancer, leukemia, AIDS, or other immune system problems, they should not receive live-virus vaccines including LAIV, MMR, varicella, and rotavirus. However, MMR and varicella may be given with asymptomatic HIV-infected children who do not show evidence of severe immunosuppression. Children should not receive any live-virus vaccines until chemotherapy or long-term steroid therapy is completed.

Importance

Communicable diseases still pose a threat, and immunization of children is paramount. Community outreach projects sponsored by the Public Health Department provide avenues for children to receive immunizations. Accurate records are crucial, and the parent or caregiver should keep a current immunization record for the child. Because a number of vaccines are recommended, several injections may be given at one time to an infant or child. Some vaccines protect the child from more than one disease. An example is the MMR. In addition, multiple vaccine administration during a visit does not increase the intensity or the number of side effects. Always remember to administer immunizations safely and efficiently. Children do not like "shots." The use of eutectic mixture of local anesthetics (EMLA) cream or a topical vapocoolant spray may help to decrease the pain at the injection site. See Chapter 3 for a discussion on injection sites and technique.

Concerns

Thimerosal, a weak antibacterial agent and mercury-containing preservative used in some childhood vaccines since the 1930s, has been criticized because of concern over the rise of mercury toxicity in children. In 1999, the American Academy of Pediatrics, Public Health Service agencies, and vaccine manufacturers agreed that thimerosal should be reduced or eliminated in vaccines as a precautionary measure. Today, thimerosal is not used with childhood immunizations.

Autism is a developmental disability caused by an abnormality in the brain (see Chapter 20 for a discussion on autism). Recently, an increase in the rate of autism has been seen. Although no one has an answer, some investigators believe that the MMR vaccine is associated with autism. However, multiple studies have failed to support an association between MMR vaccine and autism (Hornig et al., 2008). Recent research from Price and colleagues (2010) supports the findings that vaccines do not cause autism.

Get Ready for the NCLEX® Examination!

Key Points

- Nursing interventions in the treatment of communicable diseases are focused on identification, prevention of transmission, providing comfort, and prevention of complications.
- Nurses today need to be aware of indications of bioterrorism, including signs and symptoms of smallpox.
- Immunizations are an important aspect in the promotion of health for infants and children.
- By 2 years of age, the child should be protected from more than 10 different communicable diseases if proper immunizations have been given.
- Considering the consequences of morbidity and mortality, the benefits of immunizations far exceed the risks
- There is no scientific support that vaccines cause autism.

Additional Learning Resources

evolve Go to your Evolve website (*http://evolve.elsevier.com/Price/ pediatric/*) for the following FREE learning resources:
- 3-D Animations
- Answer Keys
- Appendixes
- Audio Glossary
- Spanish/English Glossary
- Video Clips

Review Questions for the NCLEX® Examination

1. Which of the following is **not** a contraindication to routine immunizations?
   1. Malignant disease
   2. Recent blood transfusion
   3. Diagnosis of autism
   4. Steroid therapy

2. Potential side effects of vaccines that parents should report to the health care provider include: (**Select all that apply.**)
   1. Temporary diarrhea
   2. Persistent high fever
   3. Local erythema
   4. Fussiness
   5. Decrease in responsiveness

3. A child is due to receive the measles, mumps, and rubella (MMR) vaccine. Which of the following allergies/ sensitivities reported by the child's parents should be brought to the attention of the health care provider?
   1. Eggs
   2. Penicillin
   3. Baker's yeast
   4. Shellfish

4. The route of administration for the Hepatitis B vaccine is:
   1. Orally
   2. Subcutaneously
   3. Intranasally
   4. Intramuscularly

5. The most frequent adverse reactions to the meningococcal vaccine (MCV) are:
   1. Pain and redness at the injection site
   2. Nausea and vomiting
   3. Low-grade fever and headache
   4. Irritability and syncope

Immune Disorders

Objectives

1. Describe nursing interventions for a child with Kawasaki disease
2. List nursing interventions for oral care for a child with Stevens-Johnson syndrome
3. Devise a nursing care plan for a 12-year-old with juvenile idiopathic arthritis, including teaching about home management
4. Identify characteristics for mononucleosis
5. Differentiate between insulin-dependent and non–insulin-dependent diabetes mellitus
6. Outline the educational needs of the child with diabetes and of the parents in the following areas: nutrition and meal planning, glucose monitoring, insulin administration, and exercise

Key Terms

antigens (ĂN-ti-gĕns; p. 355)
autoimmune (ăw-tō-ĭ-MŪN; p. 356)
cell-mediated (p. 355)
desquamation (des-kwə-MĀ-shən; p. 356)
humoral (HYÜ-mə-rəl; p. 355)

iridocyclitis (IR-ĭ-do-sə-kli-tis; p. 360)
IVIG (p. 357)
Kussmaul breathing (KOOS-moul; p. 363)
vasculitis (văs-kū-LĪ-tĭs; p. 356)

IMMUNE SYSTEM

The main function of the immune system is to protect the body by recognizing "self" from "nonself." The system launches a protective process to eliminate any foreign antigens through the function of specific cells. The process is complex and uses overlapping defense reactions. A child's immune system won't reach maturity until about 6 years of age, which makes infants and children susceptible to infectious organisms. Lymphoid tissue reaches adult size by 6 weeks of age, enlarges during the prepubertal age, and returns to normal size by puberty. The thymus reaches full size before puberty. The spleen reaches full size by adulthood. When the immune system is fully functioning, the risk of being infected by invading organisms is lower.

Antibodies are needed to fight infections. IgG is the only antibody that crosses the placenta. Full-term infants receive adult levels of IgG, which provides protection from bacterial infections. There is a physiologic drop in IgG at 6 to 8 months, and it does not return to adult levels until 7 to 8 years of age. IgM, IgE, IgA, and IgD do not cross the placenta and do not reach adult levels until later. IgM reaches adult level by 1 year of age; IgA and IgE reach adult level by 6 to 7 years of age.

The body's protective responses are either nonspecific or specific. The nonspecific response is a generalized reaction not specific to a particular antigen. The injury site produces inflammation to which phagocytes respond and ingest the antigens. If the response is effective, the inflammation clears. Should the generalized response not be successful, a more specific response is initiated. Two additional immune functions respond, the humoral and cell-mediated functions. The B lymphocytes that promote humoral response produce antibodies (IgG, IgM, IgA, IgD, and IgE) and memory cells. Each antibody has specific antigen targets; for example, IgM activates with bacterial and viral infections, and IgE is activated with allergic response. The antibodies bind with the antigen and tag it so that other components of the immune system can destroy the antigen. Phagocytes are the immune cells that destroy antigens by engulfing and digesting. The function of memory cells is to detect previously identified antigens and facilitate a quicker response to the specific antigen.

The cell-mediated response involves T lymphocyte cells. T cells are produced in the thymus. There are 3 specialized types of T cells: helper cell, killer (cytotoxic) cell, and suppressor cell. The function of T cells is to attack and destroy bacteria, viruses, and other pathogens. The killer T cells directly bind to the foreign antigen and disrupt the cell membrane. This results in the antigen's destruction. The helper T cell has several functions. It stimulates the B cell to mature and aid in the destruction of the antigen. The helper T cell retains information about specific antigens and is also able to provide that information, resulting in a quicker response. In addition, the helper T cell assists the killer cell in recognizing antigen. The suppressor T cells assist in slowing the immune response. Both the humoral and cell-mediated system work together to provide protection from infections.

Disorders of the immune system are a result of several different causes. Deficiencies of the immune cells resulting in the inability of the body to resist an infection are considered immunodeficiency. This group of disorders includes HIV/AIDS. They are discussed in Chapter 15. Other disorders are caused by an abnormal and excessive immune response to a foreign antigen. These disorders are hypersensitivity disorders such as allergies and atopic dermatitis (see Chapter 16 for further discussion on these disorders).

Disorders resulting from an abnormal and excessive response to self and these disorders are referred to as autoimmune disorders.

KAWASAKI DISEASE

Kawasaki disease (KD) is an acute severe vasculitis of all blood vessels, especially medium-sized vessels such as the coronary artery. The cause of the illness is unknown but is thought to be infectious. It is seen in children younger than 5 years of age, in boys more often than in girls, and has a higher incidence in those of Asian background. It is the leading cause of acquired heart disease in children (AAP, 2009). Coronary involvement can lead to aneurysms, ischemia, and infarcts.

Signs and Symptoms

KD progresses through three stages: acute, subacute, and convalescent. The acute stage presents with a prolonged high fever that is unresponsive to antimicrobials or acetaminophen or ibuprofen. Additional classic symptoms are conjunctival redness without drainage, strawberry tongue with oral and pharyngeal redness, red swollen hands and feet, rash on the trunk, enlarged cervical lymph nodes, and extreme irritability. The subacute stage begins after 1 to 2 weeks when the fever and acute signs resolve. Irritability, conjunctival redness, and anorexia continue with the appearance of desquamation of hands and feet, arthritis, thrombocytosis, and coronary aneurysms (Figure 19-1). This stage can last up to 4 weeks. The last stage of convalescence begins when all signs have disappeared and ends when erythrocyte sedimentation rate (ESR) and C-reactive protein (CRP) have returned to a normal value. This stage may last from 6 to 8 weeks.

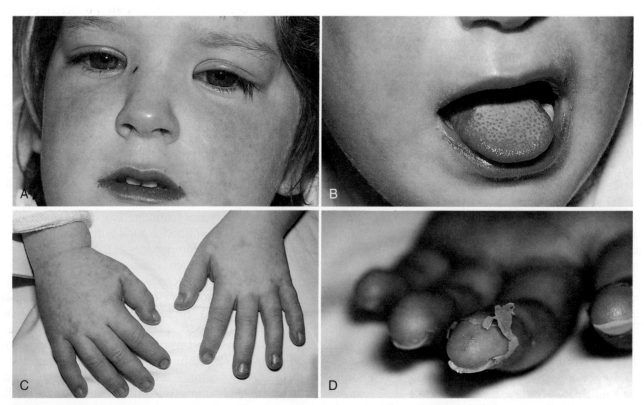

FIGURE 19-1 Kawasaki syndrome. **A,** Erythematous, cracked lips. **B,** "Strawberry tongue." **C,** Swollen, erythematous hands. Note fusiform appearance. **D.** Fingertip and toe tip peeling in subacute phase.

There is no single diagnostic test for KD. Diagnosis is made based on the clinical signs and laboratory tests (ESR, CRP, WBC, RBC, and platelet counts). A two-dimensional echocardiogram is done for cardiac evaluation.

Treatment and Nursing Care

Treatment involves reducing inflammation with intravenous immunoglobulin (IVIG) and high-dose aspirin. It has been shown that IVIG and aspirin given within the first 10 days of onset has reduced the incidence of coronary disease (AAP, 2009). The aspirin dose is reduced after fever has been controlled for 48 hours, which usually occurs at about 14 days. Aspirin administration will continue for 6 to 8 weeks and is discontinued if there are no coronary abnormalities. Most children recover without long-term complications. Low-dose aspirin is continued indefinitely for children with coronary abnormalities, and they are followed for several months or years depending on severity.

Nursing care for the acute stage focuses on relief of symptoms. Irritation of the skin may be helped with loose-fitting clothes and cool cloths. Mouth care is important. Children may not want to eat but should be encouraged to take cool liquids and soft foods. Intake and output is monitored closely. Aspirin should be in liquid form. IVIG is administered per hospital protocol.

> ⚠ **Safety Alert**
>
> IVIG administration should follow guidelines for administration of any blood product. If any reactions occur, stop the infusion immediately, and notify the physician.

The most challenging nursing issue is the extreme irritability. Providing a quiet environment may be beneficial. Parents will need a lot of emotional support as they try to find ways to comfort their child. Parents need to understand that irritability is a classic symptom for KD and they should not feel embarrassed or guilty with their child's behavior. Discharge planning should include instructing parents that they will have to administer aspirin at home for a length of time. Parents should be instructed to watch for side effects. While on antiplatelet therapy, contact activities should be avoided to prevent potential bleeding. Fevers should be reported to the physician.

STEVENS-JOHNSON SYNDROME

Stevens-Johnson syndrome is a severe form of erythema multiforme that involves lesions of the skin and mucous membranes. It is thought to be associated with a hypersensitivity reaction to certain drugs or to follow a respiratory infection. Drugs including sulfonamides, nonsteroidal antiinflammatory drugs (NSAIDs), antimicrobials, and anticonvulsants are usually the cause of the reactions.

Signs and Symptoms

This disorder presents with flulike symptoms of fever, malaise, fatigue, and sore throat. Mucosal lesions erupt in the eyes, mouth, and entire gastrointestinal tract (Figure 19-2). Pain can be severe. Lesions may appear in crops and may take weeks to heal. There is no definitive test for diagnosis. Laboratory testing may be done to assist with diagnosis.

> ⚠ **Safety Alert**
>
> If the causative agent of Stevens-Johnson syndrome is an identified medication, the medication should be immediately discontinued. The medical record and history should identify the medication as an allergy to prevent the child from being given the medication again.

Treatment and Nursing Care

Treatment is supportive. An ophthalmologist will monitor for any corneal scarring. Oral lesions benefit from mouthwashes and glycerin swabs. Topical anesthetics such as viscous lidocaine can provide pain relief. Lesions can be washed with saline or Burow's solution. Hydrogel dressings can also be soothing. If the child is not able to ingest oral intake, IV fluids may be necessary. Nutritional support may require soft foods and liquids, and severe oral lesions may require parenteral feedings. Skin should be kept clean and dry and inspected for any secondary infections. Specialty mattresses may be necessary to help with skin integrity. Corticosteroids may be used to help with inflammation. Antimicrobials are not necessary unless there is a documented infection. The disease is self-limiting and will gradually disappear without scarring. Parents should be aware that their child is at risk for recurrence, and the medical record should reflect that the child is allergic to the specific medication.

JUVENILE IDIOPATHIC ARTHRITIS

Juvenile idiopathic arthritis (JIA) is the most common arthritic condition of childhood. Formerly considered to be one disease with several subtypes, it is now classified as several different syndromes. These inflammatory diseases involve the joints, connective tissues, and viscera. JIA is seen frequently in children. The exact cause is unknown, but infections and an autoimmune response have been implicated. The symptoms mimic many of those of nonrheumatic conditions, such as Lyme disease, septic arthritis, and osteomyelitis; these conditions need to be ruled out before a diagnosis of JIA is made.

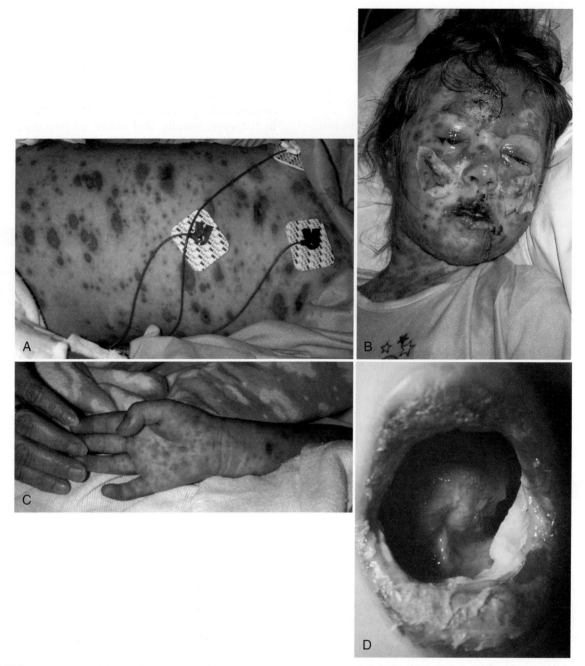

FIGURE 19-2 Stevens-Johnson syndrome. **A,** Bullous lesions of varying sizes are seen on this girl's trunk. Many are target shaped, some are hemorrhagic, and a few are denuded or eroded. **B,** Facial involvement is extensive. Some lesions have become confluent, and others have been denuded and then crusted. Note the severe conjunctival, nasal, and oral inflammation and the lid edema. **C,** This child also had numerous lesions on the proximal and distal extremities including the palms and soles. **D,** Another child has numerous vesicles and bullae of the oral mucosa along with formation of a shaggy white membrane consisting of sloughed debris.

Signs and Symptoms

The most common types of JIA are listed in Table 19-1. Symptoms vary from one child to the next, and each type has a distinct method of onset: **systemic** (acute febrile), **oligoarticular** (involving five joints or fewer), and **polyarticular** (involving more than five joints). The course is chronic, with remissions and exacerbations. Some children who present with oligoarticular progress to polyarticular. Children rarely have permanent joint deformity, although many have some functional limitations. In systemic JIA, joint symptoms may be absent at onset but do develop in most cases.

Affected joints are swollen, warm, and stiff (Figure 19-3). Joint stiffness occurs mainly in the morning or after a period of inactivity (the "gel" phenomenon). Joint effusion and thickening synovial membrane eventually erode cartilage and can cause joint destruction.

Table 19-1   Major Types of Juvenile Idiopathic Arthritis

TYPE	INCIDENCE RATE	GENDER AFFECTED	AGE	JOINTS AFFECTED	OTHER MANIFESTATIONS	PROGNOSIS
Systemic	10%-20%	Both equally	Any	Few to multiple	High fever (especially in the evening), chills, rash on trunk and extremities, enlarged liver and lymph nodes, pericarditis/pleuritis, leukocytosis, abdominal pain, anemia, arthralgias before arthritis begins	Approximately 50% develop chronic joint disease; prognosis depends on number of joints involved
Polyarticular, RF-positive	5%; may be familial	90% girls	>8 yr	Any or multiple large and small joints, upper and lower extremities, symmetrical pattern	Rapid, severe course; rheumatoid nodules (palpable near elbows); low fever; slight anemia	Early joint erosion, with many having permanent disability
Polyarticular, RF-negative	20%-30%	70%-75% girls	Early childhood, school age	Multiple large and small joints	Arthritis persists, loss of bone mass, small percentage with iridocyclitis, growth disturbances, low fever, malaise, anorexia, anemia	Small percentage have joint damage
Oligoarticular	40%-55%; may be familial	Girls: 20%-35% develop a polyarticular course after approximately 3 yr	Early childhood	Knees, ankles, elbows (<4 joints); asymmetric pattern	Chronic iridocyclitis with occasional loss of vision, malaise, low fever, slight anemia; slightly enlarged liver, spleen, and lymph nodes during active disease	More favorable prognosis regarding long-term joint function
		Boys: Many develop spondyloarthropathies	Late childhood	Large joints of lower extremities, hips, spine	Small percentage have acute iridocyclitis	

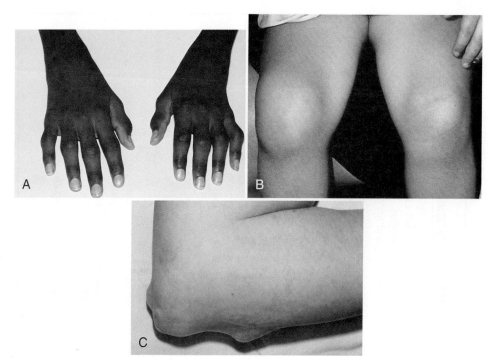

FIGURE 19-3 **A,** Child's hands show swelling and inflammation of joints with polyarticular JIA. **B,** Swollen right knee of a toddler with oligoarticular JIA. **C,** Subcutaneous nodules over the pressure points of a child's elbow.

Children with oligoarticular disease are at risk for iridocyclitis, an inflammation of the iris and ciliary body of the eye. Symptoms include redness, pain, photophobia, decreased visual acuity, and nonreactive pupils. This condition occurs most frequently in young girls. Its course is unpredictable. All children with oligoarticular arthritis need slit-lamp eye examinations several times a year for at least the first 5 years after the diagnosis of JIA. Distortion of the pupil and cataracts may occur. The long-term visual prognosis is uncertain.

Bone mass increases most during adolescence, and the process is related to weight, amount of exercise, and diet. Because children with JIA are less mobile than other children their age, they are likely to experience anorexia and reduced nutritional intake. Medications they are taking for their disease makes them more susceptible to **osteopenia** (low bone mass). If adequate bone mass is not attained during the teen years, osteoporosis in adulthood is more likely. The skeletal bone mass should be monitored closely.

There are no specific tests for JIA. The diagnosis is determined from clinical manifestations, radiographs, laboratory test results (CBC, ESR, rheumatoid factor [RF] assay, antinuclear antibody [ANA] assay), and the exclusion of other disorders. Aspirated joint fluid is yellow to green and cloudy and has a low viscosity. The goals of therapy are to reduce pain and swelling, to promote mobility, to preserve joint function, to educate the child and family, and to help the child and family adjust to living with a chronic disease.

Treatment and Nursing Care

Treatment is supportive. Drug therapy and exercise are the mainstays of therapy. First-line medications used to treat JIA are the NSAIDs, which include ibuprofen (Advil, Motrin), naproxen (Naprosyn), and tolmetin. Ibuprofen now comes in liquid form, making it easier to give to small children. Aspirin is given less frequently than previously because of its association with Reye's syndrome. These agents do not change the course of the disease but reduce pain and stiffness. Along with the NSAIDs, intraarticular long-acting corticosteroid injections may be administered to preserve joint function.

If initial treatment with NSAIDs fails after adequate trial (at least 2 to 3 months of each medication chosen), other approaches are used. Systemic corticosteroids are usually avoided unless extreme disease presents. Disease-modifying antirheumatic drugs (DMARDs) have demonstrated effectiveness; these include hydroxychloroquin (Plaquenil) and sulfasalazine (Azulfidine). Biologics (anti-TNF agents) can be effective and include etanercept (Enbrel), infliximab (Remicade), and adalimumab (Humira) (Abramson, 2008).

Regular monitoring of all medications is imperative. NSAIDs are given with meals to avoid gastric irritation. Parents should be informed of the side effects, which include tinnitus, lethargy, hyperventilation, dizziness, headaches, nausea, and vomiting.

The nurse functions as a member of a team that includes the pediatrician, rheumatologist, social worker, physical therapist, occupational therapist, psychologist, ophthalmologist, and school and community nurses. The child may be hospitalized during an acute episode or for an unrelated illness. Treatment consists of medications, warm tub baths, joint exercises, and rest. Physical and occupational therapy are included in the treatment. Their purpose is to maintain function and reduce pain. The physical therapist oversees the type and amount of exercise performed. Daily range-of-motion exercises and play activities that incorporate specific routines help preserve function, maintain muscle strength, and prevent deformities. Morning tub baths and the application of moist hot packs help lessen stiffness. Resting splints may be ordered to prevent flexion contractures and preserve functional alignment. Proper body alignment with a regular change to the prone position (unless contraindicated) facilitates comfort. Either no pillow or a small flat pillow is advocated. Measures to alleviate boredom should be undertaken.

Home Care. The child is given instructions for home care. These are reviewed with the family to determine the level of understanding. A firm mattress or bed board is necessary to prevent joints from sagging. Age-appropriate tricycles and pedal cars promote mobility and exercise. Modifications in daily living, such as elevation of toilet seats, installation of hand rails, Velcro fasteners, and so on, may be necessary. Swimming is an excellent form of exercise. Assist parents in planning nutritional meals with adequate calcium and vitamin D. Weight gain should be avoided because it places further stress on the joints. Emphasize the importance of regular eye examinations. Unnecessary physical restrictions should be avoided because these can lead to rebellion.

Facilitating School Attendance. Encourage school attendance. Excess absence from school, particularly for nonspecific symptoms, might suggest that the child is depressed or excessively preoccupied with the illness. In such cases, the meaning of the illness to the child and family and its effect on daily life need to be explored. Careful communication with the school nurse is essential for the child to have a successful school experience without interruptions in learning. The child should allow adequate preparation time in the morning to work out stiffness before arriving at school. There should be planned rest periods during the day, especially during disease flare-ups. Unobtrusive access to the school health office is important for these children so that they do not feel different from their peers.

Meeting Emotional Needs. Parents need assistance with establishing limits. Consistent negative behavior in social situations can present more problems than the actual disability. Overindulgence and preferential treatment often compromise the child's potential for happiness and independence. Siblings of chronically ill children may resent the special attention received by the child. They may also be torn between loyalty to the brother or sister and their own need to be with others. Parents need ongoing counseling and the services of various community resources. One resource is the Arthritis Foundation. The child may benefit from association with other children who have arthritis.

This disease is characterized by periods of remission and exacerbations. There is no known cure for JIA. Parents need assistance in understanding the chronic nature of the disease and the potential for recurrence of signs and symptoms. Nurses can serve as advocates for the child by recognizing the impact of the disease and by openly communicating with the child, the family, and other members of the health care team.

INFECTIOUS MONONUCLEOSIS

Infectious mononucleosis is a global disease caused by a herpes-type Epstein-Barr virus (EBV). It occurs chiefly in older children and adults; its peak incidence is in persons between 17 and 25 years of age or earlier in low socioeconomic groups. Studies suggest that the organism is transmitted by contact with saliva, either directly or on contaminated eating utensils; however, its communicability is considered low. The incubation period is from 1 to 2 months.

Signs and Symptoms

Symptoms vary from mild to moderately severe and may last for several weeks. They include low-grade fever, sore throat, headache, fatigue, skin rash, and general malaise. The lymph glands enlarge. Splenomegaly develops in approximately half the children. Liver involvement with mild jaundice occurs in a small number of persons and requires bed rest until liver function returns to normal.

The diagnosis is confirmed with the examination of peripheral blood. Lymphocytosis and the presence of atypical lymphocytes are seen. A rising titer of antibody to EBV is also indicative; the **MonoSpot** test is rapid, can detect the infection earlier than the heterophile antibody test, and is now widely used. Complications, although uncommon, include rupture of the spleen, secondary pneumonia, neurologic manifestations, and heart involvement.

Treatment and Nursing Care

Treatment is supportive because the disease is self-limiting. Acetaminophen, aspirin, or an NSAID such as ibuprofen is given as needed. An antipyretic is given to reduce fever and discomfort. An initial period of rest or restricted activities is usually needed, and returning to usual activities is based on the child's energy level. Gargling with warm saline solution and sucking on throat lozenges can be helpful for pharyngitis.

Adequate fluid intake is necessary, in particular, bland, cool liquids that are not irritating to the throat. Smoking should be discouraged. There is no special diet. Isolation is not necessary. The child is alerted to signs of secondary infection. Activities are increased as the fever and fatigue diminish. The child with an enlarged spleen is cautioned to avoid heavy lifting, trauma to the abdomen, and vigorous athletics until the splenomegaly subsides. For the athlete with an enlarged spleen, contact or collision activities should be restricted for at least 3 to 4 weeks. Severe abdominal pain is unusual, except in the presence of splenic rupture, which requires immediate attention.

The teenager with mononucleosis may be discouraged and depressed. The teenager worries about job, schoolwork, and the ability to continue extracurricular activities of importance. Open communication with school officials and classmates helps alleviate some of the anxieties. The prognosis in mononucleosis is good. It is no longer considered a prolonged, debilitating disease. Many cases go unrecognized.

DIABETES MELLITUS

Diabetes mellitus (DM) is a chronic metabolic condition in which the body is unable to metabolize and use carbohydrates, fats, and proteins properly because of a deficiency of insulin, an internal secretion of the pancreas. Insulin deficiency leads to impaired glucose transport (sugar cannot pass into the cells) and accelerated metabolism of stored fats for energy.

Diabetes is not a single entity but several different disorders. These disorders differ in cause, pathophysiology, and genetic predisposition. All result in disturbed glucose metabolism. Previously, DM was classified by treatment. The old classification was insulin-dependent DM (IDDM, or type 1) and non–insulin-dependent DM (NIDDM, or type 2). The American Diabetes Association now uses a classification system that includes type 1 and type 2 (Table 19-2).

Type 1 Diabetes Mellitus

Type 1 DM is the most common endocrine/metabolic disorder of childhood. The condition is found worldwide, affects multiple body organs, and is unique in that it requires a great deal of self-management by the person affected. The child and family education and compliance are extremely important to the successful management of the condition and the prevention of complications. Morbidity and mortality are associated with chronic complications that affect small and large blood vessels, resulting in retinopathy, nephropathy, neuropathy, ischemic heart disease, and obstruction of large vessels.

Type 1 DM was formerly known as *juvenile-onset diabetes* or *brittle diabetes*. It is characterized by partial or complete insulin deficiency. Although some insulin production may be seen during certain phases of the disease, children eventually become completely insulin deficient. Type 1 DM is a T-cell–mediated autoimmune

Table **19-2**	Classification of Types of Diabetes Mellitus		
TYPE	**ONSET**	**CLINICAL FEATURES**	**OTHER COMMENTS**
Type 1 DM	Primarily in childhood but can occur at any age	Polydipsia, polyuria, polyphagia, weight loss occurring for usually less than 1 mo Hyperglycemia: random plasma glucose above 200 mg/dL with symptoms or fasting blood glucose above 126 mg/dL and 2-hr postprandial blood glucose above 200 mg/dL with no symptoms Glycosuria, ketonuria Vaginal monilial infections in adolescent girls Elevation of antiislet or antiinsulin antibodies and presence of other indicators of immune connection	Child requires insulin to maintain life Type 1 can be diagnosed in children before symptoms appear and in family members at risk Type 1 appears to have both genetic and environmental components
Type 2 DM	Usually after age 40 yr but can occur at any age	Hyperglycemia: fasting blood glucose above 126 mg/dL and 2-hr glucose tolerance test result above 200 mg/dL on more than one occasion without precipitating factors Child is usually obese Serum insulin level can be normal or less than normal	Condition has some genetic basis Some affected children need insulin on occasion (e.g., during severe stress or illness)

disease in which the body destroys the insulin-producing islet cells in the pancreas. Environmental and genetic factors are strongly implicated. Apparently, type 1 DM is sometimes set off by seemingly harmless viruses believed to provoke the immune system into mistakenly destroying its own islet cells. The presence of islet cell antibodies (ICAs) and the evidence that associates type 1 DM with other autoimmune conditions support an autoimmune etiology.

Incidence. In the United States, surveys indicate the prevalence of type 1 DM in school-age children to be 1.9 per 1000 (Kliegman et al., 2007). The frequency increases with age. Symptoms of type 1 DM may occur at any time in childhood, but the rate of occurrence of new cases is highest among 5- to 7-year-old children and children entering puberty. In the former, the stress of school and the increased exposure to infectious diseases, particularly viral illness, may be responsible. During puberty, increased growth, increased emotional stress, and the effects of growth and sex hormones on insulin action may be implicated.

Type 1 DM occurs equally in boys and girls. Socioeconomic correlations have not been seen. The risk of type 1 DM is higher in families, particularly in the siblings and children of individuals with diabetes. Other risk factors may include psychosocial stress, increasing incidence of obesity, and viral infections as trigger mechanisms.

The disease is more severe in childhood because children are growing, they expend a great deal of energy, their nutritional needs vary, and they have to face a lifetime of diabetic management. Children with type 1 DM often do not have the typical textbook picture of the disorder; therefore the nurse must be particularly astute with subjective and objective observations.

Signs and Symptoms
Children with type 1 DM have a classic triad of symptoms: **polyuria** (excretion of large amounts of urine), **polydipsia** (excessive thirst), and **polyphagia** (constant hunger). Despite the hunger and increased food intake, the child loses weight.

The symptoms can appear insidiously, with fatigue, anorexia, nausea, lethargy, and weakness. The skin becomes dry. Vaginal yeast infections may be seen in the adolescent girl. Often the symptoms of concern in the young child are bedwetting or urine accidents during play periods in a previously trained child.

Laboratory findings indicate **hyperglycemia** (excess sugar in the blood). Glucose may be found in the urine (**glycosuria** or **glucosuria**), which occurs after the blood glucose level reaches 180 mg/dL. Other laboratory tests might include insulin levels and antibody studies.

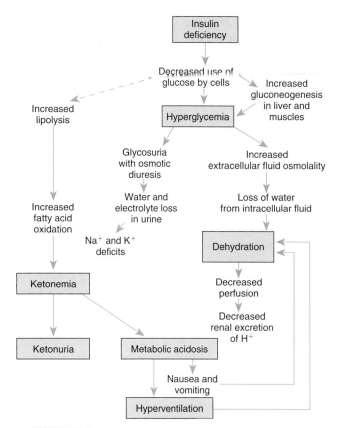
FIGURE 19-4 Pathophysiology of acidosis in diabetes mellitus.

When extremely low levels of insulin are reached, keto acids accumulate. The symptoms of **ketoacidosis** (severe hyperglycemia, ketones in the blood and urine, and acidosis) appear in children with abrupt onset, and they become very ill. Diabetic ketoacidosis (DKA) is also referred to as *diabetic coma,* although a person may have DKA with or without a coma (Figure 19-4).

Diabetic ketoacidosis can be triggered by conditions that increase insulin demand (fever, stress, infection). DKA may also affect the child with diabetes who has skipped one or more insulin doses, sometimes deliberately. The symptoms range from mild to severe and occur in hours to days. The skin is dry, and the face is flushed. The child appears dehydrated. They are thirsty but may vomit if fluids are offered. They perspire and are restless. There may be generalized pain in the abdomen and throughout the body. A characteristic fruity odor of the breath is apparent because the child expels acetone from the respiratory system. Blood pressure and pulse increase. As the condition worsens, the child becomes weak and drowsy. Breathing patterns are peculiar in that they are rapid and deep and there is no normal period of rest between inspiration and expiration; this is termed Kussmaul breathing. The child becomes unconscious. Death results unless insulin, fluids, and electrolytes are administered.

Treatment and Nursing Care

Diabetic Ketoacidosis. The correction of depleted fluids, frequent checking of vital signs, hourly blood glucose tests, regular blood chemistry measurements, and close observation of consciousness are necessary. Baseline studies include blood gases, blood glucose, serum acetone, pH, blood urea nitrogen, electrolytes, calcium, phosphate, white blood cell count, urinalysis, and appropriate cultures. Glucose levels in the blood and urine, electrolyte counts, and any other abnormal laboratory values are continuously monitored until the child's condition stabilizes. IV fluids of isotonic saline (usually 0.9% saline solution) are administered; once the circulation has been stabilized, the IV fluids are adjusted to correct serum hyperosmolality. Low doses of regular insulin are administered intravenously, and the child is observed. Only after the DKA crisis is resolved does subcutaneous injection of insulin begin. A cardiac monitor is helpful in determination of cardiac effects of changing potassium levels. If the child has an infection, the infection is treated. Cerebral edema, although rare, can be life threatening. Careful monitoring of neurologic status is essential. Careful documentation is done to record all pertinent information. Response to treatment is gradual, occurring over a period of hours.

Long-Term Management. The aims of treatment of type 1 diabetes are (1) to promote normal growth and development through metabolic control, (2) to enable the child to have a happy and active childhood, and (3) to prevent complications. Ideally, teaching begins when the diagnosis is confirmed. A planned educational program is necessary to provide a consistent body of information, which can then be individualized. Teaching sessions include the disease process itself, how to perform blood glucose monitoring, dietary information, the importance of exercise, and how to administer insulin. Sessions also include how to detect hypo- and hyperglycemia and treatment protocols. All information is given gradually and at the level of understanding of the child and the family. The child's age and financial, educational, cultural, and religious background must be considered. Continuous follow-up is extremely important.

Since the release of results from the Diabetes Control and Complication Trial (DCCT), the focus of management of diabetes is intense insulin therapy to normalize blood glucose levels. Intense therapy includes multiple insulin injections, frequent blood glucose monitoring, strict dietary intake, and exercise. The importance of glycemic control in decreasing the incidence of symptoms and complications of the disease has been established. The goal is to maintain blood glucose levels within a specific range (Table 19-3).

Insulin Administration. Insulin is used principally to control DM. Insulin was previously prepared from the pancreas of cattle or pigs. This is no longer available in the United States. Human insulin, developed with recombinant DNA technique, is the most frequently used because it is associated with a lesser incidence of allergies. When injected into the child with diabetes, insulin enables the body to burn and store sugar. Insulin is given routinely with subcutaneous injection. Insulin pumps are being used in carefully selected children. More highly purified insulins are being developed to reduce complications.

The dosage of insulin is measured in units, and special syringes are used in its administration. It is recommended to use the smallest volume syringe for the required dose to ensure accuracy. The various types of insulin and their actions are listed in Table 19-4. The main difference is in the amount of time necessary for effect and the length of coverage provided. The values listed are only guidelines. The

Table 19-3	Blood Glucose and Hemoglobin A1C Goals for Type 1 Diabetes by Age Group			
	VALUE *BEFORE MEALS	VALUE *BEDTIME/ OVERNIGHT	A1C	RATIONALE
Toddlers and preschoolers (0-6 yr)	100-180	110-200	<8.5% (but >7.5%)	High risk and vulnerability to hypoglycemia
School age (6-12 yr)	90-180	100-180	<8%	Risks of hypoglycemia and relatively low risk of complications prior to puberty
Adolescents and young adults (13-19 yr)	90-130	90-150	<7.5%	Risk of severe hypoglycemia; developmental and psychological issues; a lower goal (<7.0%) is reasonable if it can be achieved without excessive hypoglycemia

*Plasma blood glucose goal range (mg/dL)
Data from American Diabetes Association. (2010). Standards of medical care in diabetes, *Diabetes Care*, 33(suppl 1):S11-S61. Retrieved August 22, 2010, from *http://www.care.diabetesjournals.org*.

Table 19-4	Types of Insulin and Their Effects			
INSULIN TYPE	**BRAND NAME**	**ONSET**	**PEAK**	**DURATION (HRS)**
Rapid Acting				
Lispro	Humalog	5-15 minutes	30-90 minutes	3-5
Aspart	NovoLog	5-15 minutes	30-90 minutes	3-5
Glulisine	Apidra	5-15 minutes	30-90 minutes	3-5
Short Acting				
Regular	Humulin R Novolin R	30-60 minutes	2-3 hours	5-8
Intermediate Acting				
NPH	Humulin N Novolin N	2-4 hours	4-10 hours	10-16
Long Acting				
Glargine	Lantus	2-4 hours	Peakless	20-24
Detemir	Levemir	2-4 hours	6-14 hours	16-20

response of each child with diabetes to any given insulin dose is highly individual and depends on many factors, such as site of injection, local destruction of insulin by tissue enzymes, and insulin antibodies.

Regular and rapid-acting insulins are clear. NPH, an intermediate type, has small amounts of chemicals added to prolong its action and to make it more stable. This offers protection over a period of hours, enabling the child to do without repeated injections of unmodified insulin. NPH insulin is cloudy and requires mixing before extraction from the vials (Skill 19-1), which is done by rolling the bottle gently between the palms of the hands. Insulin should not be used if it is discolored. Premixed insulin preparations are now available if the family has difficulty with the insulin-mixing technique, but because they are available only in standard doses, they may not be useful for children with doses that need to be altered frequently. Among the newer insulin medications are lispro, aspart, and glargine. Lispro and aspart are both rapid-acting. Glargine is a basal insulin that most clearly imitates the human insulin as it is absorbed equally throughout the 24-hour period. Lente and Ultralente insulin have been discontinued and are no longer available.

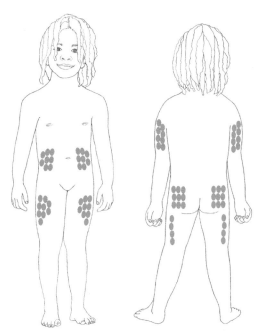

FIGURE 19-5 Sites of injection of insulin. The site of injection should be changed daily to prevent poor absorption and injury to tissues. Rotation should occur both within and among body areas.

Nursing Brief

Glargine is a clear formula unlike other long-acting insulins and cannot be mixed with any other type of insulin.

Insulin is administered **subcutaneously** at a 90-degree angle. Parents and children must be taught why it is necessary to take the hormone and how to administer it by injection. A child can generally be taught to give self-injections after 7 years of age. Proper instruction for the child is one of the most important aspects of the treatment of diabetes. The site of the injection is rotated to prevent poor absorption and injury to tissues (Figure 19-5). Children and parents should be taught to examine injection sites on a regular basis. Lumps or hardened areas should be reported to the physician. Injection model forms made from construction paper and site rotation patterns are useful. One suggested site rotation is to use one area for a week, moving to different sites within that area. The injection sites should be about 1 inch apart. The young

Skill 19-1   Mixing Insulin

1. Verify insulin label and have insulin at room temperature to assist in decreasing painful injection.
2. Wash hands and clean injection site.
3. Gently rotate insulin bottle or pen.
4. Draw back the amount of air into the syringe that equals the total dose.
5. Inject the amount of air into the long-acting (NPH) vial that equals the NPH dose. Remove the syringe from the vial.

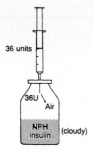

36 units

36U   Air

NPH insulin   (cloudy)

6. Inject the amount of air into the regular-acting insulin vial that equals the regular-acting dose.

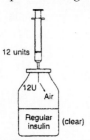

12 units

12U   Air

Regular insulin   (clear)

7. Invert the regular-acting insulin vial and withdraw the regular-acting insulin dose amount. Observe for any bubbles and remove.

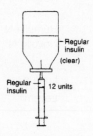

Regular insulin (clear)

Regular insulin   12 units

8. Without adding more air to the NPH vial, carefully withdraw the NPH dose.

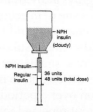

NPH insulin (cloudy)

NPH insulin
Regular insulin   36 units
48 units (total dose)

By following these steps, problems can be avoided with contamination of regular insulin with intermediate-acting or long-acting insulin. Should the regular insulin be contaminated, the action time would be affected and the insulin would not be effective in an acute situation such as DKA (American Diabetes Association, 2003).

Critical Thinking Snapshot

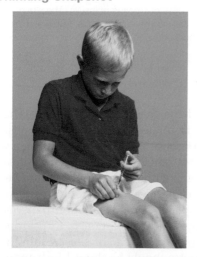

A 10-year-old newly diagnosed type 1 DM child comes to the community health clinic with his mother. He has been experiencing symptoms of hypoglycemia recently. Both he and his mother have been experiencing difficulty with blood glucose monitoring and need assistance. How would you begin working with this child and his mother? What would you include in your teaching if you discover he received only minimal education regarding type 1 DM?

child can use a doll for practice. Parents usually find the experience of injecting their own child difficult. Commercially available devices may be used for insulin administration, such as syringe-loaded injectors or pen injectors.

The goal of insulin therapy is to simulate the fluctuations in insulin levels that are normally seen in non-diabetic individuals. Two or three injections per day consisting of NPH and regular or rapid-acting insulin is an acceptable regimen for children. If a two-dose regimen is used, approximately two thirds of the daily insulin dose is given before breakfast and one third is given before dinner. It is important for the nurse to remember that the timing of the meal must be correlated to the timing and action of the insulin administered.

When multiple injections are given throughout the day, a daily dose of long-acting basal insulin and injections of rapid-acting insulin before each meal becomes the regimen. This makes meal planning less rigid because the child can adjust their insulin dosage to their mealtime carbohydrate intake. The long-term benefit of multiple injections daily helps to reduce the microvascular complications of type 1 DM.

In addition to multiple injections, children can also be taught to use an insulin pump. The pump delivers a programmed amount of basal insulin but must be programmed for delivery before each meal. The pump is usually worn on a belt. It is connected by a catheter to a needle in the subcutaneous tissue. Complications can include malfunction and skin infection.

HYPOGLYCEMIA

Hypoglycemia (low blood glucose), also known as insulin shock, occurs when the blood glucose level becomes abnormally low (below 70 mg/dL). This condition is caused by an excess of insulin in the body. Factors that may account for this imbalance include poorly planned or excessive exercise, insufficient food, inappropriate insulin dose, or errors made because of improper knowledge of insulin and the insulin syringe. Children are more prone to insulin reactions than adults because (1) the condition itself is more unstable in young people, (2) they are growing, and (3) their activities are more irregular. Mild episodes of hypoglycemia are not unusual in the child with diabetes.

The symptoms of an insulin reaction, which range from mild to severe, are generally noticed and treated in the early stages. They appear *suddenly* in the *otherwise well* person. Examination of the blood reveals a lowered blood glucose level. The child becomes irritable and may behave poorly, is pale, and may feel hungry, cold, and weak. Sweating occurs (see Did You Know?). Symptoms related to disorders of the nervous system arise because glucose is vital to the proper functioning of nerves. The child may become mentally confused and giddy and may have a headache; muscular coordination is affected. If insulin shock is left untreated, coma and convulsions can occur.

? Did You Know?

HYPOGLYCEMIA	HYPERGLYCEMIA	KETOACIDOSIS
Caused by insulin excess	Caused by inadequate insulin	Caused by insulin deficiency
Excessive activity without extra carbohydrate intake	Little or no activity, stress, illness, surgery	
Missed or delayed meal	Excessive food	
Sudden onset in healthy child	Slowly	Appears over hours or days
Blood glucose <70 mg/dL	Blood glucose >240 mg/dL	Blood glucose >240 mg/dL Urine ketones positive
Initial symptoms of sweating, tremor, feeling cold, anxiety, hunger	Initial symptoms of polyuria, polydipsia, polyphagia, fatigue, weight loss, blurred vision	Initial symptoms include those seen in hyperglycemia with abdominal pain, flushed, restless, fruity breath odor, dry skin
Late symptoms of confusion, weakness, dizziness, nausea and vomiting, headache, stupor, convulsions		Late symptoms of acidosis, dehydration, Kussmaul breathing, coma, death
Give oral carbohydrates, glucagon, intravenous glucose	Give insulin, exercise, increase oral fluids	Give insulin (intravenously), intravenous fluids, electrolyte replacement

The immediate treatment consists of administering sugar in some form, such as orange juice, cola beverages, ginger ale, hard candy, or a commercial product such as Glutose. If the child begins to feel better within a few minutes and the blood glucose level exceeds 70 mg/dL, the child may eat a small amount of protein or starch (sandwich, milk, cheese) to prevent another reaction.

Glucagon is a hormone that raises the blood glucose level by causing a rapid breakdown of glycogen into glucose in the liver. It is recommended for the treatment of severe hypoglycemia. Glucagon acts quickly to restore the child to consciousness in an emergency situation; the child is then able to consume some form of sugar. Glucagon is a hormone produced by the pancreatic islets that also produce insulin. Normally a fall in blood glucose makes the body release this substance. Because the islet cells are destroyed in children with type 1 DM, glucagon is not adequately released. Families of children on insulin therapy can be instructed to administer it subcutaneously or intramuscularly. If the child does not respond rapidly to glucagon administration, the physician should be contacted. Should a child become unconscious, they should be kept warm by covering with a blanket. Do not give anything by mouth; get medical attention.

Blood Glucose Self-Monitoring

Blood glucose self-monitoring has dramatically changed the approach to diabetes. Previously, blood tests for glucose could be carried out only in a doctor's office or laboratory. The child had to rely on urine tests, which often gave a confusing picture, particularly when the urine had been in the bladder for several hours (glucose could appear in the urine when the child's blood glucose level was actually low). Only a blood check can show the actual amount of sugar in the blood at the time of the test. Technology has made it possible for children to test their own blood glucose in the home. Although still under the supervision and consultation of the physician, the child can nonetheless make rational changes in insulin dosage, nutritional requirements, and daily exercise. This is of great psychological value to the child, teenager, and parents because it reduces feelings of helplessness and complete dependence on medical personnel.

Home glucose monitoring should be taught to all young children or their caregivers (Figure 19-6) (also see the Critical Thinking Snapshot). It is important that the child not only be skilled in the techniques but also

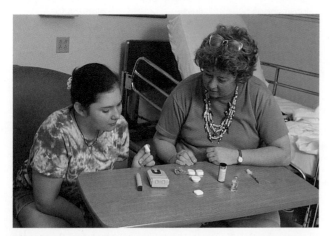

FIGURE 19-6 The school-age child can perform blood glucose monitoring at home.

understand the results and how to incorporate them into the daily regimen. The sides of the fingertips are recommended because there are fewer nerve endings and more capillary beds in these areas. The best fingers to use are the middle, ring, or little fingers on either hand. If the child washes the hands in warm water for about 30 seconds, the finger bleeds more easily. To perform the test, a drop of blood is put on a chemically treated reagent strip (Chemstrip bG or Dextrostix). Meters are available for reading blood glucose determinations. The test strip with a drop of blood is inserted, and the reading appears.

Nutritional Management

The advent of blood glucose self-monitoring has enabled more flexible nutritional plans, and yet **consistency** (amount of food and time of feeding) remains the cornerstone of appropriate nutritional management. Contrary to popular belief, no scientific evidence shows that persons with diabetes need special foods. In fact, what is good for the person with diabetes is good for the entire family. The nutrient needs of children with diabetes are essentially no different from those of children without diabetes, with the exception of the elimination of concentrated carbohydrates (simple sugars) and refined sugars. These cause a marked increase in blood glucose and generally should be avoided.

The goals of nutritional management in children are to ensure normal growth and development, to distribute food intake so that it aids metabolic control, and to individualize the diet in accordance with the child's ethnic background, age, gender, weight, activity, family economics, and food preferences. Once a diet order is received from the physician, the dietitian calculates the distribution of carbohydrates, protein, and fat. The total daily caloric intake is divided to provide 20% at breakfast, 20% at lunch, 30% at dinner, and the remaining 10% for snacks (Kliegman et al., 2007). Portion size is shown with food models and measuring cups and spoons. Regularly spaced meals and snacks are emphasized, and the family is taught how to read labels and the differences between carbohydrates, protein, and fat.

The two major approaches to nutritional management include the use of exchange lists and the constant carbohydrate diet. Exchange lists consist of foods separated into several food categories (fruit, milk, meat, bread, vegetables, fats). A food plan is developed that prescribes the amount or portion size of allowed food in each category. The child is given a choice from any number of foods in an individual category to meet the prescribed amount. In this way, the plan is flexible and according to the child's preferences.

The constant carbohydrate diet is a fairly new approach to meal planning. Children and families are provided with information regarding the carbohydrate contents of different foods and food label reading. The goal is to maintain a consistent amount of carbohydrate at each meal and snack. Regularity of meals is stressed. The amount of carbohydrate may, and usually does, vary between meals. The initial carbohydrate pattern is determined by the individual's current food intake. To calculate the number of grams of carbohydrate in food, exchange lists that divide foods according to carbohydrate content are used. This food plan appeals to young children with diabetes because of its ease in use and flexibility.

The importance of fiber in diets is well documented. In the child with diabetes, fiber has been shown to reduce blood glucose and serum cholesterol levels. Fiber appears to slow the rate of absorption of sugar by the digestive tract. Raw fruits and vegetables and whole grain breads and cereals are good sources of fiber.

Because persons with diabetes have an increased risk for heart disease, the reduction of serum cholesterol is another concern. These persons (like most of the general public) need to reduce their intake of animal fats or substitute vegetable fat for animal fat. The use of polyunsaturated fats in cooking is advised.

The form of the food is also important. An apple, apple juice, or applesauce may precipitate different blood glucose responses. Portions, the type of processing, cooking, and combinations of foods have also been shown to have a bearing on these responses.

Aspartame (NutraSweet) was approved by the U.S. Food and Drug Administration in 1981. It is used in items that do not require cooking. Aspartame is made of two amino acids. Both contain insignificant amounts of carbohydrate. One granulation form is called *Equal*. Sucralose (Splenda) is the newest low-calorie sweetener on the market. Sucralose can be used anywhere sugar can be used, such as in beverages, baked goods, and processed foods. Other artificial sweeteners are not recommended for children.

Exercise

Exercise is important for the child with diabetes because it causes the body to use sugar and promotes good circulation. It lowers the blood glucose and in this respect acts more like insulin. The child with diabetes who has planned vigorous exercise should carry extra sugar to avoid insulin reactions. The child should also carry money for candy or a drink or for a phone call. The blood glucose level is high directly after meals, so active sports can be participated in at such times. Less active games should be enjoyed directly before meals. The child with diabetes should be able to participate in almost all active sports. Poorly planned exercise, however, can lead to difficulties. Like any other child, the child with diabetes should not swim unsupervised.

Skin Care

The child should be instructed to bathe daily and dry well. Cleansing of the inguinal area, axillae, and perineum area is especially important because yeast and fungal infections tend to occur there. Inspect skin for cuts, rashes, abrasions, bruises, cysts, or boils. Treat promptly. If the skin is very dry, oil such as Alpha-Keri may be used in the bath water. Adolescents are taught to use electric razors. Avoid exposing the skin to extremes in temperatures.

Foot Care

Although circulatory problems of the feet are less common in children, proper foot hygiene habits need to be established. Instruct the child to wash and dry the feet well each day. Inspect for interdigital cracking, and check the condition of the toenails. Trim the nails straight across. Do not use corn remedies, iodine, or alcohol. Change socks daily, and avoid tight socks or large ones that bunch. Replace shoes often as the child grows. Wear boots only for short periods to minimize sweating. The child should not go barefoot. If problems arise, consult a physician or podiatrist.

Infections

Obtain immunizations against communicable diseases. Cystitis, subcutaneous nodules, and monilial vulvitis occur with greater frequency in children with diabetes. During late adolescence, females should see a gynecologist yearly.

Urine Checks

Routine urine checks for sugar have been replaced by the more accurate glucose blood monitoring. However, this procedure does not test for ketones, which the child may need to determine, particularly when the blood glucose level is high and during illness.

Glucose-Insulin Imbalances

The child is taught to recognize the signs of insulin shock and ketoacidosis. Early attention to change and daily record keeping are stressed. Many excellent teaching films and brochures are available. The child should wear a MedicAlert bracelet. Wallet cards are also available. Teachers, athletic coaches, and guidance officers should be informed about the disease and should have the phone numbers of the child's parents and physician.

Psychosocial Aspects

Children newly diagnosed with type 1 DM often go through a transitional or "honeymoon" stage. Because the body still releases small amounts of insulin until complete destruction of islet cells occurs, initial dosage requirements of insulin may decrease temporarily. This does not mean that the condition is resolving.

Parents need to understand that insulin doses vary but that the child continues to need lifelong insulin administration.

Because children with diabetes are growing, additional dimensions of the disorder and its treatment become evident. Growth is not steady but occurs in spurts and plateaus that have a bearing on treatment. Infants and toddlers may have hydration problems, especially during illness. Preschool children have irregular activity and eating patterns. School-age children may grieve over the diagnosis and ask, "Why me?" They may use the illness to gain attention or to avoid responsibilities. The onset of puberty may require adjustments in insulin as a result of growth and the antagonistic effect of the growth and sex hormones on insulin. Adolescents often resent this condition, which deviates from their concept of the body ideal. They have more difficulty in resolving the conflict between dependence and independence. This may lead to rebellion against the parents and the treatment regimen.

The impact of the disease on the rest of the family must also be considered. One mother commented, "I was so scared. I felt very strongly that whether my child lived or died depended on me. It was overwhelming. I couldn't allow myself mistakes. This was reinforced by all the do's and don'ts of the instructions." Parents may also feel guilty for having passed on the disease. Siblings may feel jealous of the child. The sharing of responsibility by parents is ideal but is not necessarily a reality. In fact the successful management of the condition greatly depends on parent involvement and family organization skills. Everyone may have difficulty accepting the diagnosis and the more regimented lifestyle it imposes. Each family member must cope with a personal reaction to the stress of the illness.

It is important that the child assume responsibility for care gradually, according to cognitive and developmental readiness, and with a minimum of pressure. Overprotection can be as detrimental as neglect. Parents who have received satisfaction from their child's dependence on them may need help letting go. An experience at a camp for children with diabetes is helpful in this respect.

Emotional upsets can be as disturbing to the child as an infection and may require food or insulin adjustments. Early detection and intervention in deteriorating personal relationships and rebellion against diabetic management decreases the severity of the effects on the child. The nurse should be attuned to little problems that are frequently veiled requests for help. Family therapy and other forms of psychotherapeutic help may be necessary. Support by caretakers helps with preventing difficulties. Table 19-5 summarizes some stresses experienced by the child with diabetes and possible nursing interventions.

Other Issues

With planning, children can enjoy travel with their families, and older adolescents can travel alone. Before traveling, the child should be seen by the physician for a checkup and prescriptions for supplies. A written statement and a card identifying the child as having diabetes should be carried. Realize that crossing time zones may affect relative mealtimes. Keep additional supplies of insulin, sugar, and food with the child. *Never* check these with luggage, especially on an airplane. If foreign travel is planned, parents need to become familiar with the food in the area so that dietary requirements can be met.

Community Considerations

Local chapters of the American Diabetes Association (*www.diabetes.org*) or the Juvenile Diabetes Research Foundation International (*www.jdrf.org*) can help vacationing families in an emergency.

The person with diabetes usually tolerates surgery well. Insulin may be given before or after the operation. If the child is NPO (nothing by mouth), calories may be supplied with intravenous glucose. Details vary according to the procedure and the child's diabetes treatment. Careful review of the child's history helps in formulating nursing care plans and provides a basis for teaching. The goal is to prevent hypoglycemia during the perioperative NPO period because the body is stressed from the surgery.

The child needs to see the physician regularly and will have frequent outpatient clinic visits to check glucose levels and monitor progress. Hemoglobin A1C will be evaluated as this test reflects the average blood glucose levels over the previous 2 to 3 months. The child should also be taught to visit the dentist regularly for cleaning of teeth and gums; appointments should be scheduled for right after meals. Brushing and flossing daily are important. Eyes should be examined regularly; blurry vision must be investigated.

Role of the Nurse

Nursing responsibilities begin with preparing the child for meals. Blood glucose is usually checked before meals and at bedtime and may need to be checked in the early morning hours if there is a problem with hypoglycemia during sleep. Because of the importance of food intake for the child with diabetes, distractions should be kept to a minimum. The child's meals and snacks are served **on time**. Children who receive regular insulin before meals may have an insulin reaction if food is not taken within 20 minutes. If nurses are scheduled for lunch when diet meals are served, they should notify the team leader and should not assume that others will feed the child. No foods or

Table 19-5   **Summary of Predictable Stress on Children with Type 1 Diabetes and Their Families**

ISSUE	NURSING INTERVENTION
Infant	
Trust versus mistrust	Stress consistency in need fulfillment
Onset and diagnosis particularly difficult during infancy; anxiety can be transmitted to baby	Involve both parents in education Avoid information overload Instill hope and confidence Focus on child rather than disease Review normal growth and development of infancy Assist in problem solving (e.g., babysitters, difficulty in obtaining specimens, baby food exchange lists)
Toddler	
Autonomy versus shame and doubt	Prepare child for procedures or separations Encourage exploration of environment Stress limit setting as a form of love
Is this a temper tantrum or high or low blood glucose?	Admit it is difficult to distinguish temper tantrums from symptoms If worsens or is prolonged or physical symptoms appear, check blood glucose; tight monitoring of blood glucose is highly recommended Provide 24-hr phone number
Preschool Child	
Initiative versus guilt	Foster sense of competence
May view injections as punishment	Educate parents to provide consistent warmth, reassurance, and love
May view denial of sweets as lack of love	Educate parents to provide consistent warmth, reassurance, and love Discuss feelings about personal life and diabetes Avoid negative connotation by words (e.g., "bad blood test," "cheating") Help parents sort out child's fantasies
"Picky eater"	Plan favorite party dishes on occasion Invite a playmate for lunch Suggest alternative nutritious snacks
Elementary School Age	
Industry versus inferiority	Assist child in how to respond to teasing from peers ("Ick, needles!")
May feel hospitalization will be cure	Explain "honeymoon" stage of disease
Grief over lack of cure	Accept child's disappointment
Rebellion over treatment regimen	Gradually have child assume self-management of insulin and specimen tests; this increases feelings of mastery and control
Rebellion over food plan	Provide lists of fast-food exchanges and resources for dining out
Anxiety about disclosure of condition to friends	Group-related education with peers who have diabetes
Embarrassed about reactions in school, missed days	Open dialogue between health personnel and teachers, school nurse, fellow students
Unpredictable effects of exercise	Continual reinforcement of treatment principles with specific regard to hypoglycemia or hyperglycemia and emergencies
At Puberty	
Bouncing blood glucose levels may make child feel out of control	Explain that growth and sex hormones affect blood glucose levels Girls, in particular, have difficulties around the time of menstruation Adjustments in insulin and food are common for most children with diabetes at this stage
Anger at the disease ("Why must I be different?")	Assist child in acceptable ways of expressing anger; discuss anger with parents, since they are often the target of it
More frequent hospitalizations	Provide encouragement and support; be alert to marital stress and sibling deprivation

Continued

Table 19-5	Summary of Predictable Stress on Children with Type 1 Diabetes and Their Families—cont'd
ISSUE	**NURSING INTERVENTION**
Teenager	
Threatens sexual identity and body image	Encourage teenager to meet other adolescents with diabetes (e.g., camps, support groups, if not tried earlier); this helps decrease isolation
Surge toward independence, risk taking, or greater than usual need for security	Provide consistency with limit setting; avoid overcontrol—listen, listen, listen
Worries about health, prospects for marriage and family	Adolescents need to have full instruction regarding pregnancy risk or male potency; provide a safe environment for discussion; make appropriate referrals
Alcohol and drug abuse	Encourage child's interest in diabetic research Share concerns and dangers with teenager

liquids, with the exception of water, are given between meals unless authorized by the physician or dietitian. Be sure that the tray is served to the **correct child**. A mistake can occur, particularly if several children are on special diets. This can happen more easily on the pediatric unit, where many children roam about freely. Foods the child especially enjoys or dislikes are noted.

When the child has finished, the nurse observes the types and amounts of foods that the child refused and charts them in the nurses' notes. These are brought to the attention of the dietitian, who determines the number of calories that need to be made up and orders a between-meal snack such as orange juice to compensate. Anorexia or vomiting is reported promptly.

Education of the child is an ongoing process. Too much information given at one time may be overwhelming to parents and discouraging to the child. Well-informed nurses can do much in the way of reinforcement and support. They can clarify such terms as *dietetic, sugar-free, juice-packed, water-packed,* and *unsweetened.* Meal trays in the hospital provide an excellent opportunity for teaching. Children should bring their own lunch to school. The nurse reinforces the interaction between nutrition, insulin requirements, and exercise and answers questions from the child or family.

Teenagers need to be advised that alcohol lowers the blood sugar. It suppresses gluconeogenesis and is high in calories. Most cocktail mixes contain sugar; however, water, sugar-free pop, club soda, and tomato juice do not. Although the consumption of alcohol is to be discouraged, if a young person of drinking age wishes to drink, it is better to drink *after* dinner or to consume the beverage with some type of food.

The Future of Research on Diabetes

Diabetic research is being conducted on many fronts. Geneticists are helping determine how diabetes is inherited so that someday they will be able to predict who will inherit the disease. If a virus is involved, a vaccine may help in its prevention. Pancreas transplantation has been performed, and the success rate is improving. β cells have been transplanted in animals, with the result that the animals have been cured. Another possibility is that of an artificial pancreas. Its precursors might be the insulin pumps being refined today. Administration of insulin via inhalation is being done. The laser beam has aided in the treatment of complicated eye conditions. Such advances hold promise for the hope of resolving or eradicating the dilemma of diabetes.

TYPE 2 DIABETES MELLITUS

Recently, physicians have noted type 2 DM increasing in incidence in children. The condition accounts for approximately one third to one half of all newly diagnosed individuals younger than 18 years of age. The diabetes appears to affect mostly children who are obese and who have Native American, African-American, or Hispanic origins. Causative factors appear to be sedentary lifestyle (increased hours in front of the television and decreased physical activity) and poor dietary habits with increased sugar consumption. Children who have a BMI greater than 95% are at risk for developing type 2 DM.

Type 2 DM arises because of insulin resistance (the body fails to use insulin properly), combined with insulin deficiency. The symptoms can present in the same manner (polydipsia, polyphagia, and polyuria). Nutritional education and improved exercise are the goals of treatment for children and adolescents with type 2 DM. While insulin may be necessary at the time of diagnosis, it can be reduced or discontinued within a few weeks of treatment. Oral agents may be prescribed because type 2 children are still producing insulin. However, the only oral medication approved for children with type 2 DM is metformin. Liver and renal function must be evaluated before therapy is initiated. Educational issues are similar to those for type 1 DM.

Get Ready for the NCLEX® Examination!

Key Points

- Irritability in the child with Kawasaki disease can be the most difficult symptom for parents to cope with.
- Home care instructions for a child with Kawasaki disease should include side effects of aspirin administration.
- Mucosal lesions can disrupt feeding in the child with Stevens-Johnson syndrome and require special techniques to meet nutritional needs.
- Any medication identified as the causative agent with Stevens-Johnson syndrome needs to be stopped.
- Pain can be a priority issue for a child with JIA.
- A child with JIA will need eye exams for at least 5 years after onset of episode.
- During the course of mononucleosis, the adolescent's emotional status should be evaluated because of the restrictions placed on them.
- The most frequently occurring pancreatic disorder is type 1 DM, which occurs with destruction of insulin-producing islet cells. Therapy is a combination of insulin, diet, and exercise.
- The goal of diabetes management is tight glucose level management. The child should be gaining self-management skills as age appropriate.
- The incidence rate of type 2 DM is increasing in children.
- Oral agents, diet, and exercise are the focus of treatment for type 2 DM.

Additional Learning Resources

e**volve** Go to your Evolve website (*http://evolve.elsevier.com/Price/pediatric/*) for the following FREE learning resources:

- 3-D Animations
- Answer Keys
- Appendixes
- Audio Glossary
- Spanish/English Glossary
- Video Clips

Review Questions for the NCLEX® Examination

1. The only antibody to cross the placenta is:
   1. IgG
   2. IgM
   3. IgE
   4. IgA

2. Which of the following children would be at the greatest risk for acquiring Kawasaki disease (KD)?
   1. A 4-year-old African-American female
   2. A 5-year-old Hispanic male
   3. A 3-year-old Asian male
   4. A 9-year-old Caucasian female

3. Stevens-Johnson syndrome is thought to be associated with:
   1. An autoimmune response.
   2. A hypersensitivity reaction to certain drugs.
   3. The Epstein-Barr virus (EBV).
   4. Disturbed glucose metabolism.

4. The following statements are true regarding systemic juvenile ideopathic arthritis: (**Select all that apply.**)
   1. 90% of those affected are girls.
   2. Prognosis depends on the number of joints involved.
   3. It occurs in children older than 8 years of age.
   4. Arthralgias are present before arthritis begins.
   5. High fever, chills, and rash on the trunk and extremities are possible manifestations.

5. The most common endocrine/metabolic disorder of childhood is:
   1. Type 1 diabetes mellitus
   2. Type 2 diabetes mellitus
   3. Hypoglycemia
   4. Diabetic ketoacidosis

Cognitive and Behavior Disorders

Objectives

1. Define the vocabulary terms listed
2. Demonstrate a positive attitude when caring for developmentally disabled children and their families
3. Relate the symptoms of a child with attention deficit/ hyperactivity disorder with corresponding social, educational, and emotional difficulties and describe strategies to help the child and family cope with the condition
4. Summarize the different characteristics that would be found in Down syndrome
5. Define the characteristics of infants with failure to thrive

6. List four kinds of child abuse, and describe the behaviors often exhibited by parent and child in each case
7. Discuss care of the hospitalized autistic child
8. Contrast the clinical presentation and nursing care of the teenager with anorexia nervosa with that of the teenager with bulimia
9. Identify health issues for substance abuse drugs
10. List four risk factors that might indicate an adolescent is contemplating suicide

Key Terms

adaptive behavior (p. 375)
anorexia nervosa (ăn-ŏ-RĔK-sē-ă něr-VŌ-să; p. 386)
bulimia (bū-LĒ-mē-ă; p. 387)
developmental disability (p. 374)
DSM-IV-TR (p. 377)

intellectual disability (p. 374)
intelligence functioning (p. 375)
mental retardation (p. 374)
translocation (tran(t)s-lō-KĀ-shən; p. 378)

OVERVIEW OF COGNITIVE AND BEHAVIOR DISORDERS

A child with an impaired cognitive ability can have significant limitation with intelligence, functioning behavior, and adaptive behavior. The limitations impact not only the child, but the family and the community. Families are confronted with medical and environmental issues that may never be solved. The focus of their care revolves around maximizing their potential and involves educational and training programs in schools and community settings.

There are several terms associated with cognitive impairment. A developmental disability is any mentally or physically disabling condition that begins during childhood and is expected to continue throughout life. This includes children with issues such as mental retardation, sensory deficits (speech, hearing, vision), orthopedic problems, and other conditions including autism and cerebral palsy. The term

for mental retardation has been changed to intellectual disability to conform with the name change for the American Association of Mental Retardation (AAMR) to American Association on Intellectual and Developmental Disabilities (AAIDD). The Centers for Disease Control and Prevention (2005) states, "intellectual disability is characterized both by a significantly below-average score on a test of mental ability or intelligence and by limitations in the ability to function in areas of daily life, such as communication, self-care, and getting along in social situations and school activities." It requires a multidimensional approach; with appropriate support, the life of the person with an intellectual disability generally improves. Many children with intellectual disabilities may have additional disabilities such as hearing loss, or attention-deficit/hyperactivity disorder.

Intellectual disability affects 2% to 3% of the population. According to Kliegman and colleagues (2007), there are two overlapping populations of intellectually disabled children. There are those with mild intellectual disability, which is associated with environmental influences, and those with severe intellectual disability, which is associated more with biological causes. Some persons have a congenital malformation of the brain; others have had damage to the brain at a critical period in prenatal or postnatal development. Conditions that can develop during the prenatal period include PKU, Down syndrome, fetal alcohol syndrome, malformations of the brain (such as microcephaly, hydrocephalus, craniosynostosis), maternal infections, and anoxia. Birth injuries or anoxia during or shortly after delivery can also cause intellectual disability. Diseases such as meningitis, lead poisoning, neoplasms, and encephalitis can cause intellectual disability in a child or adult at any age. Other causes include near-drowning and traumatic brain injury. Heredity is a factor in intellectual disability. It is also possible for children to live in such a physically and emotionally deprived environment that they develop intellectual disability. Approximately 40 to 50% of the causes have no identifiable cause (AAIDD, 2009).

The AAIDD emphasizes both intelligence functioning and adaptive behavior as criteria. Tests to measure intelligence are numerous. Intelligence is represented by intelligent quotient (IQ) scores obtained from standardized tests given by trained professionals. The IQ test score is generally 70 or below when the diagnosis of intellectual disability is made. The IQ test is only one aspect in the diagnosis; significant limitations in adaptive behavior skills and evidence that the disability was present before age 18 years are two additional elements that are critical in determining the diagnosis (AAIDD, 2008).

The Bayley Scales of Infant Development (BSID-II) is used for children 1 to 3 years of age. It assesses language, visual problem-solving skills, behavior, and fine- and gross-motor skills. Tests for adaptive behavior include the Wechsler Scales for children 3 years and older and the Woodcock-Johnson Scales (Kliegman et al., 2007). There is usually good correlation between tests for intelligence and adaptive behavior.

Signs and Symptoms

The diagnosis is determined after a thorough study by a team of experts, including a pediatrician, psychologist, psychiatrist, nurse, and social worker. Conditions such as epilepsy, cerebral palsy, severe malnutrition, emotional disturbances, blindness, deafness, and speech disorders must be ruled out. Severe intellectual disability might be noticeable at birth (see Did You Know?), and the nursery nurse must be alert to cues. Early recognition in certain cases can lessen the disability. For example, routine testing of newborns for conditions such as PKU and

congenital hypothyroidism allows for early treatment and facilitates normal intelligence.

Did You Know?

Signs Suggesting Cognitive Disability in Newborns and Infants

- Failure to suck
- Feeding difficulties
- Spasticity
- Convulsions
- Listlessness, irritability
- Floppy, hypotonic muscles
- Decreased alertness
- Unresponsive to eye contact
- Unusual clumsiness
- Jaundice
- Unusual-looking stools
- Unusual odor to urine
- Enlarged tongue
- Asian appearance in white infants
- Stubby fingers or toes
- Failure to achieve developmental milestones (e.g., smiling, rolling over, sitting)

Developmental delays with failure to meet milestones at a particular age may be an indication of intellectual disability. A child who does not smile, sit, climb stairs, stand, or walk within the usual age limits might have an intellectual disability, although these signs can be caused by other problems. A child may also be slow in speech, in learning self-care, or in toilet training. Unusual clumsiness and failure to respond to stimuli are early indications. Sometimes this disability is not discovered until the child enters school.

Even though children with intellectual disabilities are often categorized by IQ levels, each child must be frequently reevaluated according to individual progress. Many children who have received early intervention beginning in infancy outperform all expectations. A plan for each child should be devised to maximize the child's potential.

Treatment and Nursing Care

Nurses need to recognize that the pace of development is slower than that for the child without a disability. These children also lack the ability to think abstractly, so they have difficulty transferring learning from one situation to another. They learn by habit formation, which involves routine, repetition, and relaxation. Nurses working with these children must have a good understanding of the growth and developmental process. It is important that the child show a **readiness** for the task, whether it is toilet training, feeding self, or dressing. The atmosphere should be one of friendliness, and directions should be kept simple.

The nurse caring for developmentally disabled children in the hospital needs to know each child's stage of maturation and abilities. A detailed history, including a habit and care sheet, is completed. Self-help activities are documented.

Nursing Brief

A list of words, sounds, and gestures, along with their meanings, posted on the developmentally or intellectually disabled child's bed aids personnel in communicating with the child.

While communicating with the child may be difficult, it is important to follow home routines as closely as possible. The progress the child has made should not be allowed to slip during hospitalization. Good communication between parents and nurse helps make the transition from home to hospital as smooth as possible for the child.

Communication

In obtaining information about the child from the parents, a positive approach is recommended. A request such as "Tell me about Gina's eating habits" is preferable to "Does Gina feed herself?" and is likely to yield more helpful information.

Developmentally and intellectually disabled children are referred for early intervention as soon as possible after diagnosis. The American Association on Intellectual and Developmental Disabilities (AAIDD) "*Supports* approach" evaluates the specific needs of the individual and focuses on strategies and services that optimize individual functioning. *Supports* are defined as the resources and individual strategies necessary to promote individual development of the person with developmental disabilities. Support areas include home living, education, human development, community living, employment, health and safety, behavior, social, and protection and advocacy (AAIDD, 2010).

In 1975, the U.S. Congress passed the Education for All Handicapped Children Act (PL 94-142), which guarantees the right of developmentally disabled persons and other disabled persons to receive appropriate education at public expense. Recent amendments include a change in name to Individuals with Disabilities Education Act (IDEA). The amendments include 14 specific primary terms that guide how States define disability and who is eligible for free public education. Included are early intervention services for infants and toddlers (birth to 2 years of age). Developmentally disabled children who are being educated in the public schools have individual educational plans (IEP) that delineate services and specific educational adaptations to meet their needs. Many communities also have sheltered workshops in which developmentally disabled adults can work. These centers provide an opportunity for individuals to be more independent and increase their self-esteem.

Like other children, developmentally disabled children must have limits set on behavior. The adult must be firm and consistent. Correction must directly follow any offense. Love, liberal praise, respect, and infinite patience are essential in helping developmentally disabled children to develop to fullest capacity.

The parents of a developmentally disabled child need support, compassion, and understanding, not pity. For nurses to work effectively with the child and the family, they must face their own feelings and develop a positive attitude. Sharing ideas and feelings with experienced professionals who work with developmentally disabled individuals helps nurses acquire enthusiasm for what these children and families can accomplish.

The problems confronting the parents usually become more complicated as the child develops physically and chronologically but still requires constant supervision. Puberty can be a particularly difficult period. Some parents make the decision that they are no longer able to care for their child adequately at home. The decision to institutionalize the child is a difficult one. Many things must be taken into consideration, such as the health of the parents, the effect on other children in the family, the community services available, and the financial status of the family. Even when the decision is made, there are long waiting lists in many places. Facilities are overcrowded, and the tendency is to take those who are most severely developmentally disabled first.

It is important that nurses be familiar with the resources in their communities so that they can direct the family to them. The local chapter of The Arc (*www.thearc.org*) can provide information and support. The child guidance clinic or the psychological services of a nearby college or hospital may provide beneficial assistance. The visits of the public health nurse are invaluable in many cases. Children also may be eligible to obtain help from their local vocational and rehabilitation agency. Respite care workers afford needed rest and increased mobility for parents. In some communities, parent groups meet to discuss mutual problems. Arrangements for proper dental health must be made.

Developmentally disabled children can participate readily in recreational programs with supervision. The Special Olympics program, for example, facilitates participation in various individual and team sports. The enthusiasm of the children and volunteers in this program is overwhelming.

Community Considerations

Nurses play a primary role in preventing intellectual disabilities through educating the community about environmental dangers, teaching pregnant women about appropriate nutrition and prenatal care, and educating parents and children about injury prevention.

ATTENTION DEFICIT/HYPERACTIVITY DISORDER

The term **attention deficit/hyperactivity disorder (ADHD)** refers to specific patterns of behavior that include inattention and impulsivity and might or might not involve hyperactivity. Boys are affected more frequently than girls. There is increased incidence in families, suggesting a genetic etiology. Affected children usually are of normal or above-average intelligence. Boys exhibit more behavioral problems, whereas girls tend to experience more frequent academic underachievement. ADHD can lead to social, emotional, and learning problems and subsequent decreased self-esteem.

The cause of ADHD is not thoroughly understood. Proponents of a biochemical causation suggest that hyperactive children have a total lack or diminished amount of dopamine. Others attribute the problem to an alteration of the reticular activating system of the midbrain that causes the child to react to every stimulation in the environment rather than to selected ones. Newer evidence indicates that genetic factors may play an important role. These disorders have also been linked to fetal alcohol syndrome and lead toxicity.

Signs and Symptoms

The American Psychiatric Association's *Diagnostic and Statistical Manual of Mental Disorders* has repeatedly tried to precisely define and categorize symptoms of ADHD. With its most current *DSM-IV-TR* criteria, the Association identifies three major patterns of the disorder: (1) ADHD, predominantly inattentive type; (2) ADHD, predominantly hyperactive-impulsive type; and (3) ADHD, combined (American Psychiatric Association, 2004). Symptoms must be present for at least 6 months, must have appeared before 7 years of age, must be identified in more than one setting (home, school), and must cause significant impairment in psychosocial or educational adjustment and functioning (American Psychiatric Association, 2004). In addition, other causes for the behavior must be ruled out before a diagnosis can be made.

The diagnosis is difficult to establish because sometimes symptoms are subtle, and the diagnosis has become a "catch-all" for children with behavioral problems that might be the result of other causes. The diagnosis is made primarily from the child's history and interviews with family and teachers. Several screening tests are available to help with data collection.

The following are some manifestations that suggest ADHD:

- Is inattentive to details, careless with schoolwork or other activities
- Has difficulty organizing tasks
- Is unable to sustain attention for periods of time that would be appropriate for age
- Does not listen, follow instructions, or complete tasks; interrupts frequently
- Avoids activities and games that require concentration
- Is easily distracted
- Is forgetful, loses things
- Appears to have excessive energy
- Fidgety, cannot remain seated
- Cannot play quietly, excessive talking
- Runs and climbs excessively
- Blurts out answers and interrupts
- Difficulty waiting for turn
- Difficulty with social situations
- Low frustration tolerance

A child with these characteristics may have difficulties in school and in social situations. Children with ADHD are a challenge for parents, family members, and school professionals.

Treatment and Nursing Care

Children with ADHD should be managed by a multidisciplinary team consisting of a nurse, physician, social worker, psychologist, and special education teacher. Parents need support and should be referred to support groups. Family counseling may be warranted. Parents should be aware that only a physician can prescribe medication.

The ideal approach to ADHD is a combination of medications and behavioral treatment. Medications are appropriate first-line treatment for children except for preschoolers (ages 4 to 6). Behavioral therapy or parent-training programs should be considered for the preschooler. There are four categories of medications that are approved for use in children. Stimulants, selective norepinephrine reuptake inhibitors (SNRIs), alpha-2 agonists, and tricyclic antidepressants (TCAs) are all FDA-approved (Table 20-1).

In addition to medications, the American Academy of Pediatrics recommends the use of behavior therapy. Programs may use training sessions with a trained therapist in behavior modification. The goal of this approach is to assist the parents in understanding the child's behavior and learning specific techniques for altering behavior (Katragadda and Schubiner, 2007).

Initially, a careful medical history and neurologic examination are indicated. Intelligence and psychological testing may aid in determining the specific assets and liabilities of the child so that an individual learning plan can be outlined. Many schools today have special learning disability classes in which the children are helped to establish self-discipline by consistent controls, elimination of distractions, and recognition and appreciation of accomplishments. Many children with ADHD function well in the regular classroom with certain educational and behavioral modifications. These methods are reinforced by the thoughtful nurse when such a child is hospitalized.

Table 20-1 ADHD Medications

MEDICATION	APPROVED AGES	DURATION OF ACTION	COMMENTS
Alpha₂ Agonist			
Guanfacine (Intuniv)	6-17 yrs	6-12 hr	Hypotension, bradycardia
SNRIs			
Atomoxethine (Strattera)	> 6 yrs	24 hr	Suicide
Stimulants (Amphetamine and Dextroamphetamine)			
Adderall (short-acting)	> 3 yrs	4-6 hr	Monitor growth, blood
DextroStat	> 6 yrs	4-6 hr	pressure, heart rate
Dexedrine spansule	> 6 yrs	6-10 hr	
Adderall XR, Vyvanse	> 6 yrs	10-12 hr	
Stimulants (Methylphenidate)			
Ritalin, Methylin, Focalin	> 6 yrs	3-5 hr	Monitor growth, blood
Ritalin SR, Metadate ER and CD, Methylin ER	> 6 yrs	3-8 hr	pressure, heart rate
Concerta, Daytrana	> 6 yrs	8-12 hr	
Other Agents			
Wellbutrin	Not FDA	4-24+ hr	Baseline echocardiogram
Tricyclic antidepressants	approved	24 hr	Monitor blood levels

A priority in the care of these children is a careful nursing admission history, a most useful tool in dealing with children who have problems of this nature. Nurses observe the child's behavior alone and in interaction with the family. They document what they see, but they do not analyze. For example, a nurse would write, "Eric threw four crayons on the floor," not "Eric appeared distraught and misbehaved this morning." Careful attention is given to the child's attitude toward school. Other responsibilities might include education in parenting, and assisting with screening and psychological testing. Functions pertinent to the nurse's work setting might also include referral to appropriate agencies and assessment of the home and school environment.

Listening to the child and the parents and providing support are particularly important. If the child is hyperactive, opportunities for gross-motor play and screaming to externalize feelings, which can be encouraged at home, are limited in the hospital. The use of puppets, finger paints, and singing may be used to offset this imbalance.

Nursing Brief

Parents should be aware that medications will not cure ADHD.

When medications are necessary, the child and the family must understand the reasons for their use and their possible side effects. Periodic evaluation by the physician is essential. It is helpful if a behavior chart is kept and is submitted to the doctor before prescriptions are renewed. The child with a learning disability should not become a "sacrificial lamb" to the educational process, and the emphasis on education should not be disproportionate to the child's innate capabilities. Personal growth and self-esteem should be emphasized. Parents should be aware that other opportunities exist that can be adjusted to the child's abilities.

DOWN SYNDROME

Down syndrome is one of the most common genetic birth defects. The incidence of Down syndrome is approximately 1 in 800 live births; it is higher in children born of mothers 35 years of age or older. However, sometimes an infant with Down syndrome is the first child of a young mother. Depending on the cause, following children may be normal. There are three known causes of Down syndrome, all of which involve abnormalities of the chromosomes. In the most common type, **trisomy 21 syndrome**, the total chromosome count is 47 instead of the normal 46. This accounts for 95% of cases. It is a result of **nondisjunction**, or failure of a chromosome to follow the normal separation process into daughter cells. The earlier in the embryo's development this occurs, the greater the number of cells affected. With translocation, which occurs in 3% to 4% of cases, a piece of chromosome in pair 21 breaks off and attaches itself to another chromosome. Parents should have genetic counseling as translocation is usually hereditary. Mosaicism occurs in 1% to 3% of cases and results in the body cell having either normal or abnormal chromosomes. Mosaicism and trisomy 21 are not hereditary.

Prenatal testing can be done in the first or third trimester. It includes serum and ultrasound testing, with specific diagnosis using amniocentesis or chorionic villus sampling. The American Congress of

Obstetricians and Gynecologists recommends that all women be offered aneuploidy screening before 20 weeks of gestation and that all women have the option of invasive testing (ACOG, 2007).

Signs and Symptoms

The signs of this condition, which are apparent at birth, are close-set and upward-slanting eyes, small head, round face, flat nose, mouth breathing, and a protruding tongue that interferes with sucking. The hands of the infant are short and thick, and the little finger is curved. In addition, there is a deep, straight line across the palm, called the **simian crease** (Figure 20-1). There is also a wide space between the first and second toes. Undeveloped muscles (hypotonia) and loose joints enable the child to assume unusual positions. Physical growth and development may be slower than normal (Table 20-2 and Home Care Considerations box). Most children are mildly to moderately intellectually

challenged. Because of recent advances in medicine, education, and available resources, these children are able to progress further than previously possible. Many additional medical issues can accompany Down syndrome. Congenital heart deformities, gastrointestinal disorders (imperforate anus, esophageal atresia, celiac disease), pulmonary hypertension, ENT anomalies, endocrine disease (thyroid), immune dysfunction, hematologic disorders (polycythemia, leukemia), and psychiatric issues (dementia, Alzheimer's) can all be issues for the child with Down syndrome. It is important to remember that no one child exhibits all the possible physical characteristics of Down syndrome.

Table 20-2 Developmental Milestones				
	CHILDREN WITH DOWN SYNDROME		NORMAL CHILDREN	
MILESTONE	AVERAGE (MO)	RANGE (MO)	AVERAGE (MO)	RANGE (MO)
Smiling	2	1½-3	1	½-3
Rolling over	6	2-12	5	2-10
Sitting	9	6-18	7	5-9
Crawling	11	7-21	8	6-11
Creeping	13	8-25	10	7-13
Standing	10	10-32	11	8-16
Walking	20	2-45	13	8-18
Talking, words	14	9-30	10	6-14
Talking, sentences	24	18-46	21	14-32

From Carey W., Crocker, A., Elias, E., et al. (2009). *Developmental-behavioral pediatrics* (4th ed.). Philadelphia: Saunders, with permission.

Home Care Considerations

Self-Help Skills

SKILL	CHILDREN WITH DOWN SYNDROME		NORMAL CHILDREN	
	AVERAGE (MO)	RANGE (MO)	AVERAGE (MO)	RANGE (MO)
Eating				
Finger feeding	12	8-28	8	6-16
Using spoon/fork	20	12-40	13	8-20
Toilet Training				
Bladder	48	20-95	32	18-60
Bowel	42	28-90	29	16-48
Dressing				
Undressing	40	29-72	32	22-42
Putting clothes on	58	38-98	47	34-58

From Carey W., Crocker, A., Elias, E., et al. (2009). *Developmental-behavioral pediatrics* (4th ed.). Philadelphia: Saunders, with permission.

Children with Down syndrome are very lovable. However, they are restless and somewhat more difficult to teach than normal youngsters. Their resistance to infection is poor; however, with antibiotic use and ability to control infections, their life span has increased. The incidence rate of acute leukemia is higher in children with Down syndrome than in other children. They are also at risk for development of respiratory infections and otitis media. Risk for respiratory infections is primarily due to poor muscle tone and decreased ability to move secretions out of the lung. Children with Down syndrome are also prone to speech and hearing problems. Speech problems are primarily caused by the enlarged tongue, which makes it difficult to pronounce words.

Nursing Care

Nurses need to be aware of their own feelings before they can give effective support to the child with a disability and also the parents. The nurse must have patience and understanding and be able to handle a difficult situation in a positive manner. Children with

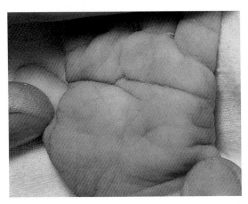

FIGURE 20-1 Bridged palmar crease, seen in some infants with Down syndrome.

Down syndrome are encouraged to help themselves within their ability, even though it may take more time. This is especially true when they are ill and hospitalized. Early infant stimulation enables children with Down syndrome to reach milestones as rapidly as possible.

With increased stimulation, love and encouragement from the family, and the utilization of community resources, the child's potential for progress has increased. The child with Down syndrome no longer needs to be institutionalized.

With an increase in funding, more and more programs and community facilities suited to the short-term and long-term needs of children with Down syndrome are becoming available. Some community facilities are group homes, foster homes, and boarding homes. The nurse should become familiar with services located in and near the community. Sometimes parents cannot accept the fact that their child is different and are ashamed to tell anyone of the infant's condition. The parents need to grieve over the loss of the normal child they do not have. This should not be interpreted as a lack of love for the child they do have. It takes exceptional strength to accept this diagnosis. Empathy from the nurse is of particular importance. Allowing parents to become involved in care and planning for the infant from the start facilitates bonding.

The staff's warm concern and care cannot be overemphasized. Pampering the infant by putting a little curl in the hair, for example, shows that others care even though this infant is different. Parents watch for evidence of rejection of their child; they are sensitive to such things as placement in the nursery.

Several organizations provide support to the child with Down syndrome, among them the National Down Syndrome Congress, The Arc, and the National Association for Down Syndrome.

FAILURE TO THRIVE

Failure to thrive is used to describe infants and children who, without specific evidence, fail to gain, and often lose, weight **(nonorganic)**. Although this condition can be caused by organic abnormalities as well, this discussion is limited to environmental causes. Infants who fail to thrive are frequently admitted to the hospital for evaluation with presenting symptoms of weight loss or failure to gain, irritability, and disturbances of food intake such as anorexia, pica, or abnormal consumption of food. Vomiting, diarrhea, and general neuromuscular spasticity sometimes accompany the condition. Children fall below the 5th percentile in growth (Figure 20-2). Their development can be delayed. These children seem apathetic, some have rag doll limpness about them (hypotonia), and they often

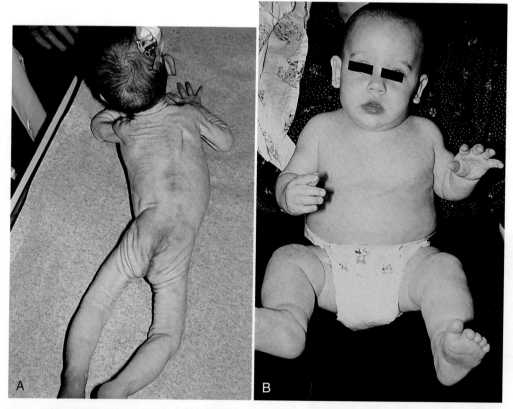

FIGURE 20-2 A, A 4½-month-old who is well below her birth weight and shows severe developmental delay. Note the loss of subcutaneous tissue manifested by wrinkled skin on the buttocks, shoulder, and upper arms. **B,** Same infant after 3½ months in foster care. Note that the infant is well nourished and is caught up developmentally.

appear wary of their caregivers. Others appear stiff and unresponsive to cuddling. The personality of the infant may be one that does not foster maternal attachment.

Although causality is sometimes obscured, there appears to be a disturbance in the mother-child or caregiver-child relationship. The situation is complex and is often associated with marital discord, economic pressures, parental immaturity and low stress tolerance, and single parenthood. Alcohol and drug abuse are often present. Many mothers feel deprived and unloved and have conflicting needs. The infant suffers from the inability to establish a sense of trust in caregivers. Coping abilities are affected by a lack of nurturing. Outward neglect and physical abuse are not uncommon.

Treatment and Nursing Care

Prevention of environmental failure to thrive consists chiefly of instituting social measures such as parenting classes, family planning, and early recognition and support of families at risk. Treatment involves a multidisciplinary approach in accordance with the circumstances; physician, nurse, social worker, family agency, and counselor may all participate. If no progress can be made, temporary or permanent placement of the child or children in a foster home may be necessary.

Treatment of the child who fails to thrive requires maturity on the part of the nurse. It is vital to support rather than reject the mother. Maternal attachment can be facilitated by listening to her and helping her to get in touch with her feelings and frustrations and explore her choices. Encourage her to assist with the daily care of her child. Stress the infant's uniqueness and responses to the mother. Point out developmental patterns, and provide anticipatory guidance in this area. Avoid lecturing. Try to understand her situation and needs. Take the initiative. Frequently, the mother's "lack of interest during visiting hours" stems from her own insecurities and feelings of rejection by hospital staff that seem critical to her. Provide parents with a 24-hour phone number, and encourage them to use it when stress mounts. Parents Anonymous and parent aides are other resources.

A consistent caregiver should be provided so that the child develops trust in the individual. The caregiver should model appropriate parenting behaviors. The parent should be praised for positive parenting. Interaction between the parent and child should be observed and documented. Nurses must be diligent about charting only objective observations. Behaviors observed and statements made by the parents meet these criteria. Nurses cannot chart their feelings or instincts about the parent-child relationship. When the child is hospitalized, nursing measures often lead to dramatic improvement in weight gain and improved social response.

The prognosis of this condition is uncertain. Emotional abuse, particularly in the early years, can be psychologically traumatic. Since maximum brain growth occurs within the first 6 months of life, inadequacies in intelligence, language, and social behavior have been documented in children who fail to thrive.

CHILD ABUSE AND NEGLECT

Because of the scope of the problem, no one definition seems entirely satisfactory, but efforts are being made to reduce ambiguity. The term *battered child syndrome* was coined by C. Kempe in his landmark paper published in 1962 in the *Journal of the American Medical Association*. The term refers to "a clinical condition in young children who have received serious physical abuse, generally from a parent or foster parent." The impact of Kempe's research was considerable and focused the attention of physicians on unexplained fractures and signs of physical abuse (Figure 20-3). Today most authorities consider this definition rather narrow and have broadened it to include neglect and maltreatment. Differences of opinion about what constitutes child abuse exist from state to state and in the criteria of various agencies concerned with this problem. Nurses must become aware of the mandates of the states and institutions in which they practice.

Statistics show that 12.1 of every 1000 children are victims of abuse or neglect (U.S. Department of Health

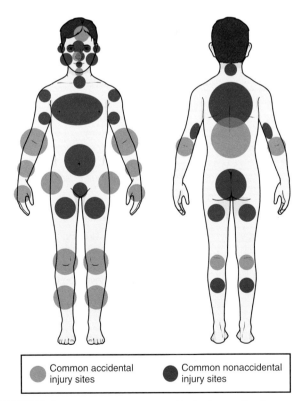

Common accidental injury sites • Common nonaccidental injury sites

FIGURE 20-3 Accidents typically cause injuries in specific sites (purple areas). The nurse should suspect physical abuse in children with injuries in nonaccidental sites (red areas).

Box 20-1   **Risk Factors for Child Abuse and Neglect**

PARENTAL/CAREGIVER RISK FACTORS
- Victim of abuse/neglect as a child
- Social isolation
- Low self-esteem, poor impulse control, antisocial behavior
- Inaccurate knowledge about child development/ unrealistic expectations
- Young parent
- Mental illness/depression/anxiety
- Substance abuse

- Domestic violence/marital conflict/single parent
- Poverty/unemployment
- Stress
- Harsh discipline

CHILD RISK FACTORS
- Infants and young children
- Adolescence (for sexual abuse)
- Physical, cognitive, and emotional disabilities
- Behavior problems, attention deficit

Data from Office on Child Abuse and Neglect, 2003; Goldman J, Salus MK, Wolcott D, et al. (2003). *A coordinated response to child abuse and neglect: the Foundation for Practice.* User Manual Series. Washington, DC: Child Welfare Information Gateway.

and Human Services, 2008). The exact number is unknown because many cases go unreported. Three children die each day as a result of abuse or neglect, and one half of all deaths are in children under 1 year of age (Box 20-1).

Federal Laws and Agencies

By 1963, the Children's Bureau had drafted a model mandatory state reporting law that has been adopted in some form in all 50 states. This law aids in establishing statistics and is based on the need to provide therapeutic help to both the child and the family. Immunity from liability is provided for persons reporting suspected cases. Most states have penalties for failure to report child abuse. Originally, only physicians were held responsible for reporting suspected cases; however, many states now include all professionals who are in contact with children, such as nurses, social workers, teachers, and clergy. Other laws state specifically that anyone may report an offense. Referrals usually go to Child Protective Services, where a caseworker is assigned to the case.

Identification and Types

The types of child abuse and means of identification are listed in the Health Promotion box. In the past, much of the treatment of child abuse was provided after the fact. Current literature stresses the need for prevention and early intervention.

Health Promotion

How to Recognize Child Abuse and Neglect

TYPE	CHILD'S APPEARANCE	CHILD'S BEHAVIOR	PARENT'S OR CAREGIVER'S BEHAVIOR
Physical abuse (injury inflicted by caregiver for any reason)	Bruises, welts, burns, bite marks, intraabdominal injuries, or fracture Injury history does not explain or fit the injury History of suspicious injuries	Displays negative behavior as viewed by caregiver May have history of prolonged neonatal hospitalization Developmentally delayed Displays a "trigger" behavior such as crying, incontinence	May have been abused as a child May use harsh discipline May misuse alcohol or other drugs Poorly prepared for child rearing Unrealistic expectation of child Low self-esteem; lacks resources
Shaken baby syndrome	Irritable, vomiting, bulging fontanel, seizures, retinal hemorrhages	Lethargic; eating poorly	Same as physical abuse
Neglect (physical, emotional)	Failure to thrive; developmentally delayed Physically dirty; tired and lethargic Comes to school without breakfast; often does not have lunch or lunch money Lacking in essential necessities Often left alone for extended periods of time Lacking medical attention	Is frequently absent from school Displays negative or unacceptable behavior May use alcohol or drugs Engages in vandalism or sexual misconduct	Misuses alcohol or other drugs May have disorganized, upset home life Noncompliant with medical treatments Fails to seek medical care May have a history of neglect as a child Isolated with few resources

Health Promotion—cont'd

TYPE	CHILD'S APPEARANCE	CHILD'S BEHAVIOR	PARENT'S OR CAREGIVER'S BEHAVIOR
Emotional abuse (often verbal)	Signs less obvious than in other forms of mistreatment	Passive and withdrawn to aggressive and acting out	Fails to provide child verbal and behavioral expressions of love and affection Determined to destroy child; poor parental self-image Unable to tolerate parental stresses
Sexual abuse	Pain or itching in the genital area Painful urination; bruising Venereal disease Pregnancy	May display regressive behavior or overly adult behavior Depends on age of child Sleeping and eating disorders Poor school performance Runs away from home	Perpetrator may have been molested as a child Usually known by child May use drugs and alcohol May threaten child if child reveals
Munchausen syndrome by proxy	History of unexplained illnesses; near-death experiences	Nondocumented symptoms only seen by caregiver	Usually caused by mother Even-tempered person with some medical education Gives false information regarding child's illness

Child abuse can be physical, sexual, or emotional (Figure 20-4). It may entail neglect. It is often difficult to determine whether an injury or situation reflects abuse. Jurgrau (1990) suggests that injuries can happen by accident—but rarely more than once. The nurse should be suspicious if there is a severe injury without evidence of a traumatic event, if there is a pattern of "accidents," or if an injury does not match the history given.

Nursing Brief

A citizen can report suspected child abuse or neglect by contacting the Child Protective Services in the Yellow Pages of the telephone directory under Social Service Organizations. This can be done with or without the use of the caller's name. After obtaining the facts, the agency informs the parents that a report is being filed and checks the condition of the child. A visit must be initiated within 72 hours. In most cases, this is accomplished within 48 hours or earlier if the situation is life threatening. All persons who report suspected abuse or neglect are given immunity from criminal prosecution and civil liability if the report is made in good faith. Many professionals, such as physicians, nurses, social workers, and so on, are mandatory reporters of child abuse.

Child abuse is not limited to abuse by parents, but parents account for 80% of the offenders. Abuse can be inflicted by babysitters, boyfriends, relatives, or casual acquaintances. Drug or alcohol abuse increases the risk for child abuse. Abuse occurs at every socioeconomic level and is often precipitated by a stressful situation within the family (unemployment, marital problems, chronic illness, poverty).

Sexual abuse is a topic that is not easy to discuss; however, it is estimated that 10% to 25% of girls and 8% to 10% of boys have been sexually abused (Kellogg, 2005). Family members and adolescent acquaintances are the most common offenders. Rarely are strangers the offenders, yet many parents focus on "bad strangers" and "good and bad touch," which can leave many children unprotected (Nelms, 2003).

Nursing Care

Prevention of child abuse is of utmost importance. One approach currently taken is identification of high-risk infants and parents during the prenatal and perinatal periods. Predictive questionnaires are used as screening tools in some clinics. Many hospitals also provide closer follow-up of mothers and neonates. The process of **maternal-infant bonding** and its significance to later parent-child relationships have recently been explored.

Nurses in obstetrical clinics have the opportunity to casually observe parents and their abilities to cope. The history of the child, the desirability of the pregnancy, the number of children already in the family, the financial and personal stability of the family, the types of support systems they have, and other factors may have a bearing on how the parents accept the new offspring. Pertinent observations include a description of parent-newborn infant interaction. Both verbal and nonverbal communications are important, as is the amount of body and eye contact. Lack of interest,

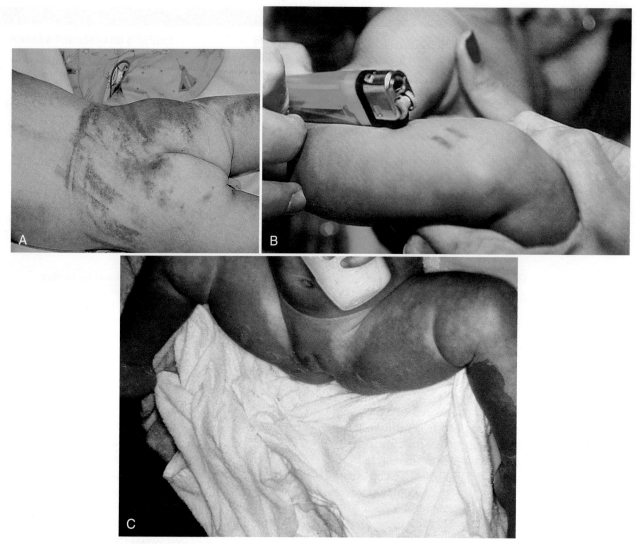

FIGURE 20-4 **A,** Lesions caused by hand, hairbrush, and a belt. **B,** Lesions caused by heated cigarette lighter wheels. **C,** Child was dipped in scalding water as a lesson for a toileting accident.

indifference, or negative comments about the gender, looks, or temperament of the infant could be significant.

In other areas, a cooperative team approach is necessary. This includes providing a wide range of services such as family planning, protective services, daycare centers, homemakers, education for parenthood classes, hotlines, self-help groups, family counseling, emergency shelters for children, child advocates, and a massive effort to reduce the incidence of preterm birth. Other related areas include financial assistance, employment services, transportation, emotional support and encouragement, and long-term follow-up. More research and data services are required, as are evaluation and reduction of violent behaviors that are prevalent in our society.

Individual nurses can help detect child abuse by maintaining a high level of suspicion in their work settings. Record keeping should be factual and objective. Pediatric nurses should make a point of reviewing old records on their patients, which may reveal repeated hospitalizations, radiographs of multiple fractures, persistent feeding problems, history of failure to thrive, and chronic absenteeism from school. Delay or neglect in seeking medical attention for a child or failure to obtain immunization and well-child care is sometimes significant. Children who seem overly upset about being discharged need to be brought to the attention of the physician.

Cultural Considerations

Although it is important to detect potential injuries, it is also important to avoid reporting innocent families. Health care providers should be aware of cultural healing practices. For example, Southwest Asians practice cupping as a means of treating fevers (Figure 20-5).

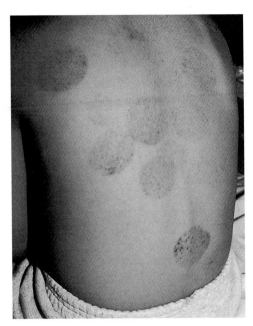

FIGURE 20-5 Cupping. These circular bruises with central petechiae are the sequelae of the Southeast Asian practice of cupping.

Nursing Brief

Bruises heal in various stages according to color (0 to 2 days, swollen, tender; 0 to 5 days, red; 5 to 7 days, green; 7 to 10 days, yellow; 10 to 14 days, brown; 14 to 28 days, clear). Does this bruise match the caregiver's explanation of what happened?

The abused child should be approached quietly, and preparation for treatments should be carefully explained in advance. The number of caregivers should be kept to a minimum. The child may be able to express some hostility and fear through play. It is not unusual for these children to be either unresponsive or openly hostile or to show affection indiscriminately. Keep direct questioning to a minimum. Use praise when appropriate. Encourage activities that promote physical and sensory development. Avoid speaking to the child about the parents in a negative manner. Consult with other professionals about setting limits for poor behavior.

The nurse must acknowledge that in cases of child abuse there are always two victims: the child **and** the abuser. Because of personal problems, the abuser often leads an isolated life. Some were themselves battered or neglected children. Many have unrealistic expectations regarding the child's intelligence and capabilities. There may be a role reversal, in which the child becomes the comforter. Although removing the child from the home is one answer, many authorities believe that this can be more detrimental in the long run. Being open to parents in this type of crisis is difficult but

essential if the nurse wishes to be part of the solution rather than part of the problem. When placement in a foster home is necessary, parents experience feelings of grief, loss, and remorse. The child also mourns the loss of the family even if there has been abuse. The nurse should be aware of the child's needs and facilitate expression of feelings of loss. The nurse who recognizes the potential for violence that lies in all persons is better able to deal with this complex problem.

In dealing with sexual abuse, parents should understand that a good parent-child relationship that fosters open communication is essential. Parents should learn good listening skills and be willing to spend time listening to their child. Parents should discuss with their child the idea of keeping secrets and that no one should have the child keep a secret from the child's parent. Parents should be aware of all individuals who spend time with their child. Many offenders are either related or a close acquaintance. The child should know that he or she can tell the parent and that the parent will protect him or her and stop the abuse.

AUTISM

Autism is described as a complex developmental disorder of the brain, most likely caused by abnormalities in brain structure or function. It is now viewed as a *spectrum disorder* and affects social interaction, language, and restrictive and repetitive behavior (Burg et al., 2006). It is estimated that about 1 per 110 children have autism (Carbone et al., 2010). Autism typically appears in the first 3 years of life. The exact cause is unknown, although many theories abound. One theory is that the measles-mumps-rubella (MMR) vaccine has led to autism in some children. Proof does not exist to support this theory. The Centers for Disease Control and Prevention has also done research in this area, and current evidence does not show a link between the two. Other theories include genetic involvement, environmental factors, pregnancy complications, and possible related medical conditions.

Early diagnosis is critical, as early treatment can be beneficial. Recommendations of early screening for all children ages 18 to 24 months can be accomplished with an autism-specific screening test. The Modified Checklist for Autism in Toddlers (M-CHAT) is a 23-question checklist that has been shown to identify a significant number of children. Surveillance of developmental milestones is also a key element in identification.

Parents may suspect that something is wrong with their child but they do not know what it is. Autistic children may exhibit bizarre characteristics. They like things to stay the same; disruption of order in their world can upset them. They may have temper tantrums. Autistic children do not interact well with others; they prefer to be alone. These children often do not maintain eye contact with another person. They may play with toys in an unusual manner and live in their "own little world." Children with autism often exhibit a delay in or lack of language development. They may use repetitive language and exhibit repetitive motor movements such as rocking. Often there is some degree of intellectual disability. On the other hand, autistic children have been known to be particularly talented in certain areas such as music, memory, and mathematics.

The prognosis has shown some improvement with an early intervention program. Comprehensive behavioral therapy begun at a young age can lead to improved cognitive, language, and adaptive skills (Carbone et al., 2010). Medications may be used to lessen some of the disturbing symptoms. While many families will include complementary and alternative medical treatments (CAM), many times there is no scientific data to support the treatment. Some children may require lifelong care, while others can function at a high level of independence.

This condition may be difficult for the family to accept. Parents may feel guilty and that they are to blame for the disorder. The entire family is affected. There is stress and added financial hardships. Referrals to a family network such as Family Voices (*www.familyvoices.org*) can help the family connect with other families. Other organizations such as The Autism Society of America (ASA) can provide information about education, treatment programs, and resources for parents.

 Community Considerations

The Autism Society of America *(www.autism-society.org)* can be reached at 800-3AUTISM or 301-657-0881.

ANOREXIA NERVOSA

In the fourth edition of the *Diagnostic and Statistical Manual of Mental Disorders* (*DSM-IV-TR*, 2000), the American Psychiatric Association defines anorexia nervosa as an eating disorder characterized by self-imposed starvation, extreme weight loss or failure to gain expected weight for growth (less than 85% of expected weight), and body image disturbance. Affected adolescents have a morbid fear of being or becoming fat. Amenorrhea (defined as the absence of three consecutive menstrual cycles) occurs in postpubertal adolescents with anorexia.

The disorder occurs primarily in girls and affects about 1% to 5% of American teenage girls and 1% of teenage boys. The adolescent sees herself as being fat, even in the stages of advanced emaciation. The term *anorexia* is misleading, for many adolescents do not have a lack of appetite. Instead, they experience intense hunger, which they deny or satisfy by eating and

purging binges. A combination of factors may cause the disease, including genetic or physiologic predisposition, sociocultural influences, and impaired psychological development.

Some theorists believe that families of these young people are dysfunctional. They may exhibit such behaviors as overprotectiveness, rigidity, lack of privacy, and inability to resolve conflicts. Affected adolescents appear to be in conflict with their parents about achieving autonomy. In addition, the child's illness may serve to maintain family balance because the parents focus on the needs of the child and thus avoid other internal conflicts.

Signs and Symptoms

Early signs and symptoms may be vague; often, in retrospect, the condition may seem to have begun with a diet or with some emotional trauma. The onset can often be pinpointed to the young girl's inability to wear some of her clothes or to life changes such as a move, parental divorce, or the death of a relative or close friend (see Did You Know?).

? Did You Know?

Anorexia Nervosa and Bulimia

DATA	ANOREXIA NERVOSA	BULIMIA
Age at onset	12-16 yr	15-20 yr
Weight	Markedly decreased below normal	Normal or slightly above normal
Body image	Distorted; person sees herself as fat even when emaciated	Realistic, but person feels eating behaviors are out of control
Underlying psychological problems	Perfectionist, unrealistic expectations of self and others, unmet needs for nurturance; desire for autonomy places the adolescent in frequent conflict with restrictive parents; decreased self-esteem	Anxiety, guilt, feelings of worthlessness and inadequacy, impulsiveness, decreased self-esteem, parents with too high expectations

Initial weight loss may be gradual or sudden, but as the child's weight drops, the sense of being overweight rises. Despite lack of intake, the child initially has a great deal of energy and may exercise strenuously to reduce more rapidly. Later, the adolescent loses the energy to participate even in activities of daily living. Adolescents with anorexia nervosa often have a preoccupation with food or with cooking for others and may exhibit bizarre eating behaviors. On physical examination, some of the following conditions become evident: emaciated appearance, dry skin, amenorrhea, lanugo hair over the back and extremities, cold intolerance, low blood pressure, low pulse, abdominal pain, and constipation. Electrolyte imbalance may be noticeable in the adolescent who induces vomiting or uses laxatives or diuretics. Elevated calcium levels indicate that osteoporosis is occurring.

Teenagers with anorexia have feelings of helplessness, lack of control, low self-esteem, and depression. Socialization with peers diminishes. Mealtime becomes a family battleground, increasing the conflict and power struggle. Some adolescents feel guilty and may go on an eating binge, which is followed by self-induced vomiting as the fear of gaining weight returns. The perception of body image becomes increasingly disturbed, and there is a lack of self-identity. The young person remains egocentric and unable to resolve normal adolescent tasks. The adolescent complains of bloating and abdominal pain after small amounts of food are ingested.

Treatment and Nursing Care

The treatment of anorexia is complex and involves several methods. A period of hospitalization may be necessary to correct electrolyte imbalance, establish minimal restoration of nutrients, and stabilize the adolsecent's weight. In addition to fluid and electrolyte imbalance, criteria for hospitalization include: severe loss of control or suicidal behavior, weight more than 25% lower than expected, too rapid weight loss, hypothermia, coexisting illness, and failure of outpatient treatment (Kliegman et al., 2007). Therapies include medical stabilization, psychotherapy, behavioral therapy, drug therapy, and family therapy. Nasogastric feedings and total parenteral nutrition are usually used only when other means have failed because they are only a temporary answer to a much larger problem. Such measures do not reflect normal eating patterns. Hospitalization is expensive and sometimes is not covered by insurance for the length of time necessary to effectively stabilize and treat the adolescent. The ongoing need for inpatient or outpatient therapy, or both, can lead to family financial stress.

The nurse can play an important role in ensuring that the atmosphere is relaxed and non-punitive while maintaining clear behavioral limits. It is important for nurses to facilitate positive coping behaviors, gradually increasing autonomy and decision making and improved body image. Some hospitals now have units that specialize in eating disorders. Continued follow-up after discharge from the unit is essential.

Nurses working with adolescents in any capacity need to be alert to the symptoms of this disease because lack of recognition is one of the biggest obstacles to treatment. Making young people aware of the seriousness of this condition is an important nursing function. Because there is a higher incidence rate of anorexia nervosa in athletes (especially gymnasts, ballet dancers, and runners), it is important for coaches and parents to recognize early signs and symptoms. Educational materials, referral sources, and counseling are available from the National Association of Anorexia Nervosa and Associated Disorders. Encouragement and support from self-help groups are also valuable.

The prognosis for children with anorexia nervosa is uncertain. Most children gain weight in the hospital regardless of the type of therapy. This may not, however, predict future success. Success rate is about 75% (Behrman et al., 2004). Complications include gastritis, cardiac arrhythmia, inflammation of the intestine, kidney problems, and others. Deaths do occur, particularly in untreated persons.

BULIMIA

Bulimia, or binge eating, is now recognized by *DSM-IV-TR* as a separate eating disorder from anorexia nervosa. It is characterized by the following behaviors: (1) regular, multiple episodes of binge eating (large amounts over a short period of time, occurring twice a week for at least 3 months) and feeling that the eating is out of control, (2) purging, or the use of methods to prevent weight gain from the binge eating (such as self-induced vomiting, laxatives, ipecac, diuretics, enemas), and (3) expressed dissatisfaction with body size or weight. It occurs more commonly in older adolescents and young women but can also be observed in men. Persons with bulimia binge periodically, usually on easily accessible high-calorie food items. These episodes are generally carried out in private. They may be followed by self-induced vomiting or the use of cathartics. Persistent vomiting can cause erosion of the enamel of the teeth, tooth decay, chronic esophagitis, chronic sore throat, inflammation, and parotitis. The person is aware that eating is out of control. Periods of binging are preceded by anxiety and followed by feelings of dejection, guilt, and self-deprecation. (See Did You Know? on p. 386 for a comparison summary of anorexia and bulimia.)

The treatment for bulimia is similar to that for anorexia but involves pharmacologic management as well. Because depression and anxiety are underlying factors, the physician may try antidepressant or anti-anxiety agents. In addition to nursing management of physical consequences, the goals of nursing care are directed toward reducing anxiety by identifying alternative methods for dealing with it, increasing effective coping mechanisms, and facilitating appropriate family interaction.

SUBSTANCE ABUSE

The problem of substance abuse is serious and complex and of great magnitude. Government effort to control the supply and distribution of dangerous drugs has generally failed. Adult society, through its widespread acceptance of self-administered pills and alcohol, has compounded the problem; in particular, the drinking patterns of teenagers appear to directly reflect those of their parents and the community.

Numerous reasons have been cited concerning why adolescents resort to drug use. Possible reasons for increased use of drugs are a decrease in perceived risks, fewer school-based substance abuse programs, media that glamorizes tobacco and alcohol use, and lenient patterns of parenting (American Academy of Pediatrics, 2005). Other reasons cited are curiosity; peer pressure; rebellion; the need to escape from loneliness, boredom, or family problems; and the desire to become more sociable and to relax. Teenagers differ from adults in a preference for **polypharmacy** (the use of several drugs together), a sense of invulnerability, and a delay in psychosocial maturation with chronic drug use. Drug-seeking behavior may include stealing (shoplifting in particular), dealing in drugs, sexual promiscuity, and prostitution. In addition, a disproportionately high number of suicides are related to substance abuse. Gender-related differences have narrowed, particularly in the use of alcohol (more girls are experimenting with drugs and alcohol in their teens).

 Nursing Brief

The use of tobacco and alcohol at an early age is a predictive factor for use of other drugs, use of greater variety of drugs, and use of more potent drugs (Figure 20-6).

Signs and Symptoms

The American Psychiatric Society has defined substance abuse as (1) a pattern of substance use that significantly interferes with normal activities of daily living, including fulfilling role obligations at home, school, or work, (2) use of substances when performing hazardous activities, (3) frequent substance-related legal difficulties, and (4) continued use despite the problems caused. Often adolescents begin by experimentation. However, there is a fine line separating use, dependence, and abuse.

Substances can cause **dependence**, an inappropriate reliance on the substance that persists despite efforts to cut down or control it. Dependence can be physiologic, marked by **tolerance**, that is, an increasing need for greater amounts of the substance to produce the same effect, and **substance withdrawal**, physical withdrawal symptoms when the substance is reduced

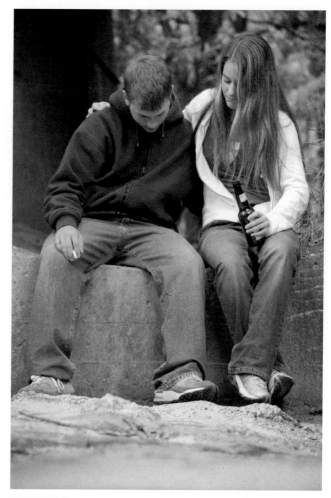

FIGURE 20-6 Cigarettes and beer are considered "gateway" substances that can lead to the use of other, illegal substances.

or stopped. Not all substances cause physiologic dependence.

Table 20-3 summarizes the characteristics of some of the drugs more commonly abused by adolescents.

Treatment and Nursing Care

Treatment and nursing care for adolescents with substance abuse problems differ, depending on the drug involved. Prevention in the community and in schools through drug and alcohol education programs, identification and referral of students known to be users or at risk, and support for drug-free communities can reduce the incidence of substance use in teens.

The prevention of alcohol and other types of substance abuse begins by helping expectant parents develop good parenting skills. It is vitally important that children learn to feel good about themselves early in life. They need adults they can trust and who serve as good role models. As orderly development proceeds, the growing child learns to interact with others and develops a sense of identity. A positive self-image

Text continued on page 394.

Table 20-3 Long-Term Effects, Tolerance, Dependence, Adulteration, and Methods of Administration for Substances Adolescents Abuse

SUBSTANCE	STREET NAME	EFFECTS	HEALTH ISSUES	METHOD OF ADMINISTRATION	TREATMENT	ISSUES
Alcohol	Booze	Sense of well-being, disinhibition, behavioral changes, impaired judgment, incoordination	Peptic ulcers, hepatitis, pancreatitis, fatty liver; damage to developing fetus	Ingestion	Behavioral treatment with psychological and pharmacologic aspects Benzodiazepines (Valium, Librium) are used during first few days to help with withdrawal. Naltrexone (Revia) is used in conjunction with counseling; lessens cravings. Disulfiram (Antabuse) discourages drinking by causing nausea and vomiting when alcohol is used.	Family involvement with treatment is important. Alcoholics Anonymous (AA) for the alcoholic, Al-Anon for spouses or significant others of alcoholics, Alateen for the children of alcoholics
Tobacco (nicotine)		Stimulates central nervous system (CNS), causing sudden release of glucose followed by depression and fatigue	Increase of chronic bronchitis, heart disease, cancer; increased number of stillbirths and prematurity for smoking pregnant women	Inhalation, ingestion (chewing)	Gradual cessation with psychological and pharmacologic support. Nicotine replacement therapies include gum, transdermal patch, nasal spray, and inhalers. Drug Zyban has been approved for use (controls nicotine craving). Future vaccine being developed. Chantix can ease withdrawal symptoms.	Heavily addictive with use; nicotine levels accumulate in body. Tolerance occurs, leading to increased dependency. Leads to preventable cause of death in the United States, and accounts for 7% of total U.S health care costs. Easily available.

Continued

Table 20-3 Long-Term Effects, Tolerance, Dependence, Adulteration, and Methods of Administration for Substances Adolescents Abuse—cont'd

SUBSTANCE	STREET NAME	EFFECTS	HEALTH ISSUES	METHOD OF ADMINISTRATION	TREATMENT	ISSUES
Methamphetamine	Speed, meth, chalk, ice, crystal, glass, beanies	Releases increased level of dopamine, resulting in increased mood and body movement, wakefulness, increased physical activity, decreased appetite	Insomnia, confusion, tremors, memory loss, convulsions, anxiety and aggressive behavior; increased heart rate and blood pressure, leading to strokes; increased hyperthermia; extreme anorexia	Inhalation, snorting, injection, oral	No pharmacologic treatments available at this time. Most effective treatment is cognitive-behavioral interventions, which increase coping mechanisms. Recovery support groups used in adjunct can be effective. Matrix Model is effective and consists of 16 weeks of intensive therapy	
Phencyclidine	Angel dust, ozone, wack, rocket fuel PCP combined with marijuana: killer joints and crystal supergrass	Feelings of strength and power, numbing effect on mind Distorts perception of sight and sound Violent behavior exhibited Muscle incoordination	Psychological effects producing violent or suicidal behavior; increased blood pressure and pulse with decrease in respirations; generalized numbness of extremities; high doses result in seizures, coma, and death; can mimic symptoms of schizophrenia	Inhalation, ingestion, snorting	No specific treatment but inpatient or cognitive-behavioral treatment can be helpful.	Addictive, leading to psychological dependence, craving, and PCP-seeking behavior. Person should be kept in a calm setting and should not be left alone.
Lysergic acid diethylamide	Acid, boomers, yellow sunshine, blotter, dots	Hallucinations, euphoria, rapid mood swings, panic, flashback	Dilated pupils, increased body temperature, increased heart rate and blood pressure, sweating, loss of appetite, sleeplessness, dry mouth, tremors	Ingestion		Effects are unpredictable and depend on amount taken, user's personality, mood, and expectations. Not considered addictive drug because does not produce drug-seeking behaviors.

Continued

3,4-methylene dioxymethamphetamine	Ecstasy, Adam, XTC, X, clarity, lover's speed, love drug, hug, beans	Hallucinations, mental alertness; used to enable individuals to dance for extended periods of time	Confusion, depression, sleep problems, drug cravings, anxiety, paranoia, muscle tension, nausea, sweating, increased heart rate and blood pressure; marked hyperthermia, cardiovascular failure, strokes, and seizures	Ingestion	No specific treatment but cognitive-behavioral treatment can be helpful.	Being used by young adults while attending clubs, raves (large, all-night dance parties), and rock concerts. Developing a rash after use may indicate future liver damage. Can be addictive.
Cocaine, crack	Coke, snow, blow, flake, C, nose candy, rock crank Cocaine or crack with heroin: speedball	Affects brain's key pleasure center by blocking removal of dopamine in synapse, causing a build-up of dopamine and results in pleasurable euphoric effects; feelings of energy; mental alertness; decreased need for sleep or food; bizarre, erratic, or violent behavior	Disturbances in heart rhythm, heart attacks, chest pain, respiratory failure, strokes, seizures and headaches, abdominal pain and nausea	Inhalation, injection, sniffing, snorting	Complex treatment including psychological, social, and pharmacologic aspects. A combination of disulfiram (a medication used with alcoholism) and buprenorphine has been effective at reducing cocaine abuse. Antidepressants have shown some benefit. Behavior treatments have proven effective with residential and outpatient facilities.	One of the oldest drugs used. Two forms: hydrochloride salt (powdered form) and "freebase." Freebase is smokable, and powder is injected or taken ntranasally.

Table 20-3   Long-Term Effects, Tolerance, Dependence, Adulteration, and Methods of Administration for Substances Adolescents Abuse—cont'd

SUBSTANCE	STREET NAME	EFFECTS	HEALTH ISSUES	METHOD OF ADMINISTRATION	TREATMENT	ISSUES
Heroin	Smack, H, skag, junk, Mexican black tar	Euphoria with warm flushing of skin, dry mouth, and heavy extremities, followed by alternating wakeful and drowsy states; mental function becomes clouded with depression of CNS	Cardiac functions slow, respirations severely decreased, collapsed veins, bacterial infections, infection of heart lining and valves, arthritis, rheumatologic problems, HIV	Injection, inhalation, sniffing, snorting	More effective with early intervention. Methadone (synthetic opiate that blocks the effects of heroin and eliminates withdrawal symptoms) has been proven effective. Naloxone and naltrexone are effective as antidotes. Now available is buprenorphine, which does not produce the same level of dependence as methadone; makes discontinuing easier. Available through a physician's office.	Highly addictive. Street heroin is "cut" with other drugs or substances such as sugar, starch, powdered milk, or quinine. Can have strychnine or other poisons included. Strength of heroin or the contents makes overdose or death a high risk.
Marijuana	Reefer, pot, weed, grass, boom, Mary Jane, gangster, chronic, ganja, widow, hash, herb, bubblegum, Northern Lights, fruity juice, Afghani #1	Euphoria, memory and learning problems, distorted perceptions, difficulty thinking or problem solving, increased appetite	Increased heart rate, panic attacks, respiratory problems such as bronchitis, chest colds, coughs, destruction of lung tissue, increased risk for cancer of head, neck, and lungs	Inhalation, ingestion	No specific treatment but cognitive-behavioral treatment can be helpful.	Can be addicting. Most commonly used illicit drug in the United States. Usually smoked as a cigarette (called a *joint* or *nail*) or in a pipe. Can be in a *blunt* (cigar emptied of tobacco and refilled with marijuana or in combination with crack).
Rohypnol	Rophies, roofies, roche, rope, "date rape" drug, forget-me pill	When combined with alcohol, produces a sedative hypnotic state with muscle relaxation and amnesia	Decreased blood pressure, drowsiness, visual disturbances, gastrointestinal disturbances, urinary retention	Ingestion	Hospitalization for detoxification and monitoring withdrawal symptoms since ingestion can be life-threatening	Can produce physical dependence on drug and cause withdrawal seizures. Odorless, colorless, and tasteless. Can be lethal with alcohol.

Drug	Street names	Effects	Health consequences	Route	Treatment	Comments
Gamma-hydroxybutyrate (GHB)	Liquid ecstasy, somatomax, scoop, grievous bodily harm, G, Georgia home boy	Euphoric, sedative effects, body-building effects; withdrawal effects of insomnia, anxiety, tremors, and sweating	Coma, seizures, especially when combined with use of methamphetamine	Ingestion	No specific treatment	Can be used as "date rape" drug in combination with alcohol. May be sold in fitness centers as synthetic steroid. Odorless, colorless, and tasteless.
Steroids (anabolic)	Arnolds, gym candy, juice, pumpers, stackers, weight trainers, roids	Performance-enhancing; designed to mimic the body-building traits of testosterone but minimizes the masculine effects; reports of "feeling good"; wide mood swings from violence to depression; paranoia, irritability, delusions, impaired judgment	Men: reduced sperm count, impotence, baldness, difficulty urinating, enlarged prostate, shrinking testicles, development of breasts. Women: facial hair growth, menstrual changes, deepened voice, breast reduction. Adolescents: premature growth halt. Liver tumors and cancer	Ingestion, injection	Being developed as more is learned about long-term effects. Supportive therapy with education about withdrawal symptoms.	Long-term users experience addiction symptoms of craving, difficulty stopping use, and withdrawal symptoms. Easily obtained on black market.
Inhalants	Butyl nitrite: bolt, bullet, climax, locker room, rush. Amyl nitrite: poppers, snappers. Balloons with nitrous oxide: whippets. Spray paint: Texas shoe shine	Quick excitement followed by drowsiness, disinhibition, staggering, agitation; body is depleted of oxygen, and death can result; heart rate is rapid and erratic	Panic attacks, emotional instability, cardiac arrhythmia, CNS depression, brain damage, liver damage, respiratory arrest; "sudden sniffing death" can occur within minutes of a prolonged session	Inhalation, sniffing, snorting		Are readily available, cheap, and can be purchased legally. Three categories: volatile solvents, nitrites, and anesthetics.

Data from National Institute on Drug Abuse. (2010). NIDA Infofax. Retrieved September 9, 2010, from www.drugabuse.gov.

and feelings of self-worth help adolescents fine-tune their adaptive coping skills. In time, they can rely on their own problem-solving abilities and, it is hoped, will not need chemicals to deal with the complexities of life. Nurses in their various settings can contribute to this process. They can also educate children about the seriousness of substance abuse.

Although it is generally true that problem drinkers cannot be helped unless they want to be, more intervention is now being done. Most adolescents involved in substance abuse do not choose to enter treatment but are coerced by family members or the juvenile justice system. Although this is a controversial issue, clinical experience in substance abuse treatment settings has shown that many adolescents become interested in treatment and make behavioral changes after they have been required to enter a treatment program.

DEPRESSION AND SUICIDE

Suicide is one of the leading causes of death among persons between 15 and 19 years of age. It ranks second as a cause of death for adolescents and college students. The incidence rate increases during spring. Completed suicide is more common among boys than girls, but girls make more attempts. Many adolescent suicides are not intended to be completed but are cries for help. The risk for death increases when there is a definite plan of action, the means are readily available (such as pills or guns), and the person has few resources for help and support. Firearms are the most common means. **Cluster suicide**, which is a situation where one suicide precipitates several others, is becoming more prevalent among adolescents and can be the result of the ideation of suicide.

Signs and Symptoms

Adolescents who do not have socially acceptable ways to express their frustrations may turn their anger and hostility inward. Their self-esteem is low and they feel trapped, rejected, and abandoned. Although each experience is individual, a group of teenagers who had attempted suicide had these common feelings: emptiness and loss, inability to experience pleasure, lack of concentration, confusion, inability to make decisions, and the sense that life lacked meaning and purpose. Physical problems revolved around eating, and sleeping disturbances also occurred. They experienced lack of appetite and insomnia or the reverse, sleeping all day. Hyperactivity was yet another symptom. Behavioral problems surfaced; these included a drop in school grades, truancy, running away, promiscuity, and other forms of acting out. Alcoholism and substance abuse were significant contributing factors, as were the breakdown of family ties and the pressure to succeed. Some felt that their own expectations and those of others significant to them were too high.

? Did You Know?

Risk Factors for Suicide

- Mood disorder
- Disruptive disorder (mostly males)
- Life stressors
- Low level of communication with family
- Maladaptive attribution and coping skills
- Substance abuse
- Family history of suicidal behavior
- Ideation of suicide
- Suicide threats
- Previous suicide attempts

Data from American Academy of Child and Adolescent Psychiatry, 2001.

More than half of suicide attempts are directly preceded by conflict with parents, ranging from misunderstandings to long-term, deep-seated problems. Some teenagers are loners, isolated from their peers and family and unable to communicate their distress. Because the symptoms are difficult to distinguish from healthy adolescent reactions to stress, they may go unrecognized. However, if the manifestations are uncharacteristic and interfere with the person's ability to function on a daily basis, further investigation is imperative. In assessment of the situation, questions to the child must be direct and specific. "Did you ever feel so upset that you wished you were not alive or wanted to die? Did you ever hurt yourself or try to hurt yourself? Are you planning to kill yourself? How? When?" Determine what coping skills the adolescent has used in the past to solve problems. Typically, when a person has a plan there is a much higher chance of the person attempting suicide. If the person has made previous serious suicide attempts, the current suicidal situation should be considered more dangerous. **Never ignore an adolescent who threatens to commit suicide. Assume the adolescent is serious, and act accordingly**.

Treatment and Nursing Care

Treatment is multidimensional. When possible, individual, group, and family therapy are provided in an outpatient setting such as a community mental health agency. Group therapy seems to be especially helpful for adolescents. The adolescent mental health or behavioral unit of a hospital provides a structured environment in which the adolescent can comfortably associate with peers in a positive way. It has the additional advantage of separating the adolescent from stressful surroundings and providing support and protection.

Depression is not always a negative experience. Often it is a reaction to a real or imagined loss. Although it is painful, it can lead to growth (Figure 20-7). The withdrawal accompanying depression is frustrating to

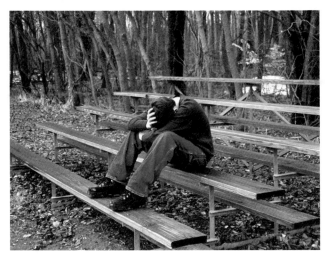

FIGURE 20-7 Adolescents are at risk for depression as they deal with the physical, emotional, and social changes that characterize this developmental stage.

many persons find it difficult to console the grieving family, which carries a heavy burden of guilt, anger, and sorrow. Self-help groups for survivors are available in most cities. The nurse needs assistance in identifying feelings toward children who express suicidal intentions.

It is usually better if the responsibility for a suicidal individual is shared by as many people as possible. A combined effort indicates to the young person that others care and are interested and ready to help. It is also beneficial for the team that their concerns can be discussed and grief can be shared in the event that the suicidal intent is carried out. In the hospital, the nurse is often the person most accessible and least threatening to the adolescent. Frequent, brief visits provide surveillance and also serve to break destructive thought patterns. The nurse must realize how sensitive the adolescent is to other people's reactions and should not add to the adolescent's guilt.

those close to the young person, and they experience a feeling of helplessness. Nevertheless, it is futile to bombard the person with platitudes such as "Cheer up" and "Nothing can be that bad." Instead, the nurse should accept adolescents where they are and help them to look at and externalize their feelings. Ask them how you can help. Remain available to them. Activities that promote physical exercise can provide hostility outlets and are therapeutic. Some days nurses may feel ineffective and need to retreat. However, they should assure the young person that they will return. This helps lessen feelings of desertion. It is important that the nurse keep in touch with his or her feelings to avoid burnout. As teenagers begin to feel more secure, they reach out and progress at their own rate.

Adults are startled and disturbed when a 15-year-old boy or girl takes his or her life. Many adults view adolescence as a carefree time and forget the painful circumstances that surrounded their own young lives. Suicide is unacceptable in Judeo-Christian society, and

Nursing Brief

When a child asks for help or to talk about "a friend" who is talking about suicide, health care providers, parents, or teachers should be alert to the possibility that the child is indirectly talking about his or her own feelings.

Crisis intervention is necessary for acute and repeated episodes. Other voluntary services such as hot lines, drop-in centers, runaway houses, and free clinics focus on the immediate needs of the child and are usually accepted by troubled youngsters. Unfortunately, there are not enough of these resources. Professionals need to be alert for warning signals of destructive behavior so that prompt intervention can be instigated; this might include earlier consideration of placement in a foster home. Community training courses for parenthood are becoming more popular and may provide another means of alleviating the complex problem of teenage suicide.

Get Ready for the NCLEX® Examination!

Key Points

- Early intervention using infant stimulation programs is essential in the care of children who are developmentally disabled.
- Attention deficit/hyperactivity disorder is difficult to establish and many times becomes a "catch-all" diagnosis for children with behavioral problems. Treatment requires a multidisciplinary team approach.
- Trisomy 21 (Down syndrome) is one of the most common forms of chromosomal abnormalities

- Parent-child interactions should be monitored when assessing an infant with failure to thrive.
- Incompatibility between the history and the injury is probably the most important indicator for suspected child abuse.
- Mandatory reporting of suspected child abuse is required for all professionals involved with children.
- Good parent-child relationships that include open communication and parental vigilance with all individuals who interact with their child are necessary to reduce the risk for sexual abuse.

- Families of children with autism need education and support.
- Eating disorders can lead to weight loss and electrolyte imbalances if not recognized and treated.
- Alcohol use, potential drug abuse, and sexual relationships are important issues that should be explored with the adolescent.
- Substance abuse is a serious growing problem in the adolescent population. When counseling the adolescent, the health care worker should be supportive, understanding, and never judgmental.
- Any adolescent who talks about suicide directly or who speaks about a friend who is contemplating suicide should be referred to a health care professional who has expertise with depression and suicide.

Additional Learning Resources

evolve Go to your Evolve website (*http://evolve.elsevier.com/Price/ pediatric/*) for the following FREE learning resources:
- 3-D Animations
- Answer Keys
- Appendixes
- Audio Glossary
- Spanish/English Glossary
- Video Clips

Review Questions for the NCLEX® Examination

1. Attention deficit/hyperactivity disorder (ADHD) refers to specific patterns of behavior that include inattention and impulsivity and might or might not involve hyperactivity. All of the following statements are true regarding ADHD **except:**
   1. Boys are affected more frequently than girls.
   2. There is increased incidence in families, suggesting a genetic etiology.
   3. Affected children usually have an accompanying intellectual disability.
   4. ADHD can lead to decreased self-esteem.

2. The most common type of Down syndrome is a result of:
   1. Heredity
   2. Translocation
   3. Mosaicism
   4. Nondisjunction

3. The highest percentage of child abuse is committed by:
   1. Casual acquaintances
   2. Babysitters
   3. Parents
   4. Relatives

4. Anorexia nervosa is an eating disorder characterized by: (**Select all that apply.**)
   1. Body image disturbance
   2. Dysmenorrhea
   3. Self-imposed starvation
   4. Lack of appetite
   5. Failure to gain expected weight for growth

5. An adolescent is being admitted to a facility to treat substance abuse. The adolescent informs the admitting nurse that he has been using "chalk" for approximately 1 year. The nurse is aware that "chalk" is a street name for:
   1. Heroin
   2. Marijuana
   3. Cocaine
   4. Methamphetamine

Hematology and Oncology Disorders

Objectives

1. Define the vocabulary terms listed
2. Recommend four food sources of iron for an infant with iron-deficiency anemia
3. Discuss how sickle cell disease is inherited
4. Describe the care of hemarthrosis in a child with hemophilia
5. List four symptoms of acute lymphoid leukemia
6. Demonstrate comfort measures for a child undergoing chemotherapy
7. Discuss pre- and postoperative care of a child with Wilms tumor
8. Compare and contrast osteosarcoma and Ewing sarcoma
9. List and describe the four stages of Hodgkin disease

Key Terms

blasts (p. 404)
hemarthrosis (hē-măr-THRŌ-sĭs; p. 408)
infarct (IN-farkt; p. 399)
neoplastic (nē-ə-PLAS-tik; p. 404)

nephroblastoma (NĔF-rō-blăs-TŌ-mă; p. 409)
neutropenic (NŪ-trō-PĒ-nik; p. 407)
thrombosis (thrŏm-BŌ-sĭs; p. 399)
transfusion (tran[t]s-FYÜ-shən; p. 405)

HEMATOLOGY

Hematology is the study of blood and blood-forming tissues. The bone marrow, blood, spleen, and lymph system are included. The red blood cells (erythrocytes), white blood cells (leukocytes), and platelets (thrombocytes) are produced in the bone marrow. The spleen produces red and white blood cells during fetal development; filters red blood cells; and stores lymphocytes, monocytes, and platelets. The lymph system contains the lymph and lymph nodes, which are responsible for fighting infection in the body.

IRON-DEFICIENCY ANEMIA

The most common nutritional deficiency of children in the United States today is anemia caused by insufficient amounts of iron in the body. The incidence rate has decreased in infants because of the use of iron-fortified formulas and cereals. Toddlers and adolescent girls remain at risk because of rapid growth and inadequate iron intake. Anemia (*an*, without; *emia*, blood) is a condition in which there is a reduction in the amount and size of the red blood cells or in the amount of hemoglobin, or both. The clinical features are related to the decrease in the oxygen-carrying capacity of the blood. Iron is needed for the manufacture of red blood cells. Iron-deficiency anemia may be caused by severe hemorrhage, the child's inability to absorb the iron received, rapid growth requirements, or an inadequate dietary intake. It is also known that whole cow's milk

can precipitate gastrointestinal (GI) bleeding in some babies, which, if left unchecked, can lead to anemia.

Prevention of iron-deficiency anemia begins with good prenatal care to ensure that the mother has a suitable intake of iron during pregnancy. For the first few months after birth, the newborn infant relies on iron that was stored during fetal development. Iron is obtained late in the prenatal period, which has an effect on the infant's iron stores. Premature infants can deplete their iron stores by as early as 2 months of age. The normal term infant who receives unfortified formula depletes iron stores by about age 4 months. Breastfed infants should be supplemented with oral iron from 4 months of age until iron-rich foods (e.g., iron-fortified cereals) are introduced (AAP Clinical Report, 2010).

The highest incidence of this type of anemia occurs from 9 to 24 months of age. During this period of rapid growth, the baby outgrows the limited iron reserve that was in the body; in addition, iron-fortified formula and infant cereals may have been eliminated from the diet. Poorly planned meals or feeding problems also contribute to this deficiency. The mother may rely too much on bottle feedings to avoid conflict at meals. Unfortunately, cow's milk contains very little iron. It is important to remember that cow's milk should not be given to children until they are over the age of 1. Instead, the amounts of solid food should be increased and the milk decreased. Boiled egg yolk; liver; green leafy vegetables; iron-fortified cereal; dried fruits (apricots, peaches, prunes, and raisins); cooked, dried beans; crushed nuts; and whole-grain bread are good sources of iron. Iron-fortified cereals eaten out of the box provide a nutritious snack.

Upon diagnosis, the child's hemoglobin level is usually less than 10 g/dL. Children may have much lower hemoglobin levels before they show signs and symptoms. Typically, blood tests are done for hemoglobin, hematocrit, morphological changes in red blood cells, and iron concentration. A dietary history is also important in the diagnosis.

Signs and Symptoms

The symptoms of iron-deficiency anemia are pallor, irritability, anorexia, and a decrease in activity. Many babies are overweight because of excess consumption of milk (so-called *milk babies*). These infants may look pale, and sometimes a slight heart murmur is heard. The spleen may be enlarged. Untreated iron-deficiency anemia progresses slowly. In severe cases, the heart muscle becomes too weak to function. If this happens, heart failure follows. Screening procedures are suggested at 9 to 24 months of age for full-term infants and earlier, at 6 to 9 months of age, for low–birth weight babies.

Treatment and Nursing Care

Iron-deficiency anemia responds well to treatment. The physician must first differentiate it from other types of anemia. The prescribed iron dosage is given orally two or three times a day between meals. Ferrous sulfate is usually prescribed; ferrous fumarate (Feostat) and ferrous gluconate (Fergon) are additional drugs that may be prescribed. Vitamin C aids in the absorption of iron; therefore juice that is enriched with vitamin C or that naturally contains vitamin C is a good choice. Strawberries, tomatoes, and orange slices are also high in vitamin C. Some liquid preparations are taken through a straw to prevent temporary discoloration of the teeth. Teeth brushing after administration of the drug may help also. Calcium interferes with the absorption of iron; therefore milk should not be given during iron supplement administration. Antacids should be avoided as well. Intramuscular iron is given in cases of malabsorption and when noncompliance with the oral route is a problem. Most children can tolerate the oral drug, and parents should be educated about the importance of compliance so the painful injections can be avoided. The injectable drug is an iron-dextran mixture (Imferon) that must be injected deep in a large muscle, with **Z-track technique** to minimize staining and irritation. Postinjection massage is not done with Z-track injections. Follow-up evaluation is important. Treatment with the iron preparation is recommended for 6 to 8 weeks after the laboratory values return to normal levels.

 Nursing Brief

Avoid iron poisoning in children by keeping preparations well out of reach. Educate parents about this hazard.

Parent Education. Parents need explicit instructions regarding the proper foods for the infant or child. The nurse stresses the importance of using iron-fortified formula throughout the first year of life. Whole milk should not be used before 12 months of age. Infants older than 6 months of age receiving formula should not take more than 32 ounces per day. For children older than 1 year of age drinking whole milk, the amount should be less—about 16 to 24 ounces per day. Infants should be started on solid foods by 6 months of age. Review solid food intake, and suggest specific iron-enriched nutrients including rice cereal. Consider financial, ethnic, and family preferences in discussions.

The stools of babies who are taking iron are tarry green in color. Absence of this finding may indicate poor compliance with therapy by the parents. **It is important to emphasize that both dietary changes and supplemental iron therapy are necessary to eradicate iron-deficiency anemia.** Dietary changes may need to be lifelong in order to maintain good health and to prevent recurrence. It is important that parents finish the prescribed medication. The main side effect of iron therapy is constipation. Reinforce to the family and child that if constipation occurs, increase water intake, bulk, and activity as permitted. Parents are encouraged to return for periodic evaluation of the child's blood status. During discussions, nurses should attempt to support parents, who usually have guilt feelings or believe they are not successful parents. It may be comforting for the nurse to reiterate that most babies are in the process of catching up on iron supplies and that the condition is not uncommon.

SICKLE CELL ANEMIA

Sickle cell anemia is one of a group of diseases in which normal Hgb (HgbA) is partly or completely replaced by abnormal sickle Hgb (HbS). Sickle cell disease (SCD) is an inherited defect in the formation of hemoglobin. It occurs mainly in populations of African descent but is also carried by some people of Arabian, Greek, Maltese, and Sicilian descent or other Mediterranean groups. Sickling caused by decreases in blood oxygen may be triggered by dehydration, infection, physical or emotional stress, or exposure to cold. Laboratory examination of the affected child's blood shows that the red blood cell has changed its shape to resemble that of a sickle blade, from which the name of the disorder is derived (Figure 21-1). These cells contain an abnormal form of hemoglobin, termed *hemoglobin* S (the sickling type). The membranes of these cells are fragile and easily destroyed. Their crescent shape makes it difficult for them to pass through

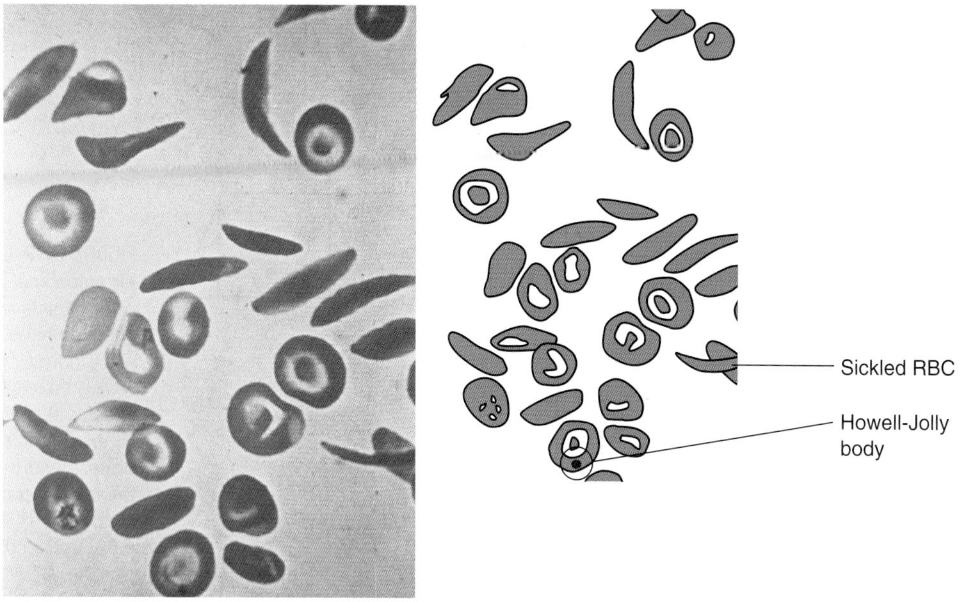

FIGURE 21-1 Peripheral blood smear from a child with hemoglobin with SCD. Note the sickle cells.

the capillaries, causing a pile-up of cells in the small vessels. This clumping together may lead to a thrombosis (clot) and cause an obstruction. Infarcts, or areas of dead tissue, may result when the tissue is denied proper blood supply. These generally develop in the spleen but may also be seen in other areas of the body, such as the brain, heart, lungs, GI tract, kidneys, and bones. The child feels pain in the affected area.

There are two types of sickle cell disorders: an **asymptomatic** (*a,* without; *symptoma,* symptom) version, referred to as **sickle cell trait**, and a much more severe form requiring intermittent hospitalization termed **sickle cell disease**. There are a variety of screening methods. Electrophoresis and high-performance liquid chromatography (HPLC) are most commonly used.

SICKLE CELL TRAIT

This form of the disease occurs in about 10% of the African-American population in the United States. The blood of the child contains a mixture of normal (hemoglobin A) and sickle (hemoglobin S) hemoglobins. The proportions of hemoglobin S are low because the disease is inherited from only one parent. The physician can distinguish sickle cell trait from the more severe form by studying the child's red blood cells and hemoglobin. In sickle cell trait, the hemoglobin and red blood cell counts are normal. Although there is no need for treatment of the mild form, the child is a carrier and genetic counseling is important. Advice might be sought from a family physician, pediatrician, or genetic specialist. The nurse encourages and supports such efforts made by the parents. The importance of regular visits to a well-child clinic or family-centered clinic is stressed.

SICKLE CELL DISEASE

This severe form of the disease results when the child inherits the abnormal gene from each parent (Figure 21-2). **Each offspring** has one chance in four of inheriting the disease (not one of four children). The incidence rate is about 1 in 600 African Americans. The symptoms generally do not appear until the last part of the first year of life, although they may occur as early as 4 months (fetal hemoglobin inhibits sickling). The first symptom may be an unusual swelling of the fingers and toes called **hand-foot syndrome** or **dactylitis** (Figure 21-3). Damage to the kidney can result, affecting the kidney's ability to concentrate urine. This can lead to increased urination in children. Small children with SCD are difficult to toilet-train and may wet the bed for several years. When this is explained to parents as a side effect of the disease, they may be more able to accept the problem. Teenagers and adults with SCD may develop painful, slow-healing ulcers on the lower legs, particularly on the ankles.

Chronic anemia is present, which is why the disease may be referred to as sickle cell anemia. The hemoglobin level ranges from 6 to 9 g/dL or lower. The child is pale, tires easily, and loses appetite. These manifestations of anemia are complicated by what is termed the **sickle cell crisis,** which can be fatal. A number of types of crises have been defined. They differ in pathology and may require somewhat different treatment (Table 21-1). Unfortunately, in some cases, the sickle cell crisis is the first evidence of the condition. For this reason, all 50 states screen all newborn infants. Parents are contacted immediately if there is a positive state screening result. Regularly scheduled health visits, penicillin prophylaxis, and immunizations including

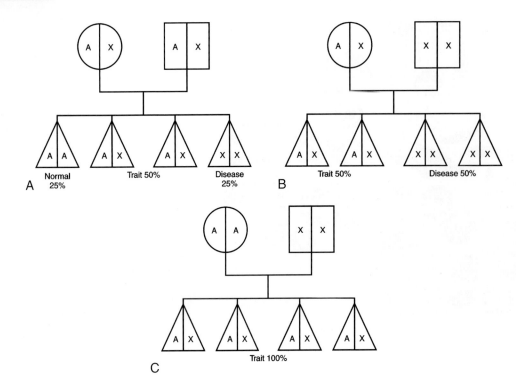

FIGURE 21-2 Inheritance patterns for autosomal genes. **A,** When both parents have a trait, offspring have a 25% chance of being normal, a 25% chance of having the disease, and a 50% chance of having the trait. **B,** When one parent has the disease and the other parent has the trait, offspring have a 50% chance of having the trait and a 50% chance of having the disease. **C,** When one parent has the disease and othe other parent is normal, all offspring will have the trait. *A,* Gene for normal hemoglobin; *X,* gene for abnormal hemoglobin.

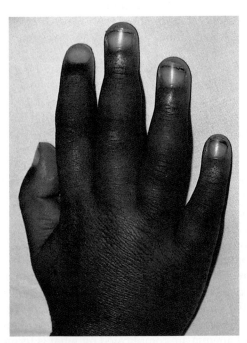

FIGURE 21-3 Hand-foot syndrome (dactylitis) in a 3-year-old child with SCD. This syndrome is primarily seen in infants and toddlers and is less frequent in the older child.

hematuria, convulsions, stiff neck, coma, or paralysis can result, depending on the organs involved. The child may be jaundiced. Cardiac enlargement and murmurs are not uncommon. Priapism is a painful penile erection that occurs in male children, adolescents, and adults. This can be a medical emergency if it is prolonged. According to Pack-Mabien and Haynes (2009), cholelithiasis (formation of gallstones) and retinopathy (disorder of the retina) resulting in blindness are additional complications to monitor for in children with sickle cell disease. The sickle cell crises recur periodically throughout childhood; however, they tend to decrease with age. Between episodes, children should be kept in good health. They should refrain from becoming overly tired. They also should avoid situations such as flying in an unpressurized airplane or exercising at high altitude because oxygen concentrations are already reduced in the blood. Added stress and exposure to cold may lower resistance, causing additional problems. Overheating, which can lead to dehydration, should also be avoided.

influenza, pneumococcal, and meningococcal vaccine should be stressed with the parents.

In a sickle cell crisis, the child appears acutely ill with severe abdominal pain. Muscle spasms, leg pains, or painful swollen joints may be seen. Fever, vomiting,

Nursing Brief

During crises, anticipate a child's need for hydration, rest, protection from infection, pain control, blood transfusions, and emotional support for life-threatening illness.

| Table 21-1 | Summary of Types of Sickle Cell Events | |
TYPE	CHARACTERISTICS	SYMPTOMS
Vaso-occlusive crisis	Most common; not life threatening; obstruction of circulation; resulting in ischemia, necrosis, and infarctions	Pain, fever, dactylitis, bone and joint pain, abdominal pain, cardiovascular accident, priapism
Acute chest syndrome	Pulmonary infarcts	Chest pain, cough, fever, hypoxia, tachypnea
Dactylitis (hand-foot syndrome)	Infarction of short tubular bones, self-limiting, occurs in children 6 months to 4 years of age	Localized swelling of hands and feet
Acute splenic sequestration	Acute, episodic, even when, for unknown reasons, blood pools in the spleen, which can result in life-threatening circulatory collapse and death; commonly preceded by acute febrile illness	Enlarged spleen, pallor, irritability, weakness, dyspnea, tachycardia, hypotension
Aplastic episodes	Diminished production of red blood cells, usually caused by viral or bacterial infection	Pallor, lethargy, faintness, anemia

Treatment and Nursing Care

When the infant or child is hospitalized during a crisis, the treatment is supportive and symptomatic. The child is often confined to bed. Heat is soothing, but cold is not used because it causes sickling and vasoconstriction. Oxygen is used short term with respiratory difficulty; however, it is not used routinely or long term with SCD. Blood transfusions may be given for anemia, but they must be given conservatively to avoid iron overload. If iron overload becomes a problem, **chelation therapy** with desferrioxamine is begun. Antimicrobials are given to all children with fever. Infection is the most common risk for infants with SCD, and this has prompted many practitioners to use penicillin prophylactically. Starting at 2 months of age, this preventive therapy has significantly reduced both morbidity and mortality from pneumococcal infections and streptococcal pneumonia. Fluid intake is increased above the maintenance level for the child's age. Analgesics are given for relief of pain. Children in a severe pain crisis should receive a continuous intravenous narcotic infusion, and morphine is the drug of choice. Meperidine (Demerol) is not routinely prescribed for children.

The nurse observes the overall appearance of the child and assesses the developmental stage, body proportions, and the relation of height and weight to age. Facial expressions, degree of restlessness, and areas of pain are noted and recorded. Signs and symptoms that may be observed and require immediate attention are signs of dehydration possibly detected by an elevated temperature; a rapid, weak pulse; a sunken fontanel in infants younger than 18 months of age; weight loss; poor tissue turgor; dry skin, lips, and mucous membranes; and a decrease in urination. If vomiting occurs, appropriate oral hygiene is provided. The nurse observes and records infusions according to unit policy. An accurate record of intake and output is kept. Careful attention is given to the skin. Jaundice (icterus) can be detected by observing whether the skin (palms and soles) and the whites of the eyes have taken on a yellowish tinge. The child's body position is changed gently due to the pain in the joints.

Because SCD can affect muscle tone, any rigidity of the muscles should be reported. Observe eye movements, swallowing, or sucking. Note whether the child is uncomfortable when the neck is flexed to have the gown changed. Watch for twitching in the face or elsewhere.

Neurologic complications such as stroke, hemiparesis, transient ischemic attack (TIA), or seizures are possible. Children should be monitored regularly. The transcranial Doppler (TCD) is effective in screening for increased blood velocity and narrowing of cerebral vessels and should be done yearly.

The prognosis is guarded. Death may result from severe anemia or secondary infection. Pregnancy may increase mortality. There is also an increased likelihood of miscarriage, premature births, and stillbirths in women with SCD. Ideally, all African-American women should be screened for the disease before pregnancy. The sickling test (Sickledex) is commonly used for screening purposes.

Surgery. The approach to splenectomy in children with SCD has been conservative. Recurrence of acute splenic sequestration becomes less likely after 5 years of age. Routine splenectomy is not recommended because the spleen generally atrophies on its own because of fibrotic changes that take place in children with SCD. However, splenectomy is indicated in selected children with multiple splenic events. Because no form of prophylaxis is foolproof and because the duration of treatment is controversial, the child should continue to be carefully observed for signs of infection. Parents should be educated on how to palpate for an enlarged spleen and monitor for signs of infections (fever).

Before elective surgery, a sickle cell screening test should be performed on all African-American children because general anesthesia places these persons at greater risk for hypoxia. With the stress of surgery and hypoxia from anesthesia, a sickle cell crisis can be precipitated.

Medication. The FDA has designated the use of hydroxyurea, an antineoplastic drug, for the palliative treatment of SCD in adults. This drug increases the production of hemoglobin F (HbF; fetal hemoglobin). HbF has a higher affinity for oxygen. Erythropoietin, which stimulates the production of red blood cells, may be used to enhance the effects of hydroxyurea. A reduction in episodes of painful vaso-occlusive crisis, fewer hospitalizations, and fewer blood transfusions have been seen. Because this is an antineoplastic drug and could possibly result in mutation of genes, child-bearing issues must be considered. Trials have been done with children between 5 and 15 years of age. These studies have positive results, but hydroxyurea use in children should be supervised by a pediatric hematologist (Hilliard and Howard, 2006).

New advances with **stem cell transplantation** have produced exciting results for the child with SCD. Ongoing investigation is continuing with stem cell and umbilical cord blood transplantation.

HEMOPHILIA

Hemophilia is one of the oldest hereditary diseases known. It has been called "the disease of kings" because of its occurrence in children of several royal families in Russia and Western Europe. In hemophilia, the blood does not clot normally, and even the slightest injury can cause severe bleeding. The clotting disorder is the result of a deficiency in specific blood clotting factors. A sex-linked genetic pattern causes most cases of hemophilia, although it can *rarely* occur with no family history of the disease. Most hemophiliacs are male. Affected males inherit the bleeding disorder from their mothers, who are the carriers. It is possible to determine the level of factor VIII in the blood with a test called the **partial thromboplastin time (PTT).** This aids in the diagnosis and assessment of the child's condition. Women who are carriers and affected fetuses can be identified.

Two types of hemophilia constitute the highest incidence of the disorder. Factor VIII deficiency, or hemophilia A, is approximately four times more common than factor IX deficiency, hemophilia B. For our purposes, this discussion is limited to classic hemophilia, or hemophilia A, which accounts for about 80% of cases.

The severity of hemophilia A depends on the level of factor VIII in the plasma of the child's blood. Hemophilia is classified as severe, moderate, or mild. In mild hemophilia, bleeding is usually only a problem after surgery or major trauma. The child with moderate hemophilia can expect bleeding episodes after trauma. Children with severe hemophilia may bleed without apparent cause. The degree of severity tends to remain constant within a given family.

Signs and Symptoms

Hemophilia often is not apparent in the newborn infant unless abnormal bleeding occurs at the umbilical cord, at sites of initial injections, or after circumcision. As the child grows older and becomes more subject to injury, the slightest bruise or cut can induce extensive bleeding. Normal blood clots in about 3 to 6 minutes. In a child with severe hemophilia, the time necessary for clotting may be an hour or more. Anemia, leukocytosis, and a moderate increase in platelets may be seen in the hemorrhaging child, who may show signs of shock. Hematuria is occasionally seen. Parents may notice that it takes a long time to stop bleeding from a cut. Death can result from excessive bleeding anywhere in the body but particularly when hemorrhage occurs into the brain or neck.

An injured knee, elbow, or ankle presents particular problems because of hemorrhage into the joint cavity (hemarthrosis) and is a cardinal sign in children with hemophilia. The earliest joint hemorrhages appear most commonly in the ankle, from instability of this joint as the toddler assumes an upright posture. Many children with severe hemophilia develop a "target" joint where repetitive bleeding episodes occur (Kliegman et al., 2007). The affected joint is stiff, warm, red, and swollen. Joint limitation occurs. Repeated hemorrhages may cause permanent deformities that could disable the child.

Treatment and Nursing Care

The mechanism of blood formation is complex. Defects in the synthesis of protein may lead to deficiencies in any of the factors in blood plasma needed for clotting to occur. The treatment of each type of hemophilia consists of replacing the deficient factor to ensure clotting. The nursing care for all types is similar.

The child's family history is of particular importance in the diagnosis of hemophilia. When hemophilia is present in the family and the child has had periods of abnormal bleeding from early childhood, the determination is relatively easy. However, in many cases the family history may be vague or unobtainable. In some instances, even careful scrutiny produces no evidence of the disease in the family.

Visible bleeding is treated immediately with the application of a cold pack and continuous, firm pressure. When possible, elevate the area above heart level to decrease blood flow. Parents should have ice packs available at all times. Nosebleeds can be controlled by tilting the head forward and applying firm pressure to the nose for 15 to 30 minutes. A nasal pack may be necessary. Mouth bleeding is usually minor, but if it cannot be controlled, an antifibrinolytic agent such as Amicar may be used to promote clot formation.

Hemarthrosis occurs most frequently in the knees, elbows, and ankles. Regardless of its location, the deficient factor should be given and the joint immobilized. Bleeding is also treated with rest, ice, compression, and elevation of the affected part (RICE). Cold packs are applied to decrease the pain, and analgesics such as acetaminophen can be given as ordered. Aspirin and nonsteroidal antiinflammatory drugs (NSAIDs), such as ibuprofen, should be avoided because they have a depressive effect on platelet function. The joint might be placed in a splint for immobilization. Therapy for muscle injuries is essentially the same. When the bleeding has ceased, the child can begin active exercises under the supervision of the physical therapist.

🔄 Nursing Brief

Instruct parents of the child with hemophilia to avoid medications that inhibit platelet function, such as aspirin and ibuprofen. Explain the importance of contacting a physician or pharmacist before giving any over-the-counter drugs to the child.

Current treatment of hemophilia includes the administration of highly purified or recombinant factor VIII concentrates to treat bleeding episodes or anticipated bleeding episodes (surgery, tooth extraction). These concentrates are in powder form and may be kept at room temperature or in the refrigerator. They are reconstituted with sterile water before IV administration. In the past, the risk for hepatitis and HIV was high in this population because concentrates were made from a pool of as many as 20,000 blood donors and were not adequately treated to eliminate viruses. Careful screening of blood donors and new techniques to make concentrate have reduced the risk for children newly diagnosed with hemophilia. Treatment ranges from four times a week (preventive regime) to three times a month.

Parents can be taught at home how to administer the factor VIII concentrate to their child. Home care and management of bleeding episodes have improved the prognosis and quality of life for children with hemophilia. The newer treatment options have also reduced the cost of treatment and decreased the risk for psychological trauma for the child. Detailed teaching is done by the physician and nurse in a specialty clinic. Instruction includes an exact explanation of the illness, with emphasis on the signs and treatment of any active bleeding. Specific procedures taught include the storage and preparation of replacement factors, venipuncture, transfusion management and possible reactions, and record keeping. Signs of complications are reviewed, and emergency numbers and other protocols are spelled out. One advantage of home treatment is its immediate availability. The earlier hemarthrosis is treated, the less severe the consequences. The goal is for the child to become independent and for the health care center to be available as a backup when a need arises. Older school-age children are able to learn self-care. Many children learn more about their disease at hemophilia camp.

Desmopressin (DDAVP) has been found to increase factor VIII levels in children with hemophilia. The increase is not enough to manage hemarthrosis or severe bleeding episodes, but it can be used to treat mild hemophilia. It is less expensive and less invasive than administration of factor VIII concentrate.

Preventing bleeding episodes is an important part of comprehensive care. When the child with hemophilia is an infant, the crib sides require padding and all toys must be checked for sharp edges. Active toddlers and preschoolers need a safe environment and close supervision in which to practice newly learned gross-motor skills. The use of protective equipment such as helmet and joint padding is essential for active children. The older child should avoid contact sports and other activities that have a high risk for injury. Swimming is an excellent competitive sport that also helps strengthen muscles and maintain joint mobility. Walking and bicycle riding are also good ways to exercise. An active, regular exercise program is beneficial. Strong muscles support joints and reduce the numbers of bleeds.

The nurse should teach the parent to carefully observe the skin at bath time for bruises or hematomas. The child's nails should be kept short. Good oral hygiene is essential. Select a toothbrush with soft bristles. The dentist needs to be consulted early in the preschool years to establish a program of preventive oral health.

The child needs well-balanced meals. Excessive weight gain should be avoided because it places additional strain on the joints. A regular exercise program strengthens muscles surrounding the joints, thus decreasing the potential for tissue injury. If the child is receiving medication via injection, or if blood work has been ordered, pressure is applied to the site immediately afterward. The site is carefully observed by the parent or nurse to ensure that all is well. The child's stools and urine are observed for blood. Vital signs are taken routinely to detect concealed bleeding. Children and adolescents are instructed to wear a Medic Alert bracelet. All children should receive routine childhood immunizations as recommended (see the Appendix on Evolve for more on immunizations).

🔄 Nursing Brief

Consult the child's physician regarding immunizations and intramuscular injections as these can cause bleeding into the muscle.

Having a child with hemophilia is a challenge to the family. The family needs to create a positive environment that allows the child to be as independent as possible. It is natural for parents to be overprotective. Parents need to understand that they can create a safe environment while still allowing the child to develop his or her full capabilities. The National Hemophilia Foundation *(www.hemophilia.org)* is a resource for financial, psychological, and medical support for the family. Research is currently under way to try to find a cure for hemophilia. Gene therapy is one promising area that continues to be explored.

ONCOLOGY

Oncology is the study of cancer. Neoplastic disorders are the leading cause of death from disease in children older than 1 year of age. Almost half of all childhood cancers involve the blood or blood-forming organs (Hockenberry and Wilson, 2009). Table 21-2 lists several childhood cancers.

LEUKEMIA

Leukemia *(leuko,* white; *emia,* blood) is a malignant disease of the blood-forming organs of the body that results in an uncontrolled growth of immature white blood cells (WBCs). There are several types of WBCs. Many are produced in the bone marrow; others are produced in the spleen and lymph nodes. The immature cells are called blasts *(blastos,* germ or formative cell). About 80% of childhood cases are **acute lymphoid leukemia (ALL),** 15% to 20% are **acute myelogenous leukemia (AML);** remaining types are rare. The survival rate of ALL is around 85%.

Generally speaking, the child's prognosis is most clearly related to age at diagnosis and initial WBC count, which could range from 50,000 to as high as 100,000 cells/mm3. In some cases, the overall WBC count is normal but the differential count may show a predominance of blast cells. The pathology of the disease comes from its ability to infiltrate and compete for metabolic elements. The reticuloendothelial system (liver, spleen, lymph glands) is most severely affected.

Other important factors include the structure of the leukemic cells **(morphology),** their reaction to different chemical agents **(cytochemistry),** their genetic makeup **(cytogenetics),** and the type of cell-surface antigens they exhibit **(immunological markers).** A classification system that identifies three major subtypes of ALL on the basis of morphology and cytochemistry (L_1 to L_3) is called the French-American-British (FAB) system. The classification of childhood leukemia has aided in the identification of prognostic factors and methods of treatment (Table 21-3).

The incidence rate of leukemia is highest in children between 3 and 4 years of age, and the disease is more common in boys than in girls. The cause of the disease is unknown. Research on the relationship of viruses to leukemia is under way. There also seems to be a genetic correlation because the incidence rate of leukemia is higher in children with Down syndrome and in twins. Investigators have associated leukemia with disorders of the immune mechanism of the body.

All tissues of the body are affected, either by direct infiltration of cancer cells or by the change in the

Table 21-2   Childhood Cancers

TYPE	DISCUSSION
Leukemia	Leukemia is the most common form of cancer in children. Acute lymphoid leukemia (ALL) is the overproduction of immature lymphocytes. ALL is the most common leukemia of childhood. Acute myelogenous leukemia (AML) is cancer of the bone marrow; it affects a group of white blood cells called the myeloid cells, which normally develop into the various types of mature blood cells, such as red blood cells, white blood cells, and platelets. It is less common than ALL.
Lymphoma	Hodgkin lymphoma originates in the lymphoid system and primarily involves the lymph nodes. Non-Hodgkin lymphoma occurs more frequently in children than Hodgkin lymphoma. It is a group of malignant tumors of B or T lymphocytes.
Wilms tumor	Nephroblastoma; the most common malignant renal and intraabdominal tumor of childhood.
Brain tumors	Most common solid tumors in children; second most common childhood cancer. Includes astrocytoma, medulloblastoma, glioma, and others.
Bone tumors	Osteosarcoma is the most common (malignant) bone cancer in children. Ewing sarcoma is the second most common malignant bone tumor in childhood. It originates in the shaft of long and trunk bones.
Neuroblastoma	Second most common solid tumor of childhood. Neuroblastoma arises from the neural crest cells that normally develop into the sympathetic nervous system and the adrenal medulla.
Rhabdomyosarcoma	Malignancy of the muscle; most common soft tissue malignancy in children.
Retinoblastoma	Rare, malignant tumor of the retina; found only in children. Presents with a white reflection (leukokoria) of the eye instead of the normal red reflection in photographs.

Table 21-3	Some Prognostic Features of ALL in Children		
PROGNOSTIC FACTOR	**POSITIVE PROGNOSIS**	**LESS POSITIVE PROGNOSIS**
Age at diagnosis	1-10 yr	<2 or >10 yr
Initial WBC count	<100,000/mm^3	>100,000/mm^3
Morphology	L1	L2 or L3
Immunologic surface markers	Pre–B-cell with CALLA	T-cell or B-cell
Cytogenetics	>50 chromosomes per cell	Presence of chromosome translocations
Other	Absent mediastinal mass or CNS involvement at diagnosis	Presence of mediastinal mass or CNS involvement at diagnosis

ALL, Acute lymphoblastic leukemia; *CALLA,* common acute lymphocytic leukemia antigen; *CNS,* central nervous system; *WBC,* white blood cell.

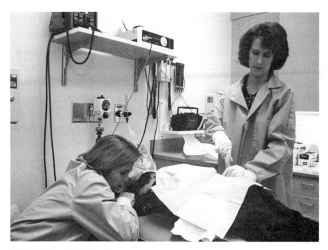

FIGURE 21-4 Child with leukemia undergoing a bone marrow aspiration.

circulating components in the blood. Because leukemia affects the bone marrow, there is also a reduction in the number of red blood cells (RBCs), which leads to anemia. In addition, the platelet count is reduced, increasing the risk of hemorrhage. Intracranial bleeding, if it occurs, can cause immediate death. Hemorrhage from other vital organs may occur. Bone and joint pain are experienced because of increased pressure within the bone marrow as blast cells continue to be produced. Physiologic fractures may also occur.

Leukemia that occurs outside the bone marrow is referred to as **extramedullary.** The most common sites for this to occur are the central nervous system (CNS) and the testicles. More cases of extramedullary leukemia are being seen because children with leukemia are surviving longer.

Signs and Symptoms

The most common symptoms during the initial phase of the illness are low-grade fever, pallor, a tendency to bruise, leg and joint pain, listlessness, and enlargement of the lymph nodes (see Critical Thinking Question and Critical Thinking Snapshot on p. 409). Abdominal pain, often attributed to other illnesses or even constipation, is a common symptom of leukemia. These symptoms may develop gradually or may be sudden in onset. As the disease progresses, the liver and spleen become enlarged. **Petechiae** (pinpoint hemorrhagic spots beneath the skin) and **purpura** (hemorrhage into the skin) may be early objective symptoms. Anorexia, vomiting, weight loss, and dyspnea are also common. The kidneys and testicles may become enlarged, and hematuria may develop.

Because the WBCs are not functioning normally, bacteria easily invade the body. Strict attention must be paid to infection control. Anemia becomes severe despite transfusions. The child may die as a direct result of the disease or of secondary infection. The symptoms are the same regardless of the type of WBC affected, yet they vary widely with each child, depending on the parts of the body involved.

Diagnosis

The diagnosis of leukemia is made on the basis of the health history, symptoms of the child, and the results of extensive blood tests that show the presence of leukemic blast cells in the blood, bone marrow, or other tissues. Because the bone marrow is where many WBCs and RBCs are formed, bone marrow is aspirated from the sternum or iliac crest with a special needle (Figure 21-4) and studied in the laboratory. Chest radiographs may also show a mediastinal mass. After the diagnosis is confirmed, a spinal tap determines if there is any CNS involvement. Kidney and liver function studies are also performed because normal function of these organs is absolutely necessary for chemotherapy to be used in treating the disease.

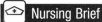 **Nursing Brief**

Repeated blood tests, especially in infants and small children with anemia, can deplete blood volume, which can lead to hypoxia and shock unless the withdrawn blood is replaced.

Treatment

The development of specific chemotherapeutic agents for treatment of ALL has changed the survival time significantly. In most cases of ALL, it is now possible to induce remissions (no evidence of leukemic cells), which are sustained for prolonged periods even after therapy is discontinued. Other varieties of leukemia show a less predictable response to therapy. Untreated leukemia results in death from infection or hemorrhage in about 6 months. Treatment of ALL consists of three phases: (1) induction, (2) consolidation, (3) and maintenance, which serves to maintain the remission phase. Therapy directed at the central nervous system is a part of each treatment plan (Burg et al., 2006).

The goal of induction therapy is to induce remission and restore normal hematopoiesis. This phase usually lasts 28 days. Chemotherapy drugs include glucocorticoids, vincristine, and l-asparaginase. Consolidation is a period of intensified therapy that uses drugs based on protocol. Methotrexate is frequently used. Maintenance is less intensive chemotherapy and includes methotrexate and 6-mercaptopurine (Burg et al., 2006).

Chemotherapy. Glucocorticoids such as prednisone have the side effects of masking the symptoms of infection, increasing fluid retention, inducing personality changes, and causing the child's face to appear moonshaped. Methotrexate is useful in maintaining remission because it acts against chemicals vital to the life of the WBC. These powerful medications produce side effects of varying degrees, such as nausea, diarrhea, rash, hair loss (alopecia), fever, anuria, anemia, and bone marrow depression. Peripheral neuropathy may be signaled by severe constipation resulting from decreased nerve supply to the bowel. Footdrop and difficulty with coordination may be seen. These complications are typically reversed once the offending drug is discontinued. The nurse should consult a pharmacology text for information on the particular drugs used for the child to anticipate potential problems.

Intrathecal chemotherapy is given for CNS prophylaxis. All children with leukemia are at risk for invasion of the CNS by the leukemic cells. Because medications cannot cross the blood-brain barrier to affect the CNS, chemotherapeutic agents must be injected directly into the spinal fluid through a lumbar puncture.

> **Nursing Brief**
>
> Nurses that administer chemotherapy receive special education and training in order to safely perform this procedure.

The various drugs used in treating leukemia may be given in cycles. Antimicrobials are administered to prevent or control infection, and transfusions of whole blood or packed cells are given to correct anemia. Sedatives necessary for the child's comfort are also administered. A pain reliever such as acetaminophen, codeine, or morphine may be ordered if the disease worsens. Medications should be administered before the pain becomes too severe. Pain control is discussed in Chapter 2.

Bone Marrow Transplants and Immunotherapy. Bone marrow transplantation is not recommended for children with ALL during the first remission because of the excellent prognosis with chemotherapy. However, it is a consideration for children with AML during their first remission and for children with ALL who have had a relapse and are in their second remission. Improvements in transplantation and supportive care, which involve specialized nursing care, have increased the number of long-term survivors of this procedure.

Immunotherapy, although still in the research stages, is another area of therapeutics. Immunotherapy may be passive or active, specific or nonspecific. The main goals of treatment are to strengthen the immune response of the child to cancer cells and, it is hoped, to prevent cancer with use of immunization.

Nursing Care
The child with acute leukemia has many needs, both physical and psychological. These vary in intensity according to exacerbations and progression of the disease. The diagnosis has such an impact on the child's family members that they are unable to focus on anything other than the child and the illness. Suppression of their own needs mounts if the disease is prolonged and can lead to illness and marital strain. Support groups, such as those provided by Ronald McDonald House and various hospice programs, aid parents in expressing and examining their concerns and give both the child and the family freedom to hurt but still remain whole.

Children's anxieties often center on their symptoms. They fear that the treatments necessary to correct their problems may be painful, as indeed some of them are (e.g., venipunctures, bone marrow aspirations, blood transfusions). Their trust in others is in precarious balance. It is important that nurses inform preschoolers of what they are about to do and why it is necessary. Child life specialists are excellent at explaining procedures to children and allowing them to "play" through their feelings (see Chapter 2). All explanations should be given honestly and in terms children can understand.

> **Communication**
>
> It may be the nurse of whom the child asks the inevitable question, "Am I going to die?" One suggested response is to reply with a question, such as "Why do you think you may be dying?" This may encourage the child to verbalize feelings.

The pediatric nurse who gives a child permission to discuss concerns finds opportunities to clear up misconceptions and decrease the child's feelings of isolation. The element of hope is conveyed and it is indispensable to continued functioning, although the nature of hope may change from that of being cured to that of additional time to live. Further information on holistic care of the dying child is discussed in Chapter 22.

Preventing Infection. As previously mentioned, upon diagnosis, induction therapy is begun. The goal is to reduce the number of leukemic cells and, preferably, to eradicate them. Careful explanations should be given to the child and family before any procedure is initiated. The disease and many of the necessary medications cause myelosuppression, which depresses the normal function of the bone marrow in addition to destroying cancer cells. The child becomes anemic, may hemorrhage, and is highly susceptible to infection, even from normally harmless environmental flora. Some of the organisms that may be hazardous to the child with leukemia are listed in Table 21-4. The choice of medication used to combat these infections varies according to the causative organism and the drug to which it is most likely to be sensitive. When fever occurs, broad-spectrum antimicrobials are begun until the offending agent is identified. Septra or Bactrim is administered to prevent the development of *Pneumocystis carinii* pneumonia, which is life threatening. WBC transfusions may also be used.

In most hospitals, children are placed in a private room for their own protection. The nurse limits visitors and any auxiliary or medical personnel who appear unhealthy. All persons must meticulously adhere to proper hand hygiene techniques. Teaching parents concurrently helps prepare them for home care—that is, protecting the child from other children with communicable diseases, using proper hand hygiene techniques, and so on. Fresh flowers or plants are not permitted if the child is neutropenic, because of bacteria they can harbor. The nurse explains to the child the purpose for the various procedures used.

Observe the child frequently for signs of infection. Particular attention should be paid to potentially infected sites, such as the child's mucous membranes and puncture breaks in the skin from laboratory or therapeutic procedures. Exudates from infection (pus) typically do not form if WBC counts are low, so it is important to observe frequently for subtle signs of inflammation and fever. Ulcerations develop about the mucous membranes of the mouth and anal region, and both have a tendency to bleed (Figure 21-5). Chemotherapy attacks all rapidly growing cells, and the skin and gastrointestinal system are both ordinarily composed of rapidly growing cells. Vital signs are observed for subtle variances because steroid therapy may mask these indicators. Turn the child often and observe for skin breakdown, particularly in the perianal area. Offer nutritious meals and supplemental feedings high in protein and calories. Teach parents and the child what to look for and to report. Chickenpox and other communicable diseases can be a particular hazard to the immunocompromised child. **Varicella zoster immune globulin (VZIG)** is given within 96 hours of an exposure to chickenpox if the child has not yet had the disease or the vaccine. Open communication among the school nurse, family, clinic nurse, and physician is paramount.

Managing Bleeding. Thrombocytopenic bleeding is a frequent complication of leukemia. The nurse observes the child's skin for petechiae and ecchymosis. Nosebleeds are common and are treated with application of cold and pressure.

The mouth is inspected daily for ulcerations and hemorrhage from the gums. Alcohol-based mouthwashes, milk of magnesia, hydrogen peroxide, and lemon glycerin swabs should be avoided. Administer antifungal drugs as ordered to prevent dissemination in immunosuppressed children. A Water Pik is helpful in massaging and toughening the gums. A soft sponge toothbrush is helpful. If the platelet count is low, the nurse may also gently clean food particles from the child's teeth with a piece of gauze wrapped around the gloved finger. Apply lip balm or petroleum jelly to dry, cracked lips.

Hemorrhagic cystitis is not uncommon because some drugs irritate the mucosa of the bladder. The

Table 21-4	Some Infectious Agents Hazardous to the Child with Leukemia

TYPE	ORGANISM
Bacterial	*Pseudomonas, E. coli, S. aureus, Klebsiella, Proteus*
Viral	*Cytomegalovirus*, varicella-zoster (chickenpox)
Protozoan	*P. carinii*
Fungal	*Candida albicans*, Histoplasma

NOTE: Overwhelming infection can lead to death in children with leukemia. The possibility of infection is high during induction therapy, immediately after radiation therapy, and during maintenance.

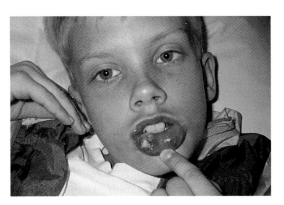

FIGURE 21-5 Mucositis (inflammation of the mucous membranes) and mouth ulcers are common side effects of chemotherapeutic drugs. Any mucous membrane can be affected.

nurse should be alert to child complaints of burning on urination or feelings of pressure, which may indicate infection. Attention is given to providing plenty of fluids and encouraging frequent voidings. The physician is notified of complications immediately so that proper adjustment in medications can be made.

The nurse observes the child for gastrointestinal bleeding. This is evidenced by **hematemesis** (bloody vomiting) and bloody or tarry stools. Hemarthrosis, or effusion of blood into a joint cavity, may develop. This makes moving about painful; therefore nursing intervention is necessary for the comfort of the child whether in or out of bed. Ensuring that the environment is free from hazards is also of importance. Emergency procedures for control of bleeding are reviewed with the child and the parents or caregiver.

Transfusions. Platelets and packed RBCs may be given to children with anemia and thrombocytopenia (decrease in platelets in blood). Hemolytic reactions caused by mismatched blood are rare. Nevertheless, the **registered** nurse should positively identify donor and recipient blood types and groups on labels and the child's chart with another professional. While the **registered** nurse initially sets up the blood transfusion (check hospital policy regarding use of a pump), the licensed practical/vocational nurse can monitor the transfusion and inform the charge nurse if any reaction occurs. Transfusions with piggyback setups are preferred. Blood is administered with **normal saline** before and after the infusion; it is also administered **slowly**. The child is observed for signs of transfusion reaction, which include chills, itching, rash, fever, headache, and pain in the back or elsewhere. If such reactions occur, **the tubing is clamped immediately and the charge nurse and physician are notified**. When blood must be stopped, tube patency can be maintained by opening the saline line. Necessary emergency medications can also be administered. If a reaction occurs, save the blood bag, tubing, and return them along with any required documentation to the blood bank. Most transfusion reactions occur within the first 10 minutes of administration; nevertheless, the child is carefully monitored throughout this treatment. Save subsequent voiding of urine for hemoglobin determination if policy dictates.

Circulatory overload is always a danger with children. Dyspnea, precordial pain, rales, cyanosis, dry cough, and distended neck veins are indicative of this complication. Apprehension can also be a warning signal of air emboli or electrolyte disturbance. The nurse must maintain a high level of alertness for such signs, particularly in children whose conditions warrant repeated transfusions.

Establish baseline data (temperature, pulse, respiration, and blood pressure [BP]) before transfusion, and monitor for changes. Always follow hospital or institution policy for blood or blood product administration. It is helpful if the parents can remain with the child during this time. Suitable diversions minimize boredom.

Tumor Lysis Syndrome

Tumor lysis syndrome often occurs in children with leukemias, lymphomas, and large solid tumors (Kliegman et al., 2007). This condition occurs when tumor cells are **lysed** or killed and the intracellular contents are dumped into the extracellular fluid. Intensive hydration with IV fluid containing bicarbonate alkalinizes the urine to help prevent uric acid formation, which damages the kidney. Oral allopurinol is also administered to decrease the uric acid level. The urine often turns milky white. Kidney failure can result if the condition is not closely monitored; careful recording of intake and output is critical.

Additional Nursing Care Considerations

- **Elimination.** Constipation is a common side effect of chemotherapy. Special care to promote normal bowel patterns is essential. Encouraging extra fluids and fiber foods is beneficial. Stool softeners may be necessary. Straining can increase the risk for bleeding.
- **Skin and hair care.** The skin should be bathed daily and whenever necessary. Thoroughly assess the skin for signs of petechiae and bruising. The rectal mucosa should be evaluated for fissures and ulcerations. Gently cleansing after each bowel movement is important. Avoid use of a rectal thermometer to prevent injury to the anal mucosa. Sitz baths promote relaxation and may lessen discomfort.
  - The child's hair is combed daily and whenever necessary. Hair loss (**alopecia**) from drug therapy is not unusual. Psychological preparation of the child and family lessens its impact. Hair returns in 3 to 6 months; meanwhile a wig or hat suitable to the child's preference and age may be worn.
  - **Skin breakdown.** Repositioning of the child is necessary to promote circulation and avoid the development of decubitus ulcers. Bone pain can be acute, and, whenever possible, coordinating administration of pain relievers with posture change is helpful. The child should be handled gently. A beanbag chair, a waterbed, or a flotation mattress may be used for comfort. Physical therapy can help prevent footdrop caused by peripheral neuropathy.
- **Nausea and vomiting.** One of the more undesirable side effects of chemotherapy in children is vomiting. In addition to monitoring the child for signs of dehydration, the nurse should administer antiemetic medications as ordered during chemotherapy. Nonpharmacologic approaches for pain control

discussed in Chapter 2 can also be implemented to manage nausea and vomiting. Maintaining IV fluids as prescribed ensures appropriate hydration.

- **Nutrition.** The child should be served well-balanced meals consisting of preferred foods. Because food may not be appealing to children with leukemia, nurses must use their ingenuity to interest them. Mealtimes should be kept pleasant. The companionship of a nurse or attendant is preferable. The nurse should note individual preferences and report them to the dietitian. Food from home may be relished. When the child is too tired or irritable to eat, between-meal feedings are given. When parents understand this, they are less anxious about what the child consumes at a particular meal. Steroid therapy often increases the appetite, which is heartening but temporary. High-calorie commercial foods are tasty and can be used as an adjunct. A low-salt diet may be ordered during chemotherapy cycles that include prednisone to reduce the side effects of the steroid. Small amounts of fluid are offered frequently. The child who is listless may receive a combination of oral and IV fluids. These children can be expected to have Hickman lines or Mediports for easy access. When parenteral fluids are given, they must be carefully monitored (see Chapter 3). A record is kept of all fluid intake and output.

WILMS TUMOR

Wilms tumor, or nephroblastoma, is one of the most common malignant diseases of early life. It is a renal tumor arising from embryonic tissue. Nephroblastoma is now known to be associated with certain congenital anomalies, particularly of the genitourinary tract. The fact that it commonly occurs in siblings and twins indicates a genetic component.

Signs and Symptoms

During the early stages of growth, as with some other malignant diseases, there are few or no symptoms. It usually occurs in children between 2 and 5 years of age. A mass in the abdomen is discovered, generally by the mother or by the physician during a routine checkup. CT scan can confirm the origin and extent of the tumor and whether the other kidney is affected. Chest radiographs to identify possible metastases (the lungs are the most common site of metastasis in this disease), ultrasonography, bone surveys, liver scan, and urinalysis may be indicated. Wilms tumor seldom affects both kidneys.

Treatment and Nursing Care

The cornerstone treatment consists of surgery, unless there is involvement in both kidneys, the child only has one kidney, or resection is not possible. Chemotherapy and radiation therapy postsurgery are based on the extent of the tumor and the histologic appearance of the tumor (Burg et al., 2006). Preoperative chemotherapy and radiation may also be considered. Wilms tumor is staged I to V (Third National Wilms Tumor Study).

- Stages I to III are confined to the kidney or abdomen.
- Stage IV involves the areas beyond the kidney including the lung, liver, bone, and/or brain.
- Stage V involves both kidneys at the time of diagnosis.

The kidney and tumor are removed as soon as possible after the diagnosis has been confirmed. It is important to prepare the parents and the child for the extent of the incision, which is considerable. Children with stages I to III have a cure rate greater than 90% (Kliegman et al., 2007). The prognosis also depends on the histologic character of the tumor and evidence of recurrence.

✶ Critical Thinking Question

1. You are caring for a 5-year-old child with ALL who is in isolation because his blood counts (WBC, RBC, and platelets) are all critically low. What nursing care will you provide because the blood counts are low? What nursing measures will you provide to help prevent boredom and foster normal growth and development?

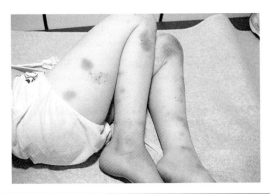

Critical Thinking Snapshot (Purpura)

In evaluating the bruising as shown here, describe two different reasons why low platelet levels occur in the child with ALL. Discuss the complications of chemotherapy and nursing care administered to a child receiving chemotherapy.

Nursing care is supportive before surgery. When the diagnosis of Wilms tumor has been made or is suspected, the *abdomen should not be palpated* because trauma to the mass could release cancer cells into the system. This is explained to the parents, and a sign is placed on the crib or child: "Do not palpate abdomen." The nurse must consider this extremely important.

In addition to preoperative teaching, the nurse teaches the parent and child about side effects such as nausea, vomiting, anorexia, and general malaise from the chemotherapy and radiation treatments. Ulceration of the mouth, alopecia, and peeling of the skin may also be seen. The nurse should anticipate such problems and should immediately report their appearance to the team leader or the nurse in charge of the unit.

Postoperative care of the child includes routine postoperative observations and specific monitoring for signs of intestinal obstruction from chemotherapy. These signs include vomiting, decreased or absent bowel sounds, and abdominal distention. Chemotherapy depresses the immune system, so the nurse must closely monitor the child for signs of infection. Bloody urine and elevated blood pressure are other symptoms that should be reported immediately.

The nurse needs to provide the family with information about protecting the remaining kidney as the child grows. Avoiding activities that risk kidney trauma is essential. Otherwise, the child should participate in activities normal for age and developmental level. Depending on the prognosis, helping the family and child face the possibility of a fatal illness is an important nursing function (see Chapter 22).

BRAIN TUMORS

Brain tumors are the second most common type of neoplasm in children. Most childhood tumors occur in the area of the brain below the cerebellum. The cause of these tumors is unknown. They occur most commonly in school-age children. The diagnosis is difficult because of the tumor's insidious onset. Metastatic tumors of the brain are rare in children. A synopsis of brain tumors in children is given in Table 21-5.

Signs and Symptoms

The signs and symptoms are directly related to the location and size of the tumor. Most tumors create increased ICP, with the hallmark symptoms of headache, vomiting, drowsiness, and seizures. Early morning headache relieved by vomiting may indicate a brain tumor. Nystagmus (constant jerky movements of the eyeball), double vision, strabismus, and decreased vision may be evident. Papilledema (edema of the optic nerve) may be seen. Other symptoms include ataxia, clumsiness, head tilt, behavioral changes, and cerebral enlargement, particularly in infants. Disturbances in vital signs are noticeable when the tumor presses on the brainstem. The diagnosis is determined from clinical manifestations, laboratory tests, magnetic resonance imaging (MRI), CT, and biopsy.

Treatment and Nursing Care

Treatment is multidisciplinary and includes surgery, radiation therapy, and, in some cases, chemotherapy. It should take place at a hospital with appropriate support. About 60% of children with brain tumors can be successfully treated using radiation, chemotherapy, and surgery (Yock and Tarbell, 2006).

Table 21-5 Most Frequently Seen Childhood Brain Tumors

TUMOR	PEAK AGE (YR)	CHARACTERISTICS
Cerebellar astrocytoma (52% of all brain tumors)	6-14 / 2-6	Slow-growing, cystic tumor; very high rate of cure with surgery (90%) / Rapidly growing, highly malignant, occurs more often in boys
Medulloblastoma (21% of all brain tumors)		*Treatment:* Surgery, craniospinal irradiation, chemotherapy *Prognosis:* 5-yr survival rate at 80% to 90%
Glioma of brainstem (19% of all brain tumors)	6-10	Slow-growing, diffuse tumor; cannot be removed with surgery; focal tumors can be removed; affects cerebral pathways and cranial nerves *Treatment:* Site radiation to shrink tumor, surgery for focal tumor *Prognosis:* Poor, but better if focal tumor is removed; 5-yr survival rate at 20%
Ependymoma (9% of all brain tumors)	5-6	Tumors grow at various speeds; because of location, invades vital centers, obstructs flow of cerebrospinal fluid *Treatment:* Partial surgical removal, irradiation of entire cerebrospinal axis *Prognosis:* Improving but related to age, location, and grade of tumor; 5-yr survival rate at 50%

In general, nursing care occurs in several phases. These phases are diagnosis, preoperative care, postoperative care, radiation therapy and chemotherapy, and convalescence. The nursing objectives in each area of care are specific but also overlap. One pervading theme is ongoing emotional support for the child and family during this taxing ordeal. "Waiting periods" for test results, surgery, and prognosis increase the anxiety levels of the entire family.

Nursing care follows the phase of treatment. Before surgery, emphasis is placed on careful explanations of various procedures and on familiarizing the child and family with the recovery room, ICU, and the hospital personnel. Of importance is that the child's head will be shaved at the incision site. The nurse should anticipate anxiety and provide empathy and support. The size of the postoperative dressing should be carefully explained. Applying a similar dressing to a doll may be helpful.

Postoperative care is the same as that given to the critically ill child. Adjuncts to care may include the use of a hypothermia blanket or a mechanical respirator. Parents must be prepared for the appearance of the child after surgery. The child may be unconscious for a while, or there may be facial edema.

In supporting the family, several common issues may need to be addressed. These are the fear of pain, truthfulness versus withholding facts, feelings of helplessness and guilt, and concerns about the future. In addition, the fear of loss is always present. Depending on the circumstances, supportive care for the terminally ill child and the family may be necessary. Oncology support groups are particularly helpful; the families identify with one another and share common concerns.

Radiation Therapy. Radiation treatment requires preparation. The radiologist outlines the areas to be treated. These marks should not be washed off. Small doses of radiation are given over a period of weeks. To develop an appropriate teaching plan, it is best to determine what the radiologist has told the child. Provide support to the child, who may feel that he or she will be burned. Advise the child that he or she will be alone in the room but will retain voice contact. Tour the facility with the child. Recognize physical symptoms of fear such as dry mouth, pupil dilation, trembling, and clinging. Tape or lotion should not be placed on the skin before or during radiation treatment in an attempt to help prevent burns. Untoward effects of treatment may begin about the end of the first week. Headaches, anorexia, nausea and vomiting, diarrhea, and general lethargy may ensue. More severe effects include leukopenia, a decreased platelet count, skin breakdown, and hair loss. Medication may be prescribed to help alleviate symptoms. Nutritious foods in small quantities should be offered. Provide a pleasant environment, one that is free of odors, sounds, and sights that might induce nausea. Radiation has been shown to impair intellectual development, affect growth, and interfere with normal hormone function. New treatments with stereotactic radiosurgery, stereotactic radiotherapy, intensity-modulated radiotherapy (IMRT), and proton radiation are providing new approaches with less damage to the normal tissue. These approaches promise fewer complications than radiation (Yock and Tarbell, 2006).

Chemotherapy. Chemotherapy regimens vary somewhat. The child and family are prepared for the possible side effects of medications. This is done initially by the physician in charge of treatment. Ongoing education by nurses is important because distraught parents can assimilate only so many facts. The nurse stresses the importance of return visits to monitor bone marrow depression and other parameters. Children need to know that the medicine is designed to make them feel better but that they may feel worse at first. The nurse should observe the sleeping child who has had nausea and frequent vomiting. The child should be positioned to avoid aspiration. Prolonged vomiting may be an indication that the medicine should be withheld or reduced. When therapy is being administered on an outpatient basis, careful instruction of parents or guardians is paramount.

The period of convalescence is punctuated by frequent clinic visits that are anxiety provoking. "Will the blood tests be all right?" "He's lost so much weight." "I hope he won't have to go back on medication." Some parents have to commute long distances to medical facilities. These problems involve all aspects of care of the chronically ill child. Many nurses try to maintain contact with discharged children by mail, reunions at the clinic, and involvement in cancer camps. The community health nurse and school nurse become significant persons on discharge. It is important that the child receive adequate nutrition and hydration. The child should be assisted in relating to a new body image. This may be augmented by the use of caps, wigs, or head scarves. Residual effects depend on the type and extent of the tumor.

It is not unusual for information such as the death of a loved child to filter back to persons who were directly involved with care. This always creates grief, which must be dealt with by the medical persons involved.

BONE TUMORS
OSTEOSARCOMA

Osteosarcoma is seen in adolescence, often during a growth spurt. This malignant bone tumor (found in the long bones) is detected because the child complains of pain, limping, and swelling. These complaints are often attributed to sports injuries and are seen in active adolescents. The diagnosis is made when injuries are ruled out. Laboratory tests include CBC and chemistry panel (usually normal) and alkaline phosphatase or lactic dehydrogenase (these are often elevated). A *sunburst pattern* is characteristic of the x-ray appearance. Bone biopsy confirms the diagnosis.

Oftentimes, preoperative chemotherapy is done to facilitate salvaging the limb. This also helps to prevent metastasis. Complete surgical resection is important for treatment. Chemotherapy is resumed after surgery. If amputation is required, early prosthetic fitting is essential. Prognosis is poor if there is bone and lung metastases.

EWING SARCOMA

Ewing Sarcoma is actually more common than osteosarcoma in children younger than 10 years of age (Kliegman et al., 2007). Symptoms include pain, swelling, limitation of motion, and tenderness over the involved bone (long bones and flat bones). Children may experience fever or weight loss and possibly respiratory distress. As with osteosarcoma, the pain may be attributed to a sports injury and diagnosis can go undetected. However, upon x-ray, there is a characteristic *onion-skinning* appearance (Figure 21-6). Bone scan, CT, and MRI are performed. Treatment includes surgery, chemotherapy, and radiation. Nursing care is provided in the same manner as for any child with cancer previously discussed. Prognosis is favorable if the tumor is small and nonmetastatic.

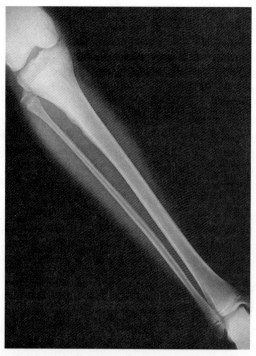

FIGURE 21-6 X-ray of tibia depicting Ewing Sarcoma; there is a characteristic *onion-skinning* appearance.

LYMPHOMAS
HODGKIN

Hodgkin disease is a malignant disease of the lymph system that primarily involves the lymph nodes. It may metastasize to the spleen, liver, bone marrow, lungs, or other parts of the body. The Reed-Sternberg cell, which can be seen on microscopic examination of lymph node tissue, contains two nuclei and is diagnostic of the disease. Hodgkin disease is rare before 10 years of age, but the incidence rate increases during late adolescence, mid to late twenties, and after age 50. It constitutes only about 6% of childhood cancers (Kliegman et al., 2007). Hodgkin is twice as common in boys as in girls. There are four subtypes, each with a different age at onset, clinical findings, and prognostic factors.

Signs and Symptoms

The presenting symptom is generally a painless lump in the cervical area or other lymph node site (supraclavicular, axillary, inguinal). Characteristically, there are few other manifestations. The swelling is generally first noted by the child or the parents. In more advanced cases, there may be high spiking fever, anorexia, weight loss, night sweats, general malaise, rash, and itching of the skin. Because this condition affects immune cells, the affected adolescent can be more prone to infection.

Infectious causes of enlarged lymph glands should be ruled out (e.g., infectious mononucleosis is common among adolescents). Blood counts may show changes in WBC differentials. A chest radiograph may show mediastinal involvement. The diagnosis is confirmed with a lymph node biopsy that reveals Reed-Sternberg cells on microscopic examination.

Determining the stage of the disease is necessary for prescribing a treatment regimen. Initially, lab tests (CBC and erythrocyte sedimentation rate or ESR), chest x-ray, and computed tomography or magnetic resonance imaging can help determine the extent of the disease. Bone scans are performed if bone pain is present or if there is an elevated alkaline phosphatase. Positron emission tomography or PET scans are analyzed.

The stages in Hodgkin disease are defined as follows:

Stage I: Disease restricted to a single, non–lymph node site or localized in a single group of lymph nodes. Asymptomatic.

Stage II: Two or more affected lymph node areas on the same side of the diaphragm, or one affected non–lymph node area and one or more affected lymph node regions on the same side of the diaphragm.

Stage III: Involvement of lymph node regions on both sides of the diaphragm; involvement of adjacent organ or spleen.

Stage IV: Diffuse disease; least favorable prognosis.

Table 21-6	Interventions for Adolescents Undergoing Cancer Chemotherapy
PROBLEM	**INTERVENTION**
Infection risk	Explain the function of the immune system and how chemotherapeutic medications affect it Use visual aids whenever applicable Review methods to prevent infection—meticulous hand hygiene, avoiding exposure to colds or illness, importance of routine checkups and immunizations
Bleeding	Advise cautious physical activity and avoid contact sports if platelet count is low Review management of nosebleeds Help the adolescent plan for low-risk social activities
Stomatitis, nausea, vomiting	Use a local anesthetic on ulcerated oral lesions before meals Advise using a soft toothbrush, Water Pik, and prescribed mouthwash Give ordered antiemetic before chemotherapy treatment; practice relaxation techniques Provide frequent small meals; discuss altered taste and foods that will appeal
Fatigue	Encourage frequent rest periods Coordinate in-school rest periods with the school nurse Explore quiet areas of interest
Body image changes	Encourage the adolescent to express feelings about changes in skin and hair and activity level Use wigs, scarves, hats, eyebrow pencils, false eyelashes, and other cosmetic devices to minimize appearance of hair loss; remind the adolescent that the hair loss is temporary Suggest clothing that minimizes body changes and enhances appearance
Enforced dependence during treatment	Involve the adolescent in decision making Advise parent not to be overprotective but to allow autonomy within treatment limits Encourage peers to visit or phone; provide Internet access
Fear	Refer the adolescent to a peer support group Allow the adolescent to express any fears, concerns, or doubts Refer adolescent and family for spiritual support Clarify information about the disease, procedures, or treatments Refer to a camp for children with cancer if the adolescent is interested

Treatment

Well-established treatment regimens are now available to combat Hodgkin disease. Both low-dose radiation therapy and chemotherapy are used in accordance with the clinical stage of the disease. The prognosis for remission is favorable. Cure is primarily related to the stage of the disease at diagnosis.

Nursing care is mainly directed toward the symptomatic relief of the side effects of radiation therapy and chemotherapy (see Table 21-6 for interventions adapted for adolescents). Education of the child and family is essential because most children are cared for in the home.

A common side effect of irradiation is malaise. The teenager tires easily and may be irritable and anorexic. The skin in the treated area may be sensitive and should be protected against exposure to sunlight and irritation, particularly during treatment. After treatment, a sun-blocking agent containing PABA (para-aminobenzoic acid) should be used to prevent burning. The attending physician may prescribe an ointment to relieve itching of the skin. Nothing should be applied to the treatment area without the recommendation of the doctor. There may be diarrhea after abdominal radiation therapy. The child **does not** become radioactive during or after therapy.

Because adolescents are cognitively able to understand the implications of serious disease, emotional support is paramount. Nurses must be prepared in particular for periods of anger, which may be directed at them. Nurses must also talk to the parents regarding this anger and come up with ways to handle this rejection and anger. Love, support, and security are what this adolescent needs. Suitable exercise, such as the use of a punching bag, allows for safe direction of anger. Routine use helps prevent the unnecessary buildup of tension. Activity in general is regulated by the child. The physician advises the child if special precautions are necessary.

NON-HODGKIN

Non-Hodgkin lymphoma (NHL) constitutes approximately 60% of all lymphomas in children and adolescents (Kliegman et al., 2007). It is seen in children between 5 and 19 years of age and has a very favorable prognosis for localized disease (90% to 95%). NHL involves the B and T lymphocytes. Diagnostic measures include lab work, chest x-rays, CT or MRI scans, PET scans, and possible bone scans. Tissue biopsy will confirm the diagnosis. Staging (I to IV) is based on the number and location of the tumors. Stage I consists of a single tumor without lymph node involvement, while stage IV includes tumors found in stages I to III as well as involvement of the CNS or bone marrow. Tumors may appear in the head and neck, mediastinum, and abdominal area. The primary treatment is chemotherapy; radiation is rarely used. Nursing care is provided in the same manner as for any child receiving chemotherapy.

Get Ready for the NCLEX® Examination!

Key Points

- Cow's milk consumption should be decreased with iron-deficiency anemia; solid and iron-enriched foods should be encouraged.
- Parental knowledge of precipitating factors that can cause a sickle cell crisis (infection, dehydration, stress, or exposure to cold) is necessary in home care management.
- Hemarthrosis is treated with RICE; aspirin and ibuprofen should be avoided.
- The focus for the child with hemophilia has shifted toward home care. Many children are treated for bleeding episodes at home by their family or with self-administration of clotting factors.
- Support groups such as the Ronald McDonald House can aid the family of the child with leukemia face significant family stressors.
- Common symptoms of ALL are fever, pallor, bruising, and lymphadenopathy.
- Chills, itching, rash, fever, headache, and pain in the back are signs and symptoms of a blood transfusion reaction. Blood transfusion is stopped immediately.
- Wilms tumors should never be palpated preoperatively.
- Signs of increased ICP may be present with brain tumors at the time of diagnosis.
- Osteosarcoma and Ewing sarcoma may initially be misdiagnosed as sports injuries.

Additional Learning Resources

evolve Go to your Evolve website (http://evolve.elsevier.com/Price/pediatric/) for the following FREE learning resources:
- 3-D Animations
- Answer Keys
- Appendixes
- Audio Glossary
- Spanish/English Glossary
- Video Clips

Review Questions for the NCLEX® Examination

1. Prevention of iron-deficiency anemia begins:
   1. By about 4 months of age
   2. With good prenatal care
   3. By encouraging mothers to breastfeed
   4. Late in the prenatal period

2. A child is suspected of having hemophilia A. The diagnostic test most likely to be used to determine the level of factor VIII in the blood is the:
   1. Partial thromboplastin time (PTT)
   2. Erythrocyte sedimentation rate
   3. Red blood cell count
   4. White blood cell count

3. The prognosis of a child diagnosed with leukemia is most clearly related to: (**Select all that apply.**)
   1. Genetic factors
   2. Age at diagnosis
   3. Initial white blood cell count
   4. Initial response to chemotherapy
   5. Presentation of symptoms

4. A 15-year old diagnosed with acute lymphoid leukemia (ALL) is about to begin induction therapy in an attempt to induce remission and restore normal hematopoiesis. The child's parents ask how long induction therapy is expected to last. The nurse correctly responds that this phase usually lasts:
   1. 1 week
   2. 28 days
   3. 40 days
   4. 3 months

5. The nurse is caring for a child with Wilms tumor (nephroblastoma). Diagnostic testing reveals involvement of areas of the lung. This would be classified as:
   1. Stage I
   2. Stage II
   3. Stage III
   4. Stage IV

End-of-Life Care for Children and Their Families

Objectives

1. Define the vocabulary terms listed
2. Discuss legal and ethical issues related to death
3. Discuss measures the nurse can take regarding palliative care
4. Discuss the child's reaction to death
5. Describe the impact death has on the different age groups
6. Discuss fears of the child related to dying
7. Discuss pain management for the dying child
8. Describe how a terminal illness affects the child and family
9. Describe cultural issues related to death
10. Discuss the benefits of hospice
11. Discuss management of symptoms the dying child may have
12. Discuss the nurse's role during the end-of-life care of a child

Key Terms

acceptance (p. 419)
anger (p. 419)
anticipatory grief (ăn-TĬS-ĭ-pă-tō-rē; p. 422)
anxiolytic (ĂNG-zī-ō-LĬ-tĭk; p. 421)
bargaining (p. 419)
bereavement (bĕ-RĒV-mĕnt; p. 422)
denial (p. 419)

depression (p. 419)
ethical (p. 415)
euthanasia (yü-thə-NĀ-zh[ē]ə; p. 416)
grief (p. 419)
legal (p. 415)
pain (p. 418)
palliative care (PĂL-ē-Ă-tĭv; p. 416)

Facing death with a child and the family is not an easy task. Nurses who become involved with dying children often express a sense of gratitude to have had the privilege of the experience. This is an area where rules fall short and patience may become stretched. While it can be tiring, discouraging, and sad, it also requires a profound look at acceptance. Nurses who deal with the dying child and his or her family undoubtedly have a special gift. Families will never forget the care provided to their dying child by their nurse.

SELF-EXPLORATION

One of the most important, if not the most important, preparations for dealing with the dying child is self-exploration. Attitudes about life and death affect our nursing practice. Those attitudes and emotions can form barriers to effective communication unless they are recognized and released. How nurses have or have not dealt with their own losses affects their ability to relate to patients. Nurses must recognize that coping is an active and ongoing process. Constructive outlets such as exercise are critical for the nurse who cares for dying children. An active support system consisting of

nonjudgmental people (professional or personal) who are not threatened by natural expressions of emotions is crucial. Taking time off periodically may be necessary. Even attending the child's funeral may help the nurse in coping and does not detract from professionalism (Hockenberry and Wilson, 2009). Proper channeling of these feelings can be a valuable part of the nurse's empathetic response to others.

LEGAL AND ETHICAL ISSUES RELATED TO DEATH

Legal issues related to death revolve around what is made a law by a legally sanctioned group. Legal issues include informed consent, role of a legal guardian, a Do Not Resuscitate (DNR) order, organ donation, and so on. In addition, each state's Nurse Practice Act regulates the practice of nursing. An ethical issue relates to what is good or moral. Ethical principles include respect for autonomy, benevolence, nonmaleficence, veracity, confidentiality, fidelity, and justice (Table 22-1). For example, life-sustaining medical treatment (such as a ventilator) may have positive and/or negative implications; ethical principles may be used to evaluate the situation. Use of these principles aids the

Table 22-1	Ethical Principles and Definitions
PRINCIPLE	**DEFINITION**
Respect for autonomy	The patient's right to self-determination and decision making
Benevolence	Doing what is good, meeting needs, balancing benefits with risk and harm, providing relief of pain and suffering
Nonmaleficence	Doing no harm
Veracity	Being honest, telling the truth
Confidentiality	Respecting privileged information; preserving rights, privacy, and dignity
Fidelity	Keeping promises
Justice	Treating fairly, ensuring distribution of resources

Box 22-1 Key Psychosocial Issues in End-of-Life Care

- Death, like birth, is a part of the natural order of things. Some die sooner than others.
- All of us have special feelings for those with whom we share our lives. There are many emotional feelings to express.
- Death is also a separation from family, friends, and siblings. The child who dies is not the only one who loses.
- The loss is never complete. Religion plays an important role in emphasizing that the child still lives on in spirit. The memory of the child is always in our hearts.
- Assure the child that he or she will not be alone in death or after death. It is very important for the child to know that the parents are there for support and love.
- At the time of death, everyone needs to know they made a difference and did all they could do with their lives.
- Assure the child that crying is acceptable and feelings of sadness may occur. It is equally all right to feel angry and resentful. Children should not feel pressured to discuss their illness. However, if a child chooses to express feelings, the support of an adult listener should be available.
- Assure the dying child that silence is acceptable, and no matter how the child chooses to express feelings, or how confused or silly it may sound, it is acceptable.
- Reassure the child that when death comes, it will not hurt. Children are very concerned about pain. They need to be reassured that the health care team will reduce their pain to a minimum.
- When someone dies, there is a need to say goodbye and to know that the arms and love of the family will surround them.
- Give the child permission to die. Saying it is "okay" to go helps put the child's mind at ease.

health care team and the family to provide the dying child with a peaceful and dignified death. Through the use of ethical principles, the unique needs of the child and family can be kept in perspective, as can assisting in resolving dilemmas that can arise during these challenging times.

PALLIATIVE CARE

Palliative care is the care and comfort given to a dying person. Palliative treatment focuses on the "relief of symptoms (e.g., pain, dyspnea) and conditions (e.g., loneliness) that cause distress and detract from the child's enjoyment of life" (American Academy of Pediatrics, 2007). Nurses provide palliative care so that the individual and the family experience a comfortable, supported, and dignified end of life. Palliative care aids the child who is experiencing death and the family to feel cared for and supported and to have this care performed in the most dignified way. The goal of palliative care is to "add life to the child's years, not simply years to the child's life" (American Academy of Pediatrics, 2007).

The American Nurses Association Code of Ethics for Nurses (2001) does not support euthanasia or "mercy killing" by nurses. However, the role of the nurse is to relieve symptoms in the dying patient even if those interventions involve the risk of hastening death (Hockenberry and Wilson, 2009).

When end-of-life care is needed for a child, it brings with it a great deal of emotional feelings. As parents and primary caregivers to a child, parents expect their children to outlive them. In the world of pediatric nursing, nurses assume that their time will be spent on curing and healing in the pediatric population. Nurses, however, must also recognize the value of caring for the child who is dying. The pediatric nurse has much to gain from working with the dying child and assisting the family in confronting issues they must face. In looking back, parents—and indeed, often the child—will look back and recall a time when living with the disease changed to preparing for death. Health care providers who work with children recognize that open and honest communication is the best approach. Broaching this subject with a child is difficult for all concerned. It is an issue that requires communication skills, empathy, and many discussions. The parent and pediatrician may consider the child's understanding of and prior experience with death, the family's religious or cultural beliefs, the developmental level of the child, how the child copes with sadness and pain, the disease experience, and the circumstances expected (American Academy of Pediatrics, 2007). Box 22-1 discusses some additional issues to consider before the discussion of death with a child.

Communication

The three main ingredients in communication are words, tone of voice, and body language. The most powerful of these is body language, followed by tone of voice, and then by the words that are actually said. If words are said with an angry tone of voice and with arms crossed, the person receiving this message perceives the sender as angry regardless of the words that are said. Children are keenly adept at reading body language and tone of voice.

For the child and family to be supported, a multidisciplinary approach is needed. A team approach is most beneficial, particularly one that allows the individual and the family to have input into the decisions that are made. At a minimum, the team includes a physician, nurse, social worker, spiritual advisor, and child life specialist. Needs that should be considered center around physical, psychological, social, and spiritual areas. Table 22-2 lists factors for each of these.

In providing care to the dying child and family, the members of the health care team should see, as a result of their efforts, a reduction of symptoms of pain or discomfort related to the disease; appropriate coping of both the child and the family; satisfaction of the child and family with the care that is being given; a sense of open and honest communication with all involved in the care; the dealing with and resolving of fears, grief, and anger; planning for future events such as the funeral; availability of quality of time for the child and family to enjoy; spiritual problems addressed and reconciled; and the family's grief being resolved after the death has occurred. This care involves a lengthy period of time and may be ongoing. There is so much to consider, and time becomes a friend as well as a foe.

Table 22-2 Physical, Psychological, Social, and Spiritual Needs

AREA	NEEDS
Physical	Pain management Management of symptoms Comfort measures
Psychological	Anxiety/stress Guilt/anger Depression Fear of dying Grief/bereavement
Social	Financial concerns Insurance concerns Role and relationship changes Social isolation
Spiritual	Meaning Religiosity Sense of despair

CHILD'S REACTION TO DEATH

Each child, like each adult, approaches death in an individual way, drawing on limited experience (Table 22-3). Nurses must become well-acquainted with children and view them within the context of their families and social culture. Children's anxiety about death often centers on symptoms. They fear that the treatments necessary to alleviate their problem may be painful, as indeed some of them are. Their sense of trust is precarious. It is important that nurses be honest and inform children of what is about to be done and why it is necessary. Information should be shared in terms that children can understand. Encourage expression of feelings, such as by saying "You seem angry." Allow sufficient time for a response. It is important that children be allowed to have as much control over what happens to them as possible. This is fostered by including them in decisions that concern their welfare. Do not, however, offer a choice when there is none. Children often communicate symbolically. **Listen** to what they are saying to you, to their toys, and to other children. Provide crayons and paper. Drawing feelings is often therapeutic.

Although age is a factor, the child's cognitive development rather than chronological age per se affects the response to death. Children younger than 5 years of

Table 22-3 Children's Concepts of Death

AGE	CONCEPT
Infant-toddler	Little understanding of death Fear and anxiety over separation
Preschooler	Something that happens to others Not permanent Curious about dead flowers and animals Magical thinking Believe that "bad thoughts" may come true, harbor guilt Believe their thoughts can cause death Death is reversible Will not happen to them
Early school years	Death is final Think they might die, but only in the distant future May understand death as a "person" Death is universal Suspect parents will die "someday" Fear of mutilation
Preadolescent-adolescent	Able to understand death in a logical manner Understand death is universal Understand death is permanent Fear of disfigurement and isolation from peers

age are mainly concerned with separation from their parents and abandonment. (Even adults are threatened by thoughts of dying alone.) Preschool children respond to questions concerning death by relying on their experience and by turning to fantasy. They may believe death is reversible or that they are in some way responsible. Children between 6 and 12 years of age are beginning to be able to make knowledgeable decisions; however, because they are able to comprehend more, they may have more fears. They need to be encouraged to discuss their feelings and have questions answered honestly. Adolescents facing death are dealing with conflicts between their treatment regimens and their need to establish independence. Teens may also not want to disappoint their parents by "giving up." This leads to anger and resentment, which are frequently displaced onto hospital staff members. An atmosphere of acceptance and nonjudgmental listening allows children freedom to express their hostility in a nonthreatening environment. Older children and teenagers also need a voice in decision-making processes, especially in a terminal condition that affords no hope with ongoing treatment.

 Nursing Brief

Brothers and sisters often feel neglected and lonely. They are frustrated because they are unable to comfort their parents and loved ones.

CHILD'S AWARENESS OF CONDITION

Surprising as it may seem, many investigators have shown that terminally ill children are generally aware of their condition even when careful concealment has been advocated. This is reflected in their drawings and play and can be detected through psychological testing. Failure to be honest with children leaves them to suffer alone, unable to express fears and sadness or even to say goodbye. The prospect of death is frightening to children; it is up to the parents and caregivers to help the child work through his or her feelings. Children need to be informed in clear, simple, age-appropriate language. They need to have honest, accurate information about their illness and prognosis.

 Communication

Wishes of the parents should be respected when it comes to talking to the child or siblings about the prognosis, unless it is decided that this is not in the child's best interest. At that point, legal involvement may be necessary.

FEARS OF THE CHILD

In dealing with death, the child most likely has two major fears: fear of pain and fear of being alone. The child should be comforted and reassured that both of these issues will be managed.

PAIN

In consideration of the child and family, **pain** should be accepted as being "whatever the experiencing person says it is, existing whenever he says it does" (McCaffery and Pasero, 1999). As discussed in Chapter 2, pain needs to be properly assessed and managed. Dying teenagers often fear symptoms of pain and suffering more than actual death, so they need reassurance that their comfort needs will be met. Narcotic analgesics such as morphine are effective pain relievers in children and adults. Studies have shown that pain is not always well controlled in children, so the nurse needs to be vigilant of the child's needs.

 Nursing Brief

In children, the intramuscular or the rectal route may be offensive, so keep this in mind when medications are changed or added.

Barriers to proper management of pain for the terminally ill child can be related to addiction or overdosing. The goal of safe and effective administration of pain medication should revolve around comfort and the ability of the child to function. As the disease worsens or as a tolerance to the medication develops, the amount of pain medication may not be as effective. The dosage may need to be adjusted, other medications added, or a stronger medication begun. Often, *complementary* methods are used along with pharmacologic approaches. Relaxation, distraction, biofeedback, or guided imagery may all be used. The dosage of narcotics can often be reduced, and the adverse effects may be diminished (Box 22-2).

Box 22-2	Complementary Methods

Relaxation is a method children can be taught to tense and relax different muscle groups. By tensing the muscle first, the child can compare how it feels when the tension is released. The child is then taught to hold the relaxed muscle for a short amount of time.

Distraction is a method used to divert attention from the main portion of an experience. Blowing bubbles is a form of distraction used with children.

Biofeedback is a method of training designed to help an individual control his or her autonomic (involuntary) nervous system.

Guided imagery is a complementary/alternative therapy that uses pleasant mental images of events, feelings, or sensations. Simple imagery entails using the sounds and sights in the imagination of the child to feel good and be less afraid. An example is having the child visualize a favorite vacation spot.

FEAR OF BEING ALONE

Reassure children that they will not be left alone. Allow the child to verbalize concerns, thoughts, and feelings. Encourage the parents and family to take the time to listen. As the child loses the ability to speak, the care and comfort given needs to be verbalized. The parents and family can also speak to the child at the bedside, reflecting on the past and discussing the present as a way of comforting the child. Children love to hear how they made an impact in a loved one's life. They need to know they made a difference.

FAMILY ROLES AND NEEDS

The impending death of a child affects every member of the family. Family dynamics and the family's ability to cope and resolve issues are of concern. Parents may be overwhelmed by the decisions they must make. Communication with the family is important, but also family members need ways to express themselves. Parents and family members need to be encouraged and given the opportunity to verbalize how they are feeling. Guilt, anger, and sadness are just some of the emotions that family members are experiencing. They need their feelings validated, and they need to be praised for the care they are giving the child. Help family members see a role they can play in the care and comfort of their loved one. Families of children who are hospitalized need to be with the dying child, even in the intensive care unit. The family may be given a pager so they can be easily contacted if they need to leave briefly. Consistency with communication, especially regarding the child's condition, is critical for families. Referrals should be made to other disciplines as the need arises. Other health care team members, such as the social worker and chaplain, can help the parents and family in dealing with social, emotional, financial, and spiritual issues.

The stages of dying as detailed by Kübler-Ross (1969)—denial, anger, bargaining, depression, and acceptance—can be applied to parents and siblings as they grieve and to the sick child. It is important to accept and support participants at whatever stage they are in and not try to direct progress. Parents should be encouraged to assist in the care of their child. It is therapeutic for children to be in their own surroundings whenever possible. Siblings involved in the child's care feel less neglected. They may be able to help with simple things, such as bringing a toy or a food item to the bedside of their dying brother or sister. Parents need to encourage siblings to be open about their own grief as well. It is common for the siblings to feel guilty because they are jealous of the attention paid to the ill child. Parents feel guilty because they cannot give equal time to all of their children. Special time with each of their children is often therapeutic. Normal parenting should not be disrupted.

Appropriate limit-setting and guidance regarding the child's behavior should continue. Normal parenting helps keep the child from feeling out of control or acting out during this difficult time (Smith and Pravikoff, 2010).

 Nursing Brief

A long illness threatens a child's independence. Do not contribute to this with overprotection.

The family's religious associations can be a source of strength and support, as can caring neighbors and friends. Statistics show a high correlation between the death of a child and divorce. Nurses should try to be alert to signs of tension between parents so that suitable interventions may be established. It is important to realize that each parent grieves in his or her own time and way, often making it impossible for spouses to be supportive of each other. The suppression of strong feelings of guilt, helplessness, and outrage can be devastating. The father may be easily overlooked because of his absence during the day or because of a need to conceal his emotions from others.

CULTURAL ISSUES

Depending on the culture, various issues may arise regarding death. Learning about different cultures is an important first step. Customs regarding death are usually unique to a given culture. For example, some cultures believe in an afterlife, and certain customs may need to be followed regarding that belief. Other cultures may have their own funeral and burial customs. Some cultures feel the dying should be protected from knowing the prognosis; some feel pain medication should be given to improve the quality of life, whereas others feel it should not (Giger and Davidhizar, 2008). Many cultures believe religion and faith are important aspects of end-of-life care. Cultural education is thus an important aspect regarding care of the dying child. See Table 22-4 for cultural considerations with death and dying.

Language barriers make it difficult to communicate in any hospital situation, especially when hospice and palliative care are involved. The use of interpreters is not always ideal, and communicating to families in stressful situations may be frustrating for all parties concerned. Patience on the part of the health care provider becomes an important virtue.

HOSPICE CARE

Hospice services are for individuals who no longer can benefit from curative care and treatment. Care is designed to provide sensitivity and support to the individual in the final phase of life. Hospice care refers to a package of palliative care services, such as durable

Table 22-4   Cultural Considerations with Death and Dying

CULTURE	BELIEF
Haitian Americans	Religious medallions, pictures of saints, talismans for protection or good luck Kinsman makes arrangements including purchase of coffin and prayer services before funeral 7 days of consecutive prayer to assist the passage of the soul to the next world
Jewish Americans	Should not be left alone Needs to be informed death is near Recite the confessional or Shema; a friend or family member may recite the confessional if the dying person is unable Eyes and mouth are closed by the nearest relative once death has occurred Body is placed on a straw mat on the floor, with the person's feet toward the door Candle is placed at the person's head to symbolize the "light" or joy and love the departed brought to others Face is covered with a sheet out of respect
Mexican Americans	Whatever is the cause of death, it is God's will Pain and suffering are common aspects in the experience Male head of the family should be consulted in health care decision making Family needs to be included in nursing care Spiritual beliefs and role of prayer very important

Data from Giger, J., and Davidhizar, R., 2008. *Transcultural nursing* (5th ed.). St. Louis: Mosby.

medical equipment, and so on. Life is seen as quality time rather than length of time. The entire family unit is considered in hospice care so that the needs of all can be met.

Global Perspectives

Hospice care began in 1974. In 1977, an 8-year-old boy was denied hospice care because he was a child. Children's Hospice International *(www.CHIonline.org)* was founded in 1983 as a nonprofit organization dedicated to the establishment of hospice care for children and adolescents with life-threatening conditions and their families. This organization's goal is quality of life for the dying child and ongoing strengthened life for the family.

Hospice care may be offered in a child's home, a hospice care facility, or a hospital. Hospice can offer many positive benefits for the dying child and the family. It is best to investigate it long before it is needed. Hospice services can be life-affirming, and parents may benefit from having this knowledge as early as possible. Children's hospice encourages day-to-day communication so that the family can look back and treasure the time spent together. The support received from hospice enables the family to cope more effectively. Grief is normal, and to cope and recover from grief requires choices. With hospice support, families can be strengthened and can return to positive and productive lives.

PREPARING FOR DEATH

The end of an individual's life is as important as the beginning of that person's life. For a birth, the family

plans and educates itself. The experience is visualized and eventually is realized. If the opportunity arises, with an expected death, an individual's preparation for death can likewise be planned. In the case of a child, wishes, dreams, and desires can be planned and accomplished if they are known. If parents and family members have time to identify what is important for them to have during the child's illness and death, then if possible, these can be arranged, leaving the parents and family with positive memories. Parents and family members need to verbalize their fears and beliefs about death. It is important to talk with the child about his or her impending death. By allowing the child to continue to express his or her wishes and emotions, he or she becomes better prepared for the inevitable. Through discussion and education, fears can often be lessened or resolved.

With a sudden and unexpected death, parents and family members do not have the opportunity to plan, and so **anticipatory grieving** rarely is able to occur. Unfortunately, some families of children do experience unexpected death. In the case of infants or very young children, they do not have the ability to communicate their wishes, making it difficult for their parents and families. Anytime the life of a child is shortened, parents, family members, health care providers, and all involved struggle to make sense of it all.

Death is a physiologic process, and there are signs and symptoms that cessation of life is occurring. Discomforts associated with the respiratory system can be distressing to the child and family. Dyspnea can be caused by worsening of the disease process, anemia, pneumonia, or heart failure. "Death rattle" or noisy chest sounds from a buildup of secretions may be heard. Nursing interventions can include elevating the head of the bed, using a cool cloth on the forehead, using oxygen, changing positions, and adding morphine. Morphine suppresses the cough reflex and also diminishes the feelings of air hunger, which is the sensation caused by dyspnea. Other medications such as a bronchodilator or an anxiolytic may be ordered.

Gastrointestinal system discomforts involve nausea or vomiting, anorexia (lack of desire to eat), dysphagia (difficulty swallowing), dehydration, and constipation. Some of these may be related to the progress of the disease, the slowing down of metabolism, or the result of medication side effects. Consider the discomfort of the child, and seek to remedy the cause. Diet and environment (sights and odors) can be adjusted. Medications may be added to the child's care to control nausea/vomiting. As the disease progresses, the child may lose his or her appetite. Help parents understand that this is to be expected and that it is okay for the child to have any food or fluid requested. Requests may occur at non–meal times. Sips of a favorite fluid, ice chips, or a Popsicle can provide comfort. Oral care is needed. Soft-bristled toothbrushes aid in cleansing and soothing the mouth, gums, teeth, and tongue. Lips may also become dry, so a topical preparation may be used. As dehydration occurs and blinking decreases, the eyes may also need moisture and artificial tears are needed.

Weakness and fatigue occur as the disease progresses. The child and family can be assisted to modify events in daily activities. Instead of doing all the care at once, plan on doing segments of it during different parts of the day. Eating is important, so plan a period of rest before and after a meal. Conserve the child's energy by the use of assistance, such as a wheelchair or a wagon for mobility. This conserves energy and yet allows the child to spend time out of the room. It is a natural process that a decrease in activity leads to weakness, so if there is an underlying problem, such as pain, depression, or poor sleeping, these issues need to be addressed for the child to remain active as long as possible.

With a decrease in activity, issues related to the skin arise. Incontinence of urine and feces add to this problem. Special care should center around providing for the child's dignity and keeping the bed linens clean and dry. Due to lack of adequate circulation to the periphery, realize that, if skin breakdown does occur, healing is difficult. Prevention of any type of skin breakdown is important. Turning, positioning, and the use of pillows or other devices to reduce pressure is essential. Assessment of the mental status of the child is valuable. If depression, fear, anxiety, or confusion occurs, these need to be addressed. Make sure there is adequate pain management.

Box 22-3 summarizes the physical signs of impending death. Parents and caregivers can recognize these. It is essential that the nurse provide dignity, comfort,

---

Box 22-3 Signs and Symptoms of Impending Death

LACK OF APPETITE
- May be seen by the family as "giving up"
- Anorexia

WEAKNESS AND FATIGUE
- Caused by disease process
- Lack of energy

DECREASE OF FLUID INTAKE
- Can be useful in keeping lungs less congested
- Care for mucous membranes if they are dry
- Decrease in circulatory perfusion
- Causes hypotension and decreased cardiac output
- Causes hands and feet to be cool
- Decrease in urine output

NEUROLOGIC DYSFUNCTION
- May lead to diminished level of consciousness
- Decreased ability to swallow
- Changes in respirations
- Loss of sphincter control
- Patient may become restless
- Key is to keep patient pain-free

---

support, guidance, and education to the parents and family members during this time. Comfort and care for the child should continue to be provided while talking to the child, even though the child may not be conscious. Because the loss of hearing cannot be reliably predicted, the parents and family can gain comfort in the fact that their loved one may still hear them.

Respect and assist the family in their spiritual and cultural needs. This is a time when prayer and the presence of family members can be profoundly meaningful. Nurses need to be sensitive to the parents' and other family members' needs. Some families need the nurse's presence; others may need their privacy. Honor their requests whenever possible. During these last few hours or moments just before death, small things have great meaning for the parents and family. Allow parents to hold and comfort their dying child (Figure 22-1). Extend to the parents and family the use of services that they may need, such as calling the spiritual advisor of their choice.

Nursing Brief

The family may be approached regarding organ donation. They need to be fully informed prior to making this decision. Support from the nurse can help the family work through issues and questions they may have.

CARE AFTER DEATH

The time of death occurs when there is absence of respiratory, cardiac, and neurologic function; pupils are fixed and dilated; body temperature falls; the

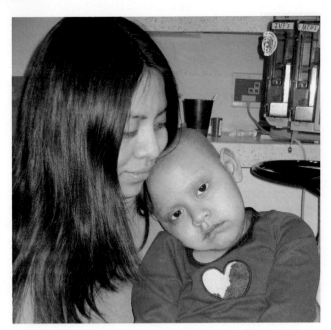

FIGURE 22-1 Parents' wishes to hold their dying child should be respected and facilitated.

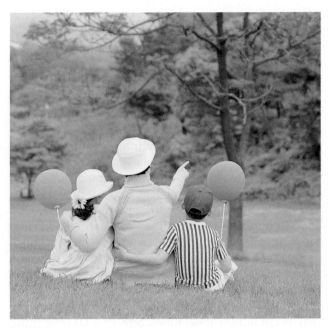

FIGURE 22-2 On the anniversary of a child's death, family members meet to send balloons (non-Mylar) with messages inside up to heaven for the deceased child.

skin is cool to the touch and pale; sphincter control is lost so there may be passing of urine and stool; and body movement ceases. There is no particular order or time frame in which these events occur. The pronouncement of death is according to the institution's policy.

Once death has occurred, the nurse and the health team members assist the family. Wishes from the parents and family need to be respected and honored. A chaplain or person of the family's choice needs to be with them during this time. Assistance may be needed in notifying other members or making decisions.

In preparing the body for viewing, the nurse should bathe and dress the child in a clean gown. The bed is changed, and the environment is cleaned and made more peaceful by removing some of the medical equipment. The parents and family are given the opportunity to view and spend time with the child. Holding the newborn, infant, or child may occur; this provides a comfort for the parents, especially if they were unable to do so before death. When the family is ready and has given permission, the body is moved. Parents may want to be present when the mortician comes to remove the body. Their requests should be honored if at all possible.

FAMILY COPING

Bereavement is a complex series of reactions that occur during and after the death of a loved one. How an individual grieves is unique. In a situation where death is expected, **anticipatory grief** may occur, which is a sense of loss and grief before death. After the actual death, bereavement can occur for a varied amount of time, and support is needed. Family members need to know that grief has no time frame and that during the first year many changes occur. With the loss of a child, there are likely to be many events that stir the feelings of loss. The first year or two after a child's death are especially difficult for the family. Parents and siblings need support systems in place. Both parents and siblings benefit from reading books about death. Making memories such as an album, quilt square, or treasure box of mementos can be therapeutic. In addition, many well-established support groups are available to assist parents and siblings in dealing with loss and grief (Figure 22-2).

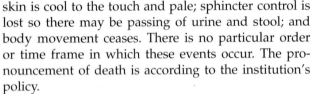 **Community Considerations**

The mission of The Compassionate Friends *(www.compassionatefriends.org)* is to assist families toward the positive resolution of grief following the death of a child of any age and to provide information to help others be supportive. Helping After Neonatal Death (HAND; *www.handonline.org*) is an organization that offers grief support for families who have lost a child (or children) through miscarriage, stillbirth, genetic abortion, or infant death.

 Nursing Brief

Grandparents, teachers, and friends are also grieving. Be alert for emotions from all significant others.

REFLECTION

Death is what occurs at the end of life. It is both normal *and* unique. In pediatrics, nurses are called on to aid children, parents, and families through the dying process, with which they may have little or no experience. Nurses are responsible for providing dignity, comfort, support, guidance, and education. Nurses must search their own values, beliefs, and judgments. Through self-reflection when feelings of conflict arise, identifying whose needs are being met becomes paramount to providing quality patient care.

In dealing with, relating to, coping with, and managing the process of death and dying, a poem by Henry Van Dyke says it very well:

Time is …
Too slow for those who wait,
Too swift for those who fear,
Too long for those who grieve,
Too short for those who rejoice,
But for those who love,
Time is eternity.

Get Ready for the NCLEX® Examination!

Key Points

- Working with a dying child and the family is a difficult task.
- Self-exploration can aid the nurse in identifying values and beliefs.
- There are many legal and ethical decisions to be made during the process of dying and death itself.
- Legal relates to laws, and ethical relates to what is good or moral.
- Palliative care involves comfort and support for physical, psychological, social, and spiritual needs.
- Palliative care is interdisciplinary and involves at least the child, parents, nurse, physician, social worker, spiritual advisor, and child life specialist.
- Communication is an essential aspect of palliative care.
- Cognitive development influences the child's needs in coping with grief and dying.
- Children with a terminal illness often recognize their condition and are aware they are dying.
- Children fear pain and dying alone.
- The stages of grief according to Kübler-Ross are denial, anger, bargaining, depression, and acceptance.
- Grief is subjective and unique for everyone.
- Hospice care provides sensitivity and support for those who are dying and their family.
- Hospice care for children is supported by CHI.
- In an expected death, planning can aid the child and family to complete goals.
- Even though the exact time of death cannot be predicted, there are physiologic signs and symptoms that allow us to know death is near.
- The care the family receives after the death of their loved one is one of their lasting memories.
- The family continues to grieve long after the death of a child, and coping mechanisms are vital for the family's welfare.

Additional Learning Resources

evolve Go to your Evolve website (*http://evolve.elsevier.com/Price/pediatric/*) for the following FREE learning resources:
- 3-D Animations
- Answer Keys

- Appendixes
- Audio Glossary
- Spanish/English Glossary
- Video Clips

Review Questions for the NCLEX® Examination

1. Legal issues related to death include: (**Select all that apply.**)
   1. Benevolence
   2. Informed consent
   3. Organ donation
   4. Fidelity
   5. Justice

2. List the three main ingredients in communication in order from most powerful to least powerful.
   1. Words
   2. Tone of voice
   3. Body language

3. All of the following are true regarding a child's reaction to death **except**:
   1. Children have a strong sense of trust.
   2. Children's anxiety about death often centers on symptoms.
   3. Children fear painful procedures.
   4. Children often communicate symbolically.

4. A complex series of reactions that occur during and after the death of a loved one is known as:
   1. Anticipatory grief
   2. Bargaining
   3. Bereavement
   4. Reflection

5. Which of the following is an example of a spiritual need?
   1. Meaning
   2. Role and relationship changes
   3. Fear of dying
   4. Comfort measures

Recommendations for Preventive Pediatric Health Care

Each child and family is unique; therefore, these Recommendations for Preventive Pdiatric Health Care are designed for the care of children who are receiving competent parenting, have no manifestations of any important health problems, and are growing and developing in satisfactory fashion. Additional visits may become necessary if circumstances suggest variations from normal.

Developmental, psychosocial, and chronic disease issues for children and adolescents may require frequent counseling and treatment visits separate from preventive care visits.

These guidelines represent a consensus by the American Academy of Pediatrics (AAP) and Bright Futures. The AAP continues to emphasize the great importance of continuity of care in comprehensive health supervision and the need to avoid fragmentation of care.

The recommendations in this statement do not indicate an exclusive course of treatment or standard of medical care. Variations, taking into account individual circumstances, may be appropriate.

TABLE KEY

• = to be performed; ★ = risk assessment to be performed, with appropriate action to follow, if positive; ← • → = range during which a service may be provided, with the symbol indicating the preferred age

American Academy of Pediatrics
DEDICATED TO THE HEALTH OF ALL CHILDREN®

Recommendations for Preventive Pediatric Health Care

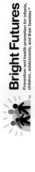

Bright Futures
Prevention and health promotion for infants, children, adolescents, and their families™

Age[a]	Prenatal[b]	Newborn[c]	3–5 d[d]	By 1 mo	2 mo	4 mo	6 mo	9 mo	12 mo	15 mo	18 mo	24 mo	30 mo	3 y	4 y	5 y	6 y	7 y	8 y	9 y	10 y	11 y	12 y	13 y	14 y	15 y	16 y	17 y	18 y	19 y	20 y	21 y
			INFANCY						EARLY CHILDHOOD							MIDDLE CHILDHOOD							ADOLESCENCE										
HISTORY Initial/interval	●	●	●	●	●	●	●	●	●	●	●	●	●	●	●	●	●	●	●	●	●	●	●	●	●	●	●	●	●	●	●	●
MEASUREMENTS																																
Length/height and weight		●	●	●	●	●	●	●	●	●	●	●	●	●	●	●	●	●	●	●	●	●	●	●	●	●	●	●	●	●	●	●
Head circumference		●	●	●	●	●	●	●	●	●	●	●																				
Weight for length		●	●	●	●	●	●	●	●	●	●	●																				
Body mass index												●	●	●	●	●	●	●	●	●	●	●	●	●	●	●	●	●	●	●	●	●
Blood pressure[e]		★	★	★	★	★	★	★	★	★	★	★	★	●	●	●	●	●	●	●	●	●	●	●	●	●	●	●	●	●	●	●
SENSORY SCREENING																																
Vision		★	★	★	★	★	★	★	★	★	★	★	★	●	●	●	●	★	●	●	●	★	★	★	★	★	★	★	●	●	★	★
Hearing	●[g]		★	★	★	★	★	★	★	★	★	★	★	★	●	●	●	★	●	★	●	●	★	●	★	●	★	★	●	★	★	★
DEVELOPMENTAL/BEHAVIORAL ASSESSMENT																																
Developmental screening[h]								●			●		●																			
Autism screening[i]											●	●																				
Developmental surveillance[j]		●	●	●	●	●	●	●	●	●	●	●	●	●	●	●	●	●	●	●	●	●	●	●	●	●	●	●	●	●	●	●
Psychosocial/behavioral assessment		●	●	●	●	●	●	●	●	●	●	●	●	●	●	●	●	●	●	●	●	●	●	●	●	●	●	●	●	●	●	●
Alcohol and drug use assessment																						★	★	★	★	★	★	★	★	★	★	★

Table row labels (rotated):

- PHYSICAL EXAMINATION[j]
- PROCEDURES[k]
- Newborn metabolic/hemoglobin screening[l]
- Immunization[m]
- Hematocrit or hemoglobin[n]
- Lead screening[o]
- Tuberculin test[q]
- Dyslipidemia screening
- STI screening
- Cervical dysplasia screening[t]
- ORAL HEALTH[u]
- ANTICIPATORY GUIDANCE[w]

a If a child comes under care for the first time at any point on the schedule, or if any items are not accomplished at the suggested age, the schedule should be brought up to date at the earliest possible time.

b A prenatal visit is recommended for parents who are at high risk, for first-time parents, and for those who request a conference. The prenatal visit should include anticipatory guidance, pertinent medical history, and a discussion of benefits of breastfeeding and planned method of feeding per AAP statement "The Prenatal Visit" (2001) [URL: http://aappolicy.aappublications.org/cgi/content/full/pediatrics;107/6/1456].

c Every infant should have a newborn evaluation after birth, breastfeeding encouraged, and instruction and support offered.

d Every infant should have an evaluation within 3 to 5 days of birth and within 48 to 72 hours after discharge from the hospital, to include evaluation for feeding and jaundice. Breastfeeding infants should receive formal breastfeeding evaluation, encouragement, and instruction as recommended in AAP statement "Breastfeeding and the Use of Human Milk" (2005) [URL: http://aappolicy.aappublications.org/cgi/content/full/pediatrics;115/2/496]. For newborns discharged in less than 48 hours after delivery, the infant must be examined within 48 hours of discharge per AAP statement "Hospital Stay for Healthy Term Newborns" (2004) [URL: http://aappolicy.aappublications.org/cgi/content/full/pediatrics;113/5/1434].

e Blood pressure measurement in infants and children with specific risk conditions should be performed at visits before age 3 years.

f If the patient is uncooperative, rescreen within 6 months per AAP statement "Eye Examination and Vision Screening in Infants, Children, and Young Adults" (1996) [URL: http://aappolicy.aappublications.org/cgi/reprint/pediatrics;98/1/153.pdf].

g All newborns should be screened per AAP statement "Year 2000 Position Statement: Principles and Guidelines for Early Hearing Detection and Intervention Programs '" (2000) [URL: http://aappolicy.aappublications.org/cgi/content/full/pediatrics;106/4/798]. Joint Committee on Infant Hearing. Year 2007 position statement: principles and guidelines for early hearing detection and intervention programs. Pediatrics. 2007;120:898–921.

h AAP Council on Children With Disabilities, AAP Section on Developmental Behavioral Pediatrics, AAP Bright Futures Steering Committee, AAP Medical Home Initiatives for Children With Special Needs Project Advisory Committee. Identifying infants and young children with developmental disorders in the medical home: an algorithm for developmental surveillance and screening. Pediatrics. 2006;118:405–420 [URL: http://aappolicy.aappublications.org/cgi/content/full/pediatrics;118/1/405].

i Gupta VB, Hyman SL, Johnson CP, et al. Identifying children with autism early? Pediatrics. 2007;119:152–153 [URL: http://pediatrics.aappublications.org/cgi/content/full/119/1/152].

j At each visit, age-appropriate physical examination is essential, with infant totally unclothed, older child undressed and suitably draped.

k These may be modified, depending on entry point into schedule and individual need.

l Newborn metabolic and hemoglobinopathy screening should be done according to state law. Results should be reviewed at visits and appropriate retesting or referral done as needed.

m Schedules per the Committee on Infectious Diseases, published annually in the January issue of Pediatrics. Every visit should be an opportunity to update and complete a child's immunizations.

n See AAP Pediatric Nutrition Handbook, 5th Edition (2003) for a discussion of universal and selective screening options. See also Recommendations to prevent and control iron deficiency in the United States. MMWR Recomm Rep. 1998;47(RR-3):1–36.

o For children at risk of lead exposure, consult the AAP statement "Lead Exposure in Children: Prevention, Detection, and Management" (2005) [URL: http://aappolicy.aappublications.org/cgi/content/full/pediatrics;116/4/1036]. Additionally, screening should be done in accordance with state law where applicable.

p Perform risk assessments or screens as appropriate, based on universal screening requirements for patients with Medicaid or high prevalence areas.

q Tuberculosis testing per recommendations of the Committee on Infectious Diseases, published in the current edition of Red Book: Report of the Committee on Infectious Diseases. Testing should be done on recognition of high-risk factors.

r "Third Report of the National Cholesterol Education Program (NCEP) Expert Panel on Detection, Evaluation, and Treatment of High Blood Cholesterol in Adults (Adult Treatment Panel III) Final Report" (2002) [URL: http://circ.ahajournals.org/cgi/content/full/106/25/3143] and "The Expert Committee Recommendations on the Assessment, Prevention, and Treatment of Child and Adolescent Overweight and Obesity." Supplement to Pediatrics. In press.

s All sexually active patients should be screened for sexually transmitted infections (STIs).

t All sexually active girls should have screening for cervical dysplasia as part of a pelvic examination beginning within 3 years of onset of sexual activity or age 21 (whichever comes first).

u Referral to dental home, if available. Otherwise, administer oral health risk assessment. If the primary water source is deficient in fluoride, consider oral fluoride supplementation.

v At the visits for 3 years and 6 years of age, it should be determined whether the patient has a dental home. If the patient does not have a dental home, a referral should be made to one. If the primary water source is deficient in fluoride, consider oral fluoride supplementation.

w Refer to the specific guidance by age as listed in Bright Futures Guidelines. (Hagan JF, Shaw JS, Duncan PM, eds. Bright Futures: Guidelines for Health Supervision of Infants, Children, and Adolescents. 3rd ed. Elk Grove Village, IL: American Academy of Pediatrics; 2008.)

Standard Precautions

HISTORICAL PERSPECTIVES

For many years, hospitals and health care providers have been struggling with infection control, trying to incorporate control procedures that prevent infection transmission not only from patient to patient but also from patient to personnel and personnel to patient. The movement of patients with infectious diseases from specialty hospitals to general hospitals during the middle of the twentieth century prompted the U.S. Department of Health and Human Services, Centers for Disease Control and Prevention (CDC), to issue detailed guidelines addressing isolation techniques to be used in the general hospital. This manual was updated twice to reflect changes in microorganisms, appearance of new organisms, new epidemiologic information, and the increase in nosocomial infection.

The identification and increasing prevalence of HIV in the early 1980s radically changed infectious disease control approaches. Because of the HIV risk to health care personnel and because of research that indicated that the asymptomatic incubation period for AIDS could be years, in 1985 the CDC published a new strategy for infection control called universal precautions (UP). The underlying premise for UP applied blood and body fluid precautions to all persons regardless of whether their infection status was known. In 1991, the Occupational Safety and Health Administration (OSHA) issued guidelines for all health care employers to prevent employee occupational exposure to blood-borne pathogens.

Confusion about definitions of contaminated fluids and substances, as well as the fact that UP and other approaches did not adequately address transmission of illnesses such as tuberculosis and newly identified diseases, prompted the CDC to work with the Hospital Infection Control Practices Advisory Committee (HIC-PAC) to revise the CDC guidelines for isolation precautions in hospitals. The new guidelines, issued in 1996, are divided into three sections: standard precautions (to be applied to all), transmission-based precautions (to reduce airborne, droplet, and contact infection), and temporary precautions (to be used for patients suspected to have certain infections).

SUMMARY OF THE RECOMMENDATIONS FOR ISOLATION PRECAUTIONS IN HOSPITALS— STANDARD PRECAUTIONS

Standard precautions are used for all patients, regardless of infection status. "Standard precautions apply to (1) blood, (2) all body fluids, secretions, and excretions except sweat, regardless of whether they contain visible blood, (3) nonintact skin, and (4) mucous membranes" (Hospital Infection Control Practices Advisory Committee and Centers for Disease Control and Prevention, 1996). Contaminated equipment or surfaces refers to contamination by the previous substances.

FUNDAMENTALS

1. Wash hands with a nonantimicrobial soap after touching blood, body fluids, secretions, excretions, and contaminated articles, regardless of whether gloves are worn. Wash hands between patients and between performing different procedures on the same patient (if appropriate). Wash hands immediately after removing gloves. Use an antimicrobial soap for special circumstances to control certain disease outbreaks.

2. Wear clean, nonsterile gloves when touching blood, body fluids, secretions, excretions, and contaminated articles, and before contacting mucous membranes or nonintact skin. Change gloves between patients and between procedures on the same patient if gloves have been in contact with an area likely to contain a high concentration of microorganisms. Remove gloves promptly after use and before touching noncontaminated articles.

3. Wear a clean gown, shoe covers, and mask, goggles, or face shield during procedures and activities likely to generate splashes or sprays of blood, body fluids, secretions, or excretions likely to cause soiling of clothing or exposure to skin and mucous membranes. Remove equipment promptly, and wash hands immediately.

4. Handle used, contaminated patient care equipment in a manner that prevents exposure to skin, mucous membranes, and clothing, and that prevents transmission of organisms to others. Properly clean and

reprocess all contaminated equipment, or properly discard all single-use articles.

5. Ensure that all hospital procedures for the cleaning and disinfection of environmental surfaces are followed.
6. Handle and process contaminated linens in a way that prevents skin and mucous membrane exposure, prevents contamination of clothing, and avoids transmission of microorganisms to others.
7. No special precautions are needed for dishes and eating utensils.
8. Follow OSHA Blood-Borne Pathogen Standards for occupational exposure and injury prevention.
   A. Use care in the handling, cleaning, and disposal of sharp instruments and devices.
   B. Never recap needles with two hands or point a needle in the direction of the body—may use a one-handed "scoop" procedure or syringes mechanically designed to cover an exposed needle after use.
   C. Do not try to break the needle after use. Dispose of all sharps in an appropriately marked puncture-resistant container placed close to the area of use.
   D. Appropriately mark and handle blood and contaminated fluids for transport (leakproof containers).
   E. Use mouthpieces, resuscitation bags, or other ventilation devices instead of mouth-to-mouth resuscitation. Keep equipment available in each patient room.
   F. Arrange to have cleaned all contaminated environmental surfaces as soon as possible after the contamination occurs.
   G. Dispose of contaminated articles in properly marked containers designed to handle regulated waste.

OSHA regulations provide for the annual review of all procedures related to the implementation of the blood-borne pathogen standard and mandates employers to provide all equipment necessary to ensure employee safety. OSHA also delineates procedures after an accidental exposure in the workplace.

SUMMARY OF THE RECOMMENDATIONS FOR TRANSMISSION-BASED PRECAUTIONS

See Box B-1 for types of precautions and patient categories.

1. Airborne precautions (5 mm or smaller)
   A. Adhere to standard precautions.
   B. Patient should be in a private room with (1) monitored negative air pressure in relation to the surrounding areas, (2) 6 to 12 air changes per hour, and (3) appropriate discharge of air outdoors or monitored high-efficiency filtration of room air before the air is circulated to other areas of the hospital. May be in room with patient who has active infection with same microorganism but no other infections. Door should stay closed, and patient should leave room only if transport is necessary. Have patient wear a mask during transport.
   C. Wear respiratory protection (N95 respirator) when entering the room of a person with known or suspected infectious pulmonary tuberculosis. Susceptible persons should not enter the room of patients known or suspected to have measles (rubeola) or varicella (chickenpox) if other immune caregivers are available. If susceptible persons must enter the room of a patient known or suspected to have measles (rubeola) or varicella, they should wear respiratory protection (N95 respirator). Persons immune to measles (rubeola) or varicella need not wear respiratory protection.
2. Droplet precautions (larger than 5 mm)
   A. Adhere to standard precautions.
   B. Patient should be in private room or in a room with a patient who has active infection with same microorganism but no other infection. Door can remain open.
   C. Wear a mask if working within 3 feet of the patient.
   D. Have patient wear a mask during transport.
3. Contact precautions
   A. Adhere to standard precautions.
   B. Patient should be in private room or with patient who has active infection with same microorganism but no other infections.
   C. In addition to wearing gloves as outlined under standard precautions, wear gloves (clean) when entering the room. During the course of providing care for the patient, change gloves after having contact with infectious material that may contain high concentrations of microorganisms (fecal material and wound drainage). Remove gloves before leaving patient's room. Wash hands immediately with an antimicrobial agent or waterless antiseptic agent. Do not touch any potentially contaminated surfaces after completing hand hygiene.
   D. Wear a gown if you anticipate patient contact, contact with environmental surfaces, or contact with items in the patient's room or if patient is incontinent or has diarrhea, an ileostomy, a colostomy, a urostomy, or wound drainage not contained by a dressing. Remove gown before leaving patient's room, but do not allow clothing to become contaminated.
   E. Avoid risk for transmission of microorganisms to other patients and equipment if transported.
   F. Adequately clean and disinfect any equipment before use by another patient.

Box **B-1** | Synopsis of Types of Precautions and Patients Requiring the Precautions

STANDARD PRECAUTIONS
Use standard precautions for the care of all patients.

AIRBORNE PRECAUTIONS
In addition to standard precautions, use airborne precautions for patients known or suspected to have serious illnesses transmitted by airborne droplet nuclei. Examples of such illnesses include:
- Measles
- Varicella (including disseminated zoster)*
- Tuberculosis[†]
- Smallpox

DROPLET PRECAUTIONS
In addition to standard precautions, use droplet precautions for patients known or suspected to have serious illnesses transmitted by large particle droplets. Examples of such illnesses include:
- Invasive *Haemophilus influenzae* type b disease, including meningitis, pneumonia, epiglottitis, and sepsis
- Invasive *Neisseria meningitidis* disease, including meningitis, pneumonia, and sepsis
- Other serious bacterial respiratory infections spread by droplet transmission, including:
  Diphtheria (pharyngeal)
  Mycoplasma pneumonia
  Pertussis
  Pneumonic plague
  Streptococcal pharyngitis, pneumonia, or scarlet fever in infants and young children
- Serious viral infections spread by droplet transmission, including:
  Adenovirus*
  Influenza
  Mumps

Parvovirus B19
Rubella

CONTACT PRECAUTIONS
In addition to standard precautions, use contact precautions for patients known or suspected to have serious illnesses easily transmitted by direct patient contact or by contact with items in the patient's environment. Examples of such illnesses include:
- Gastrointestinal, respiratory, skin, or wound infections or colonization with multidrug-resistant bacteria judged by the infection control program, based on current state, regional, or national recommendation, to be of special clinical and epidemiologic significance
- Enteric infections with a low infectious dose or prolonged environmental survival, including:
  Clostridium difficile
  For diapered or incontinent patients:
    enterohemorrhagic *Escherichia coli* o157:h7, *Shigella*, hepatitis A, or rotavirus
- Respiratory syncytial virus, parainfluenza virus, or enteroviral infections in infants and young children
- Skin infections that are highly contagious or that may occur on dry skin, including:
  Diphtheria (cutaneous)
  Herpes simplex virus (neonatal or mucocutaneous)
  Impetigo
  Major (noncontained) abscesses, cellulitis, or decubiti
  Pediculosis
  Scabies
  Smallpox
  Staphylococcal furunculosis in infants and young children
  Zoster (disseminated or in the immunocompromised host)*
- Viral/hemorrhagic conjunctivitis
- Viral hemorrhagic infections (Ebola, Lassa, or Marburg)

*Certain infections require more than one type of precaution.
[†]See CDC Guidelines for Preventing the Transmission of Tuberculosis in Health-Care Facilities.

REFERENCES

Hospital Infection Control Practices Advisory Committee and the Centers for Disease Control and Prevention. (1996). Guideline for isolation precautions in hospitals. *Am J Infect Cont*, 24(1), 24-52.
Occupational Safety and Health Act. (1991). Blood-borne pathogen standard. *Fed Register*, 56(2), 40-46.

Growth Charts

Appendix C includes several groupings of charts related to the growth of a child. The first chart, used at birth, is the Maturational Assessment of Gestational Age, also sometimes referred to as the Ballard Scoring System. This growth chart is used to determine the gestational age of a newborn by neuromuscular and physical characteristics. Using this chart aids the health care practitioner in determining the gestational development of the newborn. Those newborns who are less than 37 weeks' gestation will need further assessment and possible interventions. The second part of the Ballard Scoring System allows for the newborn's gestational age to be compared with weight, head circumference, and length. These measurements will show the newborn to be one of the following: large for gestational age, appropriate for gestational age, or small for gestational age. The newborn whose measurements are large for gestational age or small for gestational age will need further assistance and interventions.

In 2000, the Centers for Disease Control and Prevention (CDC) released new growth charts for children. These growth charts allow the health care practitioner to plot the child's measurements according to the child's age to determine how the child measures up against the national mean. The child's growth should progress, and the growth charts allow the health care practitioner and the family to quickly see how the child is growing.

The CDC growth charts begin with those for boys, birth to 36 months. The criteria that are measured in percentiles are Weight for Age, Length for Age, Head Circumference for Age, and Weight for Length.

After age 2 years, growth slows and the child is measured less frequently. The charts are still identified for boys and girls and can be used until the age of 20 years. The CDC charts for boys 2 to 20 years are Weight for Age, Stature for Age, Weight for Stature, and Body Mass Index for Age. The CDC charts for girls 2 to 20 years follow the same format as for boys. New to the growth charts is the body mass index (BMI). After age 2 years, BMI is useful in determining whether a child is progressing toward obesity.

In summary, growth charts are a quick and accurate way to measure and monitor the growth of a child as well as to compare the child's growth with the national mean. In using the growth charts, anticipatory guidance, nutrition, and health care issues can be addressed.

MATURATIONAL ASSESSMENT OF GESTATIONAL AGE (New Ballard Score)

NAME _____   SEX _____

HOSPITAL NO. _____   BIRTH WEIGHT _____

RACE _____   LENGTH _____

DATE/TIME OF BIRTH _____   HEAD CIRC. _____

DATE/TIME OF EXAM _____   EXAMINER _____

AGE WHEN EXAMINED _____

APGAR SCORE: 1 MINUTE _____ 5 MINUTES _____ 10 MINUTES _____

NEUROMUSCULAR MATURITY

NEUROMUSCULAR MATURITY SIGN	SCORE							RECORD SCORE HERE
	-1	0	1	2	3	4	5	
POSTURE								
SQUARE WINDOW (Wrist)	>90°	90°	60°	45°	30°	0°		
ARM RECOIL		180°	140°-180°	110°-140°	90°-110°	<90°		
POPLITEAL ANGLE	180°	160°	140°	120°	100°	90°	<90°	
SCARF SIGN								
HEEL TO EAR								

TOTAL NEUROMUSCULAR MATURITY SCORE

PHYSICAL MATURITY

PHYSICAL MATURITY SIGN	SCORE							RECORD SCORE HERE
	-1	0	1	2	3	4	5	
SKIN	sticky friable transparent	gelatinous red translucent	smooth pink visible veins	superficial peeling &/or rash, few veins	cracking pale areas rare veins	parchment deep cracking no vessels	leathery cracked wrinkled	
LANUGO	none	sparse	abundant	thinning	bald areas	mostly bald		
PLANTAR SURFACE	heel-toe 40-50 mm:-1 <40 mm:-2	>50 mm no crease	faint red marks	anterior transverse crease only	creases ant. 2/3	creases over entire sole		
BREAST	imperceptible	barely perceptible	flat areola no bud	stippled areola 1-2 mm bud	raised areola 3-4 mm bud	full areola 5-10 mm bud		
EYE/EAR	lids fused loosely: -1 tightly: -2	lids open pinna flat stays folded	sl. curved pinna; soft; slow recoil	well-curved pinna; soft but ready recoil	formed & firm instant recoil	thick cartilage ear stiff		
GENITALS (Male)	scrotum flat, smooth	scrotum empty faint rugae	testes in upper canal rare rugae	testes descending few rugae	testes down good rugae	testes pendulous deep rugae		
GENITALS (Female)	clitoris prominent & labia flat	prominent clitoris & small labia minora	prominent clitoris & enlarging minora	majora & minora equally prominent	majora large minora small	majora cover clitoris & minora		

Ballard JL, Khoury JC, Wedig K, et al: New Ballard Score, expanded to include extremely premature infants, *J Pediatr* 119:417-423, 1991. Reprinted by permission of Dr Ballard and Mosby.

TOTAL PHYSICAL MATURITY SCORE

SCORE

Neuromuscular _____

Physical _____

Total _____

MATURITY RATING

score	weeks
-10	20
-5	22
0	24
5	26
10	28
15	30
20	32
25	34
30	36
35	38
40	40
45	42
50	44

GESTATIONAL AGE (weeks)

By dates _____

By ultrasound _____

By exam _____

CLASSIFICATION OF NEWBORNS (BOTH SEXES)
BY INTRAUTERINE GROWTH AND GESTATIONAL AGE [1,2]

NAME _____ DATE OF EXAM _____ LENGTH _____

HOSPITAL NO. __ _____ SEX _____ HEAD CIRC. _____

RACE _____ BIRTH WEIGHT _____ GESTATIONAL AGE _____

DATE OF BIRTH _____

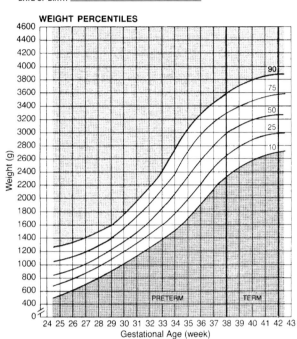

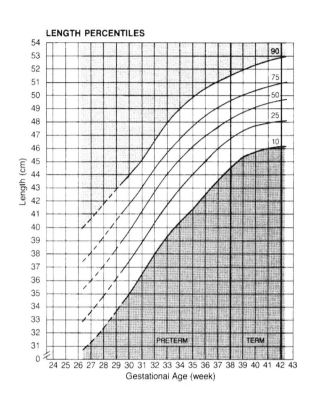

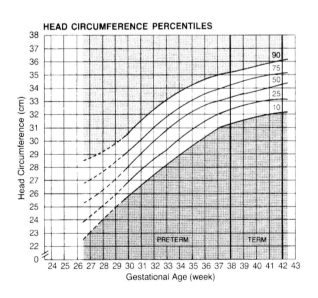

CLASSIFICATION OF INFANT*	Weight	Length	Head Circ.
Large for Gestational Age (LGA) (>90th percentile)			
Appropriate for Gestational Age (AGA) (10th to 90th percentile)			
Small for Gestational Age (SGA) (<10th percentile)			

*Place an "X" in the appropriate box (LGA, AGA or SGA) for weight, for length, and for head circumference.

1. Battaglia FC, Lubchenco LO: A practical classification of newborn infants by weight and gestational age.
   J Pediatr 71:159-163, 1967.
2. Lubchenco LO, Hansman C, Boyd E: Intrauterine growth in length and head circumference as estimated
   from live births at gestational ages from 26 to 42 weeks. Pediatrics: 37:403-408, 1966.

Birth to 36 months: Boys
Length-for-age and Weight-for-age percentiles

NAME _____

RECORD # _____

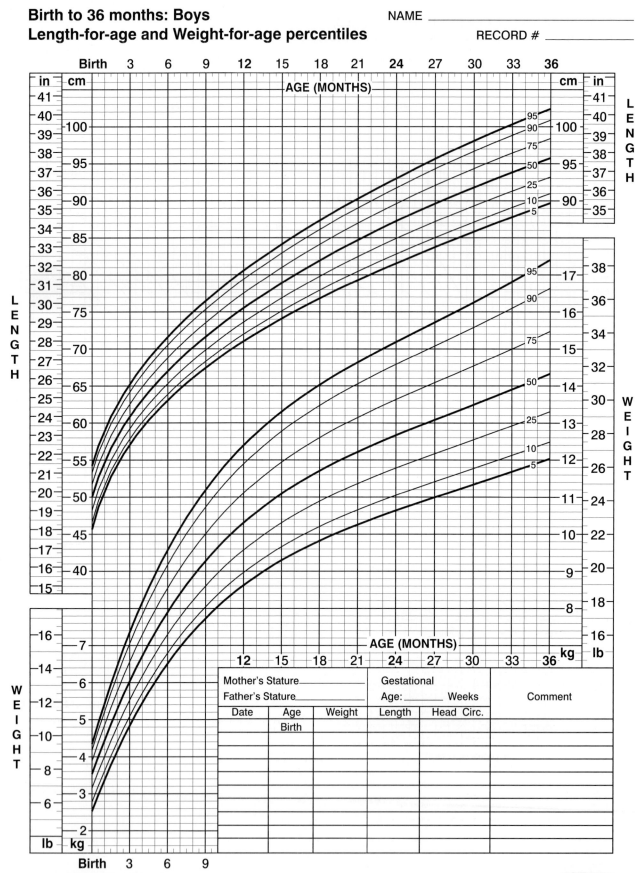

Pubished May 30, 2000 (modified 4/20/01).
SOURCE: Developed by the National Center for Health Statistics in collaboration with
the National Center for Chronic Disease Prevention and Health Promotion (2000).
http://www.cdc.gov/growthcharts

SAFER · HEALTHIER · PEOPLE™

Birth to 36 months: Girls
Length-for-age and Weight-for-age percentiles

NAME _____

RECORD # _____

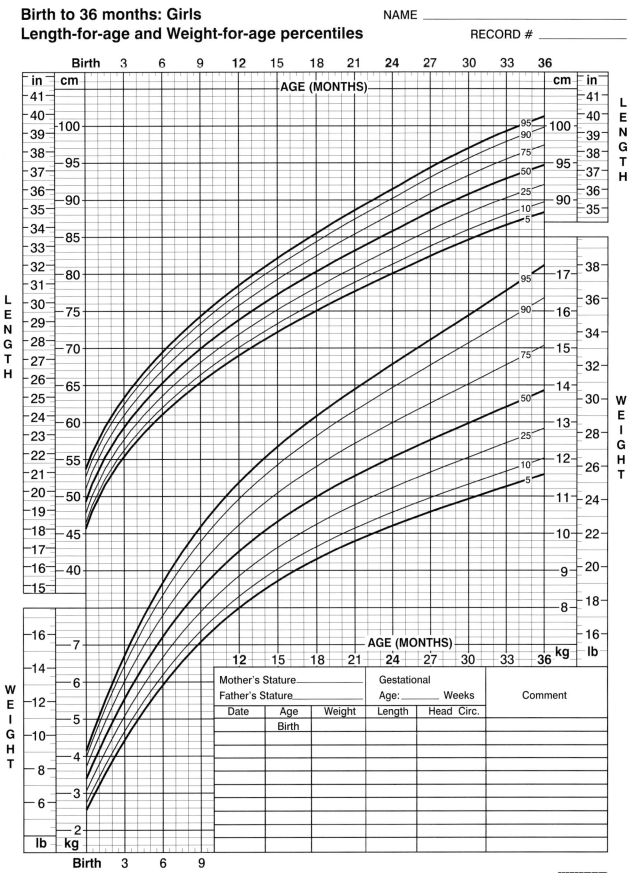

Mother's Stature_____
Father's Stature_____

Gestational
Age: _____ Weeks

Comment

Date	Age	Weight	Length	Head Circ.	
	Birth				

Published May 30, 2000 (modified 4/20/01).
SOURCE: Developed by the National Center for Health Statistics in collaboration with
   the National Center for Chronic Disease Prevention and Health Promotion (2000).
   http://www.cdc.gov/growthcharts

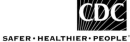

SAFER · HEALTHIER · PEOPLE™

Birth to 36 months: Boys
Head circumference-for-age and
Weight-for-length percentiles

NAME _____

RECORD # _____

AGE (MONTHS)

Head circumference percentiles (in/cm): 95, 90, 75, 50, 25, 10, 5

Weight-for-length percentiles: 95, 90, 75, 50, 25, 10, 5

LENGTH (cm / in)

Date	Age	Weight	Length	Head Circ.	Comment

Published May 30, 2000 (modified 10/16/00).
SOURCE: Developed by the National Center for Health Statistics in collaboration with
the National Center for Chronic Disease Prevention and Health Promotion (2000).
http://www.cdc.gov/growthcharts

CDC

SAFER・HEALTHIER・PEOPLE™

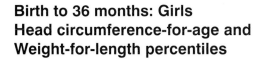

Birth to 36 months: Girls
Head circumference-for-age and
Weight-for-length percentiles

NAME _____

RECORD # _____

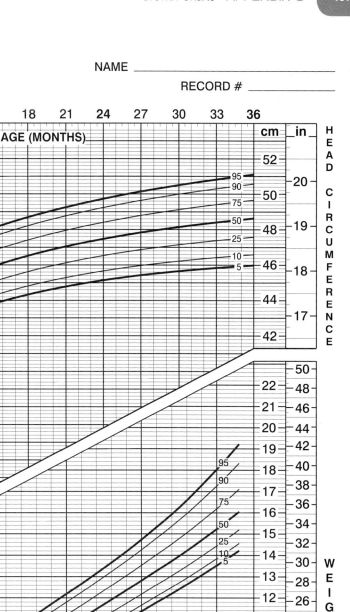

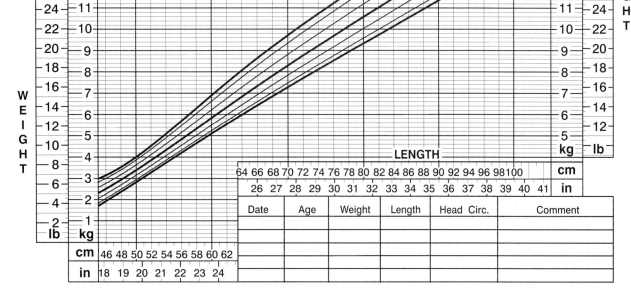

Date	Age	Weight	Length	Head Circ.	Comment

Published May 30, 2000 (modified 10/16/00).
SOURCE: Developed by the National Center for Health Statistics in collaboration with
the National Center for Chronic Disease Prevention and Health Promotion (2000).
http://www.cdc.gov/growthcharts

SAFER • HEALTHIER • PEOPLE™

2 to 20 years: Boys
Stature-for-age and Weight-for-age percentiles

NAME _____

RECORD # _____

Mother's Stature _____		Father's Stature _____		
Date	Age	Weight	Stature	BMI*

*To Calculate BMI: Weight (kg) ÷ Stature (cm) ÷ Stature (cm) x 10,000
or Weight (lb) ÷ Stature (in) ÷ Stature (in) x 703

AGE (YEARS)

12 13 14 15 16 17 18 19 20

STATURE

cm   in
190 76
185 74
180 72
175 70
170 68
165 66
     64
160 62
155 60
150

95
90
75
50
25
10
5

in   cm
62   160
60   155
58   150
56   145
54   140
52   135
50   130
48   125
46   120
44   115
42   110
40   105
38   100
36   95
34   90
32   85
30   80

3 4 5 6 7 8 9 10 11

STATURE

WEIGHT

cm   lb
105 230
100 220
95   210
90   200
85   190
80   180
75   170
     160
70   150
65   140
60   130
55   120
50   110
45   100
40   90
35   80
30   70
25   60
20   50
15   40
10   30

95
90
75
50
25
10
5

lb   kg
80   35
70   30
60   25
50   20
40   15
30   10

WEIGHT

AGE (YEARS)

kg   lb

2 3 4 5 6 7 8 9 10 11 12 13 14 15 16 17 18 19 20

Published May 30, 2000 (modified 11/21/00).
SOURCE: Developed by the National Center for Health Statistics in collaboration with
the National Center for Chronic Disease Prevention and Health Promotion (2000).
http://www.cdc.gov/growthcharts

SAFER · HEALTHIER · PEOPLE™

2 to 20 years: Girls
Stature-for-age and Weight-for-age percentiles

NAME _____

RECORD # _____

Mother's Stature		Father's Stature		
Date	Age	Weight	Stature	BMI*

*To Calculate BMI: Weight (kg) ÷ Stature (cm) ÷ Stature (cm) x 10,000
   or Weight (lb) ÷ Stature (in) ÷ Stature (in) x 703

AGE (YEARS)

12 13 14 15 16 17 18 19 20

STATURE

STATURE

WEIGHT

WEIGHT

AGE (YEARS)

2 3 4 5 6 7 8 9 10 11 12 13 14 15 16 17 18 19 20

95
90
75
50
25
10
5

Published May 30, 2000 (modified 11/21/00).
SOURCE: Developed by the National Center for Health Statistics in collaboration with
   the National Center for Chronic Disease Prevention and Health Promotion (2000).
   http://www.cdc.gov/growthcharts

SAFER · HEALTHIER · PEOPLE™

2 to 20 years: Boys
Body mass index-for-age percentiles

NAME _____

RECORD # _____

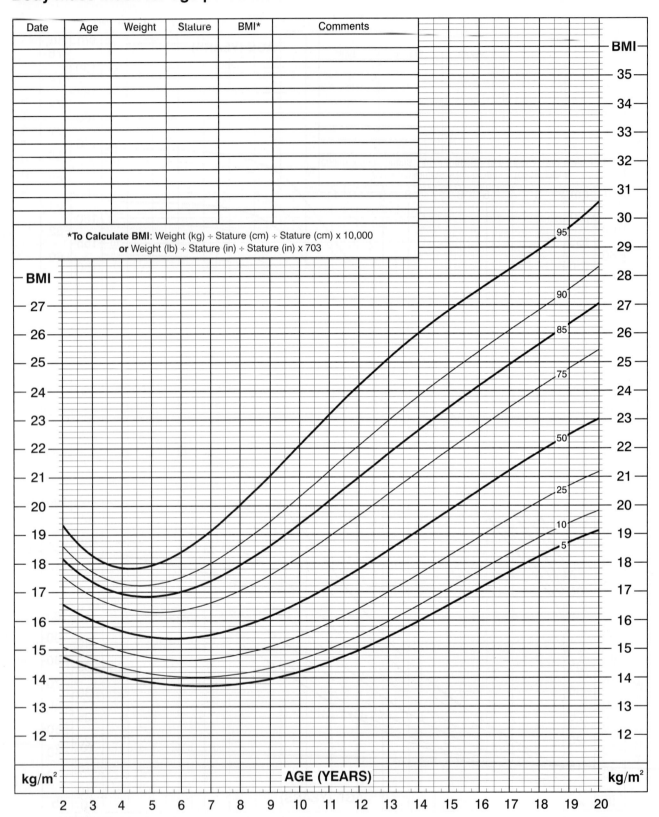

Date	Age	Weight	Stature	BMI*	Comments

*To Calculate BMI: Weight (kg) ÷ Stature (cm) ÷ Stature (cm) x 10,000
or Weight (lb) ÷ Stature (in) ÷ Stature (in) x 703

AGE (YEARS)

Published May 30, 2000 (modified 10/16/00).
SOURCE: Developed by the National Center for Health Statistics in collaboration with
the National Center for Chronic Disease Prevention and Health Promotion (2000).
http://www.cdc.gov/growthcharts

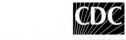

SAFER • HEALTHIER • PEOPLE™

2 to 20 years: Girls
Body mass index-for-age percentiles

NAME _____

RECORD # _____

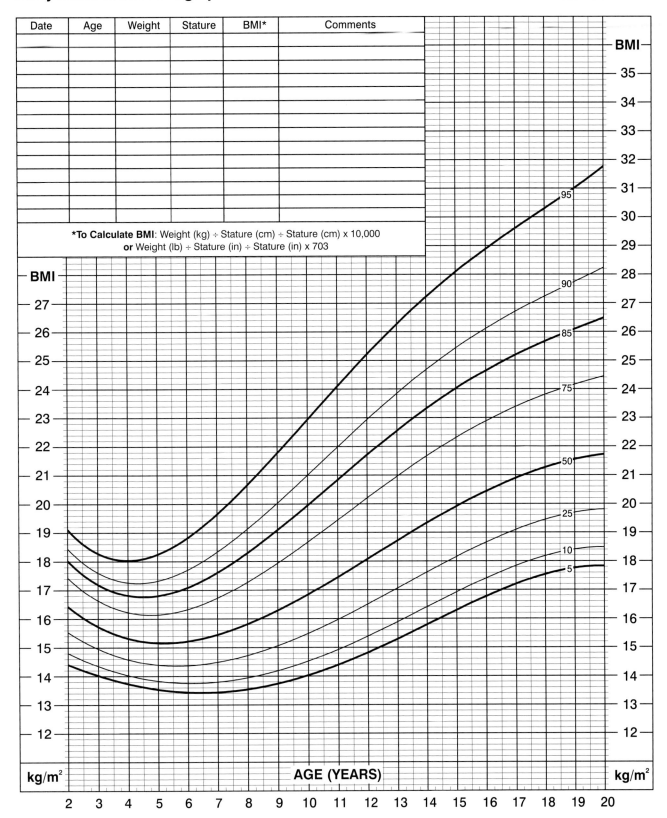

Date	Age	Weight	Stature	BMI*	Comments

*To Calculate BMI: Weight (kg) ÷ Stature (cm) ÷ Stature (cm) x 10,000
or Weight (lb) ÷ Stature (in) ÷ Stature (in) x 703

AGE (YEARS)

kg/m²

Published May 30, 2000 (modified 10/16/00).
SOURCE: Developed by the National Center for Health Statistics in collaboration with
the National Center for Chronic Disease Prevention and Health Promotion (2000).
http://www.cdc.gov/growthcharts

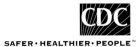

SAFER · HEALTHIER · PEOPLE™

NAME _____

RECORD # _____

Weight-for-stature percentiles: Boys

Date	Age	Weight	Stature	Comments

STATURE

cm   80   85   90   95   100   105   110   115   120

in   31 32 33 34 35 36 37 38 39 40 41 42 43 44 45 46 47

Published May 30, 2000 (modified 10/16/00).
SOURCE: Developed by the National Center for Health Statistics in collaboration with
the National Center for Chronic Disease Prevention and Health Promotion (2000).
http://www.cdc.gov/growthcharts

SAFER · HEALTHIER · PEOPLE™

Weight-for-stature percentiles: Girls

NAME _____

RECORD # _____

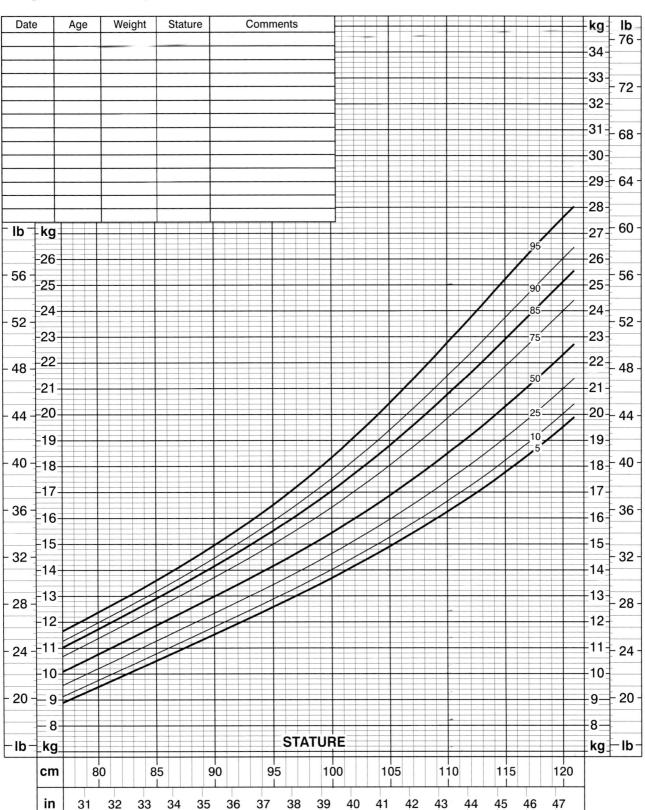

Date	Age	Weight	Stature	Comments

STATURE

cm	80	85	90	95	100	105	110	115	120

| in | 31 | 32 | 33 | 34 | 35 | 36 | 37 | 38 | 39 | 40 | 41 | 42 | 43 | 44 | 45 | 46 | 47 |

Published May 30, 2000 (modified 10/16/00).
SOURCE: Developed by the National Center for Health Statistics in collaboration with
the National Center for Chronic Disease Prevention and Health Promotion (2000).
http://www.cdc.gov/growthcharts

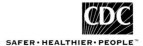

SAFER · HEALTHIER · PEOPLE™

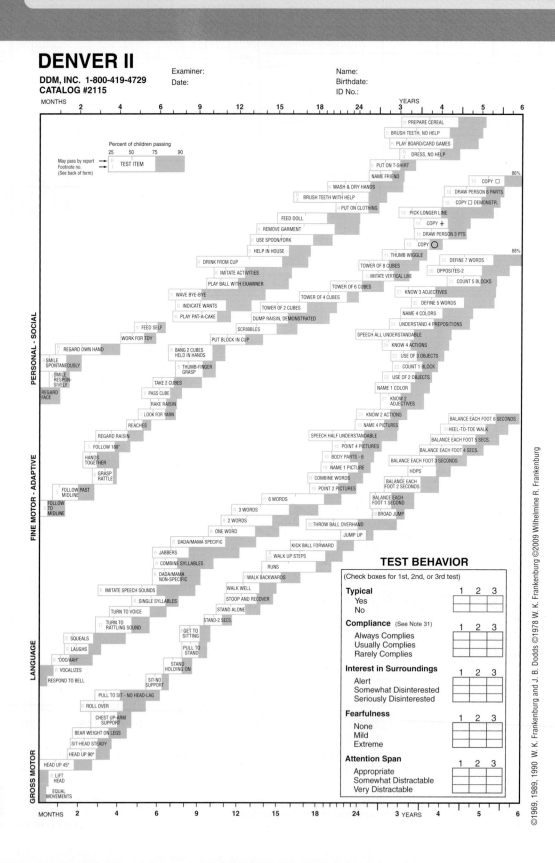

DENVER II

DDM, INC. 1-800-419-4729
CATALOG #2115

Examiner:
Date:

Name:
Birthdate:
ID No.:

DIRECTIONS FOR ADMINISTRATION

1. Try to get child to smile by smiling, talking or waving. Do not touch him/her.
2. Child must stare at hand several seconds.
3. Parent may help guide toothbrush and put toothpaste on brush.
4. Child does not have to be able to tie shoes or button/zip in the back.
5. Move yarn slowly in an arc from one side to the other, about 8" above child's face.
6. Pass if child grasps rattle when it is touched to the backs or tips of fingers.
7. Pass if child tries to see where yarn went. Yarn should be dropped quickly from sight from tester's hand without arm movement.
8. Child must transfer cube from hand to hand without help of body, mouth, or table.
9. Pass if child picks up raisin with any part of thumb and finger.
10. Line can vary only 30 degrees or less from tester's line. /
11. Make a fist with thumb pointing upward and wiggle only the thumb. Pass if child imitates and does not move any fingers other than the thumb.

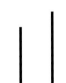

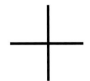

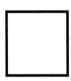

12. Pass any enclosed form. Fail continuous round motions.

13. Which line is longer? (Not bigger.) Turn paper upside down and repeat. (pass 3 of 3 or 5 of 6)

14. Pass any lines crossing near midpoint.

15. Have child copy first. If failed, demonstrate.

When giving items 12, 14, and 15, do not name the forms. Do not demonstrate 12 and 14.

16. When scoring, each pair (2 arms, 2 legs, etc.) counts as one part.
17. Place one cube in cup and shake gently near child's ear, but out of sight. Repeat for other ear.
18. Point to picture and have child name it. (No credit is given for sounds only.)
    If less than 4 pictures are named correctly, have child point to picture as each is named by tester.

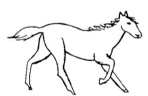

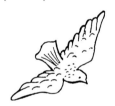

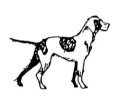

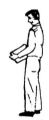

19. Using doll, tell child: Show me the nose, eyes, ears, mouth, hands, feet, tummy, hair. Pass 6 of 8.
20. Using pictures, ask child: Which one flies?...says meow?...talks?...barks?...gallops? Pass 2 of 5, 4 of 5.
21. Ask child: What do you do when you are cold?...tired?...hungry? Pass 2 of 3, 3 of 3.
22. Ask child: What do you do with a cup? What is a chair used for? What is a pencil used for?
    Action words must be included in answers.
23. Pass if child correctly places <u>and</u> says how many blocks are on paper. (1,5).
24. Tell child: Put block **on** table; **under** table; **in front of** me, **behind** me. Pass 4 of 4.
    (Do not help child by pointing, moving head or eyes.)
25. Ask child: What is a ball?...lake?...desk?...house?...banana?...curtain?...fence?...ceiling? Pass if defined in terms
    of use, shape, what it is made of, or general category (such as banana is fruit, not just yellow). Pass 5 of 8, 7 of 8.
26. Ask child: If a horse is big, a mouse is ___? If fire is hot, ice is ___? If the sun shines during the day, the moon shines
    during the ___? Pass 2 of 3.
27. Child may use wall or rail only, not person. May not crawl.
28. Child must throw ball overhand 3 feet to within arm's reach of tester.
29. Child must perform standing broad jump over width of test sheet (8 1/2 inches).
30. Tell child to walk forward, ∞∞∞∞→ heel within 1 inch of toe. Tester may demonstrate.
    Child must walk 4 consecutive steps.
31. In the second year, half of normal children are non-compliant.

OBSERVATIONS:

Denver Developmental Materials, Inc.
P.O. Box 371075
Denver, Colorado 80237-5075
Tele. #: (303) 355-4729
(800) 419-4729

Conversion Charts

Weight and Length Conversion

WEIGHT				LENGTH			
lb	kg	kg	lb	in	cm	cm	in
1	0.5	1	2.2	1	2.5	1	.4
2	0.9	2	4.4	2	5.1	2	.8
4	1.8	3	6.6	4	10.2	3	1.2
6	2.7	4	8.8	6	15.2	4	1.6
8	3.6	5	11.0	8	20.3	5	2.0
10	4.5	6	13.2	12	30.5	6	2.4
20	9.1	8	17.6	18	46	8	3.1
30	13.6	10	22	24	61	10	3.9
40	18.2	20	44	30	76	20	7.9
50	22.7	30	66	36	91	30	11.8
60	27.3	40	88	42	107	40	15.7
70	31.8	50	110	48	122	50	19.7
80	36.4	60	132	54	137	60	23.6
90	40.9	70	154	60	152	70	27.6
100	45.4	80	176	66	168	80	31.5
150	68.2	90	198	72	183	90	35.4
200	90.8	100	220	78	198	100	39.4

1 lb = 0.454 kg; 1 in = 2.54 cm; 1 kg = 2.204 lb; 1 cm = 0.3937 in.

Temperature Equivalents (Celsius and Fahrenheit)*

C	F	C	F
0	32.0	39.0	102.2
20	68.0	39.2	102.6
30	86.0	39.4	102.9
31	87.8	39.6	103.3
32	89.6	39.8	103.7
33	91.4	40.0	104.0
34	93.2	40.2	104.4
35	95.0	40.4	104.7
36	96.8	40.6	105.1
37	98.6	40.8	105.4
37.2	99.0	41.0	105.8
37.4	99.3	41.2	106.2
37.6	99.7	41.4	106.5
37.8	100.1	41.6	106.9
38.0	100.4	41.8	107.2
38.2	100.8	42	107.6
38.4	101.2	43	109.4
38.6	101.5	44	111.2
38.8	101.8	100	212.0

*To convert Celsius (centigrade) readings to Fahrenheit, multiply by 1.8 and add 32. To convert Fahrenheit readings to Celsius, subtract 32 and divide by 1.8.

The Joint Commission Lists of Dangerous Abbreviations, Acronyms, and Symbols

A "minimum list" of dangerous abbreviations, acronyms, and symbols has been approved by The Joint Commission (TJC). The items in Table F-1 must be included on each accredited organization's "Do Not Use" list. Other items being considered for inclusion are listed in Table F-2.

As a recommended precaution, two nurses must double-check the following before administration: heparin, insulin, parenteral chemotherapeutic agents, patient-controlled analgesia, and epidural pumps.

HIPAA privacy requirements state that patient information concerning name, age, diagnosis, and other personal information should not be posted. Charts and medication records must be kept in a confidential area. Also, the Institute for Safe Medication Practices (ISMP) has published a list of dangerous abbreviations relating to medication use that it recommends should be explicitly prohibited. This list is available on its website: *http://www.ismp.org*.

Table F-1 Official "Do Not Use" List*

DO NOT USE	POTENTIAL PROBLEM	USE INSTEAD
U (for unit)	Mistaken for 0 (zero), 4 (four), or cc.	Write "unit."
IU (for international unit)	Mistaken for IV (intravenous) or the number 10 (ten).	Write "international unit."
Q.D., QD, q.d., qd (daily) Q.O.D., QOD, q.o.d., qod (every other day)	Mistaken for each other. Period after the Q mistaken for I and the O can be mistaken for I.	Write "daily." Write "every other day."
Trailing zero (X.0 mg)† Lack of leading zero (.X mg)	Decimal point is missed.	Write "X mg." Write "0.X mg."
MS MSO_4 and $MgSO_4$	Can mean morphine sulfate or magnesium sulfate. Confused for one another.	Write "morphine sulfate." Write "magnesium sulfate."

*Applies to all orders and all medication-related documentation that is handwritten (including free-text computer entry) or on preprinted forms.
†Exception: A trailing zero may be used only where required to demonstrate the level of precision of the value being reported, such as for laboratory results, imaging studies that report size of lesions, or catheter/tube sizes. It may not be used in medication orders or other medication-related documentation.

Table F-2 Additional Abbreviations, Acronyms, and Symbols*

DO NOT USE	POTENTIAL PROBLEM	USE INSTEAD
> (greater than) < (less than)	Misinterpreted as the number 7 (seven) or the letter L. Confused for one another.	Write "greater than." Write "less than."
Abbreviations for drug names	Misinterpreted due to similar abbreviations for multiple drugs.	Write drug names in full.
Apothecary units	Unfamiliar to many practitioners. Confused with metric units.	Use metric units.
@	Mistaken for the number 2 (two).	Write "at."
cc	Mistaken for U (units) when poorly written.	Write "mL" or "ml" or "milliliters" ("mL" is preferred).
μg	Mistaken for mg (milligrams), resulting in 1000-fold dosing overdose.	Write "mcg" or "micrograms."

*For possible future inclusion in the Official "Do Not Use" List.
From the Joint Commission, 2011.

The Fourth Report on the Diagnosis, Evaluation, and Treatment of High Blood Pressure in Children and Adolescents

Blood Pressure Levels for Boys by Age and Height Percentile*

AGE (YEAR)	BP PERCENTILE	SYSTOLIC BP (mm Hg) ←PERCENTILE OF HEIGHT→							DIASTOLIC BP (mm Hg) ←PERCENTILE OF HEIGHT→						
		5th	10th	25th	50th	75th	90th	95th	5th	10th	25th	50th	75th	90th	95th
1	50th	80	81	83	85	87	88	89	34	35	36	37	38	39	39
	90th	94	95	97	99	100	102	103	49	50	51	52	53	53	54
	95th	98	99	101	103	104	106	106	54	54	55	56	57	58	58
	99th	105	106	108	110	112	113	114	61	62	63	64	65	66	66
2	50th	84	85	87	88	90	92	92	39	40	41	42	43	44	44
	90th	97	99	100	102	104	105	106	54	55	56	57	58	58	59
	95th	101	102	104	106	108	109	110	59	59	60	61	62	63	63
	99th	109	110	111	113	115	117	117	66	67	68	69	70	71	71
3	50th	86	87	89	91	93	94	95	44	44	45	46	47	48	48
	90th	100	101	103	105	107	108	109	59	59	60	61	62	63	63
	95th	104	105	107	109	110	112	113	63	63	64	65	66	67	67
	99th	111	112	114	116	118	119	120	71	71	72	73	74	75	75
4	50th	88	89	91	93	95	96	97	47	48	49	50	51	51	52
	90th	102	103	105	107	109	110	111	62	63	64	65	66	66	67
	95th	106	107	109	111	112	114	115	66	67	68	69	70	71	71
	99th	113	114	116	118	120	121	122	74	75	76	77	78	78	79
5	50th	90	91	93	95	96	98	98	50	51	52	53	54	55	55
	90th	104	105	106	108	110	111	112	65	66	67	68	69	69	70
	95th	108	109	110	112	114	115	116	69	70	71	72	73	74	74
	99th	115	116	118	120	121	123	123	77	78	79	80	81	81	82
6	50th	91	92	94	96	98	99	100	53	53	54	55	56	57	57
	90th	105	106	108	110	111	113	113	68	68	69	70	71	72	72
	95th	109	110	112	114	115	117	117	72	72	73	74	75	76	76
	99th	116	117	119	121	123	124	125	80	80	81	82	83	84	84
7	50th	92	94	95	97	99	100	101	55	55	56	57	58	59	59
	90th	106	107	109	111	113	114	115	70	70	71	72	73	74	74
	95th	110	111	113	115	117	118	119	74	74	75	76	77	78	78
	99th	117	118	120	122	124	125	126	82	82	83	84	85	86	86
8	50th	94	95	97	99	100	102	102	56	57	58	59	60	60	61
	90th	107	109	110	112	114	115	116	71	72	72	73	74	75	76
	95th	111	112	114	116	118	119	120	75	76	77	78	79	79	80
	99th	119	120	122	123	125	127	127	83	84	85	86	87	87	88
9	50th	95	96	98	100	102	103	104	57	58	59	60	61	61	62
	90th	109	110	112	114	115	117	118	72	73	74	75	76	76	77
	95th	113	114	116	118	119	121	121	76	77	78	79	80	81	81
	99th	120	121	123	125	127	128	129	84	85	86	87	88	88	89

Blood Pressure Levels for Boys by Age and Height Percentile—cont'd

AGE (YEAR)	BP PERCENTILE	SYSTOLIC BP (mm Hg) ←PERCENTILE OF HEIGHT→							DIASTOLIC BP (mm Hg) ←PERCENTILE OF HEIGHT→						
		5th	10th	25th	50th	75th	90th	95th	5th	10th	25th	50th	75th	90th	95th
10	50th	97	98	100	102	103	105	106	58	59	60	61	61	62	63
	90th	111	112	114	115	117	119	119	73	73	74	75	76	77	78
	95th	115	116	117	119	121	122	123	77	78	79	80	81	81	82
	99th	122	123	125	127	128	130	130	85	86	86	88	88	89	90
11	50th	99	100	102	104	105	107	107	59	59	60	61	62	63	63
	90th	113	114	115	117	119	120	121	74	74	75	76	77	78	78
	95th	117	118	119	121	123	124	125	78	78	79	80	81	82	82
	99th	124	125	127	129	130	132	132	86	86	87	88	89	90	90
12	50th	101	102	104	106	108	109	110	59	60	61	62	63	63	64
	90th	115	116	118	120	121	123	123	74	75	75	76	77	78	79
	95th	119	120	122	123	125	127	127	78	79	80	81	82	82	83
	99th	126	127	129	131	133	134	135	86	87	88	89	90	90	91
13	50th	104	105	106	108	110	111	112	60	60	61	62	63	64	64
	90th	117	118	120	122	124	125	126	75	75	76	77	78	79	79
	95th	121	122	124	126	128	129	130	79	79	80	81	82	83	83
	99th	128	130	131	133	135	136	137	87	87	88	89	90	91	91
14	50th	106	107	109	111	113	114	115	60	61	62	63	64	65	65
	90th	120	121	123	125	126	128	128	75	76	77	78	79	79	80
	95th	124	125	127	128	130	132	132	80	80	81	82	83	84	84
	99th	131	132	134	136	138	139	140	87	88	89	90	91	92	92
15	50th	109	110	112	113	115	117	117	61	62	63	64	65	66	66
	90th	122	124	125	127	129	130	131	76	77	78	79	80	80	81
	95th	126	127	129	131	133	134	135	81	81	82	83	84	85	85
	99th	134	135	136	138	140	142	142	88	89	90	91	92	93	93
16	50th	111	112	114	116	118	119	120	63	63	64	65	66	67	67
	90th	125	126	128	130	131	133	134	78	78	79	80	81	82	82
	95th	129	130	132	134	135	137	137	82	83	83	84	85	86	87
	99th	136	137	139	141	143	144	145	90	90	91	92	93	94	94
17	50th	114	115	116	118	120	121	122	65	66	66	67	68	69	70
	90th	127	128	130	132	134	135	136	80	80	81	82	83	84	84
	95th	131	132	134	136	138	139	140	84	85	86	87	87	88	89
	99th	139	140	141	143	145	146	147	92	93	93	94	95	96	97

BP, Blood pressure

*The 90th percentile is 1.28 SD, 95th percentile is 1.645 SD, and the 99th percentile is 2.326 SD over the mean. For research purposes, the standard deviations in Appendix Table B-1 allow one to compute BP Z-scores and percentiles for boys with height percentiles given in Table 3 (i.e., the 5th, 10th, 25th, 50th, 75th, 90th, and 95th percentiles). These height percentiles must be converted to height Z-scores given by (5% = −1.645; 10% = −1.28; 25% = −0.68; 50% = 0; 75% = 0.68; 90% = 1.28; 95% = 1.645) and then computed according to the methodology in steps 2 to 4 described in Appendix B. For children with height percentiles other than these, follow steps 1 to 4 as described in Appendix B.

Blood Pressure Levels for Girls by Age and Height Percentile*

AGE (YEAR)	BP PERCENTILE	SYSTOLIC BP (mm Hg) ←PERCENTILE OF HEIGHT→							DIASTOLIC BP (mm Hg) ←PERCENTILE OF HEIGHT→						
		5th	10th	25th	50th	75th	90th	95th	5th	10th	25th	50th	75th	90th	95th
1	50th	83	84	85	86	88	89	90	38	39	39	40	41	41	42
	90th	97	97	98	100	101	102	103	52	53	53	54	55	55	56
	95th	100	101	102	104	105	106	107	56	57	57	58	59	59	60
	99th	108	108	109	111	112	113	114	64	64	65	65	66	67	67
2	50th	85	85	87	88	89	91	91	43	44	44	45	46	46	47
	90th	98	99	100	101	103	104	105	57	58	58	59	60	61	61
	95th	102	103	104	105	107	108	109	61	62	62	63	64	65	65
	99th	109	110	111	112	114	115	116	69	69	70	70	71	72	72
3	50th	86	87	88	89	91	92	93	47	48	48	49	50	50	51
	90th	100	100	102	103	104	106	106	61	62	62	63	64	64	65
	95th	104	104	105	107	108	109	110	65	66	66	67	68	68	69
	99th	111	111	113	114	115	116	117	73	73	74	74	75	76	76
4	50th	88	88	90	91	92	94	94	50	50	51	52	52	53	54
	90th	101	102	103	104	106	107	108	64	64	65	66	67	67	68
	95th	105	106	107	108	110	111	112	68	68	69	70	71	71	72
	99th	112	113	114	115	117	118	119	76	76	76	77	78	79	79
5	50th	89	90	91	93	94	95	96	52	53	53	54	55	55	56
	90th	103	103	105	106	107	109	109	66	67	67	68	69	69	70
	95th	107	107	108	110	111	112	113	70	71	71	72	73	73	74
	99th	114	114	116	117	118	120	120	78	78	79	79	80	81	81
6	50th	91	92	93	94	96	97	98	54	54	55	56	56	57	58
	90th	104	105	106	108	109	110	111	68	68	69	70	70	71	72
	95th	108	109	110	111	113	114	115	72	72	73	74	74	75	76
	99th	115	116	117	119	120	121	122	80	80	80	81	82	83	83
7	50th	93	93	95	96	97	99	99	55	56	56	57	58	58	59
	90th	106	107	108	109	111	112	113	69	70	70	71	72	72	73
	95th	110	111	112	113	115	116	116	73	74	74	75	76	76	77
	99th	117	118	119	120	122	123	124	81	81	82	82	83	84	84
8	50th	95	95	96	98	99	100	101	57	57	57	58	59	60	60
	90th	108	109	110	111	113	114	114	71	71	71	72	73	74	74
	95th	112	112	114	115	116	118	118	75	75	75	76	77	78	78
	99th	119	120	121	122	123	125	125	82	82	83	83	84	85	86
9	50th	96	97	98	100	101	102	103	58	58	58	59	60	61	61
	90th	110	110	112	113	114	116	116	72	72	72	73	74	75	75
	95th	114	114	115	117	118	119	120	76	76	76	77	78	79	79
	99th	121	121	123	124	125	127	127	83	83	84	84	85	86	87

Blood Pressure Levels for Girls by Age and Height Percentile—cont'd

AGE (YEAR)	BP PERCENTILE	SYSTOLIC BP (mm Hg) ←PERCENTILE OF HEIGHT→							DIASTOLIC BP (mm Hg) ←PERCENTILE OF HEIGHT→						
		5th	10th	25th	50th	75th	90th	95th	5th	10th	25th	50th	75th	90th	95th
10	50th	98	99	100	102	103	104	105	59	59	59	60	61	62	62
	90th	112	112	114	115	116	118	118	73	73	73	74	75	76	76
	95th	116	116	117	119	120	121	122	77	77	77	78	79	80	80
	99th	123	123	125	126	127	129	129	84	84	85	86	86	87	88
11	50th	100	101	102	103	105	106	107	60	60	60	61	62	63	63
	90th	114	114	116	117	118	119	120	74	74	74	75	76	77	77
	95th	118	118	119	121	122	123	124	78	78	78	79	80	81	81
	99th	125	125	126	128	129	130	131	85	85	86	87	87	88	89
12	50th	102	103	104	105	107	108	109	61	61	61	62	63	64	64
	90th	116	116	117	119	120	121	122	75	75	75	76	77	78	78
	95th	119	120	121	123	124	125	126	79	79	79	80	81	82	82
	99th	127	127	128	130	131	132	133	86	86	87	88	88	89	90
13	50th	104	105	106	107	109	110	110	62	62	62	63	64	65	65
	90th	117	118	119	121	122	123	124	76	76	76	77	78	79	79
	95th	121	122	123	124	126	127	128	80	80	80	81	82	83	83
	99th	128	129	130	132	133	134	135	87	87	88	89	89	90	91
14	50th	106	106	107	109	110	111	112	63	63	63	64	65	66	66
	90th	119	120	121	122	124	125	125	77	77	77	78	79	80	80
	95th	123	123	125	126	127	129	129	81	81	81	82	83	84	84
	99th	130	131	132	133	135	136	136	88	88	89	90	90	91	92
15	50th	107	108	109	110	111	113	113	64	64	64	65	66	67	67
	90th	120	121	122	123	125	126	127	78	78	78	79	80	81	81
	95th	124	125	126	127	129	130	131	82	82	82	83	84	85	85
	99th	131	132	133	134	136	137	138	89	89	90	91	91	92	93
16	50th	108	108	110	111	112	114	114	64	64	65	66	66	67	68
	90th	121	122	123	124	126	127	128	78	78	79	80	81	81	82
	95th	125	126	127	128	130	131	132	82	82	83	84	85	85	86
	99th	132	133	134	135	137	138	139	90	90	90	91	92	93	93
17	50th	108	109	110	111	113	114	115	64	65	65	66	67	67	68
	90th	122	122	123	125	126	127	128	78	79	79	80	81	81	82
	95th	125	126	127	129	130	131	132	82	83	83	84	85	85	86
	99th	133	133	134	136	137	138	139	90	90	91	91	92	93	93

BP, Blood pressure

*The 90th percentile is 1.28 SD, 95th percentile is 1.645 SD, and the 99th percentile is 2.326 SD over the mean. For research purposes, the standard deviations in Appendix Table B-1 allow one to compute BP Z-scores and percentiles for girls with height percentiles given in Table 4 (i.e., the 5th, 10th, 25th, 50th, 75th, 90th, and 95th percentiles). These height percentiles must be converted to height Z-scores given by (5% = −1.645; 10% = −1.28; 25% = −0.68; 50% = 0; 75% = 0.68; 90% = 1.28; 95% = 1.645) and then computed according to the methodology in steps 2 to 4 described in Appendix B. For children with height percentiles other than these, follow steps 1 to 4 as described in Appendix B.

Answers to Review Questions for the NCLEX® Examination

Go to your Evolve website *(http://evolve.elsevier.com/Price/pediatric/)* for rationales.

Chapter 1
1. 4
2. 3
3. 2
4. 3
5. 4

Chapter 2
1. 3
2. 2
3. 3
4. 1, 2, 3
5. 2

Chapter 3
1. 2, 3, 4, 5
2. 4
3. 4
4. 4
5. 2, 3

Chapter 4
1. 3
2. 1
3. 4
4. 2
5. 2, 5

Chapter 5
1. 3
2. 4
3. 1, 2
4. 1
5. 2

Chapter 6
1. 3
2. 1, 2, 3
3. 4
4. 3
5. 1

Chapter 7
1. 4
2. 2
3. 2, 4, 5, 6
4. 1
5. 3

Chapter 8
1. 4
2. 1
3. 4
4. 3, 5
5. 3

Chapter 9
1. 2
2. 3
3. 4
4. 1
5. 2, 5

Chapter 10
1. 1
2. 4
3. 2, 3, 5
4. 3
5. 2

Chapter 11
1. 3, 4
2. 4
3. 4
4. 4
5. 2

Chapter 12
1. 2, 3, 5
2. 1
3. 2
4. 4
5. 1

Chapter 13
1. 4
2. 3
3. 1
4. 2
5. 1, 2, 3, 4, 5

Chapter 14
1. 1
2. 1, 2, 3, 6
3. 3
4. 2
5. 4

Chapter 15
1. 2
2. 4
3. 2, 3, 5
4. 1
5. 4

Chapter 16
1. 2
2. 2
3. 1
4. 4, 5
5. 2

Chapter 17
1. 1, 2, 4, 5
2. 2
3. 4
4. 2
5. 1

Chapter 18
1. 3
2. 2, 5
3. 1
4. 4
5. 1

Chapter 19
1. 1
2. 3
3. 2
4. 2, 4, 5
5. 1

Chapter 20
1. 3
2. 4
3. 3
4. 1, 3, 5
5. 4

Chapter 21
1. 2
2. 1
3. 2, 3
4. 2
5. 4

Chapter 22
1. 2, 3
2. 3, 2, 1
3. 1
4. 3
5. 1

Bibliography

Chapter 1

Heron, M., Sutton, P., Xu, J., et al. (2010). Annual summary of vital statistics: 2007. *Pediatrics*, 125, 4-15.

U.S. Department of Health and Human Services. Healthy People 2010. Retrieved May 18, 2010, from *http://www. healthypeople.gov/2010/LHI/Priorities.htm*.

U.S. Department of Health and Human Services. Healthy People 2020. The road ahead (last revised November 3, 2009). Retrieved May 18, 2010, from *http://www.healthypeople. gov/hp2020/*.

 Online Resources

American Academy of Pediatrics: *http://aap.org*
Healthy Start Program: *http://hrsa.gov*
National Center for Health Statistics: *http://www.cdc.gov/nchs/ fastats/infmort.htm*
The Society of Pediatric Nursing: *http://www.pedsnurses.org*
United Nations Children's Fund: *http://www.unicef.org*
U.S. Department of Health and Human Services: *http://www. hhs.gov/news*
World Health Organization: *http://www.who.int/en*

Chapter 2

Giger, J., & Davidhizar, R. (2008). *Transcultural nursing* (5th ed.). St Louis: Mosby.

Hockenberry, M., & Wilson, D. (2009). *Wong's essentials of pediatric nursing* (8th ed.). St. Louis: Mosby.

Merkel, S. I., Voepel-Lewis, T., Shayevitz, J. R., et al. (1997). The FLACC: a behavioral scale for scoring postoperative pain in young children. *Pediatr Nurs*, 23(3), 293-297. Used with permission. © The Regents of the University of Michigan and the University of Michigan Health System. Can be reproduced for clinical and research use.

National Center for Complementary and Alternative Medicine (NCCAM) Fact Sheets. 2005-2006. National Institutes of Health. Updated 2008. Retrieved from *http://nccam.nih.gov/ health/herbsataglance.htm*.

The National Pain Foundation. Using complementary therapy to relieve pain. Retrieved June 12, 2006, from *http://www. nationalpainfoundation.org/MyTreatment/News_Complementary. asp*.

Potter, A., & Perry, A. (2009). *Fundamentals of nursing* (7th ed.). St. Louis: Mosby.

Wong, D. I., & Baker, C. M. (1988). Pain in children: comparison of assessment scales. *Pediatric Nurs*, 14(1), 9-17.

 Online Resources

American Academy of Pediatrics: *http://aappolicy. aappublications.org*
Centers for Disease Control and Prevention: *http://www.cdc.gov*
Child Life Specialists: *www.childlife.org*
Children's health: *http://www.kidshealth.org*
The Joint Commission 2010 National Patient Safety Goals: *http://www.jointcommission.org/PatientSafety/ NationalPatientSafetyGoals*
National Center for Complementary and Alternative Medicine (NCCAM) Fact Sheets. National Institutes of Health: *http:// nccam.nih.gov/health/herbsataglance.htm*

Quality and Safety Education for Nurses (QSEN): *http://qsen. org*

Chapter 3

Cook, I. F., & Murtagh, J. (2006). Ventrogluteal area—a suitable site for intramuscular vaccination of infants and toddlers. *Vaccine*, 24(13), 2403-2408. Date of electronic publication: December 20, 2005.

Hockenberry, M., & Wilson, D. (2009). *Wong's essentials of pediatric nursing* (8th ed.). St. Louis: Mosby.

Kliegman, R. M., Jenson, H. B., Behrman, R. E., et al. (2007). *Nelson textbook of pediatrics* (18th ed.). Philadelphia: Saunders.

National High Blood Pressure Education Program (NHBPEP) Working Group on High Blood Pressure in Children and Adolescents. (2004). The fourth report on the diagnosis, evaluation, and treatment of high blood pressure in children and adolescents. *Pediatrics*, 114(2), 555-576.

Schmitt, B. (2009). Enemas: how to give. CRS—Pediatric Advisor: p. 1-1.© 2009 Relay Health and/or its affiliates. All rights reserved.

U.S. Department of Health and Human Services, National Institutes of Health, National Heart, Lung, and Blood Institute, and National High Blood Pressure Education Program. (2005). The fourth report on the diagnosis, evaluation, and treatment of high blood pressure in children and adolescents. NIH Publication No. 05-5267. Originally printed September 1996. Revised May 2005. Washington, DC: U.S. Government Printing Office.

 Online Resources

High blood pressure in children:
http://www.nhlbi.nih.gov/health/dci/Diseases/Hbp/HBP_WhatIs. html
http://www.mayoclinic.com
www.nlm.nih.gov/medlineplus/highbloodpressure.html

Chapter 4

Baker, J. L. (2007). Childhood body-mass index and the risk of coronary heart disease in adulthood. *N Engl J Med*, 357(23), 2329-2337.

Centers for Disease Control and Prevention. (2009). Growth charts. Retrieved June 10, 2010, from *www.cdc.gov/ growthcharts/Default.htm*.

Centers for Disease Control and Prevention. (2010). Obesity prevalence among low-income, preschool-aged children 1998-2008. Retrieved June 2, 2010, from *www.cdc.gov/ nccdphp/dnpa/obesity/trend/index.htm*.

Hockenberry, M. J., & Wilson, D. (2007). *Wong's nursing care of infants and children* (8th ed.). St. Louis: Mosby.

James, S. R., & Ashwill, J. W. (2007). *Nursing care of children: principles and practice*. Philadelphia: Saunders.

Kliegman, R. M., Behrman, R. E., Jenson, H. B., et al. (2007). *Nelson textbook of pediatrics* (18th ed.). Philadelphia: Saunders.

March of Dimes. (2010). Quick reference fact sheets: newborn screening. Retrieved June 2, 2010, from *www.marchofdimes. com*.

 Online Resources

Abraham Maslow: *www.webspace.ship.edu/cgboer/maslow.html*
Erik Erikson: *www.webspace.ship.edu/cgboer/erikson.html*
Genetic disease information: *www.cdc.gov/genomics/*
Growth charts: *www.cdc.gov/nchs/about/major/nhanes/ growthcharts/clinical_charts.htm*
Jean Piaget: *www.webspace.ship.edu/cgboer/piaget.html*
Major personality theories: *www.webspace.ship.edu/cgboer/ perscontents.html*
March of Dimes: *www.marchofdimes.org*
National Center for Health Statistics: *www.cdc.gov/nchs/*
National Newborn Screening and Genetics Resource Center: *www.genes-r-us.uthscsa.edu/*
New York Online Access to Health (NOAH): *http://www. noah-health.org*

Chapter 5

American Academy of Pediatrics Policy Statement. (2007). Cord blood banking for potential future transplantation. Retrieved July 8, 2010, from *http://www.pediatrics.org*.
American Academy of Pediatrics Policy Statement. (2005). The changing concept of sudden infant death syndrome: diagnostic coding shifts, controversies regarding the sleeping environment, and new variables to consider in reducing risk. *Pediatrics*, 116(5), 1245-1255 (doi: 10.1542/ peds.2005-1499). Reaffirmation statement published January 1, 2009. Retrieved July 8, 2010, from *http://aappolicy. aappublications.org/cgi/content/full/pediatrics;116/5/1245*.
American Academy of Pediatrics Clinical Practice Guideline. (2004). Management of hyperbilirubinemia in the newborn infant 35 or more weeks of gestation. *Pediatrics*, 114(1), 297-316. Retrieved November 14, 2010, from *http://pediatrics. aappublications.org/cgi/content/full/114/1/297*.
Association of Women's Health, Obstetric and Neonatal Nurses. National standards for newborn screening. May, 2005.
Association of Women's Health, Obstetric and Neonatal Nurses. Breastfeeding position statement (and the role of the nurse in the promotion of breastfeeding position statement). Combined and reaffirmed December, 2007.
Boyd, C. D., & Starino, A. T. (2006). Acute respiratory distress syndrome. In F. D. Burg, J. R. Ingelfinger, R. A. Polin, et al. (Eds.), *Current pediatric therapy* (18th ed.). Philadelphia: Saunders.
Burke, M. (2006). A pacifier reduces the risk of SIDS. *Contemp Pediatr*, January 1, 2006. Retrieved from *http://www. contemporarypediatrics.com/contpeds/content/*.
Caplan, M. S. (2009). Probiotic and prebiotic supplementation for the prevention of neonatal necrotizing enterocolitis. *J Perinatol*, 29(suppl 2), S2-S6.
Chiang, M. F., & Flynn, J. T. (2006). Retinopathy of prematurity. In F. D. Burg, J. R. Ingelfinger, R. A. Polin, et al. (Eds.), *Current pediatric therapy* (18th ed.). Philadelphia: Saunders.
Hirji, H., Charlton, R., & Sarmah, S. (2005). Male circumcision: a review of the evidence. *J Men's Health & Gender*, 2(1), 21-30.
Hockenberry, M., & Wilson, D. (2007). *Wong's nursing care of infants and children* (8th ed.). St. Louis: Mosby.
Joint Committee on Infant Hearing. (2000). Year 2000 position statement: principles and guidelines for early hearing detection and intervention programs. *Pediatrics*, 106(4), 798-817.

Kliegman, R. M., Jenson, H. B., Behrman, R. E., et al. (2007). *Nelson textbook of pediatrics* (18th ed.). Philadelphia: Saunders.
Lin, J. C., & Carcillo, J. A. (2006). Management of sepsis and septic shock. In F. D. Burg, J. R. Ingelfinger, R. A. Polin, et al. (Eds.), *Current pediatric therapy* (18th ed.). Philadelphia: Saunders.
March of Dimes. (2006). Quick reference fact sheets: Chorionic villus sampling. Retrieved June 2, 2006, from *http://www. marchofdimes.com*.
McKinney, E. S., James, S. R., Murray, S. S., et al. (2009). *Maternal-child nursing* (3rd ed). St. Louis: Saunders.
National Center for Missing and Exploited Children (2009). *For healthcare professionals: guidelines on prevention of and response to infant abductions* (9th ed.). Office of Juvenile Justice and Delinquency Prevention (U.S. Department of Justice).
National Institutes of Health: National Institute of Child Health and Human Development. (2005). SIDS Back to Sleep Campaign. Retrieved from *http://www.nichd.nih.gov/ sids/sids.cfm*.
Schmitt, B. (2006). Caffeine therapy for apnea of prematurity. *N Engl J Med*, 354(20), 2112-2121.
Soll, R. F., & Pfister, R. H. (2006). Special problems in the infant and neonate. In F. D. Burg, J. R. Ingelfinger, R. A. Polin, et al. (Eds.), *Current pediatric therapy* (18th ed.). Philadelphia: Saunders.
Uys, L. R. (2009/2010). Prevention is the only cure. *Nursing Update*, December/January.
Wagner, C. L., Greer, F. H., & the Section on Breastfeeding and Committee on Nutrition. (2008). Prevention of rickets and vitamin D deficiency in infants, children, and adolescents. American Academy of Pediatrics. Retrieved from *www. pediatrics.org/cgi/doi/10.1542/peds.2008-1862*.

 Online Resources

American Academy of Pediatrics: *http://aap.org*
Back to Sleep Campaign, National Institutes of Health (NIH): *http://nih.gov*
Brazelton Behavioral Assessment Scale: *http://www.brazelton- institute.com/intro.html*
Joint Committee on Infant Hearing (JCIH): *http://www.jcih.org*
La Leche League for breastfeeding mothers: *http://www. lalecheleague.org*
March of Dimes: *http://www.marchofdimes.com*
S.T.A.B.L.E: *http://www.stableprogram.com/contact.php*

Chapter 6

American Academy of Pediatrics. (2010). Car safety seats: Information for families for 2010. Retrieved from *http:// www.healthychildren.org*.
Hockenberry, M., & Wilson, D. (2007). *Wong's nursing care of infants and children* (8th ed.). St. Louis: Mosby.
Mahan, L. K., & Escott-Stump, S. (2007). *Krause's food, nutrition, and diet therapy* (11th ed.). Philadelphia: Saunders.
Peckenpaugh, N. (2007). *Nutrition essentials and diet therapy* (9th ed.). St. Louis: Saunders.

 Online Resources

American Academy of Pediatrics: *http://aap.org*

Chapter 7

American Academy of Pediatrics Policy Statement. (2007). The use and misuse of fruit juice in pediatrics (RE0047). *Pediatrics*, 107(5), 1210-1213. Retrieved July 26, 2010, from *http://aappolicy.aappublications.org/cgi/content/full/ pediatrics;107/5/1210*.

American Academy of Pediatrics. (2008). Healthy children fun in the sun: keep your family safe. Last updated June 10, 2010. Retrieved July 26, 2010, from *http://www.healthychildren.org/English/safety-prevention/at-play/Pages/Sun-Safety.aspx*.

American Academy of Pediatrics. (2010). Car safety seats: information for families for 2010. Retrieved July 28, 2010, from *http://www.healthychildren.org/English/safety-prevention/on-the-go/Pages/Car-Safety-Seats-Information-for-Families.aspx*.

American Academy of Pediatrics. (2011). AAP updates recommendation on car seats. Retrieved March 21, 2011, from *http://www.aap.org/advocacy/releases/carseat2011.htm*.

Burg, F. D., Ingelfinger, J. R., Polin, R. A., et al. (Eds.), (2006). *Current pediatric therapy* (18th ed.). Philadelphia: Saunders.

Hockenberry, M., & Wilson, D. (2007). *Wong's nursing care of infants and children* (8th ed.). St. Louis: Mosby.

Kliegman, R. M., Jenson, H. B., Behrman, R. E., et al. (2007). *Nelson textbook of pediatrics* (18th ed.). Philadelphia: Saunders.

Peckenpaugh, N. (2007). *Nutrition essentials and diet therapy* (10th ed.). Philadelphia: Saunders.

Schmitt, B. (2010). *Discipline basics.* © 2010 Relay Health and/or its affiliates. All rights reserved.

U.S. Department of Agriculture: Center for Nutrition Policy and Promotion, April 2005. retrieved July 2010 from *http://www.MyPyramid.gov*.

Online Resources

American Academy of Pediatrics: *http://www.aap.org*

MyPyramid Plan for Preschoolers: *http://www.mypyramid.gov/preschoolers/Plan/index.html*

National Resource Center for Health and Safety in Child Care and Early Education: *http://nrckids.org/providers.htm*

National Safe Kids Campaign: *http://www.safekids.org*

Poison prevention: *http://www.aapcc.org*

SafetyBeltSafe USA: *http://www.carseat.org*

U.S. Department of Agriculture: *http://www.usda.gov*

Chapter 8

American Academy of Pediatrics: Committee on Communication and Media. (2009). Policy revision statement: media violence. *Pediatrics*, 124(5), 1495-1503.

American Academy of Pediatrics: Committee on Hospital Care. (2006). Policy Statement: Child life services. *Pediatrics*, 118(4), 1757-1763.

American Academy of Pediatrics: Committee on Injury and Poison Prevention. (2006). Policy reaffirmation statement: trampolines at home, school, and recreational centers. *Pediatrics*, 117(5), 1846-1847.

American Academy of Pediatrics: Committee on Injury, Violence, and Poison Prevention. (2009). Policy statement: role of pediatrician in youth violence prevention. *Pediatrics*, 124(1), 393-402.

American Academy of Pediatrics: Committee on Public Education. (2001). Policy statement: children, adolescents, and television. *Pediatrics*, 107(2), 423-426.

American Academy of Pediatrics: Committee on Psychosocial Aspects of Child and Family Health. (2004). Policy reaffirmation statement: guidance for effective discipline. *Pediatrics*, 114(4), 1126.

American Academy of Pediatrics: Council on Communication and Media. (2009). Policy statement: Impact of music, lyrics, and music videos on children and youth. *Pediatrics*, 124(5), 1488-1494.

Anderson, J. (2006). Sibling rivalry: when a family circle becomes a boxing ring. *Contemp Pediatr*. Retrieved June 12, 2010, from *http://contemporarypediatrics.modernmedicine.com/contpeds/content/printContentPopup.jsp?id=306594*.

Carey, W., Crocker, A., Elias, E., et al. (2009). *Developmental-behavioral pediatrics* (4th ed.). Philadelphia: Saunders.

Driessnack, M. (2006). Children's drawings as facilitators of communication: a meta-analysis. *J Pediatr Nurs*, 20(6), 415-423.

Helms, D., & Turner, J. (1978). *Exploring child behavior: basic principles* (p. 447). Philadelphia: Saunders.

Hockenberry, M. J., & Wilson, D. (2007). *Wong's nursing care of infants and children* (8th ed.). St. Louis: Mosby.

Kliegman, R. M., Behrman, R. E., Jenson, H. B., et al. (2007). *Nelson textbook of pediatrics* (18th ed.). Philadelphia: Saunders.

Larsen, M., & Tentis, E. (2003). The art and science of disciplining children. *Pediatr Clin North Am*, 50(4), 817-840.

Schmitt, B. (2010). Discipline basics. RelayHealth. Retrieved June 10, 2010, from *www.mdconsult.com/das/patient/body/205175410-2/0/10068/18763.html*.

U.S. Department of Agriculture. MyPyramid. Retrieved June 10, 2010, from *www.mypyramid.com*.

Online Resources

Bright Futures: *http://www.brightfutures.org*

Chapter 9

American Academy of Pediatrics: Committee on Injury and Poison Prevention. (2007). Statement of reaffirmation for policy statement: All-terrain vehicle injury prevention in two, three, four wheeled unlicensed motor vehicles. *Pediatrics*, 119(5), 1031.

American Academy of Pediatrics: Committee on Injury and Poison Prevention. (2006). Statement of reaffirmation for policy statement: In-line skating injuries in children and adolescents. *Pediatrics*, 117(5), 1846-1847.

American Academy of Pediatrics: Committee on Injury and Poison Prevention. (2004). Statement of reaffirmation for policy statement for firearm related injuries affecting the pediatric population. *Pediatrics*, 114(4), 1126.

American Academy of Pediatrics: Committee on Psychosocial Aspects of Child and Family Health. (2001). The new morbidity revisited: a renewed commitment to the psychosocial aspect of pediatric care. *Pediatrics*, 108(5), 1227-1230.

American Academy of Pediatrics: Committee on Public Education. (2006). Policy statement: children, adolescents, and advertising. *Pediatrics*, 107(2), 423-426.

American Academy of Pediatrics: Council on Communication and Media. (2007). Policy revision statement: media violence. *Pediatrics*, 124(5), 1495-1503.

Bradford, N. F. (2009). Overweight and obesity in children and adolescents. *Primary Care*, 36(2), 319-339.

Chen, T. L., Brenner, R. A., Wright, J. L., et al. (2004). Children's violent television viewing: Are parents monitoring? *Pediatrics*, 114(1), 94-99.

Cohen, G. J. (2002). Helping children and families deal with divorce and separation. *Pediatrics*, 110(5), 1019-1023.

Hockenberry, M. J., & Wilson, D. (2007). *Wong's nursing care of infants and children* (8th ed.). St. Louis: Mosby.

Howard, B. J., Broughton, D. D., & Committee on Psychosocial Aspect of Child and Family Health. (2004). The pediatrician's role in prevention of missing children. *Pediatrics*, 114(4), 1100-1105.

Kliegman, R. M., Behrman, R. E., Jenson, H. B., et al. (2007). *Nelson textbook of pediatrics* (18th ed.). Philadelphia: Saunders.

Marx, J., Hockberger, R., & Walls, R. (2009). *Rosen's emergency medicine* (7th ed.). Philadelphia: Mosby.

Schmitt, B. (2005a). Divorce: helping children cope. Pediatric Advisor. McKesson Corporation. Retrieved June 10, 2010, from *http://home.mdconsult.com.*

Schmitt, B. (2005b). Television: reducing the negative impact. Pediatric Advisor. McKesson Corporation. Retrieved June 10, 2010, from *http://home.mdconsult.com.*

Schmitt, B. (2005c). Video games. Pediatric Advisor. McKesson Corporation. Retrieved June 10, 2010, from *http://home.mdconsult.com.*

Schuman, A. J. (2008). An obesity action plan for children. *Contemp Pediatr*, 25(4), 37-38, 41-42, 45-46.

Scott, J. U., Hague-Armstrong, K., & Downes, K. L. (2003). Teaching and bullying: what can pediatricians do? *Contemp Pediatr*, 20(4), 105-120.

U.S. Department of Agriculture. MyPyramid. Retrieved March 2, 2011, from *www.mypyramid.com.*

U.S. Department of Justice: National Criminal Justice Reference Service. (2002). Preventing school shootings: a summary of a U.S. secret service safe school initiative report. Retrieved June 12, 2010, from *www.ncjrs.gov/pdffile/jr000248c.pdf.*

Wolak, J., Mitchell, K., & Finkelhor, D. (2006). Online victimization of youth: five years later. National Center for Missing and Exploited Children. Alexandria, VA. Retrieved June 12, 2010, from *www.missingkids.com/en_us/publications/NC176.pdf.*

 Online Resources

American Academy of Pediatrics: *www.aap.org*
Bright Futures: *www.brightfutures.org*
Entertainment Software Rating Board: *www.esrb.org*
Missing children: *www.pollyklaas.org*
National Resource for Safe Schools: *www.safetyzone.org*
U.S. Department of Agriculture: *www.usda.gov*
U.S. Department of Agriculture Food Pyramid: *www.mypryamid.com*

Chapter 10

American Academy of Pediatrics. (2006). Academy lends expertise on web safety service for children. *AAP News*, 27(5), 17.

American Academy of Pediatrics: Committee on Adolescence. (2005). Adolescent pregnancy—current trends and issues. *Pediatrics*, 116(1), 218-286.

American Academy of Pediatrics: Committee on Adolescence. (2007). Contraception and adolescents. *Pediatrics*, 120(5), 1135-1148.

American Academy of Pediatrics: Committee on Injury, Violence and Poisoning and Committee on Adolescence. (2006). The teen driver. *Pediatrics*, 118(6), 2570-2581.

American Academy of Pediatrics: Committee on Injury, Violence and Poisoning. (2009). Role of the pediatrician in youth violence prevention. *Pediatrics*, 124(61), 393-402.

American Academy of Pediatrics: Committee on Substance Abuse. (2010). Revised policy statement: alcohol use by youth and adolescents: a pediatric concern. *Pediatrics*, 125(5), 1078-1087.

American Academy of Pediatrics: Committee on Nutrition. (2006). Revised policy statement: optimizing bone health and calcium intakes of infants, children, and adolescents. *Pediatrics*, 117(2), 578-585.

Anderson, J., & Martel, S. (2002). Decorating the "human canvas": body art and your patients. *Contemp Pediatr*, 8, 86. Retrieved June 18, 2010, from *http://www.contemporarypediatrics.com/contpeds/.*

Broughton, D. D. (2005). Keeping children safe in cyberspace. *AAP News*, 26(8), 11.

Carakushansky, M., O'Brien, K., & Levine, M. (2003). Vitamin D and calcium: strong bones for life through better nutrition. *Contemp Pediatr*, 3, 37. Retrieved June 15, 2010, from *http://www.contemporarypediatrics.com/contpeds/.*

Centers for Disease Control and Prevention. (2010). Youth risk behavior surveillance USA—2009. *MMWR*, 59(SS-5), 1-142.

Fallat, M., & Ignacio, R. (2008). Breast disorders in children and adolescents. *J Pediatr Adolesc Gynecol*, 21(6), 311-316.

Hockenberry, M. J., & Wilson, D. (2007). *Wong's nursing care of infants and children* (8th ed.). St. Louis: Mosby.

James, S. R., & Ashwill, J. W., (Eds.), (2007). *Nursing care of children*. Philadelphia: Saunders.

Kliegman, R. M., Behrman, R. E., Jenson, H. B., et al. (2007). *Nelson textbook of pediatrics* (18th ed.). Philadelphia: Saunders.

Nall, J., Shenk, C., Barnes, J., et al. (2009). Childhood abuse, avatar choices, and other risk factors associated with Internet-initiated victimization of adolescent girls. *Pediatrics*, 123(6), 1078-1083.

Oski, J. (2009). Counseling adolescents on contraceptive choices. Retrieved June 15, 2010, from *www.modernmedicine.com/modernmedicine/article/articleDetail.jsp?id=609778&pageID=1&sk=&date=.*

Scott, J. U., Hague-Armstrong, K., & Downes, K. L. (2003). Teasing and bullying: what can pediatricians do? *Contemp Pediatr*, 20(4), 105-120.

Selekman, J. (2003). A new era of body decoration: what are kids doing to their bodies? *Pediatr Nurs*, 29(1), 77-79.

Verkler, E. (2005). Upping the ante: poker craze puts glamorous spin on gambling, but betting is not risk-free for youths. *AAP News*, 26(5), 1.

Walsh, J., Mitchell, K., & Finkelhor, D. (2007). Unwanted and wanted exposure to online pornography in a national sample of youth Internet users. *Pediatrics*, 119(2), 247-257.

Ybarra, M., Diener-West, M., Markov, D., et al. (2008). Linkages between internet and other media violence with seriously violent behavior by youth. *Pediatrics*, 122(5), 929-937.

 Online Resources

American Academy of Pediatrics: *www.aap.org*
Bright Futures: *www.brightfutures.org*
Safe Sitter: *http://www.safesitter.org*
Teen gambling: *www.nati.org*

Chapter 11

Allen, J. L. (2006). Bronchitis and bronchiolitis. In F. D. Burg, J. R. Ingelfinger, R. A. Polin, et al. (Eds.), *Current pediatric therapy* (18th ed.). Philadelphia: Saunders.

American Academy of Pediatrics. (2000). Policy statement: infection control in the physician's office. *Pediatrics*, 10(6), 1361-1369.

American Academy of Pediatrics and American Academy of Family Physicians. (2004). Clinical practice guidelines: subcommittee on management of acute otitis media: diagnosis and management of acute otitis media. *Pediatrics*, 113(5), 1451-1465.

American Academy of Pediatrics: Committee on Infectious Diseases. (2009). Modified recommendations for the use of palivizumab for prevention of respiratory syncytial virus. *Pediatrics*, 124(6), 1694-1701.

American Academy of Pediatrics: Subcommittee on Diagnosis and Management of Bronchiolitis. (2006). Diagnosis and management of bronchiolitis. *Pediatrics*, 118(4), 1774-1793.

American Academy of Pediatrics: Task Force on SIDS. (2005). Reaffirmation of policy statement: the changing concept of sudden infant death syndrome: diagnostic coding shifts, controversies regarding the sleep environment, and new variable to consider in reducing risk. *Pediatrics*, 116(5), 1245-1255.

Askin, D., & Diehl-Jones, W. (2009). Pathogenesis and prevention of chronic lung disease in the neonate. *Crit Care Nurs Clin North Am*, 21(1), 11-25.

Banasiak, N. (2009). Childhood asthma practice guideline part 3: update of 2007 national guidelines for diagnosis and treatment of asthma. *J Pediatr Health Care*, 23(1), 59-61.

Belcastro, M. R. (2004). Bronchopulmonary dysplasia: a new look at an old problem. *NAINA*, 4(2), 121-125.

Carrier, C. (2009). Back to sleep: a culture change to improve practice. *Newborn Infant Nurs Rev*, 9(3), 163-168.

Centers for Disease Control and Prevention. (2009). CDC reported tuberculosis in the U.S., 2008. U.S. Department of Health and Human Services. Retrieved July 2, 2010, from *wwwcdc.gov/tb/statistics/reports/2008/default.htm*.

Centers for Disease Control and Prevention. (2010). Division of Tuberculosis fact sheet: treatment of drug susceptible tuberculosis disease in persons not infected with HIV. Retrieved March 11, 2011, from *www.cdc.gov/tb/publications/factsheet/treatment/treatmentHIVnegative.htm*.

Charsha, D. (2009). Gently caring: supporting the first few critical hours of life for the extremely low birth weight infant. *Crit Care Nurs Clin North Am*, 21(1), 57-65.

Cunha, B. (2010). Swine influenza (H1N1) pneumonia: clinical considerations. *Infect Dis Clin North Am*, 24(1), 203-228.

Durbin, W., & Stille, C. (2008). Pneumonia. *Pediatr Rev*, 29(5), 147-158.

Hockenberry, M. J., & Wilson, D. (2007). *Wong's nursing care of infants and children* (8th ed.). St. Louis: Mosby.

Kliegman, R. M., Behrman, R. E., Jenson, H. B., et al. (2007). *Nelson textbook of pediatrics* (18th ed.). Philadelphia: Saunders.

Malveaus, F. (2009). The state of childhood asthma: introduction. *Pediatrics*, 123(1), S129-S130.

Martin, J. (2010). Pharyngitis and streptococcal throat infections. *Pediatr Ann*, 39(11), 22-27.

Martinez, F. (2009). Managing childhood asthma: challenge of preventing exacerbations. *Pediatrics*, 123(suppl 3), S146-S150.

Messner, A. (2003). Treating pediatric patients with obstructive sleep disorders: an update. *Otolaryngol Clin North Am*, 36(3), 519-530.

Morris, P. (2009). Acute and chronic otitis media. *Ped Clin North Am*, 56(16), 1383-1399.

Morris, P. S. (2009). Upper respiratory tract infections (including otitis media). *Pediatr Clin North Am*, 56(1), 101-117.

National Asthma Education and Prevention Program. (2007). Expert panel report 3: guidelines for the diagnosis and management of asthma. Full report 2007. U.S. Department of Health and Human Services. Retrieved July 2, 2010, from *www.nhlbi.nih.gov/guidelines/asthma*.

National Institute of Child Health and Human Development. (2009). Study links factors to choice of infant sleep position. *NIH News*, National Institute of Health. Retrieved July 2, 2010, from *nichd.nihlgov/news/releases/120709-infant_sleep_position.cfm*.

Rance, K. (2008). Understanding and implementing the new NHLBI asthma guidelines. *JNP*, 4(4), 254-261.

Robinson, L., & El-Sadr, W. M. (2006). Tuberculosis. In F. D. Burg, J. R. Ingelfinger, R. A. Polin, et al. (Eds.), *Current pediatric therapy* (18th ed.). Philadelphia: Saunders.

Sexton, S. (2009). Risk and benefits of pacifiers. *Am Fam Phys*, 79(8), 681-685.

Shaikh, N., & Hoberman, A. (2010). Update: acute otitis media. *Pediatr Ann*, 39(1), 28-33.

Sobol, S. E. (2008). Epliglottitis and croup. *Otolarygol Clin North Am*, 41(3), 551-566.

U.S. Food and Drug Administration. (2010). Public health advisory: FDA recommends that over-the-counter (OTC) cough and cold products not be used for infants and children under 2 years of age. Retrieved July 2, 2010, from *www.fda.gov/drugs/drugsafety/publichealthadvisories/ucm051137.html*.

Van Riper, C. (2010). Position of the American Dietetic Association: providing nutrition services for people with developmental disabilities and special health care needs. *J Am Diet Assoc*, 110(2), 296-307.

Wald, E. (2010) Croup: common syndromes and therapy. *Pediatr Ann*, 39(1), 15-21.

Zorc, J. (2010). Bronchiolitis: recent evidence on diagnosis and management. *Pediatrics*, 125(2), 342-349.

 Online Resources

American Academy of Pediatrics: *http://www.aap.org/*
Centers for Disease Control and Prevention: *http://www.cdc.gov/*
Cystic Fibrosis Foundation: *http://www.cff.org/*
National Institute of Child Health and Human Development: *http://www.nichd.nih.gov/*
National Institutes of Health: *http://www.nih.gov/*

Chapter 12

Bailey, P., & Jobes, D. (2009). The fontan patient. *Anesthesiol Clin*, 27(2), 258-300.

Bryant P. (2009). Some of the people, some of the time susceptibility to acute rheumatic fever. *Circulation*, 119(5), 742-753.

Carapetis, J. (2010). Prevention of rheumatic fever. *Pediatr Infect Dis J*, 29(1), 91-92.

Ferri, F. (2010). *Ferri's clinical advisor* (1st ed.). Philadelphia: Mosby Elsevier.

Fraisse, A., Losay J., Bourlan, F., et al. (2008). Efficiency of transcatheter closure of atrial septal defects in small and symptomatic children. *Cardiol Young*, 18(3), 343-347.

Gerber, H., Baltmore, R., Eaton, C., et al. (2009). Prevention of rheumatic fever and diagnosis and treatment of acute Streptococcal pharyngitis: a scientific statement from the American Heart Association Rheumatic Fever, Endocarditis, and Kawasaki Disease Committee of the Council on Cardiovascular Disease in the Young, the Interdisciplinary Council on Functional Genomics and Translational Biology, and the Interdisciplinary Council on Quality of Care and Outcomes Research: endorsed by the American Academy of Pediatrics. *Circulation*, 119(11), 1541-1551. Retrieved October 12, 2010, from *http://circ.ahajournal.org/cgi/reprint/CIRCULATIONAHA.109.191959v1?maxtohow=&HITS=108&hits=10&RESULTFORMAT=gerber&searched_1&FIRSTINDEX=0&resourcetype=HWCIT*.

Hartas, G., Tsounia, S., & Gupta-Malhotra, M. (2009). Approach to diagnosing congenital cardiac disorders. *Crit Care Nurs Clin North Am*, 21(1), 27-36.

Hockenberry, M. J., & Wilson, D. (2007). *Wong's nursing care of infants and children* (8th ed.). St. Louis: Mosby.

Kliegman, R. M., Behrman R. E., Jenson, H. B., et al. (2007). *Nelson textbook of pediatrics* (18th ed.). Philadelphia: Saunders.

Park, M. (2008). *Pediatric cardiology for practitioners* (5th ed.). Philadelphia: Mosby.

Lancet Neurology. (2010). Neurological burden of acute rheumatic fever and rheumatic heart disease: the case for action. *Lancet Neurol*, 9(5), 447.

Steer, A., & Carapetis, J. (2009). Acute rheumatic fever and rheumatic heart disease in indigenous populations. *Pediatr Clin North Am*, 56(6), 1401-1409.

Sadowski, S. L. (2009). Congenital cardiac disease in the newborn infant: past, present, and future. *Crit Care Nurs Clin North Am*, 21(1), 37-48, vi.

Singh, A. (2010). Acute rheumatic fever: subcutaneous nodules and carditis. *Circulation*, 121(7), 946-947.

 Online Resources

American Academy of Pediatrics: *www.aap.org*

Birth Defects: *www.cdc.gov/ncbddd/birthdefects*

Children's Heart Institute: *www.childrenheartinstitute.org*

Congenital Heart Defects: *www.congenitalheartdefects.com www.americanheart.org*

Congenital Heart Information Network: *www.tchin.org*

Pediatric Heart: *www.pediheart.org*

U.S. National Library of Medicine: *www.nlm.nih.gov*

Chapter 13

Hockenberry, M., & Wilson, D. (2007). *Wong's nursing care of infants and children* (8th ed.). St. Louis: Mosby.

Hockenberry, M., & Wilson, D. (2009). *Wong's essentials of pediatric nursing* (9th ed.). St. Louis: Mosby.

Kliegman, R. M., Jenson, H. B., Behrman, R. E., et al. (2007). *Nelson textbook of pediatrics* (18th ed.). Philadelphia: Saunders Elsevier.

National Institute of Neurological Disorders and Stroke Fact Sheet. (2006). U.S. Department of Health and Human Services: National Institutes of Health. Retrieved from *www.ninds.nih.gov*.

Nordi, D. R. (2006). In F. D. Burg, J. R. Ingelfinger, R. A. Polin, et al. (Eds.), *Current pediatric therapy* (18th ed.). Philadelphia: Saunders.

 Online Resources

The American Speech-Language-Hearing Association: *http://www.asha.org*

Epilepsy Foundation of America: *http://www.epilepsyfoundation.org*

The National Hydrocephalus Foundation: *http://www.nhfonline.org*

Chapter 14

American Academy of Pediatrics: Committee on Nutrition Policy Statement. (2003). Prevention of pediatric overweight and obesity. *Pediatrics*, 112(2), 424-430.

American Academy of Pediatrics: Council on Sports Medicine and Fitness and Council on School Health. (2006). Policy statement: active healthy living: prevention of childhood obesity through increased physical activity. *Pediatrics*, 117(5), 1834-1842.

Amieva, M. R. (2005). Important bacterial gastrointestinal pathogens in children: a pathogenesis perspective. *Pediatr Clin North Am*, 52(3), 749-777.

Belongia, E., Irving, S. A., Shui, I. M., et al. (2010). Real-time surveillance to assess risk of intussusception and other adverse events after pentavalent bovine-derived rotavirus vaccine. *Pediatr Infect Dis J*, 29(1), 1-5.

Campbell, A., Costello, B., & Ruiz, R. (2010). Cleft lip and palate surgery: an update of clinical outcomes for primary repair. *Oral and Maxillofacial Surgery Clinics North Am*, 22(1), 43-58.

Cleft Palate Foundation. (2001). *Cleft lip and palate: the first four years*. Chapel Hill, NC: Author.

Cleft Palate Foundation. (2002). *Feeding an infant with a cleft*. Chapel Hill, NC: Author.

Cohen, H., Greene, E., & Boulden, T. (2010). The vomiting neonate or young infant. *Ultrasound Clin*, 5(1), 97-112.

Craig, W., Hanlon-Dearman, A., Sinclair, C., et al. (2010). Metoclopramide, thickened feedings, and positioning for gastro-esophageal reflux in children under two years. *Cochrane Database Syst Rev*, 18(4), CD003502.

Creasy, R., Resnik, R., & Iams, J. (2008). *Creasy and Resnik's maternal-fetal medicine* (6th ed.). Philadelphia: Saunders.

Crowles, R. A., & Stolar, C. J. (2006). Abdominal wall defects and disorders of the umbilicus. In F. D. Burg, J. R. Ingelfinger, R. A. Polin, et al. (Eds.), *Current pediatric therapy* (18th ed.). Philadelphia: Saunders.

Dennehy, P. H. (2005). Acute diarrheal disease in children: epidemiology, prevention, and treatment. *Infect Dis Clin North Am*, 19(3), 585-602.

Donn, S., & Senha, S. (2006). *Manual of neonatal respiratory care* (2nd ed.). Philadelphia: Mosby.

Durkin, E., & Shaaban, A. (2009). Commonly encountered surgical problems in the fetus and neonate. *Pediatr Clin North Am*, 56(3), 647-669.

Feldman, M., Friedman, L., & Brandt, L. (2006). *Sleisenger and Fordtran's gastrointestinal and liver disease* (9th ed). Philadelphia: Saunders.

Frankowski, B. L., & Weiner, L. B. (2002). Head lice. *Pediatrics*, 110(3), 638-643.

Goday, P. (2009). Short bowel syndrome: how short is too short? *Clin Perinatal*, 36(1), 101-110.

Grimwood, K., & Forbes, D. (2009). Acute and persistent diarrhea. *Pediatr Clin North Am*, 56(6), 1343-1361.

Hockenberry, M. J., & Wilson, D. (2007). *Wong's nursing care of infants and children* (8th ed.). St. Louis: Mosby.

Huelsing, J., Kanafoni, N., Mao, J., et al. (2010). Camp jump start: effects of a residential summer weight-loss camp for older children and adolescents. *Pediatrics*, 125(4), e884-e890.

James, S., & Ashwill, J. (2007). *Nursing care of children: principles and practice* (3rd ed.). St. Louis: Saunders.

Kaster, E., Schmidt, S., Zickler, C., et al. (2008). Team care of the patient with cleft lip and palate. *Curr Probl Pediatr Adolesc Health Care*, 38(5), 138-135.

Keating, J. (2006). Intussusception. In F. D. Burg, J. Ingelfinger, R. A. Polin, et al. (Eds), *Current pediatric therapy* (18th ed.). Philadelphia: Saunders.

Kerkar, N., & Emre, S. (2007). Issues unique to pediatric liver transplantation. *Clin Liver Dis*, 11(2), 323-335.

Klein, J., Sesslberg, T., Johnson, M., et al. (2010). Adaption of body mass index guidelines for screening and counseling in pediatric practice. *Pediatrics*, 125(2), 265-272.

Kliegman, V., Behrman, R., Jenson, H. B., et al. (2007). *Nelson textbook of pediatrics* (18th ed.). Philadelphia: Saunders.

Kliegman, R. M., Jenson, H. B., Marcdante, K. J., et al. (2006). *Nelson essentials of pediatrics* (5th ed.). Philadelphia: Saunders.

Louie, J. (2007). Essential diagnosis of abdominal emergencies in the first year of life. *Emerg Med Clin North Am*, 25(4), 1009-1040.

Malcomb, W., Gantx, M., Martin, R. et al. (2008). Use of medications for gastroesophageal reflux at discharge among extremely low birth weight infants. *Pediatrics*, 121(1), 22-27.

Masi, P. (2008). Pediatric anorectal disorders. *Gastroenterol Clin North Am*, 37(3), 709-730, x.

McCallough, M. (2006). Abdominal pain in children. *Pediatr Clin North Am*, 53(1), 107-137.

Miniate, D. N., & Albanese, C. T. (2004). Pyloric stenosis. *OTGS*, 6(4), 296-306.

Morin, K. (2004). Infant nutrition: solids—when and why. *MCN*, 29(4), 259.

Morin, K. (2005). Infant nutrition: preparing baby food at home safely. *MCN*, 30(1), 67.

Muir, T. L. (1999). Successful feeding interventions for infants with cleft lip and palate and craniofacial anomalies. Presented at the 56th Annual Meeting of the American Cleft Palate-Craniofacial Association, Scottsdale, AZ.

Niewinski, M. (2008). Advances in celiac disease and gluten-free diet. *J Am Diet Assoc*, 108(4), 661-672.

Olieman, J., Penning, C., Ijsselstijn, H., et al. (2010). Enteral nutrition in children with short-bowel syndrome: current evidence and recommendations for the clinician. *J Am Diet Assoc*, 110(3), 420-426.

Pearlman, D. L. (2004). A simple treatment for head lice: dry-on, suffocation-based pediculicide. *Pediatrics*, 114(3), e275-e279.

Reilly, S., Reid, J., Skeat, J., & Academy of Breastfeeding Medicine Clinical Protocol Committee. (2007). ABM clinical protocol #17: guidelines for breastfeeding infants with cleft lip, cleft palate or cleft lip and palate. *Breastfeed Med*, 2(4), 243-250.

Schnitzer, J. J. (2006). Hernias and hydroceles. In F. D. Burg, J. R. Ingelfinger, R. A. Polin, et al. (Eds.), *Current pediatric therapy* (18th ed.). Philadelphia: Saunders.

Tipnis, N., & Tipnis, S. (2009). Controversies in the treatment of gastroesophageal reflux disease in preterm infants. *Clin Perinatal*, 36(1), 153-164.

Tobia, N. (2008). Management principles of organic causes of childhood constipation. *J Pediatr Health Care*, 22(1), 12-33.

Townsend, C., Beauchamp, R., Evers, R., et al. (2007). *Sabiston textbook of surgery* (18th ed). Philadelphia: Saunders.

Verklan, M., Walden, M., & AWHONN. (2009). Core curriculum for neonatal intensive care (4th ed). London: Saunders.

 Online Resources

American Academy of Pediatrics: *www.aap.org*
Celiac Disease Foundation: *www.celiac.org*
Celiac Sprue Association: *www.csaceliacs.org*
Centers for Disease Control and Prevention: *www.cdc.gov*
Cleft Palate Foundation: *www.cleftline.org*

Chapter 15

American Academy of Pediatrics: Committee on Infectious Disease. (2006). *Red book: 2006 report of the Committee on Infectious Diseases* (27th ed.). Elk Grove Village, IL: American Academy of Pediatrics.

Centers for Disease Control and Prevention: Sexually Transmitted disease curriculum for clinical educators, Retrieved October 5, 2010, from at *www.cdc.gov/stdtraining/readytouse*.

Greenbaum, L., & Mesrobian, H. (2006). Vesicoureteral reflux. *Pediatr Clin North Am*, 53(3), 413-427.

Hockenberry, M. J., & Wilson, D. (2009). *Wong's essentials of pediatric nursing* (8th ed.). St. Louis: Mosby.

Hockenberry, M. J., & Wilson, D. (2007). *Wong's nursing care of infants and children* (8th ed.). St. Louis: Mosby.

Kliegman, R. M., Jenson, H. B., Behrman, R. E., Stanton, B. F. (2007). *Nelson's textbook of pediatrics* (18th ed.). Philadelphia: Saunders.

Polizzotto, M. J. (2005). Prevention of sexually transmitted diseases. *Clin Fam Pract*, 7(1), 127-137.

 Online Resources

AIDS and STDs: *http://nih.gov*
http://aap.org

Chapter 16

Cardona, I., Boguniewics, M., & Leung, D. Y. (2006). Atopic dermatitis. In F. D. Burg, J. R. Ingelfinger, R. A. Polin, et al. (Eds.), *Current pediatric therapy* (18th ed.). Philadelphia: Saunders.

Duffy, B., McLaughlin, P., & Eichelberger, M. (2006). Assessment, triage, and early management of burns in children. *Clin Pediatr Emer Med*, 7(2), 82-93.

Kliegman, R. M., Jenson, H. B., Behrman, R. E., et al. (2007). *Nelson textbook of pediatrics* (18th ed.). Philadelphia: Saunders.

McKinney, E., James, S., Murray, S., et al. (2009). *Maternal-child nursing* (3rd ed). St. Louis: Saunders.

U.S. Food and Drug Administration. (2009). Consumer health information: treating head lice.

Online Resources

American Burn Association: *http://ameriburn.org*
Burn Survivor: *http://www.burnsurvivor.com*
Head lice information from the CDC: *http://www.cdc.gov/lice/head*
Skin rashes: *http://www.nlm.nih.gov/medlineplus/ency/article/003220.htm*

Chapter 17

American Academy of Neurology. (1997). Practice parameter: the management of concussion in sports (summary statement). Report of the Quality Standards Subcommittee. *Neurology*, 48(3), 581-585.

Brenner, J. (2007). Overuse injuries, overtraining, and burnout in child and adolescent athletes. *Pediatrics*, 119(6), 1242-1245.

Bullough, P. (2010). *Orthopaedic pathology* (5th ed.). Philadelphia: Mosby.

Burg, F. D., Ingelfinger, J. R., Polin, R. A., et al. (Eds.), (2006). *Current pediatric therapy* (18th ed.). Philadelphia: Saunders.

Canale, S., & Beaty, J. (2008). *Campbell's operative orthopaedics* (11th ed.). Philadelphia: Mosby.

Committee on Sports Medicine and Fitness. (2008). Policy statement revision: strength training by children and adolescents. *Pediatrics*, 121(4), 835-840.

Cruz, A., & Smith, B. (2010). Scoliosis in children and adolescents: an update. *Contemp Pediatr*, 27(1), 42-53.

Diokno, E., & Rowe, D. (2010). Medical and orthopedic conditions and sports participation. *Pediatr Clin North Am*, 57(3), 839-847.

Dodge, N. (2008). Cerebral palsy: medical aspects. *Pediatr Clin North Am*, 55(5), 1189-1207.

Garfunkel, L., Kaczarowski, J., & Christy, C. (2007). *Pediatric clinical advisor* (2nd ed.). Philadelphia: Mosby.

Grady M. (2010). Concussion in the adolescent athlete. *Curr Probl Pediatr Adolesc Health Care*, 40(7), 154-169.

Halstead, M., Walter, K., Council on Sports Medicine and Fitness. (2010). Clinical report: sport related concussion in children and adolescents. *Pediatrics*, 126(3), 597-615.

Howard, P., & Steinmann, R. (2009). *Sheehy's emergency nursing: principles and practice* (6th ed.). St. Louis: Mosby.

Hockenberry, M. J., & Wilson, D. (2007). *Wong's nursing care of infants and children* (8th ed.). St. Louis: Mosby.

Horn, B., & Davidson, R. (2010). Current treatments of clubfoot in infancy and childhood. *Foot and Ankle Clin*, 15(2), 235-243.

Haufmann, P. (2009). Missed opportunities for Duchenne muscular dystrophy. *J Pediatr*, 155(3), 309-310.

Kliegman, R. M., Behrman R. E., Jenson, H. B., et al. (2007). *Nelson textbook of pediatrics* (18th ed.). Philadelphia: Saunders.

Lovell, M. (2009). The management of sports-related concussion: current status and future trends. *Clin Sport Med*, 28(1), 95-111.

Mercier, L. (2008). *Mercier: Practical orthopedics*. Philadelphia: Mosby.

National Institute of Arthritis and Musculoskeletal and Skin Disease (NIAMS). (2009). Handout on health: childhood sports injuries and their prevention: a guide for parents with ideas for kids. Retrieved November 1, 2010, from *www.niams.nih.gov/Health_Info/Sports_Injuries/child_sports_injuries.asp*.

National Institute of Neurological Disorders and Stroke. (2010). Cerebral palsy: hope through research. Retrieved November 1, 2010, from *www.ninds.nih.gov/disorders/cerebral_palsy/cerebral_palsy.htm*.

Patel, D., & Reddy, V. (2010). Sport related concussion in adolescents. *Emerg Med Clin North Am*, 57(3), 649-670.

Peele M. (2000). Management of adolescent idiopathic scoliosis. *Neurosurg Clin N Am*, 18(4), 575-583.

Quintero, A., Wright, V., Fu, F. et al. (2009). Stem cells for the treatment of skeletal muscle injury. *Clin Sports Med*, 28(1), 1-11.

Rice, S. (2008). Policy revision: medical conditions affecting sports participation. *Pediatrics*, 121(4), 841-848.

Waite, B., & Krabak, B. (2008). Examination and treatment of pediatric injuries of the hip and pelvis. *Phys Med Rehabil Clin N Am*, 19(2), 305-318.

Zitelli, B., & Davis, H. (2007). *Atlas of pediatric physical diagnosis* (5th ed.) Philadelphia: Mosby.

 Online Resources

Cerebral palsy: *www.ninds.nih.gov/disorders/cerebral_palsy/cerebral_palsy.htm*

Duchenne muscular dystrophy: *www.mda.org/disease/dmd.html*

Scoliosis: *www.scoliosis.org*

Chapter 18

American Academy of Pediatrics. (2009). In Pickering, L., Baker, C., Kimberlin, D., et al. (Eds.), *Red book: 2009 report of the Committee on Infectious Diseases* (28th ed.). Elk Grove Village, Illinois: American Academy of Pediatrics. Retrieved November 5, 2010, from *http://aapredbook.aappublications.org*.

Centers for Disease Control and Prevention. (2011). Updated recommendations for use of tetanus toxoid, reduced diphtheria toxoid, and acullular pertussis (Tdap) vaccine from the advisory committee immunizations practices, 2010. *MMWR*, 60(1) 13-15. Retrieved March 18, 2011, from *http://www.cdc.gov/mmwr/preview/mmwrhtml/mm6001a4.htm?s_cid=mm6001a4_w*.

Centers for Disease Control and Prevention. (2010a). FDA licensure of quadrivalent human papillomavirus vaccine (HPV4, gardasil) for use in male and guidance from the Advisory Committee on Immunization Practice (ACIP). *MMWR*, 59(20), 630-632.

Centers for Disease Control and Prevention. (2010b). Vaccines and immunizations. Retrieved August 19, 2009, from *www.cdc.gov/vaccines*.

Centers for Disease Control and Prevention: Department of Health and Human Services. (2010). Recommended immunization schedules for persons aged 0 to 18 years—United States 2010. Retrieved July 20, 2010, from *http://www.cdc.gov/vaccines/recs/schedules/child-schedule.htm*.

Centers for Disease Control and Prevention: Department of Health and Human Services. (2009). Guide to vaccine contraindications and precautions. Retrieved July 20, 2010, from *http://www.cdc.gov/vaccines/recs/vac-admin/contraindications.html*.

Centers for Disease Control and Prevention: Department of Health and Human Services. (2008). *Your baby's first vaccines: what you need to know*. Vaccine information statement.

Hornig M, Briese T, Buie T, et al. (2008). Lack of association between measles virus vaccine and autism with enteropathy: a case-control study. *PLoS ONE*, 3(9), e3140. Retrieved November 5, 2010, from *www.plosone.org/article/info%3Adoi%2F10.1371%2Fjournal.pone.0003140*.

Hockenberry, M. J., & Wilson, D. (2007). *Wong's nursing care of infants and children* (8th ed.). St. Louis: Mosby.

Kliegman, R. M., Behrman R. E., Jenson, H. B., et al. (2007). *Nelson textbook of pediatrics* (18th ed.). Philadelphia: Saunders.

Knudtson, M., Tiso, S., & Phillips, S. (2009). Human papillomavirus and the HPV vaccine: are the benefits worth the risks? *Nurs Clin North Am*, 44(3), 293-299.

Price, C., Thompson, W., Goodson, B., et al. (2010). Prenatal and infant exposure to thimerosal from vaccines and immunoglobulins and risk of autism. *Pediatrics*, 126(4), 656-664.

 Online Resources

American Academy of Pediatrics: *http://aap.org*

Centers for Disease Control and Prevention: *http://www.cdc.gov*

Immunization Action Coalition: *http://www.immunize.org*

Vaccine Adverse Events Reporting System (VAERS): *http://www.vaers.org*

Chapter 19

Abramson, L. (2008). Arthritis in children. Retrieved November 5, 2010, from *www.rheumatology.org/practice/clinical/patients/diseases_and_conditions/juvenilearthritis.pdf#search="juvenileideopathicarthritis"*

American Academy of Pediatrics. (2009). In L. Pickering, C. Baker, D. Kimberlin, et al. (Eds.), *Red book: 2009 report of the Committee on Infectious Diseases* (28th ed.). Elk Grove Village, IL: American Academy of Pediatrics. Retrieved November 5, 2010, from *http://aapredbook.aappublications.org*.

American Diabetes Association. (2010). Standards of medical care in diabetes, *Diabetes Care*, 33(suppl 1), 511-561. Retrieved August 22, 2010, from *http://www.care.diabetesjournals.org*.

Claudius, I., & Baraff, L. (2010). Pediatric emergencies associated with fevers. *Emerg Med Clin North Am*, 28(1), 67-84.

Hockenberry, M. J., & Wilson, D. (2007). *Wong's nursing care of infants and children* (8th ed.). St. Louis: Mosby.

Custa, J., & Rau, R. (2009). *Harriet Lane handbook: a manual of pediatric house officers*. Philadelphia: Mosby.

Kliegman, R. M., Behrman R. E., Jenson, H. B., et al. (2007). *Nelson textbook of pediatrics* (18th ed.). Philadelphia: Saunders.

Knudtson, M., Tiso, S., & Phillips, S. (2009). Human papillomavirus and the HPV vaccine: are the benefits worth the risks? *Nurs Clin North Am*, 44(3), 293-239.

Mercier, L. (2008). *Practical orthopedics* (6th ed.). Philadelphia: Mosby.

Zitelli, B., & Davis, H. (2007). *Atlas of physical diagnosis* (5th ed.). Philadelphia: Mosby.

Weiss, J., & Ilowite, N. (2007). Juvenile idiopathic arthritis. *Rheum Dis Clin North Am*, 33(3), 441-470.

Willis, E., & Hahn, T. (2010). Refusal to walk and stiff neck in toddler boy. *Contemp Pediatr*, 27(9), 47-52.

Online Resources

American College of Rheumatology: *www.rheumatology.org*
American Diabetes Association: *www.diabetes.org/home.jsp*
Arthritis Foundation: *www.arthritis.org*
Juvenile Diabetes Research Foundation International: *www.jdrf.org*
Kawasaki Disease Foundation: *www.kdfoundation.org/*
Stevens-Johnson Syndrome Foundation: *www.sjsupport.org*

Chapter 20

American Academy of Child and Adolescent Psychiatry. (2009). ADHD resource center. Retrieved September 11, 2010, from *www.aacap.org/cs/ADHD. Resource Center.*

American Association for Intellectual and Developmental Disabilities. (2008). Policy statement: education. Retrieved September 11, 2010, from *www.aaidd.org.*

American Association for Intellectual and Developmental Disabilities. (2008). Policy statement: early childhood service. Retrieved September 11, 2010, from *www.aaidd.org.*

American Congress of Obstetricians and Gynecologists. (2007). New recommendations for Down syndrome: screening should be offered to all pregnant women. Retrieved September 11, 2010, from *www.acog.org/from_home/ publications/press_releases/nr01-02-07-1.cfm.*

American Psychiatric Association. (2004). *Diagnostic and statistical manual of mental disorders (DSM-IV-TR)* (4th ed.). Washington, DC: American Psychiatric Association.

Bertoglio, K., & Hendren, R. (2009). New development in autism. *Psychiatr Clin North Am*, 32(1), 1-14.

Bloss, D., & Krugman, R. (2009). Child maltreatment law and policy as a foundation for child advocacy. *Pediatr Clin North Am*, 56(2), 429-439.

Bope, E., Rakel, R., & Kellerman, R. (2010). *Conn's current therapy* (1st ed.). Philadelphia: Saunders Elsevier.

Burg, F. D., Ingelfinger, J. R., Polin, R. A., et al. (2006). *Current pediatric therapy* (18th ed.). Philadelphia: Saunders.

Carbone, P., Farley, M., & Davis, T. (2010). Primary care of children with autism. *Am Fam Physician*, 81(4), 453-460.

Centers for Disease Control and Prevention. (2005). Department of Health and Human Services: Intellectual disabilities. Retrieved September 11, 2010, from *www.cdc.gov/ncbddd/dd/mr2htm.*

Fanton, J., & Gleason, M. (2009). Psychopharmacology and preschoolers: a critical review of current conditions. *Child Adolesc Psychiatr Clin N Am*, 18(3), 159-173.

Goldman, J., Salus, M., Wolcott, D., et al. (2003). *Office on Abuse and Neglect: a coordinated response to child abuse and neglect.* The Foundation for Practice. User manual series. Washington, DC, Child Welfare Information Gateway, 2003.

Grange, D., & Eilser, I. (2009). Family intervention in adolescent anorexia nervosa. *Child Adolesc Psychiatr Clin N Am*, 18(1), 753-771.

Greenhill, L., Posner, K., Vaughan, B., et al. (2008). Attention deficit hyperactivity disorder in preschool children. *Child Adolesc Psychiatr Clin N Am*, 17(2), 347-366.

Herpertz-Dahlmann, B. (2009). Adolescent eating disorders: definition, symptomatology, epidemiology, and comorbidity. *Child Adolesc Psychiatr Clin N Am*, 18(1), 31-47.

Harris, T. (2010). Bruises in children: normal or child abuse? *J Pediatr Health Care*, 24(4), 216-221.

Hockenberry, M. J., & Wilson, D.(2007). *Wong's nursing care of infants and children* (8th ed.). St. Louis: Mosby.

Johnson, C. (2008). Recognition of autism before age 2 years. *Pediatr Rev*, 29, 86-96.

Jurgrau, A. (1990). How to spot child abuse. *RN*, 53(10), 26-32.

Katragadda, S., & Schubiner, H. (2007). ADHD in children, adolescents and adults. *Prim Care*, 32(2), 317-341.

Kellog, N. (2005). The evaluation of sexual abuse in children. *Pediatrics*, 116(2), 506-512.

Kempe, C. (1962). The battered child syndrome. *JAMA*, 181, 17-24.

Kratochvil, C., Vaughan, B., Barker, A., et al. (2009). Review of pediatric attention deficit/hyperactivity disorder for the general psychiatrist. *Psychiatr Clin North Am*, 32(1), 39-56.

Kliegman, R. M., Behrman R. E., Jenson, H. B., et al. (2007). *Nelson textbook of pediatrics* (18th ed.). Philadelphia: Saunders.

Leder, M., Knight, J., & Emans, J. (2001). Sexual abuse: management strategies and legal issue. *Contemp Pediatr*, 5, 77. Retrieved September 11, 2010, from *www.modernmedicine. com/modernmedicine/Features/Sexual-abuse-Management- strategies-and-legal-issue/ArticleStandard/Article/detail/ 131423.*

Mcvoy, M., & Findling, R. (2009). Child and adolescent psychopharmacology update. *Psychiatr Clin North Am*, 32(1), 111-133.

Nicholls, D., & Bryant-Waugh, R. (2009). Eating disorders of infancy and childhood: definition, symptomology, epidemiology, and comorbidity. *Child Adolesc Psychiatr Clin N Am*, 18(1), 17-30.

Pratt, H. D., & Greydanus, D. E. (2007). Intellectual disability (mental retardation) in children and adolescents. *Prim Care*, 34(2), 375-386.

Schmidt, U. (2009). Cognitive behavior approaches in adolescent anorexia and bulimia nervosa. *Child Adolesc Psychiatr*, 18(1), 147-158.

Shevell, M. (2008). Global developmental delay and mental retardation or intellectual disability: conceptualization, evaluation, and etiology. *Pediatr Clin North Am*, 55(5), 1071-1084.

U.S. Department of Health and Human Services. (2008). *Child maltreatment 1990-2006: reports from the states to the National Child Abuse and Neglect Data System.* Washington DC: U.S. Government Printing Office.

Williams, P., Goddie, J., & Motsinger, C. (2008). Treating eating disorders in primary care. *Am Fam Physician*, 77(2), 187-195, 195-197.

Zitelli, B., & Davis H. (2007). *Atlas of pediatric physical diagnosis* (5th ed.). Philadelphia: Mosby.

 Online Resources

American Academy of Child and Adolescent Psychiatry: *www. aacap.org*
American Association on Intellectual and Developmental Disabilities: *www.aamr.org*
American Association of Suicidology: *www.suicidology.org*
American Foundation for Suicide Prevention: *www.afsp.org*
Child Abuse Prevention Network: *www.child-abuse.com*
Child Welfare Information Gateway: *www.childwelfare.gov*
Individuals with Disabilities Education Act: *http:idea.ed.gov*
National Association for Retarded Citizens (ARC of the United States): *www.thearc.org/*
National Dissemination Center for Children with Disabilities (NICHCY): *www.nichcy.org*

Chapter 21

Baker, R. D., Greer, F. R., Committee on Nutrition. (2010). Diagnosis and prevention of iron deficiency and iron deficiency anemia in infants and young children (0-3 years of age). American Academy of Pediatrics Clinical Report. *Pediatrics*, 126(5), 1040-1050. Retrieved December 4, 2010, from *http://aappolicy.aappublications.org/cgi/content/full/pediatrics;126/5/1040.*

Burg, F. D., Ingelfinger, J. R., Polin, R. A., et al. (Eds.), (2006), *Current pediatric therapy* (18th ed.). Philadelphia: Saunders.

Hilliard, L., & Hovard, T. (2006). Sickle cell disorders. In F. D. Burg, J. R. Inglefinger, R. A. Polin, et al. (Eds), *Current pediatric therapy* (17th ed.). Philadelphia: Saunders.

Hockenberry, M., & Wilson, D. (2007). *Wong's nursing care of infants and children* (8th ed.). St. Louis: Mosby.

Kliegman, R. M., Jenson, H. B., Behrman, R. E., et al. (2007). *Nelson textbook of pediatrics* (18th ed.). Philadelphia: Saunders.

Pack-Mabien, A., & Haynes, J. (2009). A primary care provider's guide to preventive and acute care management of adults and children with sickle cell disease. *J Am Acad Nurse Pract*, 21(5), 250-257. Retrieved August 29, 2010, from *http://ezp.tccd.edu:2358/login.aspx?direct=true&db=c8h&AN=2010277051&site=ehost-live&scope=site*

Yock, T. I., & Tarbell, N. J. (2006). Pediatric brain tumors. In F. D. Burg, J. R. Ingelfinger, R. A. Polin, et al. (Eds.), *Current pediatric therapy* (17th ed.). Philadelphia: Saunders.

Online Resources

American Cancer Society: *http://www.cancer.org/*
Centers for Disease Control and Prevention: *http://www.cdc.gov*
National Hemophilia Foundation: *http://www.hemophilia.org*

Ronald McDonald House: *http://rmch.org*
Sickle Cell Disease: *http://www.sicklecelldisease.org/*

Chapter 22

American Academy of Pediatrics. (2007). Policy statement. Palliative care for children. *Pediatrics*, 106(2), 351-357.

Giger, J., & Davidhizar, R. (2008). *Transcultural nursing* (5th ed.). St. Louis: Mosby.

Hockenberry, M., & Wilson, D. (2009). *Wong's essentials of pediatric nursing* (8th ed.). St. Louis: Mosby.

Kübler-Ross, E. (1969). *On death and dying*. New York: Macmillan.

McCaffery, M., & Pasero, C. (1999). *Pain: clinical manual*. St. Louis: Mosby.

Smith, N., & Pravikoff, D. (2010). Terminally ill children: caring for the dying child and the family of the dying child. CIHAHL Nursing Guide, April 2, 2010. Retrieved July 2, 2010, from Nursing Reference Center at: *http://ezp.tccd.edu:2321/nrc/detail?vid=4&hid=10&sid=e7b2d98a-a7f3-40e2-8f9e-f51d78af66a6%40sessionmgr12&bdata=JnNpdGU9bnJjLWxpdmU%3d#db=nrc&AN=5000011594.*

Online Resources

Children's Hospice International: *http://www.chionline.org*
The Compassionate Friends: *http://compassionatefriends.org*
Helping After Neonatal Death (HAND): *http://www.handonline.org*
National Hospice and Palliative Care Organization: *http://www.nhpco*

Illustration Credits

Chapter 1

Figure 1-1: From Hockenberry, M. J., & Wilson, D. (2011). *Wong's nursing care of infants and children* (9th ed.). St. Louis: Mosby.

Chapter 2

Figure 2-1: From Harkreader, H., Hogan, M. A., & Thobaben, M. (2008). *Fundamentals of nursing: Caring and clinical judgement* (3rd ed.). St. Louis: Saunders.

Figures 2-2, 2-12, 2-14: From Hockenberry, M. J., & Wilson, D. (2011). *Wong's nursing care of infants and children* (9th ed.). St. Louis: Mosby.

Figures 2-3, 2-15, 2-16: From Hockenberry, J. (2009). *Wong's essentials of pediatric nursing* (8th ed.). St. Louis: Mosby.

Figures 2-4, 2-8, 2-9, 2-17: From Bowden, V., Dickey, S., & Greenberg, C. (2010). *Children and their families: the continuum of care* (2nd ed.). Philadelphia: Wolters Kluwer Health.

Figure 2-5: From Cincinnati Children's Hospital.

Figure 2-6: Copyright Jupiter Images.

Figure 2-7: From Potter, P., & Perry, A. (2010). *Basic nursing* (7th ed.). St. Louis: Mosby.

Figure 2-10: From Zitelli, B., & Davis, H. (2008). *Atlas of pediatric physical diagnosis* (5th ed.). Philadelphia: Mosby.

Figure 2-11: From Cook Children's Medical Center, Ft. Worth, Texas. Used with permission.

Chapter 3

Figures 3-1, 3-7: From Hockenberry, M. J., & Wilson, D. (2011). *Wong's nursing care of infants and children* (9th ed.). St. Louis: Mosby.

Unnumbered Figure 3-1: From Hockenberry, M., Wilson, D., Winkelstein, M., & Kline, N. (2003). *Wong's nursing care of infants and children* (7th ed.). St. Louis: Mosby.

Figure 3-2: From Bonewit-West, K., Hunt, S., & Applegate, E. (2009). *Today's medical assistant* (1st ed.). St. Louis: Saunders.

Unnumbered Figure 3-2: Courtesy Parkland Health and Hospital System, Dallas, Texas. In Hockenberry, M., Wilson, D., Winkelstein, M., & Kline, N. (2003). *Wong's nursing care of infants and children* (7th ed.). St. Louis: Mosby.

Figure 3-3: From Christensen, B., & Kockrow, E. (2011). *Foundations of nursing* (6th ed.). St. Louis: Mosby.

Figures 3-4, 3-11, 3-16: From James, S., & Ashwill, J. (2007). *Nursing care of children: principles and practice* (3rd ed.). Philadelphia: Saunders.

Figure 3-5: Nomogram modified from data of E. Boyd by C.D. West. From Behrman, R., Kliegman, R., & Jenson, H. (2004). *Nelson's textbook of pediatrics* (17th ed.). Philadelphia: Saunders.

Figure 3-6: From Lilley, L., Collins, S., Harrington, S., & Snyder, J. (2011). *Pharmacology and the nursing process* (6th ed.). St. Louis: Mosby.

Figures 3-8, 3-19: From Hockenberry, J. (2009). *Wong's essentials of pediatric nursing* (8th ed.). St. Louis: Mosby.

Figure 3-9: From Kee, J., Hayes, E., & McCuistion, L. (2009). *Pharmacology: a nursing process approach* (6th ed.). St. Louis: Elsevier.

Figure 3-10: From Kee, Joyce Lefever. (2008). *Clinical calculations: with applications to general and specialty areas* (6th ed.). St. Louis: Saunders.

Figure 3-12: Courtesy Gwen Martin.

Figures 3-13, 3-14, 3-15, Unnumbered Figure 3-3: From Perry, S., Hockenberry, M., Lowdermilk, D., & Wilson, D. (2010). *Maternal child nursing care* (4th ed.). St. Louis: Mosby.

Figure 3-20: From National Institutes of Health, National Heart, Lung, Blood Institute. (Sept. 1996). Update on the Task Force Report (1987) on High Blood Pressure in Children and Adolescents: a working group report from the National High Blood Pressure Education Prog.

Chapter 4

Figure 4-1: From U.S. National Library of Medicine (2011). Handbook: help me understand genetics. Department of Health and Human Services. Accessed from *http://ghr.nlm.nih.gov/*.

Figure 4-2: From Duderstadt, K. (2007). *Pediatric physical examination* (1st ed.). St. Louis: Mosby.

Figure 4-3, 4-4: Copyright Jupiter Images.

Chapter 5

Figure 5-1: From Thompson, E. (1995). *Introduction to maternity and pediatric nursing* (2nd ed.). Philadelphia: Saunders.

Figures 5-2, 5-3: Courtesy Johanna Rosser.

Figures 5-4, 5-25: From Murray, S., McKinney, E., & Gorrie, T. (2002). *Foundations of maternal-newborn nursing* (3rd ed.). Philadelphia: Saunders.

Figure 5-5A: From Korones, S. B. (1986). *High-risk newborn infants: the basis for intensive care* (4th ed.). St. Louis: Mosby.

Figure 5-5B: Modified from Battaglia, F. C., & Lubchenko, L. C. (1967). A practical classification of newborn infants by weight and gestational ages. *J Pediatr*, 71, 159.

Figures 5-6, 5-9, 5-10, 5-11, 5-12, 5-14: From Zitelli, B., & Davis, H. (2008). *Atlas of pediatric physical diagnosis* (5th ed.). Philadelphia: Mosby.

Figures 5-7, 5-13, 5-16, 5-20, 5-22: From Murray, S., & McKinney, E. (2010). *Foundations of maternal-newborn and women's health nursing* (5th ed.). St. Louis: Saunders.

Figure 5-8: From Hockenberry, J. (2009). *Wong's essentials of pediatric nursing* (8th ed.). St. Louis: Mosby.

Figures 5-15, 5-23: From Hockenberry, M. J., & Wilson, D. (2011). *Wong's nursing care of infants and children* (9th ed.). St. Louis: Mosby.

Figure 5-17: Copyright Respironics Inc., Phillips/Norelco. Phillips Children's Medical Ventures. BiliTX Phototherapy System.

Figure 5-18: From Hockenberry, M., Wilson, D., Winkelstein, M., & Kline, N. (2003). *Wong's nursing care of infants and children* (7th ed.). St. Louis: Mosby.

Figure 5-19: Modified From the American Academy of Pediatrics; and Silverman, W., & Andersen, D. (1956). A cold clinical trial of effects of water mist on obstructive respiratory signs, death rate, and necropsy findings among premature infants. *Pediatrics*, 17, 4.

Figure 5-21: From Peckenpaugh, N. (2003). *Nutrition essentials and diet therapy* (9th ed.). St. Louis: Saunders.

Figure 5-24: From James, S., & Ashwill, J. (2002). *Nursing care of children: principles and practice.* (2nd ed.). Philadelphia: Saunders.

Chapter 6

Figure 6-1: From Mahan, K., & Escott-Stump, S. (2007). *Krause's food and nutrition therapy* (12th ed.). St. Louis: Saunders.

Unnumbered Figures 6-1, 6-2, 6-6, 6-7: From Zitelli, B., & Davis, H. (2008). *Atlas of pediatric physical diagnosis* (5th ed.). Philadelphia: Mosby.

Figures 6-2, 6-4, Unnumbered Figures 6-4, 6-5, 6-9, 6-12: From James, S., & Ashwill, J. (2007). *Nursing care of children: principles and practice* (3rd ed.). Philadelphia: Saunders.

Unnumbered Figure 6-8: Copyright Jupiter Images

Unnumbered Figure 6-10: From Hockenberry, J. (2009). *Wong's essentials of pediatric nursing* (8th ed.). St. Louis: Mosby.

Unnumbered Figure 6-11: From Hockenberry, M. J., & Wilson, D. (2011). *Wong's nursing care of infants and children* (9th ed.). St. Louis: Mosby.

Chapter 7

Figures 7-2, 7-3, 7-6, 7-9: Copyright Jupiter Images.

Figures 7-4, 7-8, 7-14: From Hockenberry, J. (2009). *Wong's essentials of pediatric nursing* (8th ed.). St. Louis: Mosby.

Figure 7-5: Copyright U.S. Department of Agriculture Food and Nutrition Service.

Figure 7-7: From McKinney, E. S., James, S., Murray, S., & Ashwill, J. (2009). *Maternal-child nursing* (3nd ed.). Philadelphia: Saunders.

Figure 7-11: From James, S., & Ashwill, J. (2002). *Nursing care of children: principles and practice* (2nd ed.). Philadelphia: Saunders.

Chapter 8

Figures 8-1, 8-2A, 8-3, 8-4, 8-5: Copyright Jupiter Images.

Figure 8-2B: From McKinney, E. S., James, S., Murray, S., & Ashwill, J. (2009). *Maternal-child nursing* (3nd ed.). Philadelphia: Saunders.

Chapter 9

Figures 9-1, 9-2, 9-3, 9-4, 9-5, 9-6, 9-8: Copyright Jupiter Images.

Figure 9-7: From Hockenberry, M., Wilson, D., Winkelstein, M., & Kline, N. (2003). *Wong's nursing care of infants and children* (7th ed.). St. Louis: Mosby.

Figure 9-9: From Hockenberry, M. J., & Wilson, D. (2011). *Wong's nursing care of infants and children* (9th ed.). St. Louis: Mosby.

Figure 9-10: From Hockenberry, J. (2009). *Wong's essentials of pediatric nursing* (8th ed.). St. Louis: Mosby.

Figure 9-11: From Bowden, V., Dickey, S., & Greenberg, C. (1998). *Children and their families: the continuum of care.* Philadelphia: Wolters Kluwer Health.

Chapter 10

Figures 10-1, 10-2, 10-3, 10-5, 10-6 , 10-7 , 10-8 , 10-10: Copyright Jupiter Images.

Unnumbered Figures in Table 10-1: From James, S., & Ashwill, J. (2007). *Nursing care of children: principles and practice* (3rd ed.). Philadelphia: Saunders.

Figure 10-4: From Hockenberry, M., Wilson, D., Winkelstein, M., & Kline, N. (2003). *Wong's nursing care of infants and children* (7th ed.). St. Louis: Mosby.

Figure 10-9: From National Association of Emergency Medical Technicians. (2007). *PHTLS: Prehospital Trauma Life Support* (6th ed.). St. Louis: Mosby.

Chapter 11

Figure 11-1: From Hockenberry, M. J., & Wilson, D. (2011). *Wong's nursing care of infants and children* (9th ed.). St. Louis: Mosby.

Unnumbered Figure 11-1: Courtsey of Electromed, Inc. SmartVest.

Figures 11-2, 11-3, 11-4, 11-9, 11-10: From James, S., & Ashwill, J. (2007). *Nursing care of children: principles and practice* (3rd ed.). Philadelphia: Saunders.

Unnumbered Figure 11-2: From Hockenberry, M., Wilson, D. (2007). *Wong's nursing care of infants and children* (8th ed.). St. Louis: Mosby.

Unnumbered Figure 11-3: From Perry, A., & Potter, P. (2009). *Clinical nursing skills and techniques* (7th ed.). St. Louis: Mosby.

Figure 11-5: Copyright Jupiter Images.

Figures 11-6, 11-7: From Hockenberry, M., Wilson, D., Winkelstein, M., & Kline, N. (2003). *Wong's nursing care of infants and children* (7th ed.). St. Louis: Mosby.

Figure 11-8: From Lilley, L., Collins, S., Harrington, S., & Snyder, J. (2011). *Pharmacology and the nursing process* (6th ed.). St. Louis: Mosby.

Chapter 12

Figure 12-2: From Hockenberry, J. (2009). *Wong's essentials of pediatric nursing* (8th ed.). St. Louis: Mosby.

Figures 12-3, 12-4, 12-6, 12-8, 12-9, 12-10, 12-11, 12-12: From James, S., & Ashwill, J. (2007). *Nursing care of children: principles and practice* (3rd ed.). Philadelphia: Saunders.

Figure 12-5: Copyright AGA Medical Corporation, Plymouth, Minnesota.

Unnumbered Figure 12-1: From Zitelli, B., & Davis, H. (2008). *Atlas of pediatric physical diagnosis* (5th ed.). Philadelphia: Mosby.

Chapter 13

Figure 13-1: From James, S., & Ashwill, J. (2002). *Nursing care of children: principles and practice* (2nd ed.). Philadelphia: Saunders.

Figure 13-2: From Hockenberry, J. (2009). *Wong's essentials of pediatric nursing* (8th ed.). St. Louis: Mosby.

Figure 13-3: From Zitelli, B., & Davis, H. (2008). *Atlas of pediatric physical diagnosis* (5th ed.). Philadelphia: Mosby.

Figure 13-4: Courtesy Albert Biglan, MD, Children's Hospital of Pittsburgh. From Zitelli, B., & Davis, H. (2002). *Atlas of pediatric physical diagnosis* (4th ed.). Philadelphia: Mosby.

Figure 13-6: From James, S., & Ashwill, J. (2007). *Nursing care of children: principles and practice* (3rd ed.). Philadelphia: Saunders.

Figures 13-7, 13-8, 13-9: From Zitelli, B., & Davis, H. (2002). *Atlas of pediatric physical diagnosis* (4th ed.). Philadelphia: Mosby.

Chapter 14

Figure 14-1: From Townsend, C., Beauchamp, R., Evers, M., & Mattox, K. (2008). *Sabiston textbook of surgery* (18th ed.) Philadelphia: Saunders.

Figure 14-2: Courtesy Paul Vincent Kuntz, Texas Children's Hospital. From Hockenberry, M., & Wilson, D. (2007). *Wong's nursing care of infants and children* (8th ed.). St. Louis: Mosby.

Figure 14-3: From McKinney, E. S., Ashwill, J., Murray, S. S., James, S. R., Gorrie, T. M., & Droske, S. C. (2000). *Maternal-child nursing*. Philadelphia: Saunders.

Figure 14-4A: From Schoenwolf, G., Bleyl, S., Brauer, P., & Francis-West, P. (2009). *Larsen's human embryology* (4th ed.). Philadelphia: Churchill Livingstone.

Figure 14-4B. From Gilbert-Barness, E., Kapur, R., Oligny, L., & Siebert, J. (2008). *Potter's pathology of the fetus, infant and child* (2nd ed.). Edinburgh: Mosby.

Figure 14-5: From Kliegman, R., Marcdante, K., Jenson, H., & Behrman, R. (2006). *Nelson's essentials of pediatrics* (5th ed.). Philadelphia: Saunders.

Figure 14-6: From Christensen, B., & Kockrow, E. (2011). *Foundations of nursing* (6th ed.). St. Louis: Mosby.

Figures 14-7, 14-8, 14-11: From Liebert, P. S. (1996). *Color atlas of pediatric surgery* (2nd ed.). Philadelphia: Saunders.

Figure 14-9: From Zitelli, B., & Davis, H. (2002). *Atlas of pediatric physical diagnosis* (4th ed.). Philadelphia: Mosby.

Figure 14-10: From Black, J., & Hawks, J. H. (2009). *Medical-surgical nursing: clinical management for positive outcomes* (8th ed.). St. Louis: Saunders.

Figure 14-12: From McCance, K., & Huether, S. (2010). *The biologic basis for disease in adults and children* (6th ed.) St. Louis: Mosby.

Chapter 15

Unnumbered Figures 15-1, 15-3: From Zitelli, B., & Davis, H. (2002). *Atlas of pediatric physical diagnosis* (4th ed.). Philadelphia: Mosby.

Figures 15-2, 15-3, 15-4: From James, S., & Ashwill, J. (2007). *Nursing care of children: principles and practice* (3rd ed.). Philadelphia: Saunders.

Unnumbered Figures 15-2, 15-4: From Shah, B. R., & Laude, T. A. (2000). *Atlas of pediatric clinical diagnosis*. Philadelphia: Saunders.

Chapter 16

Figures 16-1, 16-7: From Hockenberry, J. (2009). *Wong's essentials of pediatric nursing* (8th ed.). St. Louis: Mosby.

Unnumbered Figure 16-1: From Weston, W. L., Lane, A. T., & Morelli, J. G. (2002). *Color textbook of pediatric dermatology* (3rd ed.). St. Louis, Mosby.

Figures 16-2A, 16-4, 16-9: From Zitelli, B., & Davis, H. (2002). *Atlas of pediatric physical diagnosis* (4th ed.). Philadelphia: Mosby.

Figure 16-2B: From Fireman, P., & Slavin, R. G. (1991). *Atlas of allergies*. New York: Gower.

Unnumbered Figures 16-2, 16-3, 16-4, 16-5, 16-6: Modified from McKinney E., et al. (2009). *Maternal-child nursing* (3rd ed.). Philadelphia: Saunders.

Figure 16-3: From Shah, B. R., & Laude, T. A. (2000). *Atlas of pediatric clinical diagnosis*. Philadelphia: Saunders.

Figure 16-5: From Zitelli, B., & Davis, H. (1998). *Atlas of pediatric physical diagnosis* (3rd ed.). Philadelphia: Mosby.

Figure 16-6: Courtesy Michael Sherlock, MD. In Zitelli, B. & Davis, H. (2002). *Atlas of pediatric physical diagnosis* (4th ed.). St. Louis: Mosby.

Figure 16-8: From Hockenberry, M. J., & Wilson, D. (2011). *Wong's nursing care of infants and children* (9th ed.). St. Louis: Mosby.

Chapter 17

Figure 17-1: From Kliegman, et al. (2007). *Nelson's textbook of pediatrics* (18th ed.). Philadelphia: Saunders.

Figure 17-2: From Tachdjean, M. (1999). *Pediatric orthopedics*. Philadelphia: Saunders.

Figure 17-3: Courtesy Wheaton Brace, Carol Stream, Illinois. From Canale, S. T., Beaty, J. (2008). *Campbell's operative orthopaedics* (vol. 2) (11th ed.). Philadelphia: Mosby.

Figure 17-4, Unnumbered Figures 17-1, 17-2: From McKinney, E. S., Ashwill, J., Murray, S. S., James, S. R., Gorrie, T. M., & Droske, S. C. (2000). *Maternal-child nursing*. Philadelphia: Saunders.

Unnumbered Figures 17-3, 17-5, 17-6, 17-9, 17-10: McKinney, E. S., James, S., Murray, S., & Ashwill, J. (2009). *Maternal-child nursing* (3rd ed.). Philadelphia: Saunders.

Unnumbered Figure 17-4: From Beare, P. G., Myers, J.L. (1998). *Principles and practice of adult health nursing* (3rd ed.). St. Louis, Mosby.

Unnumbered Figure 17-7: From Sorrentino, S., & Gorek, B., (2007). *Mosby's textbook for long-term care nursing assistants* (5th ed.). St. Louis: Mosby.

Unnumbered Figure 17-8: From Perry, S., Hockenberry, M., Lowdermilk, D., & Wilson, D. (2010). *Maternal child nursing care* (4th ed.). St. Louis: Mosby.

Figures 17-5, 17-6, 17-9: From Zitelli, B., & Davis, H. (2002). *Atlas of pediatric physical diagnosis* (4th ed.). Philadelphia: Mosby.

Figure 17-7: From James, S., & Ashwill, J. (2007). *Nursing care of children: principles and practice* (3rd ed.). Philadelphia: Saunders.

Figure 17-8: From Hockenberry, M. J., & Wilson, D. (2011). *Wong's nursing care of infants and children* (9th ed.). St. Louis: Mosby.

Figure 17-10: Copyright The National Scoliosis Foundation.

Figure 17-11: From Hockenberry, J. (2009). *Wong's essentials of pediatric nursing* (8th ed.). St. Louis: Mosby.

Unnumbered Figure 17-11: Courtesy Parkland Health and Hospital System, Dallas, Texas. In James, S., & Ashwill, J. (2007). *Nursing care of children: principles and practice* (3rd ed.). Philadelphia: Saunders.

Chapter 19

Figures 19-1, 19-2, 19-3: From Zitelli, B., & Davis, H. (2008). *Atlas of pediatric physical diagnosis* (5th ed.). Philadelphia: Mosby.

Figure 19-4: From Hockenberry, M., Wilson, D. (2007). *Wong's nursing care of infants and children* (8th ed.). St. Louis: Mosby.

Figures 19-5, 19-6: From James, S., & Ashwill, J. (2007). *Nursing care of children: principles and practice* (3rd ed.). Philadelphia: Saunders.

Unnumbered Figure 19-5: From Hockenberry, M. J., & Wilson, D. (2011). *Wong's nursing care of infants and children* (9th ed.). St. Louis: Mosby.

Chapter 20

Figures 20-1, 20-2, 20-4: From Zitelli, B., & Davis, H. (2002). *Atlas of pediatric physical diagnosis* (4th ed.). Philadelphia: Mosby.

Figure 20-5: Courtesy Dr. Robert Hickey, Children's Hospital of Pittsburgh, Pa. In Zitelli, B., & Davis, H. (2008). *Atlas of pediatric physical diagnosis* (5th ed.). Philadelphia: Mosby.

Figures 20-6, 20-7: Copyright Jupiter Images.

Chapter 21

Figures 21-1, 21-3: From Zitelli, B., & Davis, H. (2002). *Atlas of pediatric physical diagnosis* (4th ed.). Philadelphia: Mosby.

Figure 21-2: From Buttaro, T., Trybulski, J., Bailey, P., Sandberg-Cook, J. (2008). *Primary care: a collaborative practice* (3rd ed.). St. Louis: Mosby.

Figure 21-4: From Hockenberry, M. J., & Wilson, D. (2011). *Wong's nursing care of infants and children* (9th ed.). St. Louis: Mosby.

Figure 21-5, Unnumbered Figure 21-1: From James, S., & Ashwill, J. (2007). *Nursing care of children: principles and practice* (3rd ed.). Philadelphia: Saunders.

Figure 21-6: From Behrman, R., Kliegman, R., & Alvin, A. (2007). *Nelson's textbook of pediatrics* (18th ed.). Philadelphia: WB Saunders.

Chapter 22

Figure 22-1: From Hockenberry, J. (2009). *Wong's essentials of pediatric nursing* (8th ed.). St. Louis: Mosby.

Figure 22-2: Copyright Jupiter Images.

Glossary

A

acceptance The act or process of taking something offered. The condition of being accepted or acceptable. The final stage in Elizabeth Kübler-Ross's stages of grief and dying.

acquired immunity Antibody production resulting from exposure to antigen (e.g., having communicable disease).

acrocyanosis Peripheral blueness of the hands and feet, which is normal in newborn infants.

acromion The lateral, triangular projection of the spine of scapula, forming the point of the shoulder and articulating with the clavicle.

acholic Deficiency or absence of bile.

active immunity Antibody production is stimulated without causing disease (e.g., by a vaccine).

acute rheumatic fever A systemic disease that involves the joints, heart, central nervous system, skin, and subcutaneous tissues. It follows an infection by certain strains of group A, B-hemolytic streptococci.

adaptive behavior Behavior that fosters effective individual interaction with the environment, including activities of daily living.

adolescence The period from the beginning of puberty until maturity.

adventitious Accidental or acquired; not natural or hereditary.

AIDS (acquired immune deficiency syndrome) Characterized by depression of the immune system and opportunistic infection. Seen in neonates and infants who live in high-risk populations and in children with hemophilia and other conditions who have received contaminated blood products.

alimentation The process of nourishing the body, which includes mastication, swallowing, digestion, absorption, and assimilation.

alkalosis Excessive alkalinity of body fluids from accumulation of alkalis or reduction of acids.

allergen A substance, such as pollen, that causes an allergic reaction.

allograft Skin is obtained from human cadavers that have been screened for communicable disease and serves as a temporary graft.

amblyopia (lazy eye) A decrease in or loss of vision, usually in one eye.

amniocentesis A needle is placed into the uterus of an expectant mother to obtain a specimen of amniotic fluid for analysis. This is done to determine possible damage to the fetus by Rh incompatibility, to determine Down syndrome, and for other tests.

anastomosis A natural communication between two vessels or surgical or pathological connection of two tubular structures.

androgen Any steroid hormone that promotes male characteristics. The two main androgens are androsterone and testosterone.

anger A feeling of extreme hostility, indignation, or exasperation; rage; wrath. The second stage in Elizabeth Kübler-Ross's stages of grief and dying.

angioma A tumor, usually benign, that is made up chiefly of blood and lymph vessels.

animism A period of cognitive development in which the child attributes life to inanimate objects.

anorexia nervosa A syndrome most often seen in adolescent girls, characterized by an extreme form of poor appetite or self-starvation. Although its onset may be acute, the underlying emotional problem develops over a relatively long period of time.

antibody A protein that combines with antigens to assist with the body's destruction of antigen.

anticipatory grief Grief that occurs before a loss or a perceived loss.

anticipatory guidance Providing families with information on normal growth and development and nurturing child-rearing practices before the child enters that stage of development. Injury prevention is an area of anticipatory guidance typically addressed in the care of children.

antigen A cell marker that identifies the cell as foreign.

anuria The cessation of urine production or a urinary output of less than 100 mL/day.

anxiolytic A classification of drugs used to decrease anxiety. The action of these drugs decreases anxiety and does not cause excessive sedation.

Apgar scoring chart A standardized chart used to evaluate the condition of the neonate immediately after delivery. The following five objective signs are evaluated: heart rate, respiration, muscle tone, reflexes, and color.

aplastic anemia Anemia caused by deficient red blood cell production because of bone marrow dysfunction.

*From Chabner, D-E. (2001). *The language of medicine* (6th ed.). Philadelphia: Saunders.

arthroscopy A surgical procedure designed to assess joint damage. A small scope is inserted into the joint for visualization of joint structures.

artificialism A period of cognitive development in which the child believes the world and everything in it are created by human beings.

ascariasis Roundworm infestation.

asplenia Absence of the spleen.

associative play Children play together in a similar or the same activity, but there is no organization or leadership

asymmetry One side of the body looking different from the other.

asynchrony Lack of concurrence in time. The appearance of a growing child may be gangling because of asynchrony of growth (i.e., different body parts maturing at different rates).

ataxia Failure of muscular coordination.

atelectasis Incomplete expansion of the lungs at birth or a collapse after expansion because of a mucous plug, a tumor, pressure from organs, or other causes.

atresia A congenital anomaly in which a normal opening is absent (e.g., atresia of the esophagus).

attention-deficit hyperactivity disorder (ADHD) Refers to specific patterns of behavior that include inattention and impulsivity, which may or may not involve hyperactivity.

audiometry Measurement of hearing.

Auditory Brainstem Response (ABR) An electrophysiologic test used to measure hearing sensitivity and evaluate the integrity of ear structures from the auditory nerve through the brainstem.

aura A subjective sensation or motor phenomenon that precedes and marks the onset of an episode of a neurological condition, particularly an epileptic seizure or a migraine.

autism A mental state in which the child becomes absorbed in the self, excluding reality.

autograft Permanent grafts are obtained from an undamaged area of the individual's body.

autoimmunity A condition in which antibodies are produced against the body's own tissues.

autonomy The state of functioning independently, without extraneous influence.

autosome Any of the chromosomes other than the sex (X and Y) chromosomes.

azotemia The presence of nitrogenous bodies in the blood.

B

baby bottle tooth decay Damage to teeth as a result of exposure to sugary acids (from constant access to a bottle of milk or juice).

Back to Sleep Program created to reduce the incidence of sudden infant death syndrome (SIDS).

bacterial agent Pertaining to bacteria (in former systems of classification, a division of the kingdom *Procaryotae*, including all prokaryotic organisms except the blue-green algae).

bargaining To negotiate the terms or conditions of a transaction. The third stage in Elizabeth Kübler-Ross's stages of grief and dying.

barrier technique A method of medical asepsis with use of various types of isolation.

bereavement An acute state of intense psychological sadness experienced after the loss of a loved one or some prized possession.

bilirubin An orange-yellow pigment in the bile that forms as a product of hemoglobin.

blast Immature stage in cellular development before appearance of the definitive characteristics of the cell.

bleb An irregular shaped elevation of the epidermis; a blister or bulla.

body mass index (BMI) An index for estimating obesity.

bonding Attachment; the process whereby a unique relationship is established between two people. Used in conjunction with parent-newborn infant ties.

bone marrow transplant Transplantation of bone marrow from one person to another. Currently used to treat aplastic anemia and leukemia.

booster injection Administration of a substance to renew or increase the effectiveness of a prior immunization injection (e.g., a tetanus booster).

Bradford frame A special oblong frame made of 1-inch pipe, covered with canvas strips, and supported by blocks to raise it from the mattress. The canvas strips are movable; thus the patient can urinate and defecate without moving the spine.

Broviac catheter A central venous line used in small children who need total parenteral or continuous intravenous infusion.

Bryant traction A type of traction apparatus commonly used for toddlers with a fractured femur. Vertical suspension is used. Child may not weigh more than 32 pounds.

bulimia A neurotic disorder seen in female adolescents and young women who wish to remain thin. Characterized by overeating and induced vomiting, fasting, and use of purgatives. Also called *bulimorexia*.

C

cafe-au-lait spots Light brown patch spots on the skin, characteristic of neurofibromatosis (condition of tumors of various sizes on peripheral nerves).

caput succedaneum A localizing, pitting edema in the scalp of a fetus that may overlie sutures of the skull.

cardiac decompression Heart failure.

cariogenic Conducive to caries or decay.

case manager One (generally a nurse) who provides appropriate services to individuals and families through a problem-solving process.

catecholamines A group of compounds, including epinephrine and dopamine, that have a marked effect on nervous, cardiovascular, and other systems.

celiac syndrome An inability to absorb fats, which results in malnutrition, vitamin deficiency, foul bulky stools, and a distended abdomen.

cell-mediated Refers to part of the immune response that is mediated primarily by the T-cells.

cellulitis A bacterial infection of the skin, which can spread.

centering The tendency to concentrate on a single outstanding characteristic of an object while excluding its other features.

cephalhematoma Swelling caused by subcutaneous bleeding and accumulation of blood.

cephalocaudal development The orderly development of muscular control, which proceeds from head to foot and from the center of the body to the periphery.

cerebral palsy A term used to describe a group of nonprogressive disorders that affect the motor centers of the brain.

cerumen Ear wax.

chemoprophylaxis The administration of a medication for the purpose of preventing disease or infection.

chickenpox A communicable disease of childhood, also known as *varicella*. It is caused by a virus and is characterized by successive crops of macules, papules, vesicles, and crusts.

Children's Bureau Government agency for child welfare.

chordee A congenital anomaly in which a fibrous strand of tissue extends from the scrotum of the penis, preventing urination with the penis in the normal elevated position. Commonly associated with hypospadias.

chorionic villi sampling (CVS) A procedure by which a sample of chorionic villa is obtained, which can provide information used in evaluation of the chromosomal, enzymatic, and DNA status of the fetus.

choroid plexus A highly vascularized area that protrudes into the lateral ventricle of the brain. Similar areas are present in the third ventricle.

chromosome A DNA-containing structure found in the nuclei of plant and animal cells and responsible for the transmission of hereditary characteristics.

chronic ulcerative colitis A serious chronic inflammatory disease of the large intestine.

circumcision The surgical removal of the foreskin of the penis.

cleft lip and palate Congenital anomalies caused by failure of the embryonic structures of the face to unite. Characterized by an opening in the upper lip or palate.

clubfoot A congenital orthopedic anomaly, characterized by a foot that has been twisted inward or outward.

cluster suicide A situation in which one suicide precipitates several others; this is becoming more prevalent in the adolescent population.

coarctation of the aorta A constriction of the aortic arch or of the descending aorta.

cognition The mental process by which knowledge is acquired; awareness with perception, reasoning, judgment, intuition, and memory.

cold stress A condition that can occur in a newborn due to the inability to produce or conserve heat; can result in metabolic and physiologic problems.

comedo A skin lesion caused by a plug of keratin, sebum, and bacteria. The two types are blackheads and whiteheads.

communicable An infection that has been transmitted by direct or indirect contact, vehicle or vector, or airborne route.

compartment syndrome Pressure on tissues from edema or swelling, resulting in compromised circulation.

compulsive overeating An eating disorder in which people eat not because they are hungry but because they use food to satisfy emotional, rather than physical, needs.

congenital anomaly A malformation present at birth.

congenital syphilis Syphilis passed from an infected mother to the fetus. Causes multiple organ system problems including growth retardation and mucocutaneous, skeletal, hematologic, central nervous system, and ocular involvement.

contaminated Soiled, stained, or polluted; rendered unfit for use through introduction of a substance that is harmful or injurious.

contractures Degeneration or shortening of the muscles because of lack of use.

cooperative play An organized form of play; children play with other children and there is a goal and leadership

corrosive A caustic agent.

cover test One eye is covered, and movement of the uncovered eye is observed while the child looks at a distant object. If the uncovered eye does not move, it is aligned. Both eyes are checked. This test is used to detect strabismus.

cradle cap A common seborrheic dermatitis of infants that consists of thick, yellow, greasy scales on the scalp.

craniosynostosis Premature closure of the cranial sutures that produces a head deformity and damage to the brain and eyes; also called *craniostenosis*.

cretinism A congenital defect in the secretion of the thyroid hormones, characterized by physical and mental retardation.

critical pathway Multidisciplinary plan that schedules clinical interventions over an anticipated time frame for high-risk, high-volume, high-cost types of cases. Also called *clinical pathway*.

critical thinking Advanced way of thinking that emphasizes process, inquiry, reasoning, creativity, and ingenuity. It is a form of analyzing and problem solving.

Crohn's disease (regional enteritis) Inflammation most often found in the anus and ileum.

croup A nonspecific term applied to a number of conditions, the chief symptom of which is a brassy (croupy) cough and varying degrees of inspiratory stridor.

cryptogenic Idiopathic (of unknown cause or spontaneous origin).

cryptorchidism Failure of the testicles to descend into the scrotum.

currant jelly stool Stool that is composed of mucus and blood; a finding with a diagnosis of intussusception.

cyber bullying Online harassment.

cystic fibrosis A generalized disorder of the exocrine glands, especially the mucous and sweat glands. The lungs and pancreas in particular are involved.

cystic hygroma A lymphangioma most frequently seen in the neck and the axillae.

D

DDST (Denver Developmental Screening Test) Used to assess the developmental status of a child during the first 6 years of life in five areas: personal, social, fine motor adaptive, language, and gross motor activities.

deciduous teeth Baby teeth.

defecation Elimination of wastes and undigested food as feces from the rectum.

denial An unconscious defense mechanism used to allay anxiety and to deny the existence of important conflicts or troublesome impulses. The first stage in Elizabeth Kübler-Ross's stages of grief and dying.

Denis Browne splint Two separate footplates attached to a crossbar and fitted to a child's shoes, used in the correction of clubfeet.

Denver II Test used to assess the developmental status of children during their first 6 years of life.

depression A temporary mental state characterized by feelings of sadness, loneliness, despair, low self-esteem, and self-reproach; accompanying signs include psychomotor retardation, withdrawal from social contact, and loss of appetite and insomnia. The fourth stage in Elizabeth Kübler-Ross's stages of grief and dying.

desquamation The shedding of the outer layers of the skin.

development Growth to full size or maturity.

developmental disability Any mentally or physically disabling condition that begins during childhood and is expected to continue throughout life.

diagnosis-related groups (DRGs) A group of patients classified for measuring a medical facility's delivery of care. These classifications determine Medicare insurance payments for inpatient care.

diaphoresis Profuse sweating.

disinfected Free of pathogenic organisms.

disseminated intravascular coagulation (DIC) A secondary disease characterized by abnormal overstimulation of the coagulation process.

DNA (deoxyribonucleic acid) A complex protein believed to be the storehouse of hereditary information. It is present in the chromosomes of cell nuclei.

domestic mimicry Imitation of activities parents perform, such as doing the dishes.

Down syndrome A form of mental retardation caused by chromosomal defects; formerly known as *mongolism*.

dramatic play Play in which children act out roles and experiences that may have happened to them, that they fear will happen to them, or that they have observed happening to someone else.

DSM-IV-TR Classification system for mental disorders that is clinically focused. Allows for the clinicians to diagnose, study, and treat mental disorders. It is also used for reimbursement.

Duchenne muscular dystrophy A genetically determined progressive muscular disorder.

ductus arteriosus A congenital anomaly in which the opening between the aorta and the pulmonary artery fails to close after birth.

ductus venosus Shunts a significant majority (80%) of the blood flow of the umbilical vein directly to the inferior vena cava in the fetus.

dysarthria A speech disorder consisting of imperfect articulation due to loss of muscular control after damage to the central or peripheral nervous system.

dyscrasia A disease that is usually undefined and associated with blood disorders.

dysfunctional Inadequate; abnormal.

dysmenorrhea Pain in association with menstruation.

E

eczema An inflammation of the skin, frequently associated with an allergy to food protein or environment.

egocentrism A kind of thinking in which a child has difficulty seeing anyone else's point of view; this self-centering is normal in young children.

emancipated minor A term that generally refers to an adolescent less than 18 years of age who is no longer under parental authority.

empyema Pus, especially in the chest cavity.

encephalitis An inflammation of the brain.

encephalopathy Any degenerative disease of the brain.

encopresis The passage of stools in a child's underwear or other inappropriate place after the age of 4 years. Some children display concurrent behavioral problems.

endemic Diseases that occur in expected cycles or continuously.

enteral A method of nutrient delivery in which fluid is given directly into the gastrointestinal tract.

enuresis Abnormal inability to control urine; may be the result of organic, allergic, or psychological problems.

epidemic Disease that attacked many people at the same time in the same geographic location.

epidemiology Study of factors that determine and influence the frequency and distribution of disease, injury, and other health-related events and their causes in a defined human population for the purpose of establishing programs to prevent and control their development and spread.

epiglottitis Inflammation and swelling of the tissues above the vocal cords. Can be life-threatening to children.

epilepsy A convulsive disease, characterized by seizures and loss of consciousness.

epiphyseal plate The ends of the bones that continue to grow throughout childhood and adolescence.

epispadias A congenital anomaly in which the urethral meatus is located on the upper (dorsal) surface of the penis.

Erikson Erik Erikson, who developed a psychosocial theory that focused on the interrelationship between emotional and physical variables.

erythroblastosis fetalis Physiological hemolytic anemia as the result of blood incompatibility. Associated with babies born of Rh-positive fathers and Rh-negative mothers.

eschar Burned tissue.

esotropia An inward deviation of one or both eyes.

estrogen A generic term for estrus-producing compounds; the female sex hormones, including estradiol, estriol, and estrone.

ethical Pertaining to what is good or moral; in accordance with accepted principles governing the conduct of a group.

euthanasia The act of putting to death painlessly or allowing to die.

evidence-based practice A problem-solving approach to clinical decision-making within a health care organization that integrates the best available scientific evidence with the best available experiential evidence.

Ewing sarcoma Endothelioma that occurs in long bones and in flat bones such as pelvis, ribs, and scapulae.

exanthema Eruption on the skin occurring as a symptom of a disease.

exogenous Artificial.

exotropia Outward deviation of one or both eyes.

extravasation Escape of fluid or blood from a blood vessel into body tissue.

extrusion reflex Reflex that occurs in infancy when food is pushed out of the mouth by the tongue; generally disappears by about 4 months.

F

fat embolism Condition in which fat globules are released from the marrow of the broken bone into the bloodstream, migrate to the lungs, and cause pulmonary hypertension.

fetoscopy A procedure that utilizes an optical scope to visualize the fetus in the uterus.

fluorosis Condition caused by exposure to excessive amounts of fluorine or its compounds.

fontanels Openings at the point of union of skull bones, often referred to as "soft spots."

foramen ovale A septum connection between the right and left atrium

foreskin The fold of loose skin covering the end of the penis; also called *prepuce*.

fulminating Occurring rapidly; usually refers to a disease.

fundoplication Wrapping the top of the stomach around the lower esophageal sphincter (LES).

G

gavage Feeding the patient with a stomach tube or with a tube passed through the nose, pharynx, and esophagus into the stomach.

"gel" phenomenon Joint stiffness that occurs mainly in the morning or after a period of inactivity.

gender Sex; the category to which an individual is assigned on the basis of sex.

genetics The study of heredity.

geographic tongue Unusual patterns of papilla formation and denuded areas on the tongue.

glioma Sarcoma involving the support tissue or glial cells of the brain.

glomerulus A tuft or cluster; used in anatomic nomenclature as a general term to designate such a structure, such as one composed of blood vessels or nerve fibers.

glucometer A meter used to measure blood glucose.

gluten The protein of wheat and other grains; gives dough its tough, elastic character.

Gower maneuver A characteristic way of rising from the floor.

grasp reflex Reflex that occurs in infancy when the palms of the infant's hands are touched and flexion occurs; generally disappears by about 3 months of age.

greenstick fracture An incomplete fracture in which one side of the bone is broken and the other is bent. A common type of fracture in children.

grief Deep sadness, as over a loss. An emotional response to an external loss.

growth The progressive development or increase in size of a living thing.

grunting Abnormal short, deep, hoarse sounds in exhalation; grunting occurs because the glottis briefly stops the flow of air.

guarding Tightening or rigidity of the abdominal muscles when the abdomen is palpated.

Guiac stool test Used to determine if blood is present in stool.

H

habilitation A term used to describe a treatment on a patient who is handicapped from birth and therefore is learning, not relearning, a task.

Healthy People 2010 Government document listing health-related objectives for Americans.

hemangioma A benign tumor of the skin that consists of blood vessels.

hemarthrosis Extravasation of blood into a joint or its synovial cavity.

hemodynamics A study of the forces involved in circulating blood through the body.

hemophilia A hereditary disease, characterized by an abnormal tendency to bleed.

Henoch-Schönlein purpura An allergic purpura generally seen in children between the ages of 2 and 8 years; may be caused by medication, insect bites, or other factors.

heparin lock A type of intermittent intravenous device for the administration of heparin. It does not require a continuous flow of fluids; the intravenous flow can be disconnected and the heparin lock filled with a heparin solution that maintains patency of the needle.

hernia Protrusion of an organ through an abnormal opening in the muscle wall of the cavity that surrounds it.

Hickman catheter A tiny rubber catheter that is inserted into a chest vein to establish a long-term or short-term central venous line. Used mainly in adults and teenagers. *See* Broviac catheter.

high risk Any neonate, regardless of birth weight, size, or gestational age, who has a greater than average chance of morbidity or mortality, especially within the first 28 days of life.

HIPAA (Health Insurance Portability and Accountability Act) A 1996 act designed to ensure health insurance portability for workers and families when they change or lose jobs; the main focus is protection of privacy.

Hirschsprung's disease Megacolon; enlargement of the colon without evidence of mechanical obstruction. There is a congenital absence of ganglionic cells in the distal segment of the colon.

holistic An approach to caring for a child that recognizes and adapts to the physical, intellectual, emotional, and spiritual natures; a way of relating to the patient as a whole or biopsychosocial individual rather than just a person with an ailment.

homeostasis State of equilibrium of the internal environment of the body that is maintained by dynamic processes of feedback and regulation.

hospice A facility that provides palliative and supportive care for terminally ill patients and their families, either directly or on a consulting basis.

humoral Refers to the part of the immune system that includes antibodies and immunoglobulins in the blood serum, which arise from B-lymphocytes.

hyaline membrane disease Respiratory distress often seen in premature babies in which a membranous substance lines the alveoli of the lungs, preventing the exchange of gases.

hydrocarbon An organic compound that contains carbon and hydrogen only.

hydrocele An abnormal collection of fluid that surrounds the testicles, causing the scrotum to swell.

hydrocephalus A congenital anomaly, characterized by an increase of cerebrospinal fluid in the ventricles of the brain, which results in an increase in the size of the head and in pressure changes in the brain.

hyperalimentation The administration or ingestion of unusually large amounts of nutrients

hyperbilirubinemia Excessive amount of bilirubin in the blood.

hypercapnia Increased amount of carbon dioxide in the blood.

hypernatremia Excess sodium in the blood.

hyperpnea Energetic (deep and rapid) respiration that occurs normally after exercise or abnormally with fever or various disorders.

hyperthermia Body temperature exceeding the set point, such as from heat stroke or seizures.

hypertonic Having lost more fluids than electrolytes.

hypertrophy An abnormal increase in the size of an organ or part

hypnosis A state of altered consciousness, usually artificially induced, characterized by focusing of attention; heightened responsiveness to suggestions and commands; suspension of disbelief with lowering of critical judgment; the potential of alteration in perceptions, motor control, or memory in response to suggestions; and the subjective experience of responding involuntarily.

hypokalemia Potassium deficit in the blood.

hypospadias A developmental anomaly in which the urethra opens on the lower surface of the penis.

hypotonic Pertinent to defective muscular tone or tension. A solution of lower osmotic pressure than that of a reference solution or of an isotonic solution.

I

icterus neonatorum Jaundice; golden yellow skin color caused by deposition of bile pigments.

identification A defense mechanism by which an individual unconsciously takes as his or her own the characteristics, postures, achievements, or other identifying traits of other persons or groups.

identity The aggregate of characteristics by which an individual is recognized by herself or himself and others.

idiopathic Of unknown cause or spontaneous origin.

imaginary friends Made-up friends to which preschoolers talk and behave as though they are really present in the room.

immunization Induction of immunity, which is protection against infectious disease.

imperforate anus A congenital anomaly in which there is no anal opening.

impetigo An infectious disease of the skin, caused by staphylococci or streptococci.

in vitro fertilization Test tube fertilization in which the ripe ovum is collected and fertilized in vitro (glass) with sperm. The embryo is then transferred to the woman's uterus.

incarcerated Confined; constricted.

incest Sexual activities among family members. Often seen in father-daughter relationships; less frequently in mother-son or sibling relationships.

incubation period Period of time between exposure to infection and the appearance of first symptoms.

infant mortality rate The ratio between the number of deaths of infants less than 1 year of age during any given year and the number of live births occurring in the same year.

infanticide The killing of an infant.

infarct An area of tissue in an organ or part that undergoes necrosis after cessation of blood supply.

infective endocarditis (IE) A form of endocarditis caused by infectious agents.

infectious mononucleosis A generalized disease that causes enlargement of the lymph tissues throughout the body. The number of mononuclear leukocytes in the blood is increased. It occurs mainly in older children and adolescents.

informed consent Written approval needed in order for surgery or a procedure to be performed.

intellectual disability A significantly below-average score on a test of mental ability or intelligence and limitations in the ability to function in areas of daily life, such as communication, self-care, and getting along in social situations and school activities.

intelligence functioning The level of an individual's ability to learn or understand and the ability to apply knowledge to situations.

intention tremor When beginning a voluntary movement, a resultant trembling that affects the body part being used and worsens as the individual gets nearer to the desired object; often seen in patients with cerebral palsy.

interatrial septal defect An abnormal opening between the right and left atria of the heart. Blood that contains oxygen is forced from the left to the right atrium.

intertrigo A superficial dermatitis in the folds of the skin.

interventricular septal defect An opening between the right and left ventricles of the heart. Blood passes directly from the left to the right ventricle.

intimacy Of a very personal, private nature.

intussusception The slipping of one part of the intestine into another part just below it, often noted in the ileocecal region.

iridocyclitis An inflammation of the iris and ciliary body of the eye.

isotonic Having lost equal amounts of fluids and electrolytes.

IVIG Intravenous immunoglobulin.

J

Jones criteria Cluster of major and minor manifestations that help in the diagnosis of acute rheumatic fever.

juvenile rheumatoid arthritis (JRA) A collection of inflammatory diseases that involve the joints, connective tissues, and viscera.

K

karyotype The chromosomal makeup of a normal body cell.

kernicterus A grave form of jaundice of the neonate, accompanied by brain damage.

ketogenic diet Diet used in seizure patients in which a state of ketosis is developed.

Kohlberg Lawrence Kohlberg, a theorist who described moral development in children.

Kussmaul breathing Rapid and deep breathing patterns with no normal period of rest between inspiration and expiration.

kwashiorkor Extreme protein malnutrition seen in infants and children living in poverty.

L

lanugo Soft downy hair covering a normal fetus beginning in the fifth month of gestation and almost entirely shed by the ninth month.

laryngotracheobronchitis Inflammation of the larynx, trachea, and bronchi.

latchkey child A child who comes home to an empty house (after school) because the parent(s) is (are) at work.

latent Dormant or concealed; not manifest.

lecithin/sphingomyelin (L/S) ratio The ratio of two components of amniotic fluid; used for predicting fetal lung maturity.

legal Of or relating to the law. Authorized or based on law. Established by law. In conformity with or permitted by law.

Legg-Calvé-Perthes disease Inadequate blood supply to the head of the femur, characterized by pain in the hip joint; also called *flat hip*.

lichenification Cutaneous thickening and hardening of the skin as a result of continual irritation.

Logan bow (bar) Device to reduce tension on a suture line.

Lonalac Low-salt formula.

lumbar puncture Insertion of a hollow needle into the subarachnoid space between the third and fourth vertebrae; also called *spinal puncture* and *spinal tap*.

lupus erythematosus A chronic inflammatory disease of collagen or connective tissue that may be life-threatening.

M

macrosomia Abnormally large size.

Maslow's hierarchy of needs Abraham Maslow was a humanistic theorist who theorized that basic human needs are organized into a hierarchy of relative priority from lower order requirements to higher order needs.

maturation The full development of adult characteristics (e.g., the development of adult organs or tissue); the development of emotional maturity.

mature minor doctrine Recognizes that individuals mature at different rates.

Meckel's diverticulum A congenital blind pouch, sometimes seen in the lower part of the ileum. A cord may continue to the umbilicus, or a fistula may open at the umbilicus. An intestinal obstruction may occur if the cord becomes strangulated. Corrected with surgery.

meconium The first stool of the newborn; a mixture of amniotic fluid and secretions of the intestinal glands.

meconium ileus A deficiency of pancreatic enzymes in the intestinal tract of the fetus in which the meconium becomes excessively sticky and adheres to the intestinal wall, causing obstruction. Occasionally seen in babies born with cystic fibrosis.

mediastinum The mass of tissues and organs separating the two pleural sacs, between the sternum anteriorly and the vertebral column posteriorly and from the thoracic inlet superiorly to the diaphragm inferiorly. It contains the heart and pericardium, the bases of the great vessels, the trachea and bronchi, esophagus, thymus, lymph nodes, thoracic duct, phrenic and vagus nerves, and other structures and tissues.

megacolon *See* Hirschsprung's disease.

menarche Establishment or beginning of the menstrual function.

meningocele A congenital anomaly, characterized by a protrusion of the meninges or membranes through an opening in the spinal column.

meningomyelocele A congenital anomaly, characterized by a protrusion of the membranes and spinal cord through an opening in the spinal column.

mental retardation A level of intelligence functioning that is well below average and impacts an individual's ability to perform activities of daily living.

metabolic rate The rate of utilization of energy.

microcephaly A congenital anomaly in which the head of the newborn infant is abnormally small.

midstream specimen Urine specimen collected after the first few milliliters of urine have been voided.

miliaria Prickly heat; an inflammation of the skin caused by sweating.

mittelschmerz Abdominal pain midway between menstrual periods, occurring at the time of ovulation and from the ovulation site.

modeling A behavior modification technique in which the patient is taught to imitate the desired behavior of another.

molding Occurs as the fetal head conforms to the size and shape of the mother's pelvis.

mongolism *See* Down syndrome.

morbidity Illness, chronic disease, or disability.

Moro reflex When newborn infants are jarred, they draw the legs up and fold the arms across the chest in an embrace position.

mucoviscidosis *See* Cystic fibrosis.

multifactorial The result of many factors (e.g., a disease resulting from the combined action of several conditions).

murmur A sound heard when listening to the heart, caused by blood leaking through openings that have not closed before birth as they normally do.

muscular dystrophy Wasting away and atrophy of muscles. There are several forms, all with some common characteristics.

mutation A change in genetic material.

myelinization Production of myelin around an axon (of certain nerve fibers).

N

negativism Opposition to suggestions or advice; an attitude or behavior opposite to that appropriate to a specific situation.

neonatal intensive care unit An intensive care unit specifically for neonates; also called *NICU.*

neonate A newborn infant from birth to 28 days of age.

neoplastic Refers to an abnormal mass of tissue such as a tumor.

nephroblastoma Kidney tumor.

neural tube defects (NTDs) Defective closures of the neural tube during early embryogenesis. Included are fetal anencephaly, spina bifida, lumbar meningomyelocele, and meningocele.

neutropenic Having a decreased number of neutrophils (mature granular leukocytes) in the blood.

nevus (pl. nevi) A congenital discoloration of an area of the skin, such as a strawberry mark or mole.

Niemann-Pick disease A hereditary disease in which there is a disturbance in the metabolism of lipids (substances resembling fats), causing physical and mental retardation.

nomogram Representation by graphs, diagrams, or charts of the relationship between numerical variables.

nonbilious vomitus Contains mucus and may be blood streaked but does not contain bile.

nonshivering thermogenesis The oxidiation of brown fat in the neonate to produce heat to keep warm.

nuchal Pertaining to the neck.

nurse practitioner A registered nurse who has well-developed competencies in utilization of a broad range of cues. These cues are used for prescribing and implementing both direct and indirect nursing care and for articulating nursing therapies with other planned therapies. They demonstrate expertise in nursing practice and ensure ongoing development of expertise through clinical experience and continuing education.

Nursing Interventions Classification (NIC) A comprehensive, standardized grouping of interventions or actions that nurses perform.

Nursing Outcomes Classification (NOC) Outcomes that serve as criteria against which to judge the success of nursing interventions.

nystagmus Constant, involuntary, cyclical movement of the eyeball.

O

occlusion Obstruction.

olecranon A large process of the ulna projecting behind the elbow joint and forming the bony prominence of the elbow.

oliguria Decreased urine output.

omphalocele A herniation of the abdominal contents through the umbilicus.

open reduction A surgical insertion of fixation devices, such as pins, to maintain alignment while healing occurs.

ophthalmia neonatorum Acute conjunctivitis of the newborn infant, often caused by *Neisseria gonorrhoeae* and *Chlamydia trachomatis.*

opisthotonic A form of spasm in which the head and heels are bent backwards and body is bowed forward. Caused by titanic spasm.

orthopnea A disorder in which the patient has to sit up to breathe.

Ortolani's sign When the physician can actually feel and hear the femoral head slip into the acetabulum under gentle pressure.

Osgood-Schlatter disease Tendinitis of the knee, seen in adolescents and adults who participate in sports.

ossification Formation of bone substance.

osteochondroma Benign tumor composed of cartilage and bone.

osteogenesis imperfecta A congenital bone disease in which the bones fracture easily.

osteomyelitis Infection of the bone.

osteosarcoma The malignant bone tumor most frequently encountered in children.

ostomy Surgical procedure that creates an opening into a body structure.

otitis media Inflammation of the middle ear.

ototoxic Causing damage to the vestibulocochlear nerve or the organs of hearing and balance.

P

pain An unpleasant sensation arising from injury, disease, or emotional disorder. Pain is whatever the person experiencing it says it is and exists whenever he or she says it does.

palliative care Care and comfort at the end of life. Reducing the severity of the symptoms. Alleviation of symptoms without curing the underlying disease.

palpation The act of feeling with the hand; the application of the fingers with tight pressure to the surface of the body for the purpose of determining the consistency of the parts beneath in physical diagnosis.

pandemic A disease that is epidemic in different parts of the world.

papilledema Edema and inflammation of the optic nerve at its point of entrance into the eyeball.

parachute reflex Protective arm extension that occurs when an infant is suddenly thrust downward when prone.

parallel play A type of play that emerges in toddlerhood when children play side by side with similar or different toys, demonstrating little or no social interaction.

paraphimosis Impaired circulation of the uncircumcised penis caused by improper retraction of the foreskin.

passive immunity Antibodies produced by another person and given to the child (e.g., maternal antibodies transferring across the placenta to the fetus).

patent ductus arteriosus One of the most common cardiac anomalies, in which the ductus arteriosus fails to close. Blood continues to flow from the aorta into the pulmonary artery.

Pavik harness Device used in the treatment of developmental dysplasia of the hip (DDH); consists of straps that maintain hip flexion and abduction.

peak expiratory flow rate (PEFR) The force of expiration from maximum lung inflation.

pectus excavatum A variation in the normal configuration of the chest in which the lower portion of the sternum is depressed.

pediatric nurse practitioner Master's-prepared nurse that cares for children, generally in an outpatient setting; often collaborates with the physician.

pediatrics Branch of medicine that deals with children.

percutaneous umbilical blood sample (PUBS) A procedure that involves the aspiration of a sample of fetal blood from the umbilical vein of the fetus.

period of communicability Period of time the infected individual can pass the infectious agent to another person.

peristalsis Intestinal motility.

peritonitis A generalized infection caused by the appendix rupturing and the infected contents spilling into the abdominal cavity.

petechiae Small, purplish, hemorrhagic spots on the skin that appear with certain severe fevers and are indicative of great prostration. May be caused by an abnormality of blood-clotting mechanisms.

phagocytosis The engulfing of microorganisms or other cells and foreign particles by phagocytes (any cell capable of ingesting particulate matter).

phenylketonuria (PKU) An inborn error of metabolism causing retardation; the body is unable to use phenylalanine, an amino acid.

phimosis A tightening of the prepuce of the uncircumcised penis.

physiologic anorexia A decrease in appetite manifested when the extremely high metabolic demands of infancy slow to keep pace with the more moderate growth of toddlerhood.

Piaget Swiss philosopher and psychologist Jean Piaget (1896-1980) whose work provided understanding of how children's thinking differs from adults' and of how children learn.

pica Abnormal appetite for or compulsive ingestion of nonfood substances such as paint, clay, or crayons.

pincer grasp The thumb and index finger are coordinated, and grasping is achievable.

play therapy A technique used in child psychotherapy in which play is used to reveal unconscious information.

plumbism Lead poisoning.

poliomyelitis An acute infectious disease of the brain stem and spinal cord.

polycythemia When the body determines there is hypoxemia (decreased oxygen in blood), it compensates by increasing the number of red blood cells to carry oxygen to the tissues.

polydactyly A developmental anomaly characterized by the presence of extra fingers or toes.

polyhydramnios An excess of amniotic fluid in pregnancy.

Ponseti method A manipulative technique used in the correction of clubfoot. Serial casting was developed by Dr. Ignacio Ponseti.

portal of entry Route by which an organism enters a host

portal of exit Route by which an organism leaves the reservoir.

postictal Occurring after a seizure.

prehension Use of hands to pick up small objects; grasping.

premenstrual syndrome (PMS) A syndrome that occurs several days before the onset of menstruation and ends a short time after the onset of menstruation.

previability Fetus incapable of extrauterine existence.

primary dysmenorrhea Painful menstruation associated with the menstrual cycle in the absence of organic pelvic disease.

prodromal (symptoms) Indicating the onset of disease.

prognosis A forecast of the probably outcome of an attack of disease.

projectile vomiting The force of vomiting progressing until most of the food is ejected several inches from the mouth.

proximodistal development Directional pattern of growth in which development proceeds from the center of the body to the periphery.

pseudohypertrophy Enlargement at the site of an organ or body part, resulting from an increase in size or number of a separate tissue.

puberty Period in life at which members of both genders become functionally capable of reproduction.

pulmonary function test Measures the vital and expiratory capacity.

pulse oximetry Measured by a pulse oximeter, a means of determining the amount of oxygen in the blood. Infrared light measures the amount of saturated arterial hemoglobin (oxyhemoglovin)during a pulse. Accuracy is influenced by adequate blood flow.

pyloric stenosis A congenital narrowing of the pylorus of the stomach as the result of an enlarged muscle.

pyloromyotomy The surgery performed for pyloric stenosis.

R

rapport Harmonious relationship.

reactive airway disease *See* Asthma.

reconciled To check against another for accuracy.

rectal prolapse A dropping or protrusion of the mucosa of the rectum through the anus.

regurgitation Gentle ejection of the stomach contents into the mouth without nausea or retching.

reservoir An environment in which a microorganism exists and multiplies.

respiratory distress syndrome (RDS) An acute lung disease of the newborn, caused by a deficiency of pulmonary surfactant.

respiratory syncytial virus (RSV) A virus that induces formation of syncytial masses in infected cell cultures. A major cause of acute respiratory disease in children.

respite care Health care providers who assist parents in the home setting to care for children with chronic or developmental illness.

retractions Abnormal "sucking in" of the chest wall during inspiration, indicating respiratory distress.

retrolental fibroplasia Blindness usually found in preterm infants that is associated with high oxygen concentrations and in which the blood vessels of the retina become damaged.

Reye syndrome Acute encephalopathy with fatty degeneration of the liver, characterized by fever and impaired consciousness.

rhabdomyosarcoma Extremely malignant neoplasm that originates in skeletal muscle.

RICE *R*est, *i*ce, *c*ompression, and *e*levation; used to treat soft tissue injury.

rickets A disease of the bones, caused by lack of calcium or vitamin D.

ritual In psychiatry, a series of repetitive acts performed compulsively to relieve anxiety, as in obsessive-compulsive neurosis.

rooting reflex The infant turns the head toward anything that touches the cheek as a means of reaching food.

roseola Self-limited infection manifested by high fever followed by maculopapular rash. The child appears well otherwise and usually remains active.

rubella German measles.

rubeola Measles.

S

scoliosis Lateral curvature of the spine.

scurvy A disease caused by the lack of vitamin C in the diet and characterized by joint pains, bleeding gums, loose teeth, and lack of energy.

sebum A fatty secretion of the sebaceous glands of the skin.

self-image How a person views himself or herself.

shunt A bypass.

sibling rivalry Emotional conflict between siblings (brothers and sisters) that arises from a competition for the love, attention, and approval of one or both parents.

sickle cell anemia A disease associated with an inherited defect in the synthesis of hemoglobin, producing sickled cells.

SIDS (sudden infant death syndrome) The sudden and unexpected death of an apparently healthy infant, typically occurring between the ages of 3 weeks and 5 months and not explained by careful postmortem studies; also called *crib death* or *cot death.*

Snellen alphabet chart A device used to measure near and far vision; a variation is the Snellen E chart.

spina bifida A congenital defect in which there is an imperfect closure of the spinal canal.

squatting position A crouching position with knees bent and buttocks on or near the floor; in children with congenital heart disease, a position they may assume to decrease blood flow to the lower extremities and assist with increasing blood flow to the essential organs, including the brain.

standard precautions Guidelines recommended by the Centers for Disease Control and Prevention (CDC) to reduce the risk for transmission of bloodborne and other pathogens in the hospital.

stridor Emission of a shrill sound during respiration; caused by air passing through a narrowed portion of the respiratory tract.

subacute bacterial endocarditis (SBE) A bacterial infection of the endocardium and heart valves that can lead to deformities or destruction of the valve leaflets.

subluxation Dislocation.

surface area The exterior of the human body (also called *body surface area* [BSA]).

syndrome of inappropriate antidiuretic hormone (SIADH) Increased ADH activity in spite of reduced plasma osmolarity. First recognized by a relative hyponatremia; most commonly associated with central nervous system disorders, various tumors, and drugs.

T

talipes equinovarus *See* Clubfoot.

tantrum A violent display of temper.

Tay-Sachs disease A degenerative, fatal brain disease caused by a lack of hexosaminidase A in all body tissues. Seen mostly in Eastern European Jews, it is genetically transmitted.

tenesmus Spasmodic contraction of the anal or vesical sphincter with pain and persistent desire to empty the bowel or bladder, with involuntary ineffectual straining efforts.

tetralogy of Fallot A congenital heart defect involving pulmonary stenosis, ventricular septal defect, dextroposition of the aorta, and hypertrophy of the right ventricle.

thalassemia A hereditary blood disorder in which the patient's body cannot produce sufficient hemoglobin.

thelarche The beginning of breast development.

therapeutic holding A secure, comfortable, temporary holding position that provides close physical contact with the parents or caregivers.

thermoregulation Regulation of heat.

thoracentesis Surgical removal of fluids using a large-bore needle.

thrombosis The formation, development, or existence of a blood clot or thrombus within the vascular system.

thrush An infection of the mucous membranes of the mouth or throat caused by the fungus *Candida.*

tinea A contagious fungus infection; ringworm.

TORCH Acronym used to describe a group of infections that represent potentially severe fetal problems if infection occurs during pregnancy. *TO,* Toxoplasmosis; *R,* rubella; *C,* cytomegalovirus; and *H,* herpesvirus.

torticollis A condition in which the head inclines to one side because of a shortening of either sternocleidomastoid muscle. Also called *wryneck.*

total parenteral nutrition (TPN) Providing for all nutritional needs by administration of liquids into the blood; used in life-threatening conditions. Also called *hyperalimentation.*

toxin A poison; frequently used to refer specifically to a protein produced by some higher plants, certain animals, and pathogenic bacteria, which is highly toxic for other living organisms.

tracheoesophageal fistula The esophagus, instead of being an open tube from the throat to the stomach, is closed at some point. A fistula between the trachea and the esophagus is common.

tracheostomy A surgical procedure in which an opening is made in the trachea to enable the child to breathe.

transfusion The introduction of whole blood or blood components directly into the bloodstream.

transillumination Inspection of a cavity or organ by passing a light through its walls. When pus or a lesion is present, the transmission of light is diminished or absent.

transitional object A child's favorite possession brought from home to ease the transition into the hospital and promote the child's sense of control.

translocation When a piece of chromosome in pair 21 breaks off and attaches itself to another chromosome.

transport team A team or group of health care professionals that move a patient from one place to another.

Trendelenburg gait Pelvic drops on the side of the affected hip joint when standing on one leg

triage The sorting out and classification of casualties to determine priority of need and proper place of treatment.

tripod position Posturing that a child uses when in respiratory distress; the child sits upright, leaning forward, with the chin up and mouth open while leaning on the arms.

truncus arteriosus A single arterial trunk leaves the ventricular portion of the heart and supplies the pulmonary, coronary, and systemic circulations.

tuberculosis A disease caused by the tubercle bacillus and characterized by inflammatory infiltration, formation of tubercles, caseation, necrosis, abscesses, fibrosis, and calcification. Commonly affects the respiratory system but can affect other body parts.

turgor Elasticity of the skin.

tympanography Process of recording the relative compliance and impedance of the tympanic membrane and ossicles (small bones) of the middle ear.

tympanometry Measurement of mobility of the tympanic membrane of the ear and estimation of middle ear pressure.

tympanostomy tubes Small tubes inserted into the ear drum to prevent accumulation of fluid in the middle ear; commonly used with persistent, chronic middle ear infections.

U

uncover test Test in which the eye is covered and the child looks at a light source. When the eye is quickly uncovered, it should not move; this indicates alignment. Used to detect strabismus.

V

varicella Chickenpox.

variola Smallpox.

vasculitis Inflammation of the blood vessels.

vector A carrier that transfers an infectious agent from one host to another.

ventriculography Radiographic examination of the ventricles of the brain after the injection of air into the ventricles.

vernix caseosa A cheeselike substance that covers the skin of a newborn infant.

vesicostomy A surgical procedure that brings the bladder out to the abdominal wall, facilitating continuous urinary drainage.

viral agent One of a group of minute infectious agents (with certain exceptions, such as poxviruses) not resolved in the light microscope; characterized by a lack of independent metabolism and by the ability to replicate only within living host cells.

virulence Strength of effect produced by a pathogen

volvulus A twisting of the loops of the small intestine, causing obstruction.

W

weaning Discontinuation of breastfeeding of an infant, with substitution of other feeding habits.

wheal Large, slightly raised red or blistered area of skin; may itch.

White House Conference on Children and Youth Government commission that issued recommendations for children and their well-being.

Wilms tumor A malignant tumor of the kidneys.

Z

zygote A fertilized egg.

Index

Page numbers followed by *b*, *t*, and *f* indicate boxes, tables, and figures, respectively.

477

Child Health Evolution

Student Name _____ Date _____

Matching Questions

1. ____ evidence-based practice
2. ____ emancipated minor
3. ____ pediatrics
4. ____ State Children's Health Insurance Program
5. ____ morbidity
6. ____ WIC
7. ____ Healthy People 2010
8. ____ anticipatory guidance

a. food program that provides nutritious food and nutrition education to low-income women and children
b. illness, chronic disease, and disability
c. health promotion and disease prevention objectives for the future
d. examines research literature and focuses on important evidence for quality of care
e. provides families with information on normal growth and development and nurturing child-rearing practices before the child enters that stage of development
f. insures children who are ineligible for Medicaid
g. an adolescent who is younger than 18 years of age and is no longer under his or her parents' authority
h. branch of medicine that deals with children and their development and care

Multiple Choice

1. The infant mortality rate in the United States is decreasing. Which of the following describes the infant mortality rate?
   1. number of infant deaths per 1000 live births
   2. number of infant deaths per 10,000 live births
   3. annual number of infant deaths
   4. number of infants with fatal illnesses

2. In the United States, the leading cause of death in children younger than 1 year of age is:
   1. congenital anomalies
   2. respiratory illness
   3. accidents
   4. suicide

3. Which of the following is a major contributor to infant mortality in developed countries?
   1. low birth weight
   2. communicable diseases
   3. contaminated water supply
   4. under-immunization

4. A 26-year-old single mother with one child, age 7 years, meets the guidelines for low-income families. Which of the following programs could this mother access for her child to ensure adequate nutrition?
   1. Social Security
   2. Children and Youth Project
   3. National School Lunch Program
   4. Head Start

5. Which of the following provides screening, diagnosis, and treatment for low-income children?
   1. Medicaid EPSDT
   2. WIC
   3. SCHIP
   4. UNICEF

6. A family that does not qualify for Medicaid would generally be eligible for which of the following?
   1. FMLA
   2. SCHIP
   3. WIC
   4. Head Start

Community Search

1. Attend a Pediatric Nurse Society meeting in your area, and discuss the role of this organization. (Reference section: Current Practice)

2. Investigate a local WIC center. Observe various aspects of the program, and determine its major objectives. (Reference section: Evolution of Child Health)

Case Studies with Critical Thinking Questions

An 18-month-old toddler is seen by the nurse practitioners at a local community clinic. Her diagnosis is failure to thrive, and she is behind on her immunizations. Her mother is a single parent who earns minimum wage at a grocery store.

1. What criteria does the family have that make them eligible for assistance?

2. Which programs would be available for this family?

Internet Activities

1. Investigate the Maternal and Child Health Bureau (MCHB), part of the U.S. Dept of Health and Human Services *(www.hrsa.gov)* to find out what programs are available.

2. Explore *http://brightfutures.aap.org*. Locate at least one reference that could be used for parent education.

Care of the Child with Medical/Surgical Needs

Student Name _____   Date _____

Matching Questions

1. ____ discharge
2. ____ playroom
3. ____ case manager
4. ____ hospital unit
5. ____ adventitious
6. ____ critical pathway
7. ____ cross-contamination
8. ____ patient's room
9. ____ disposable mask
10. ____ hand hygiene

a. considered a "safe place" for the child
b. pediatric setting differs from adult setting
c. variety of toys available for play
d. begins on admission
e. protects from respiratory droplets
f. accidental or acquired
g. used to achieve outcomes within a specific time frame
h. oversee a continuum of patient care
i. most important barrier against transmission of disease
j. the spread of germs from one child to another

Multiple Choice

1. The nurse understands that safety is important because of which of the following reasons?
   1. sets a good example for parents
   2. keeps the playroom in order
   3. ensures that accidents will never happen
   4. guarantees that errors will never be made

2. All invasive procedures should be performed in which location?
   1. patient's bed
   2. treatment room
   3. playroom
   4. surgery

3. A 2-year-old with pyelonephritis is admitted to your hospital unit. Her mother needs to go home this evening to be with her other children. Which of the following reactions do you anticipate when her mother leaves?
   1. laughter
   2. silence
   3. crying and screaming
   4. quiet conversation with her doll from home

4. A 4-year-old preschooler is screaming for a Band-Aid after a capillary blood sample is obtained. Which of the following fears of the preschooler explains the reason for this?
   1. their hearts will stop beating
   2. their insides will leak out
   3. they were responsible for their illness
   4. the injury will be permanent

5. A preschooler who received an injection specifically requested a Band-Aid with the picture of a popular fictional hero. What is the purpose of fantasy with preschool children?
   1. helps them avoid reality
   2. diminishes guilt
   3. decreases nightmares
   4. helps them cope with their environment

6. The nurse understands that a major fear of school-age children is which of the following?
   1. that their parents will abandon them
   2. bodily harm
   3. loss of sexual function
   4. not being able to play

7. Which of the following herbs would a mother give to her child for anxiety and insomnia?
   1. kava
   2. St. John's wort
   3. gingko
   4. echinacea

8. In which culture is touching the head forbidden?
   1. African American
   2. Mexican American
   3. Vietnamese American
   4. Navajo

9. What are hospital-acquired infections called?
   1. nosocomial
   2. disinfection
   3. medical asepsis
   4. contamination

10. Which of the following is the most appropriate restraint to use when a 5-year-old child receives venipuncture for laboratory work?
    1. therapeutic holding
    2. jacket restraint
    3. mummy restraint
    4. elbow restraints

Study Questions

1. Compile a list of safety measures that would be effective on the children's unit of your hospital. Perform an audit to determine if those safety measures are being done. (Reference section: Safety)

2. Describe the differences in performing a systems review with a child, compared to an adult. (Reference section: The Nurse's Role)

3. The charge nurse has just told you to prepare Room 101 for a new admission who is suspected of having meningitis. The patient is 6 years old. How would you do this? (Reference section: Safety)

4. Discuss how you would evaluate a 4-year-old child for pain. (Reference section: The Child in Pain)

Case Study with Critical Thinking Questions

A 7-year-old boy is admitted to the outpatient surgery section of the hospital where you work.

1. How will you discuss his surgery with him?

2. What will you need to do before surgery?

3. What are the types of things to consider after surgery with a 7-year-old?

A 3-year-old is brought to the pediatrician's office. During the history, the mother states she occasionally gives her child herbs.

1. What questions should be asked of the mother?

2. What are the pros and cons of using herbs and other forms of complementary and alternative medicine?

Internet Activities

1. Visit *www.kidshealth.org* and click on Parents. Under "What's New for Parents," review the section on "Preparing Your Child for Anesthesia." If the article is not in the featured list, type in a key word or two (e.g., *anesthesia*) in the Search box. Make a list of all the helpful suggestions you can offer parents.

2. Investigate *http://qsen.org,* and select an activity that involves pediatrics.

Pediatric Procedures

Student Name _____ Date _____

Matching Questions

1. ____ metabolic rate
2. ____ nomogram
3. ____ tepid baths
4. ____ gastrostomy feeding
5. ____ infant bath water
6. ____ nasopharyngeal culture
7. ____ fever
8. ____ 1 mL
9. ____ enema
10. ____ half-strength hydrogen peroxide
11. ____ rectal temperature
12. ____ apical heart rate

a. should take 20 to 25 minutes to complete
b. temperature should not exceed 38° C
c. rules out pertussis
d. maximum volume (IM) administered to deltoid muscle
e. used for hyperthermia
f. body temperature above 38° C
g. increases 10% for every 1° C
h. calculates body surface area
i. used to clean tracheal stoma
j. should be administered over 10 to 15 minutes
k. counted for 1 full minute
l. contraindicated in newborns

Multiple Choice

1. The age group that benefits most from explanations through drawings, pictures, and contact with equipment is the:
   1. toddler group
   2. preschooler group
   3. school-age group
   4. adolescent group

2. The nurse monitors urine output for a child utilizing which of the following?
   1. 0.5 to 2 mL/kg/hr
   2. 3 to 4 mL/kg/hr
   3. 5 to 6 mL/kg/hr
   4. 10 to 12 mL/kg/hr

3. The nurse monitors a child for which of the following after a lumbar puncture?
   1. fever, CSF leakage, and headache
   2. use of playtime, headache, and urine output
   3. urine output, fever, and headache
   4. naptime, headache, and decrease in appetite

4. The nurse is preparing to administer a subcutaneous injection. Which syringe will be used?
   1. 21-gauge, 1-inch needle
   2. 23-gauge, ⅝-inch needle
   3. 25-gauge, ½-inch needle
   4. 27-gauge, 1-inch needle

5. The best procedure for the nurse to follow if an infant clenches the eyes shut when administering eyedrops is to:
   1. call the doctor
   2. apply the drops in the nasal corner where the lids meet
   3. try to open the eyelids and administer
   4. notify the charge nurse

6. The injection site that is well developed at birth, has relatively few major nerves and blood vessels, and is the largest muscle mass in infants is the:
   1. dorsogluteal
   2. ventrogluteal
   3. vastus lateralis
   4. deltoid

7. Thrombosis, hyperglycemia, and contamination are all potential complications of which therapy?
   1. total parenteral nutrition
   2. intravenous infusion
   3. gastrostomy feedings
   4. IM medications

8. During a lumbar puncture procedure, the nurse should be constantly assessing the child's:
   1. spine alignment
   2. respiratory status
   3. blood pressure
   4. temperature

9. When the nurse is suctioning a tracheostomy, suction should be held no longer than:
   1. 5 seconds
   2. 15 seconds
   3. 25 seconds
   4. 35 seconds

10. The nurse recognizes that signs of inadequate oxygenation include:
    1. increased restlessness, decreased pulse oximetry, and increased respiratory rate
    2. decreased restlessness, increased pulse oximetry, and increased respiratory rate
    3. increased restlessness, increased pulse oximetry, and increased respiratory rate
    4. increased restlessness, decreased pulse oximetry, and decreased respiratory rate

11. When the nurse chooses a blood pressure cuff:
    1. it should cover one third of the upper arm
    2. it should be long enough to encircle the extremity
    3. it should cover the entire upper arm
    4. it should encircle one half of the extremity

12. A 2-year-old is seen in the clinic with a respiratory rate of 28. The nurse understands that:
    1. this is a normal finding
    2. this is diminished for a 2-year-old
    3. this is too rapid for a 2-year-old

Study Questions

1. What special precaution must be taken when giving medications to children? Explore a drug circular and the information provided for administering this drug to a child. Is the information adequate for your purposes? Discuss how and where medications are charted in your hospital. Are there differences between documentation of a medication to a child and an adult? (Reference section: Administering Medications)

2. A 6-month-old has an order for obtaining a sterile urine culture. The mother is extremely anxious and tearful. This is her first child and the child's first hospitalization. Discuss what you will need to explain to the mother regarding the procedure. How can you reduce the mother's anxiety? Outline the steps for obtaining a culture from this infant. (Reference section: Collection of Specimens [urine])

3. Discuss the approach and methodology the nurse uses for obtaining a blood pressure on a 2-year-old versus an 8-year-old. Include differences in results in your discussion. (Reference section: Measurement of Vital Signs)

Case Study with Critical Thinking Questions

A 12-month-old girl is scheduled for a lumbar puncture. The child is extremely fearful of any health care providers. She screams and kicks and bites. The mother is very anxious and tearful.

1. What approach is needed for the child?

2. What approach is needed for the mother?

3. What steps are necessary during this procedure?

Growing Children and Their Families

Student Name _____   Date _____

Matching Questions

1. ___ growth
2. ___ development
3. ___ maturation
4. ___ anticipatory guidance
5. ___ preoperational stage
6. ___ BMI (body mass index for age)
7. ___ initiative/guilt

a. thinks egocentrically (everyone sees the world as he or she does)
b. an increase in physical size, measured in pounds or kilograms
c. questions everything, explores environment and own body, understands gender differences
d. the total way in which a person grows and develops, as dictated by inheritance
e. providing information regarding expectations of an age group, a potential problem or issue, or future occurrence
f. calculated with height and weight measurements
g. a progressive increase in the function of the body (e.g., a baby's ability to digest solids as he or she matures)

Multiple Choice

1. A normal karyotype is made up of:
   1. 23 pairs of chromosomes
   2. 47 chromosomes
   3. 22 pairs of sex chromosomes
   4. 49 individual chromosomes

2. An example of a sex-linked genetic disorder is:
   1. phenylketonuria
   2. hemophilia
   3. cystic fibrosis
   4. Down syndrome

3. Growth occurs in all of the following ways **except:**
   1. cephalocaudal
   2. proximodistal
   3. general to specific
   4. posterior to anterior

4. Birth weight usually triples by age:
   1. 1 year
   2. 2 years
   3. 3 years
   4. 6 months

5. Knowledge of developmental theories is useful for the nurse because it:
   1. allows the nurse to know exactly what to do
   2. provides a framework to guide the nurse in caring for the patient
   3. is a set of facts that each child follows in a prescribed method
   4. is predictable and aids in controlling the child's development

6. BMI is used in children to:
   1. estimate the child's height when fully grown
   2. identify underweight, at risk for overweight, and overweight
   3. identify children who will have a heart attack
   4. evaluate the need to change formula calories

7. Using the growth charts in Appendix C, plot the measurements for a 24-month-old girl who weighs 13 kilograms. What is the percentile for weight for this child?
   1. 5th percentile
   2. 50th percentile
   3. 25th percentile
   4. 75th percentile

8. List factors that influence growth and development. **(Select all that apply.)**
   1. third child
   2. male
   3. rapid growth
   4. blond hair
   5. single parent

Study Questions

1. Identify the different disorders that can be identified with prenatal screening in your area.

Community Search

1. Research what specific programs for homeless families are available in your area.

Case Study with Critical Thinking Questions

A pregnant couple is seen in the genetic clinic because they have family history of sickle cell disease. They are scheduled to have genetic testing.

1. How is the sickle cell trait carried?

2. If both parents have the trait, what is the possible risk for their fetus to have the disease?

Internet Activities

1. With a web browser such as *www.google.com,* search for any of the following topics:
   • Genetics
   • Moral development
   • Erikson's developmental theory
   • Maslow's hierarchy of needs

2. Visit the CDC website *(www.cdc.gov/nccdph/dnpa/ growthcharts/)* and explore the CDC Growth Chart Training Modules and Resources.

The Newborn Infant

Student Name _____   Date _____

Matching Questions

1. ____ Moro reflex
2. ____ tonic neck reflex
3. ____ retracting
4. ____ atelectasis
5. ____ lanugo
6. ____ anterior fontanel
7. ____ gestational age
8. ____ level of maturation
9. ____ cold stress
10. ____ desquamation
11. ____ meconium
12. ____ acrocyanosis

a. a bluish discoloration of the extremities
b. unexpanded lung alveoli
c. closes by 12 to 18 months of age
d. fine, downy hair
e. pulling in of tissue above, between, or below the ribs with each respiratory effort
f. how well the baby is developed at birth
g. the first stool
h. actual time from conception to birth
i. may be seen when an infant's crib is bumped
j. peeling of the skin
k. the "fencing" position
l. can cause metabolic and physiologic problems

Multiple Choice

1. A low-birth weight infant is one who is:
   1. less than 2500 g
   2. less than 2000 g
   3. less than 1500 g
   4. less than 1000 g

2. The most effective prevention of infection in the newborn is:
   1. administration of antibiotics on time
   2. use of disposable items
   3. keeping others away
   4. proper hand hygiene by staff and family

3. Because of the neonate's sterile intestinal flora at birth, the newborn receives an injection of:
   1. vitamin K
   2. erythromycin
   3. vitamin C
   4. tetracycline

4. The reason for the development of respiratory distress syndrome in the preterm infant is:
   1. lack of surfactant
   2. too much surfactant
   3. lack of vitamin K
   4. unknown at present

5. Neonatal apnea may be treated with which of the following medications?
   1. erythromycin
   2. ampicillin
   3. caffeine
   4. vitamin K

6. Necrotizing enterocolitis can be a complication of:
   1. breastfeeding
   2. elevated oxygen levels
   3. hypoglycemia
   4. prematurity

7. The best nursing action in response to an alarming apnea monitor would be to:
   1. suction the nose
   2. begin the treatment for cardiac arrest
   3. silence the alarm
   4. assess for respiratory distress and color

8. If the fluid needs of a preterm infant are 100 mL/kg/24 hr and the weight of the newborn is 1200 g (1.2 kg), what is the infant's hourly intravenous rate?
   1. 0.5 mL/hr
   2. 5 mL/hr
   3. 50 mL/hr
   4. 120 mL/hr

9. In the NICU, discharge planning begins:
   1. at birth
   2. on admission to the transitional area
   3. 2 days before discharge
   4. when the parents are completely comfortable

10. The infant of a mother with diabetes is most likely to:
    1. be small for gestational age
    2. be appropriate for gestational age
    3. be large for gestational age
    4. have intrauterine growth retardation

11. Of the following, the description of the most likely sign of infection in the newborn is:
    1. temperature of 96.6° F, vomiting, and lethargy
    2. temperature of 97.8° F, alert, and fussy about every 4 hours
    3. temperature of 98° F, central cyanosis, and fatigue with feedings
    4. temperature of 98.4° F, ruddy pink coloring, and active with stimulation

12. Which of the following responses most indicates that bonding is occurring?
    1. The mother speaks to her newborn while holding and stroking him.
    2. The mother allows her newborn to cry for a minimum of 10 minutes before checking on him.
    3. The mother is reluctant to hold her newborn and describes her role of mother as burdensome.
    4. The mother desires others to always care for the newborn.

Community Search

1. Visit a parenting class at a local hospital and be able to discuss content covered. (Reference section: Care of the Newborn Infant)

2. Visit a breastfeeding class at a local hospital and be able to discuss tips and techniques given to parents planning to breastfeed. (Reference section: Care of the Newborn Infant, Nutrition)

Study Questions

1. What differences occur in caring for the circumcision done with the Gomco clamp versus the Plastibell? (Reference section: Characteristics of the Newborn, Genitourinary System)

2. Discuss behavioral states in the newborn and their importance. (Reference section: Infant Behavior)

3. List the risks related to preterm births. (Reference section: Preterm Infants)

Case Studies with Critical Thinking Questions

A young expectant mother has attended a breastfeeding class but was unable to attend a parenting class. She is in labor and is asking what happens to the baby after birth.

1. What procedures are done immediately after birth?

2. What procedures are done prior to discharge?

After the birth, she has additional questions about providing cord care and about bathing the baby.

3. How will she provide cord care?

4. What advice needs to be given regarding bathing the baby?

A 32-week-gestation female is born to a mother who had preterm labor for 2 weeks. The mother received Celestone. The baby weighed 1.54 kg at birth.

1. Using the Ballard maturational assessment (Appendix C), determine this newborn's classification for gestational age.

2. What care will be needed for this preterm infant?

3. An intravenous (IV) line is needed, and the order is for 80 mL/kg/24 hr. What will be the amount for 24 hours? What will be the amount for each hour?

Internet Activity

1. Find sources of information for parents or health care providers related to the premature infant. Investigate the March of Dimes (http://www.marchofdimes.com).

The Infant

Student Name _____   Date _____

Matching Questions

1. ____ baby teeth
2. ____ grasp reflex
3. ____ Moro reflex
4. ____ pincer reflex
5. ____ prehension reflex

a. flexion of the fingers or toes in response to pressure
b. intentional grasping of objects between thumb and all the fingers
c. coordination of index finger and thumb
d. generalized response to noise or loss of balance
e. deciduous

Multiple Choice

1. If the needs of the infant are met in a consistent manner, the infant will develop:
   1. independence
   2. responsibility
   3. trust
   4. love

2. The first year of life involves a great deal of growth and development. Parents need to anticipate what their child will be doing next, not only to enjoy their child's accomplishments but also for the child's:
   1. love
   2. freedom
   3. dependence
   4. safety

3. When teaching parents, the nurse explains that the ability to hold the head erect in mid-position occurs during which month of age?
   1. first
   2. second
   3. fourth
   4. sixth

4. Speech begins with cooing. Parents are taught to expect this at which age?
   1. 2 months of age
   2. 4 months of age
   3. 6 months of age
   4. 8 months of age

5. Anticipatory guidance for crawling includes teaching parents to expect this at which age?
   1. 4 months of age
   2. 6 months of age
   3. 8 months of age
   4. 12 months of age

6. Walking around objects for support can be observed in the infant who is:
   1. 4 months of age
   2. 6 months of age
   3. 8 months of age
   4. 10 months of age

7. The nurse explains to new parents that by 12 months of age, the infant's birth weight will:
   1. double
   2. triple
   3. quadruple

8. When teaching parents about nutrition, the nurse explains that the first solid food item to be introduced into an infant's diet is:
   1. vegetables
   2. meat
   3. fruit
   4. cereal

9. When parents inquire about teething, the nurse explains that the infant's first tooth is usually anticipated around which month of age?
   1. second
   2. fourth
   3. sixth
   4. twelfth

Study Questions

1. Why must the pediatric nurse be able to recognize the various stages of growth and development in the infant? (Reference section: General Characteristics and Development)

2. Discuss the needs of the newborn infant. How do these needs change during the first year? (Reference section: Physical Development, Social Behavior, Care, and Guidance)

3. What is the value of attending to the needs of an infant promptly and cheerfully during the first year? (Reference section: General Characteristics and Development)

4. A mother has been bringing her 4-month-old daughter to the well-child clinic since she was 1 month old. What services are provided by a well-child clinic? (Reference section: Health Promotion and Maintenance)

5. How does the infant's environment affect physical growth and development? Mental health? (Reference section: General Characteristics and Development)

Case Study with Critical Thinking Questions

A 4-month-old infant is brought to the well-child clinic. He weighs 15 pounds 11 ounces and is 25 inches long. He is being breastfed and eats every 3 to 4 hours.

1. Using a growth chart in Appendix C, what is this infant's percentile for weight and length?

2. What type of information does the mother need for anticipatory guidance?

Internet Activity

1. Explore the Internet and review normal growth and development for an infant.

The Toddler

Student Name _____   Date _____

Matching Questions

1. ____ ritualism
2. ____ right and wrong
3. ____ egocentric thinking
4. ____ anal phase
5. ____ autonomy versus shame or doubt
6. ____ negativism
7. ____ autonomy
8. ____ ambivalence

a. Freud's stage of personality development
b. Erikson's developmental task
c. Kohlberg's moral development
d. self-confidence
e. fluctuation of emotions
f. increases a toddler's sense of security
g. opposition to suggestion or advice
h. difficulty seeing anyone else's point of view

Multiple Choice

1. At which age would the nurse expect a child to throw a ball overhand without falling and build a tower of three to four cubes?
   1. 15 months of age
   2. 18 months of age
   3. 24 months of age
   4. 30 months of age

2. The nurse explains to the parent of a 2-year-old whose weight was 20 pounds 1 year ago and is now 25 pounds that the toddler:
   1. gained too much weight
   2. gained too little weight
   3. gained the right amount
   4. needs a nutritional consult

3. Which does the nurse describe to the parent as appropriate for a 2-year-old's sentence?
   1. five-word complex sentences
   2. two-word noun-verb simple sentences
   3. use of adjectives when describing nouns
   4. cannot speak in sentences

4. The nurse explains to a parent that the most effective discipline for a 2-year-old is which of the following?
   1. spanking works best
   2. a 5-minute time out
   3. a 2-minute time out
   4. no method is effective

5. Physiologic anorexia is a phenomenon of toddlerhood that occurs because of:
   1. decreased appetite and increased nutritional need
   2. increased appetite and lack of food preferences
   3. increased appetite and strong food preferences
   4. decreased appetite and decreased nutritional need

6. The nurse teaches the parent that one indication the toddler is ready to toilet-train is:
   1. the ability to climb onto the toilet
   2. the ability to stay dry for 1 hour
   3. the ability to communicate needing to urinate or defecate
   4. the willingness to sit on the potty for 2 to 3 minutes

7. Toddlers playing side by side with dolls exhibit which type of play?
   1. associative
   2. team
   3. solitary
   4. parallel

8. Toys that promote growth and development of toddlers include:
   1. toys with small, removable parts
   2. wind-up toys
   3. toys that can be pushed or pulled
   4. balloons because they often come in bright colors

9. A 2-year-old comes to the emergency department with an accidental overdose of acetaminophen. The nurse anticipates the doctor will begin treatment with:
   1. mucomyst
   2. gastric lavage
   3. syrup of ipecac
   4. chelation therapy

10. The nurse is evaluating a child with a lead level of 30 mcg/dL and explains to the parents that treatment will consist of:
    1. IM injections of BAL
    2. oral administration of succimer
    3. medical evaluation and environmental investigation
    4. a review of educational materials

Study Questions

1. Prepare a day's menu for a toddler. Include between-meal snacks. (Reference section: Nutrition Counseling)

2. Define parallel play. Of what value is play to the child? (Reference section: Play)

3. Review your newspaper for 1 week. Bring to class accounts of various accidents that occurred to children during that week. Be prepared to discuss how they might have been prevented. (Reference section: Injury Prevention)

Case Study with Critical Thinking Questions

You are the nurse in a community clinic. A 2-year-old boy comes in for a routine physical. The mother states he is very healthy and "all boy." On examination, the physician states he is "doing well" physically. Routine immunizations are ordered. After you administer them, the mother asks you why her child is such a "picky eater" and when he will be ready to "potty train."

1. What anticipatory guidance needs to be provided to this child's mother in regard to nutrition and toileting?

2. What other anticipatory guidance is needed for a child of this age?

Internet Activities

1. Explore the Internet and find sites that provide information on concepts of growth and development related to the toddler, including safety, nutrition, and daycare.

2. Explore the USDA MyPyramid website and investigate the nutritional needs of a 2-year-old.

The Preschool Child

chapter

8

STUDY
GUIDE

Student Name _____   Date _____

Matching Questions

1. ____ preoperational phase
2. ____ artificialism
3. ____ speech
4. ____ sense of initiative
5. ____ phallic phase
6. ____ 3-year-old
7. ____ 4-year-old
8. ____ 5-year-old
9. ____ stuttering
10. ____ centering

a. posturing repetition of sounds
b. a stage in Erikson's development theory
c. reflected in child beginning to make friends outside of the family
d. a stage in Freud's theory of the psyche
e. more responsible, have more patience
f. boisterous, stormy age
g. a stage in Piaget's developmental theory
h. the world and everything in it are created by human beings
i. tendency to concentrate on a single characteristic of an object while excluding its other features
j. utterance of vocal sounds conveying ideas

Multiple Choice

1. Thumb sucking is considered:
   1. normal in the preschool child
   2. detrimental to the preschool child
   3. normal until 8 years of age
   4. dangerous and must not be allowed

2. Masturbation in the preschool child is viewed as:
   1. disruptive to the family
   2. embarrassing to the parents
   3. normal behavior that can best be dealt with by ignoring the behavior and providing distraction
   4. abnormal behavior that needs to be dealt with immediately

3. An important aspect of the preconceptual stage is:
   1. the increasing development of language and symbolic functioning
   2. the development of moral thinking
   3. the development of spiritual thinking
   4. the development of socialization of the individual

4. Three-year-olds will:
   1. play cooperatively for long periods of time
   2. play well with new friends
   3. revert to parallel play if placed in a strange situation with children they do not know
   4. share toys eagerly when others want them

5. The presence of an imaginary friend generally occurs around which age?
   1. 3 years of age
   2. 4 years of age
   3. 5 years of age

6. The play activity best suited to a 4-year-old is:
   1. pretending
   2. any game with numbers or letters
   3. riding a two-wheeler
   4. hopscotch

7. An effective means of establishing rapport with the hospitalized preschooler is through:
   1. lengthy discussion
   2. explanation with drawings and models
   3. play
   4. silence

8. A sexually abused child may be able to express feelings best through:
   1. therapeutic play
   2. play therapy such as dramatic play
   3. talking quietly with the nurse
   4. drawing a picture

9. A preschooler pretending to do the dishes is an example of:
   1. centering
   2. artificialism
   3. magical thinking
   4. domestic mimicry

10. A warning sign of speech development that could indicate the need for further evaluation of a 24-month-old would be
    1. does not follow simple instructions
    2. is difficult to understand by outside people
    3. is able to imitate sounds
    4. is able to use four words

Study Questions

1. How do you think the preschool child would react to hospitalization? Give reasons for your answer. (Reference section: Theories of Development)

2. A 4-year-old's father dies unexpectedly. What special problems will this present to the preschool child? (Reference section: The 4-Year-Old Child)

3. Visit a preschool. Evaluate a child based on observations listed in Box 8-1. (Reference section: Preschool)

Case Study with Critical Thinking Questions

You are the nurse in a preschool clinic, working with a nurse practitioner. A 4-year-old girl comes in for a well checkup. The parents state she is "doing great." Their only concerns are occasional "bad language" and that she still sucks her thumb.

1. What advice needs to be given?

2. What other anticipatory guidance is needed for a child of this age?

Internet Activity

1. Explore the Internet and find sites that provide information on the concepts of growth and development related to the preschooler, including safety, play, and preschool advice.

The School-Age Child

Student Name _____   Date _____

Matching Questions

1. ____   6 years
2. ____   7 years
3. ____   8 years
4. ____   9 years
5. ____   10 years
6. ____   11 to 12 years
7. ____   sibling rivalry
8. ____   self-image

a. emotional conflict between brothers and sisters
b. period of complete disorganization
c. can be bossy, rude, sensitive to criticism
d. beginning of preadolescence
e. easiest age to teach
f. group fads begin, hero worship is evident
g. how a person perceives himself or herself
h. worries, compulsions, and nervous habits may be common

Multiple Choice

1. Erikson believes that the school-age child is in the stage of:
   1. self-esteem versus shame and doubt
   2. identity versus identity confusion
   3. industry versus inferiority
   4. autonomy versus inferiority

2. According to Piaget (cognitive development), the school-age child:
   1. thinks and reasons in concrete terms
   2. thinks and reasons in abstract terms
   3. thinks and reasons in philosophical terms
   4. thinks and reasons in preoperational terms

3. The best guidelines to use when answering children's questions related to sex include:
   1. answering questions simply and at the child's level of understanding
   2. answering questions with complex terms because the school-age child is old enough to understand
   3. answering questions in a matter-of-fact way so that the child does not become embarrassed
   4. deferring questions back to the child's teachers because they are better at answering these types of questions

4. The American Academy of Pediatrics suggests how much television viewing per day by school-age children?
   1. none
   2. 1 to 2 hours
   3. 2 to 3 hours
   4. 3 to 4 hours

5. An advantage of playing video games includes:
   1. dominating leisure time
   2. promoting eye-hand coordination
   3. teaching acceptance of violence
   4. promoting competition among friends

6. A 7-year-old girl is caught stealing. Which course of recommended action should her mother take?
   1. tell her how wrong she was and what a bad child she is
   2. tell her what she did wrong and that she must return the item to the store with an apology
   3. tell her it is okay to steal only when she really needs something and cannot afford it
   4. tell her in front of the store manager that she has done a terrible thing and certainly was not brought up this way

7. A 9-year-old boy has been repeatedly biting his fingernails at school. His mother wants advice on how to handle this problem. The best advice is to tell her:
   1. this is a normal nervous habit that will disappear when tension disappears
   2. this is a dangerous habit, and she should discuss the problem with her physician
   3. she should ignore the problem because "all kids do it"
   4. this is not normal for a child this age, and he must be having emotional problems

8. A 10-year-old child whose parents are going through a divorce will likely demonstrate:
   1. open grieving
   2. uncontrollable crying in the classroom
   3. hatred toward the teacher
   4. school performance problems

509

9. Children in which of the following age groups begin to use the clock for practical purposes and to use cursive writing?
   1. 6 years
   2. 7 years
   3. 8 to 9 years
   4. 10 to 12 years

10. Children in which of the following age groups can think about social problems and see others' points of view?
   1. 6 years
   2. 7 years
   3. 8 to 9 years
   4. 10 to 12 years

Study Questions

1. Discuss activities enjoyed by the child of 8 years. What diversion would you suggest for the long-term patient of this age? (Reference section: Eight Years)

2. Plan a day's menu for the school-age child. What foods should be included? (Reference section: Nutrition)

3. Investigate after-school programs in your community. What types of guidance/activities are provided? What is the cost involved? (Reference section: Latchkey Children)

Case Study with Critical Thinking Questions
You are the elementary school nurse.

1. How will you determine whether health needs are being met for children in your school? What resources are available if needs are not being met?

2. Develop a teaching plan for a parent who wants to introduce measures to prevent child abduction for a specific age group.

3. What signs might a child demonstrate when being bullied? What are some of the interventions that the school nurse could initiate?

Internet Activity
1. Using the Internet, investigate drug abuse prevention in your community.

The Adolescent

Student Name _____ Date _____

Matching Questions

1. _____ asynchrony
2. _____ adolescence
3. _____ sense of identity
4. _____ preadolescence
5. _____ puberty
6. _____ menarche
7. _____ androgens
8. _____ estrogens

a. developmental stage in Erikson's theory
b. male hormones
c. onset of menstruation
d. different body parts mature at different rates
e. to "grow up"
f. female hormones
g. marked by rapid changes in the structure and function of various parts of the body
h. reproductive organs become functional

Multiple Choice

1. The years of greatest turmoil for most families include those of:
   1. preadolescence
   2. early adolescence
   3. middle adolescence
   4. late adolescence

2. Which of the following statements is true regarding puberty?
   1. Puberty begins at around 15 years of age in both boys and girls.
   2. Puberty occurs about 2 years earlier in girls than in boys.
   3. Puberty occurs about 2 years earlier in boys than in girls.
   4. Puberty begins at around 14 years of age in boys.

3. The first sign of puberty in boys is usually:
   1. enlargement of the testes
   2. the beginning of nocturnal emissions
   3. production of sperm
   4. changes in the voice

4. Which of the following statements best describes how parents should act with regard to limit setting during adolescence?
   1. Limit setting is not necessary because teens are very responsible individuals.
   2. Limit setting is essential because teens still need guidance.
   3. Limit setting is a waste of time because most teens will do what they want anyway.
   4. Limit setting is necessary only in certain situations.

5. When adolescents can see a situation from many points of view and can imagine or organize unseen or unexperienced possibilities, they are said to be in the stage of:
   1. concrete operations
   2. postconventional thinking
   3. identity versus role confusion
   4. formal operations

6. Iron is an essential element in a teenager's diet. Which of the following are good sources of iron?
   1. oysters and nuts
   2. milk and cheese
   3. hamburgers and french fries
   4. fish and dried beans

7. A healthy lunch that meets mineral needs and avoids high fat intake for a teenager would include:
   1. skim milk, tuna on wheat bread, and salad
   2. chocolate milkshake, hamburger on a bun, and french fries
   3. cola drink, roast beef sandwich, and chips
   4. whole milk, hamburger on a bun, and salad

8. Confidentiality cannot be maintained by the physician if:
   1. the adolescent has questions about birth control
   2. the adolescent has questions regarding nocturnal emissions
   3. the adolescent is so angry that he or she is considering running away
   4. the adolescent has questions regarding HIV

9. A 15-year-old girl is taller than everyone in her class. During a health examination, she tells the nurse that she feels everyone is always staring at her and she does not want to go to school anymore. The nurse's best response would be to say:
   1. "That is okay. It will not be that way forever."
   2. "Everyone feels that way at some point during adolescence."
   3. "Just ignore everyone. That will make you feel better."
   4. "Tell me more about your feelings."

10. Which of the following are potential risks for the pregnant adolescent? (**Select all that apply.**)
    1. low birth infant
    2. overweight infant
    3. maternal hypertension
    4. sudden infant death syndrome
    5. continuing school during pregnancy

Study Questions

1. A boy and a girl are each beginning to establish a sense of identity. What does this mean? How may this development be reflected in their behavior? (Reference section: Development Theories)

2. Investigate a babysitting course in your area and discuss what information is presented to adolescents regarding babysitting skills. (Reference section: Responsibility)

3. Plan a day's menu for a 15-year-old girl and a 17-year-old boy. What are the nutritional requirements in terms of calories, protein, calcium, and iron? (Reference section: Nutrition)

Case Study with Critical Thinking Questions

You are the high school nurse.

1. What are the needs of the pregnant teenagers in your school?

2. What resources do you have to help meet their needs?

Internet Activity

1. Explore the Internet and find sites that provide information on anticipatory guidance with the adolescent.

Respiratory Disorders

Student Name _____   Date _____

Matching Questions

1. ____ TB
2. ____ cystic fibrosis
3. ____ SIDS
4. ____ myringotomy
5. ____ otitis media
6. ____ bronchiolitis
7. ____ Haemophilus influenzae
8. ____ peak expiratory flow meter

a. common causative organism is RSV (respiratory syncytial virus)
b. most common cause of epiglottitis
c. force of expiration from maximum lung inflation
d. middle ear infection
e. inherited disease involving the exocrine glands
f. causative organism is the mycobacterium
g. small incision into the eardrum
h. higher incidence in African-American population

Multiple Choice

1. When a child has otitis media and begins therapy with an antibiotic, this medication should be taken:
   1. until the symptoms go away
   2. until the entire prescription is gone
   3. only when the child has symptoms
   4. as long as fever persists

2. When an oral pancreatic extract is given, which of the following should be considered?
   1. give the medication with meals or snacks
   2. give the medication even if the child is ill or not eating
   3. the enteric-coated tablets may be crushed or chewed
   4. give the medication between meals

3. Infants and young children can become dehydrated from a respiratory infection because of:
   1. loss of fluids through increased temperature and respirations
   2. decreased intake resulting from anorexia
   3. vomiting
   4. all of the above

4. When collecting data about a child with suspected epiglottitis, the nurse keeps in mind that, unlike croup, epiglottitis:
   1. has a brassy cough
   2. develops rapidly
   3. occurs in infants
   4. is worse at night

5. When the nurse is planning care for the child who has had surgery to remove the tonsils and adenoids, a major goal is to:
   1. prevent hemorrhage
   2. decrease dehydration
   3. prevent pneumonia
   4. control activity

6. A 6-year-old is admitted to the hospital with wheezing. He was well until a few days ago, when he developed a cold. Which of the following signs and symptoms suggest that he has respiratory distress?
   1. cough, fever, sore throat
   2. flushed, skin, thirst, increased breathing
   3. decreased pulse, restlessness, clammy skin
   4. retractions, increased respirations, pallor

7. A child is diagnosed with asthma. The nurse needs to administer albuterol via nebulizer every 20 minutes. Albuterol is:
   1. a bronchodilator
   2. an antiinflammatory
   3. a cough suppressant
   4. an antiallergenic agent

8. Which of the following is a long-term nursing goal for a child with asthma?
   1. maintaining hydration
   2. appropriate home monitoring of respiratory status
   3. decreasing exercise
   4. oxygen saturation of 92%

9. Transmission of TB is by:
   1. direct contact of the organism on the skin
   2. handling of feces or urine
   3. ingestion of the organism
   4. inhalation of an infected droplet

10. The plan of care for a child with bronchitis should include:
    1. bedrest and minimal oral fluid intake
    2. keeping room air cool and dry
    3. expectorants and coughing to clear secretions
    4. shallow inspiration to decrease chest pain

Study Questions

1. Describe what factors could precipitate an asthma attack. (Reference section: Asthma)

2. Demonstrate how to measure the PEFR, and explain what the results may mean. (Reference section: Asthma)

3. Discuss the preoperative teaching and postoperative care for the child who is undergoing tonsillectomy and adenoidectomy. (Reference section: Tonsillitis and Adenoiditis)

4. An 18-month-old has been seen in the office by the family pediatrician. He has been diagnosed with croup. List the home care instructions for caring for this child. (Reference section: Croup)

5. List the symptoms for epiglottitis. Why do these symptoms occur with this disease? (Reference section: Epiglottitis)

6. Discuss the method for treatment of a child who has TB. Include the family support that will also be needed with this child. (Reference section: Tuberculosis)

Case Study with Critical Thinking Questions

A 2-year-old child is admitted with pneumonia.

1. List the problems that would be expected for a child with this diagnosis.

2. What nursing interventions are appropriate?

3. What discharge instructions would be expected with this child?

Internet Activity

1. Go to the National Institute of Child and Health Development website (http://nichd.nih.gov) and find information regarding teaching objectives for discussing SIDS prevention in the community.

Cardiac Disorders

chapter

12

STUDY
GUIDE

Student Name _____   Date _____

Matching Questions

1. ____ infective endocarditis
2. ____ patent ductus arteriosus
3. ____ cardiac catheterization
4. ____ hypoplastic left heart
5. ____ digoxin
6. ____ ventricular septal defect
7. ____ coarctation of the aorta
8. ____ tetralogy of Fallot
9. ____ transposition of the great vessels
10. ____ foramen ovale
11. ____ Jones criteria

a. a congenital heart defect resulting in increased pulmonary blood flow
b. a tool used to assist with diagnosis of rheumatic fever
c. an example of a congenital heart defect resulting in mixed blood flow
d. fetal shunt that closes after birth
e. a congenital heart defect resulting in obstructive blood flow
f. a tool used to evaluate heart chamber pressures, blood flow, and oxygen saturations
g. may be closed by administering indomethacin (prostaglandin inhibitor)
h. potassium levels need to be monitored, which can effect drug action
i. requires a septostomy prior to corrective surgery
j. inflammation of the heart lining that may result from cardiac surgery
k. the leading cause of death from cardiac defects

Multiple Choice

1. The nurse realizes that a family needs further teaching regarding digoxin when the mother states:
   1. "If our child vomits the digoxin, we should not give another dose."
   2. "The purpose of digoxin is to speed up the heart rate."
   3. "We should always use the oral syringe to measure the amount."
   4. "We should encourage foods such as bananas."

2. While caring for a child with rheumatic fever, the nurse knows which laboratory test is helpful?
   1. antistreptolysin O titer
   2. glucose tolerance test
   3. sodium level
   4. bilirubin

3. An infant in congestive heart failure shows signs of accumulating fluids when the nurse observes:
   1. sunken fontanel
   2. bradycardia
   3. crackles heard on auscultation
   4. capillary refill time of 2 seconds

4. The most common cardiac condition is:
   1. patent ductus arteriosus (PDA)
   2. pulmonary stenosis
   3. tetralogy of Fallot
   4. truncus arteriosus

5. Of the following congenital heart defects, the one least likely to present initially with cyanosis is:
   1. tetralogy of Fallot
   2. truncus arteriosus
   3. transposition of the great vessels
   4. ventricular septal defect (VSD)

6. Tetralogy of Fallot has four defects. Which of the following are parts of this defect?
   1. left ventricular hypertrophy, atrial septal defect, aortic stenosis, and overriding aorta
   2. aortic hypertrophy, left ventricular hypertrophy, pulmonary atresia, and pulmonary hypertension
   3. right ventricular hypertrophy, ventricular septal defect, pulmonary stenosis, and overriding aorta
   4. hypoplasia of aorta, atrial septal defect, mitral valve insufficiency, and right ventricular hypertrophy

7. The mother of a child with transposition of the great arteries asks what the reason is for giving prostaglandin to her child.
   1. prevents infective endocarditis
   2. maintains patency of ductus arteriosus to provide oxygenation
   3. to prevent infection before cardiac catheterization
   4. closes the foramen ovale to improve cardiac output

8. An infant with tetralogy of Fallot begins to get cyanotic after a blood draw. The nurse knows that the mother understands the hypercyanotic spell when she:
   1. holds the child in an upright position
   2. provides a pacifier to calm the infant
   3. immediately calls the nurse for help
   4. places the child in a knee-chest position

9. Dehydration in a child with a cyanotic heart defect is a risk for:
   1. pneumonia
   2. clubbing of fingers
   3. cerebral vascular accident
   4. hypokalemia

10. A child who is 1 hour post–cardiac catheterization has a wet dressing. The nurse should:
    1. recheck the dressing in 15 minutes
    2. apply pressure above the insertion site
    3. apply more dressing to the site
    4. elevate the affected leg

Study Questions

1. Discuss the nursing goals in caring for a child with a heart defect. Also include the care for the family. (Reference section: Nursing Goals and Treatment in Congenital Heart Disease)

2. Develop a teaching plan for a 6-year-old who is undergoing a cardiac catheterization. (Reference section: Cardiac Catheterization)

3. Review home care of a school-age child with rheumatic fever. (Reference section: Rheumatic fever)

Case Study with Critical Thinking Questions

A male child who is term (40 weeks' gestation) is delivered to first-time parents. He was cyanotic at birth and has been diagnosed with hypoplastic left heart (HPLH). The parents are distraught.

1. What will be the first concern for this newborn?

2. What resources are available for his parents?

3. What can the nurse do to help with the bonding process for this family?

4. What will the course of treatment involve for this infant?

Internet Activity

1. Go to several websites that provide information on cardiac defects and explore the child-focused materials that are available.

Neurologic and Sensory Disorders

Student Name _____   Date _____

Matching Questions

1. ____ meningitis
2. ____ hydrocephalus
3. ____ spina bifida
4. ____ meningocele
5. ____ meningomyelocele
6. ____ decerebrate
7. ____ postictal
8. ____ opisthotonos
9. ____ SIADH
10. ____ cover test
11. ____ aura
12. ____ occlusion

a. posturing indicating injury to the midbrain
b. involve the membranes and cerebrospinal fluid
c. spinal tap used as a diagnostic procedure
d. covering or obstruction
e. diagnostic exam for strabismus
f. precedes seizure activity
g. increase of cerebrospinal fluid in the ventricles of the brain
h. head and heels bend backwards; body bows forward
i. occurring after a seizure
j. embryonic neural tube defect
k. increased ADH activity resulting in hyponatremia
l. involves the membranes, the spinal cord, and cerebrospinal fluid

Multiple Choice

1. The nurse caring for a patient with bacterial meningitis understands that the disease:
   1. may be preceded by cold or upper respiratory tract infection
   2. has declined as a result of the *H. influenzae* type b vaccine
   3. causes the patient to be overly sensitive to stimuli
   4. all of the above

2. The nurse realizes that one of the first signs of increasing intracranial pressure in a nonverbal toddler is:
   1. decreasing blood pressure
   2. behavior changes
   3. seizures
   4. increasing heart rate

3. The nurse explains to a parent that the most severe form of spina bifida is:
   1. meningomyelocele
   2. meningocele
   3. spina bifida occulta
   4. lipoma

4. The nurse teaches a parent that patching the unaffected eye is a method of treatment for amblyopia because it:
   1. forces the weaker eye to function
   2. automatically enlarges the pupil of the opposite eye
   3. decreases abnormal eye muscle movement
   4. decreases sensory input to the brain

5. First aid measures during a tonic-clonic seizure are based on the understanding that the child:
   1. is aware of what is happening
   2. might injure others
   3. is unconscious
   4. has control over muscle action

6. Nursing care for a child with encephalitis includes which of the following?
   1. monitoring intravenous fluids
   2. providing a quiet environment
   3. providing seizure precautions
   4. all of the above

7. A nurse instituting seizure precautions includes all of the following **except:**
   1. padding the side rails of the bed
   2. maintaining oxygen and suction equipment
   3. keeping a padded tongue blade at the bedside
   4. having emergency airway equipment available

8. The priority of care for a 5-year-old child admitted with *H. influenzae* meningitis is:
   1. begin ordered antibiotics
   2. place the child in isolation
   3. order a full liquid diet
   4. teach meningitis prevention

Study Questions

1. List the symptoms of increased intracranial pressure. (Reference section: Increased Intracranial Pressure)

2. Discuss the nursing goals in caring for a child with a myelomeningocele. (Reference section: Myelodysplasia/Spina Bifida)

3. Visit a pediatrician's office and observe hearing and vision testing. Summarize your findings. (Reference section: Sensory Disorders)

Case Study with Critical Thinking Questions

A 3-year-old is admitted to your hospital unit with tonic-clonic seizure disorder.

1. What are the precautions taken for this child in the hospital?

2. What resources are available for the parents?

3. What teaching is done prior to discharge?

Internet Activity

1. Visit the Epilepsy Foundation at *www.epilepsyfoundation.org* and investigate ongoing research.

Gastrointestinal Disorders

Student Name _____   Date _____

Matching Questions

1. ____ inguinal hernia
2. ____ currant jelly stool
3. ____ silastic silo
4. ____ polyhydramnios
5. ____ McBurney's point
6. ____ Haberman Feeder
7. ____ guiac stool test
8. ____ gluten
9. ____ intussusception
10. ____ rotovirus
11. ____ aganglionic megacolon

a. midway between the umbilicus and the right iliac crest
b. excessive amniotic fluid associated with fetal anomalies
c. most common cause of gastroenteritis
d. telescoping of bowel
e. protein in wheat, barley, and rye
f. Hirschsprung's disease
g. specialized device used to feed cleft lip and/or palate infants
h. stools with mucus and blood
i. keeps abdominal contents protected during replacement
j. more common in boys than in girls
k. identifies blood in stool

Multiple Choice

1. The most common surgical condition of the digestive tract in infancy is:
   1. pyloric stenosis
   2. umbilical hernia
   3. intussusception
   4. meconium ileus

2. A symptom of Hirschsprung's disease is:
   1. reflux
   2. hyperactive bowel sounds
   3. constipation
   4. diarrhea

3. When a family is treated for pinworm infestation, the nurse recommends which of the following additional actions?
   1. washing all kitchen utensils in the dishwasher
   2. washing underwear and bed linens in very hot water
   3. airing out blankets and pillows
   4. throwing away all "dress-up" clothes

4. A nurse is caring for a newborn with gastroschisis. Which is the priority nursing diagnosis at this time?
   1. risk for infection
   2. risk for impaired urinary elimination
   3. risk for delayed development
   4. risk for caregiver role strain

5. The infant who has returned from surgery for repair of a cleft lip should be placed in which position?
   1. prone position
   2. supine position
   3. left side position
   4. right side position

6. Which symptom might indicate a tracheoesophageal fistula in a newborn?
   1. continuous crying
   2. coughing at nighttime
   3. choking with feedings
   4. severe projectile vomiting

7. Which symptom would the parents describe if their infant has been hospitalized for pyloric stenosis?
   1. explosive watery diarrhea
   2. refusal to breastfeed
   3. light yellow but odorous urine
   4. projectile vomiting

8. When discussing home instructions for an infant with GER, which of the following would be included?
   1. placing the infant upright in an infant seat for 45 minutes after feeding
   2. limiting the amount of burping during a feeding
   3. thickening the feeding with a small amount of rice cereal
   4. thinning the feeding with a small amount of water

9. The nurse will know that the parents understood instructions regarding food choices for celiac disease when they select which choices for breakfast?
   1. waffles with syrup and strawberries
   2. scrambled eggs with hash browns and orange juice
   3. Cheerios cereal with milk and bananas
   4. sausage, cheese, and egg biscuit with apple juice

10. The nurse is caring for a 9-year-old who is 5 hours post appendectomy. What would be the nursing priority with this child?
1. providing the child with acetaminophen every 4 hours
2. asking the parents if the child needs a pain shot
3. placing the child in a comfortable position and darkening the room
4. instructing the child how to use the PCA pump

Study Questions

1. List the symptoms of pyloric stenosis. Why must infants with pyloric stenosis be fed so carefully? (Reference section: Pyloric Stenosis)

2. You are working with a 9-year-old who has just been diagnosed with celiac disease. Her favorite foods are hamburger, French fries, and Coca-Cola. What nutritional principles would you discuss with her? (Reference section: Celiac disease)

3. A nurse in the newborn nursery notes that a 4-hour-old newborn has heart sounds on the right side and bowel sounds in the chest. She also notes that the respiratory rate has increased to 60 and there are moderate retractions. What are the priority nursing interventions and rationales for this infant? (Reference section: Diaphragmatic hernia)

4. During a 2-month-old's well infant visit, the mother reports that her mother-in-law is pressuring her to start giving the infant cereal and fruits to help the infant sleep at night. How should the nurse handle this situation, and what information should be given to the mother? (Reference section: Description)

Case Study with Critical Thinking Questions

A 13-year-old is being seen in the clinic for a well child checkup prior to the beginning of school. All of her vital signs are normal, but her weight is 145 pounds. She is 5 feet 3 inches tall. She is enrolled in the local middle school. She is very quiet and only responds with short answers. Her mother says she spends most of her time watching television or playing computer games. Her mother is a very large woman who has diabetes and high blood pressure.

1. What additional information would the nurse gather in the history assessment?

2. The mother expresses concern about her child getting diabetes. What information can the nurse share with the mother about her fears?

3. What nutritional principles should the nurse discuss with the child and the mother regarding the child's weight?

4. How does "being fat" alter the child's psychological development?

Internet Activity

1. Use the Internet to find programs that are available for weight management in your area. What is the focus and the plan of action for each program? What other resources can be accessed for this child?

Fluid Balance, Renal, and Reproductive Disorders

Student Name _____   Date _____

Matching Questions

1. ____ cryptorchidism
2. ____ anuria
3. ____ dysmenorrhea
4. ____ homeostasis
5. ____ hypertonic
6. ____ oliguria
7. ____ hypotonic
8. ____ vesicoureteral reflux

a. a uniform state
b. undescended testicles
c. the child has lost more fluids than electrolytes
d. urine moves upward into the ureters
e. the child has lost more electrolytes than fluids
f. suppression of urine formation
g. decreased urine output
h. painful menstruation

Multiple Choice

1. Which of the following symptoms are present in a child with severe dehydration?
   1. Decreased heart rate and respiratory rate
   2. Pink and moist mucous membranes
   3. No urine output for the past few hours
   4. Capillary refill time less than 2 seconds

2. Further teaching is needed for the adolescent with HSV who states which of the following?
   1. "I am more at risk for human immunodeficiency virus."
   2. "The virus cannot be passed if I am asymptomatic."
   3. "Condoms may not fully prevent transmission."
   4. "I need to abstain from sex while symptomatic."

3. When teaching parents about home management of the child with nephrotic syndrome, the nurse emphasizes:
   1. daily blood pressure measurements
   2. strict activity restrictions
   3. low protein diet
   4. accurate testing for urine protein

4. Which of the following symptoms might indicate urinary tract infection in an infant?
   1. frequency, urgency
   2. poor feeding, unexplained fever
   3. flank pain, chills
   4. incontinence, foul-smelling urine

5. Which of the following is an important nursing intervention for a child with enuresis?
   1. reprimand the child for wetting the bed
   2. teach parents never to punish the child
   3. administer diuretics as ordered
   4. encourage parents to limit daytime fluids

6. Which of the following is an important nursing intervention for a child who is post-op from a hypospadias repair?
   1. Change the dressing as needed
   2. Restrict fluid intake for 48 hours
   3. Encourage a diet high in protein
   4. Monitor the child's temperature

7. The nurse identifies the symptoms of nephrotic syndrome based on the following:
   1. hyperproteinemia, hyperlipidemia, proteinuria
   2. hyperproteinemia, hypolipidemia, hematuria
   3. hypoproteinemia, hyperlipidemia, proteinuria
   4. hypoproteinemia, hypolipidemia, hematuria

8. The common symptoms for acute poststreptococcal glomerulonephritis are:
   1. increased urine output with marked periorbital edema
   2. urine may be clear but child has painful urination
   3. diarrhea, nausea, and vomiting accompanied by a high fever
   4. bloody or smoky urine that is decreased in output

9. The nurse is aware that the most frequently seen sexually transmitted disease in the United States is which of the following?
   1. syphilis
   2. gonorrhea
   3. chlamydia
   4. genital herpes

10. When reviewing the prevention of STDs with sexually active adolescent girls, it is important to tell them that:
    1. all STDs can be prevented through condom use
    2. if their sexual partner is not symptomatic, disease is unlikely
    3. having sex with only one partner usually is safe
    4. multiple sexual partners will increase their risk

Study Questions

1. Compare and contrast nephrotic syndrome and acute glomerulonephritis. (Reference section: Acute Glomerulonephritis and Nephrotic Syndrome)

2. Discuss care of the adolescent with an STD and the social stigma that may be involved. (Reference section: Sexually Transmitted Diseases)

3. Discuss care of the child with HIV. (Reference section: Acquired Immunodeficiency Syndrome)

Case Study with Critical Thinking Questions

A 6-year-old with HIV is being cared for by the child's aunt and uncle. The couple has also adopted a 2-year-old foster child with HIV.

1. The aunt who is the caretaker of the 6-year-old with HIV asks the nurse, "When and what should I tell her about HIV?" She relates that her child has been asking her questions about why she always has to have her blood checked and why she has to take so many pills. What is the nurse's best response?

2. The 2-year-old foster child with HIV is being placed in daycare. What issues should be discussed with the family before the child begins attending the daycare?

Internet Activity

1. Explore sites for teens/children with an STD or HIV. What resources are available? How can health care professionals provide support for these teens/children?

Integumentary Disorders

Student Name _____   Date _____

Matching Questions

1. ____ autograft
2. ____ pediculosis
3. ____ Accutane
4. ____ eschar
5. ____ comedo
6. ____ eczema
7. ____ allograft
8. ____ impetigo

a. systemic treatment for severe acne
b. atopic dermatitis
c. area of undamaged skin used to cover a burn wound
d. caused by staphylococci
e. burned tissue
f. head lice
g. plug of keratin, sebum, and bacteria
h. skin from cadavers

Multiple Choice

1. The nurse teaches that head lice can be transmitted by:
   1. sitting next to a child with lice
   2. wearing the headphones of a child with lice
   3. spraying hairspray used by child with lice
   4. using the shampoo used by child with lice

2. A toddler with atopic dermatitis is seen in the clinic. The mother is taught by the nurse that this disorder is:
   1. seen only after 2 years of age
   2. seen more frequently in breastfed infants
   3. an allergic response to a substance
   4. more frequent in summer

3. Which of the following nursing interventions is recommended for a child with facial cellulitis?
   1. apply cold packs to affected area prn
   2. perform range of motion exercises three times a day
   3. complete oral antibiotics at home
   4. assess IV site frequently for signs of infiltration

4. The nurse is providing acne education for a 17-year-old girl. Which of the following statements shows that the adolescent understands the teaching?
   1. "I will need to avoid chocolate, potato chips, and colas."
   2. "Daily use of sunscreen is important with certain products."
   3. "The best way to eliminate pimples is to gently squeeze them."
   4. "I will not need to take my birth control pills if I am put on Accutane."

5. Which of the following nursing interventions is recommended for a child with pediculosis?
   1. avoid sharing caps and brushes
   2. apply Lindane liberally and frequently
   3. launder bedding in warm water
   4. cut the child's hair so it is easier to manage

6. The nurse is reviewing instructions with a parent for a child with impetigo. What instructions should be included? (**Select all that apply.**)
   1. clean lesions 3 to 4 times a day with soap and water
   2. prescribed oral antibiotics need to be completed
   3. good hand hygiene will help prevent the spread of infection
   4. the topical application of nystatin will promote healing

7. Fluid volume must be restored in a patient with major burns in order to prevent:
   1. burn shock
   2. infection
   3. airway obstruction
   4. scarring

8. A 2-year-old child just admitted with full thickness burns on the torso and partial thickness burns on the face requires which of the following nursing interventions?
   1. fluid replacement with D5W at keep open rate
   2. monitoring of urine output by carefully weighing diapers
   3. careful monitoring of airway, breathing, and circulation
   4. ordering a full liquid diet that includes favorite liquids

Study Questions

1. Determine the discharge needs of a burn victim who experienced 50% full thickness burns (Reference section: Burns, Treatment and Nursing Care)

2. Design a home care instruction pamphlet for the child with atopic dermatitis. (Reference section: Atopic Dermatitis, Nursing Care)

3. Compare and contrast the nursing care of babies with diaper dermatitis and diaper rash from candidiasis. (Reference section: Diaper Dermatitis, Treatment and Nursing Care)

Case Study with Critical Thinking Questions

A 5-year-old has full-thickness burns on his legs after mimicking his older brother by stomping out a campfire. He weighs 24 kg.

1. Discuss the initial ABCs of this child's care.

2. Devise a nursing care plan for his care, including wound management, nutrition, and pain control.

Internet Activity

1. Explore the Internet for home care instructions for patients with pediculosis.

Musculoskeletal Disorders

Student Name _____   Date _____

Matching Questions

1. ____ dysarthria
2. ____ idiopathic
3. ____ dyskinetic
4. ____ arthroscopy
5. ____ epiphyseal plate
6. ____ Gower maneuver
7. ____ *S. aureus*
8. ____ Pavik harness
9. ____ compartment syndrome

a. found at the end of long bones
b. common causative organism for osteomyelitis
c. characteristic movement of children with muscular dystrophy
d. problems with coordination of muscles needed for speech
e. device that maintains abduction of the hips
f. no known cause
g. resulting from edema and swelling in the tissue
h. procedure to assess joint damage
i. involuntary, purposeless movements

Multiple Choice

1. One of the major goals when caring for children with cerebral palsy is to:
   1. prevent further brain damage
   2. maximize their physical and intellectual potential
   3. recommend they be placed in special classes
   4. keep them from taking undue physical risks

2. A young child with a lower extremity cast has swelling of the toes. The toes are bluish in color, and capillary refill is slow. The child is crying. The parents are worried. The nurse first:
   1. calls to have the cast removed
   2. reassures the child's parents that this is normal
   3. notifies the charge nurse or physician
   4. takes measures to stop the child's crying

3. A serious complication for children with fractures is:
   1. discoloration of the skin
   2. injury to the epiphyseal plate
   3. a greenstick fracture
   4. swelling over the fracture

4. Duchenne muscular dystrophy:
   1. is a random occurrence
   2. is sex-linked, with the mother as the carrier
   3. only occurs in girls
   4. can be contagious

5. An important nursing goal for the adolescent required to be in a shell brace for the treatment of scoliosis is:
   1. restoring normal spine curvature
   2. maintaining normal activity levels
   3. decreasing pain
   4. ensuring compliance

6. Talipes equinovarus is the most common form of a:
   1. cleft palate
   2. clubfoot
   3. cleft lip
   4. defect of the hand

7. When screening for scoliosis, the nurse looks at the child from front and back to determine:
   1. symmetry
   2. degree of curve
   3. flexibility
   4. muscle spasm

8. Which of the following situations could be an indication of potential risk for sport injury?
   1. the coach requiring all team members to sit on the ground when an athlete has been injured
   2. 6-year-old boys and girls playing on the same sport team
   3. a limping player being removed from the game for the day
   4. 9-year-old and 14-year-old boys playing on the same sport team

9. A child has been admitted with a diagnosis of possible osteomyelitis. Which of the following lab reports would support this diagnosis?
   1. decreased white blood cell (WBC) count
   2. elevated C-reactive protein
   3. elevated BUN
   4. decreased hematocrit

10. The nurse is instructing parents on home care of an infant with a Pavik harness. Which statement indicates the need for more teaching?
    1. "We should check the baby's skin frequently."
    2. "A light T-shirt should be worn under the harness."
    3. "The harness should be worn for 6 hours a day."
    4. "Since this was caught early, our child may not need surgery."

Study Questions

1. A 2-year-old in traction needs diversional activities. What toys/activities are appropriate for a child of this age? (Reference section: Care of the Child in Traction).

2. A young male wants to join the high school swimming team. What health factors need to be considered in investigating this possibility? (Reference section: Sports Injuries)

3. Discuss the multidisciplinary team approach needed in the treatment of a child with the diagnosis of Duchenne muscular dystrophy. (Reference section: Duchenne Muscular Dystrophy)

4. Review cast care and anticipate potential problems associated with a pediatric patient who has a cast. (Reference section: Cast Care)

5. Discuss the special needs of a family who has a child with cerebral palsy. (Reference section: Cerebral Palsy)

Case Study with Critical Thinking Questions

A 13-year-old who has been diagnosed with scoliosis is being admitted to the hospital. Admission information indicates that she was identified with this problem at 10 years of age and that she has been wearing a brace for the past 3 years. She has indicated that she does not like to wear the brace because it makes her "look funny," and her mother has indicated that compliance with wearing the brace has been a problem. Her orthopedic physician has decided to perform a surgical procedure (TSRH) on the patient because of the progressive curvature. She is scheduled for the surgical procedure in 2 days. You are to develop a preoperative teaching plan.

1. What preoperative, intraoperative, and postoperative issues should be covered during this part of the teaching?

2. After her surgical procedure, what issues should be addressed in preparing the child for discharge?

Internet Activities

1. Go to the National Institute of Neurological Disorders' website *(www.ninds.nih.gov)* and search the links to other organizations to compile information for a family who has a child with cerebral palsy.

2. Using Google, explore some of the different websites or blogs that parents of children who have Duchenne muscular dystrophy have posted. What are some of the common issues that these parents have discussed?

Communicable Diseases

Student Name _____   Date _____

Matching Questions

1. ____ smallpox
2. ____ rubeola
3. ____ chain of infection
4. ____ prodrome
5. ____ VAERS
6. ____ thimerosal
7. ____ fifth disease
8. ____ lyme disease
9. ____ rubella
10. ____ pertussis
11. ____ contraindicated with a history of intussusception
12. ____ administered to the newborn in the hospital
13. ____ contraindicated with immunodeficiency

a. serious disease for a small infant
b. Rotavirus vaccine
c. required to break to prevent infections
d. time immediately before the onset of a communicable disease
e. MMR vaccine
f. mercury-containing preservative rarely used in vaccines
g. hepatitis B vaccine
h. measles
i. caused by a tick
j. slapped face
k. risk for causing fetal anomalies
l. potential bioterrorism agent
m. Vaccine Adverse Events Reporting System

Multiple Choice

1. The polio vaccine, diphtheria-tetanus-pertussis, and *Haemophilus influenzae* type b immunizations are begun at which age?
   1. 1 month of age
   2. 2 months of age
   3. 3 months of age
   4. 4 months of age

2. The initial MMR (mumps, measles, rubella) vaccination is recommended at which age?
   1. 12 to 15 months of age
   2. 6 months of age
   3. 6 weeks of age
   4. 9 months of age

3. A 12-month-old infant has recently been diagnosed with leukemia. Which of the following immunizations will the nurse administer?
   1. MMR
   2. LAIV
   3. varicella
   4. none of the above

4. A preschooler was exposed to chickenpox at daycare. After the nurse explains about chickenpox, which statement indicates that the mother needs more information?
   1. "My child should not visit my pregnant sister at this time."
   2. "My child can spread chickenpox several days before there are any skin lesions."
   3. "I should not use aspirin for fever since Reye syndrome can be a complication."
   4. "During the prodomal period, my child will have lesions all over his body."

5. A mother of a 1-year-old says breastfeeding is providing sufficient immunity so she does not need to be immunized. What would be the best approach for the nurse to use when discussing this topic?
   1. discuss active and passive immunity
   2. explain that immunizations are legally mandatory
   3. discuss the mother's diet
   4. administer the needed immunizations without her permission

6. A mother asks the nurse why it is important to know the incubation period for a communicable disease. The nurse should include which of the following information?
   1. identifies the period when the child might be contagious
   2. determines the severity of the infection
   3. varies with the age of the child
   4. identifies a time period when medications can prevent development of symptoms

7. A mother calls to report that her 8-year-old has chickenpox. Her children have not been immunized. She wants to know about how long it will be before his 5-year-old sister gets it. You tell her:
   1. 7 to 10 days
   2. 2 to 6 days
   3. 14 to 48 days
   4. 10 to 21 days

8. A child with rubeola is being admitted to the hospital. The nurse should anticipate placing the child in which precaution?
   1. contact
   2. enteric
   3. airborne
   4. protective

Study Questions

1. Compare the symptoms and rash characteristics of the following communicable diseases: chickenpox, measles, German measles, roseola, and fifth disease. (Reference section: Communicable Diseases and Table 18-1)

2. Identify the home care for a child who has skin issues with a communicable disease. (Reference section: Communicable Diseases)

3. Discuss the immunizations that an adolescent should have. (Reference section: Immunizations)

Case Study with Critical Thinking Questions

A 4-month-old infant is brought to the well-child clinic. He weighs 15 pounds 11 ounces and is 25 inches long. He is being breastfed and eats every 4 to 6 hours. At 2 months of age, he received the second Hep B and the first dose of the DTaP, HIB, IPV, Rotavirus, and PCV.

1. What immunizations will he need to receive at this visit?

2. What instructions need to be given to the mother related to the reactions the infant may have regarding the immunizations?

Internet Activity

1. Explore the Immunization Action Coalition website (www.immunize.org) and review the parent/patient information sheets (vaccine information statements) on various immunizations. Be prepared to discuss how you would explain various immunizations to parents.

Immune Disorders

Student Name _____   Date _____

Matching Questions

1. ____ hyperglycemia
2. ____ autoimmune
3. ____ EBV
4. ____ IVIG
5. ____ antigen
6. ____ glargine
7. ____ iridocyclitis
8. ____ polydipsia

a. long-acting insulin that cannot be mixed with other insulin
b. given early to help with Kawasaki disease
c. thirst
d. identifies cells as either self or non-self
e. high blood sugar
f. inflammation of the iris
g. disorders in which self fails to recognize self
h. causative organism for mononucleosis

Multiple Choice

1. A child is admitted to the hospital with the diagnosis of juvenile idiopathic arthritis. Which of the following symptoms would **not** be seen?
   1. stiffness in the morning or after rest
   2. swelling and redness of the involved joint
   3. normal CBC with normal ESR
   4. Positive rheumatoid factor and antinuclear antibody assay

2. The nurse recognizes that an adolescent with mononucleosis needs additional discharge teaching if which of the following statements was made?
   1. "I can return to football practice next week."
   2. "I will need to continue to monitor my temperature and take ibuprofen if needed."
   3. "If I feel tired, I should make sure I take a nap."
   4. "I can eat anything that I want."

3. Which of the following is an activity that would be appropriate for a child with juvenile idiopathic arthritis?
   1. volleyball
   2. tennis
   3. bicycle riding
   4. swimming

4. Which of the following is a priority nursing action when administering IVIG?
   1. keeping the head of the bed elevated
   2. checking the ESR level
   3. taking vital signs before beginning administration
   4. administering antihistamine prior to administration

5. A 12-year-old girl has juvenile idiopathic arthritis, polyarticular type. Which of the following is the best advice to give to help her cope successfully with the school day? Tell her to:
   1. not go to school when she does not feel well
   2. allow plenty of extra time in the morning to get ready for school
   3. get up and walk around the classroom if she feels stiff
   4. take a warm shower after gym

6. The major pathophysiologic difference between type 1 and type 2 diabetes is that:
   1. children with type 2 never need insulin
   2. children with type 1 can take insulin orally
   3. type 1 results from pancreatic islet cell destruction
   4. affected children with type 1 are obese

7. When the nurse reviews nutritional management with a school-age child with type 1 diabetes, which of the following would be an expected outcome?
   1. strict adherence to the prescribed diet
   2. complete avoidance of sweets
   3. appropriate choices of a wide variety of foods
   4. no episodes of hypoglycemia

8. Which of the following statements about home care for a child with Kawasaki disease indicates the parents have an understanding?
   1. "Our child may be irritable for several weeks."
   2. "We can stop giving aspirin in 2 days."
   3. "The IVIG that was given will prevent our child from ever getting this again."
   4. "We will not have to monitor our child's cardiac status."

Study Questions

1. What factors would you consider when determining whether a 9-year-old is ready to administer her own insulin? How would you best teach her this skill? (Reference section: Insulin-Dependent Diabetes Mellitus)

2. A young girl has joined the school softball team, which practices twice a week after school. How will this affect her diabetes? What factors would you consider when providing anticipatory guidance to her and her parents regarding this new activity? (Reference section: Insulin-Dependent Diabetes Mellitus)

3. A 3-year-old has been hospitalized for a reaction to his seizure medication. He has severe oral lesions, and his hands and feet are blistered and oozing. The parents are extremely upset. Develop a nursing care plan and include the emotional needs of both parents and child. (Reference section: Stevens-Johnson Syndrome)

Case Study with Critical Thinking Questions

A 9-year-old girl has been recently admitted to the hospital for juvenile idiopathic arthritis. Her parents are very concerned with the drugs she is receiving. They have heard over the years that children should not take aspirin, but their daughter is receiving this medication.

1. What information can you tell the parents to relieve their anxiety?

2. The parents also express concern about how they are going to take care of their daughter when she is discharged. Develop a home care plan for this child, including activities.

Internet Activity

1. Use the Internet to find information about juvenile arthritis. Visit *www.arthritis.org* and select the section on juvenile arthritis. What information did you find? Is there information that would be helpful to parents?

Cognitive and Behavior Disorders

Student Name _____   Date _____

Matching Questions

1. ____ failure to thrive
2. ____ bulimia
3. ____ polypharmacy
4. ____ cupping
5. ____ child abuse
6. ____ intellectual disability
7. ____ IDEA
8. ____ trisomy 21

a. guarantees the right of developmentally disabled persons to receive appropriate education
b. total of 27 chromosomes
c. cultural practice that can be misidentified as child abuse
d. below the 5th percentile in growth
e. replacing mental retardation
f. binge eating
g. more common in boys than in girls
h. using several drugs together

Multiple Choice

1. An important intervention for infants who have developmental disabilities is to:
   1. have them institutionalized as soon as possible
   2. help the parents realize that their child will never develop further
   3. stress the importance of early infant stimulation programs
   4. have children reevaluated at 2 years to confirm the diagnosis

2. The three hallmarks of attention-deficit/hyperactivity disorder are:
   1. organization, intelligence, and distractibility
   2. impulsivity, excess energy, and inattention
   3. poor school performance, dyslexia, and poor gross-motor skills
   4. learning disability, below-average IQ, and difficulty communicating

3. When failure to thrive is the result of an environmental cause, which of the following statements is correct?
   1. A sense of trust is missing in the child.
   2. The growth of the child is above the 50th percentile.
   3. The mother cannot be helped.
   4. The mother has the ability to tolerate high levels of stress.

4. A major difference in the clinical manifestations of adolescents with anorexia nervosa and those with bulimia is:
   1. binge eating
   2. body image distortion
   3. purging
   4. decreased self-esteem

5. A teacher in a school where you are the school nurse shows you a poem written as a class assignment by a student. In the poem, the student has expressed a desire to "end it all." Your first action should be to:
   1. ignore it because it is just poetry
   2. ask the student, "Are you planning to kill yourself?"
   3. alert the student's parents
   4. ask the teacher whether the student is really suicidal

6. When assessing an adolescent with bulimia nervosa, which of the following would most likely be observed?
   1. dry skin
   2. dental caries
   3. low body weight
   4. amenorrhea

7. The nurse is caring for an 8-year-old child who is a potential child abuse patient. Which of the following could be a flag for abuse?
   1. a fractured bone
   2. bruising on the knees and elbows
   3. displaying anger and hyperactivity
   4. a burn that has not been treated

8. The nurse is caring for a 4-year-old with autism who has been admitted with a UTI. Which of the following behaviors would the nurse expect for a child with autism?
   1. conversing with others without shyness
   2. displaying repetitive activities such as rocking back and forth
   3. playing with other children but unable to share
   4. putting together a very complex puzzle

Study Questions

1. Discuss the special needs of a family who has a child with Down syndrome. (Reference section: Down Syndrome)

2. An 18-year-old girl has anorexia nervosa. Define this condition and its causes. What approach would you take when meeting with her for the first time? Discuss the reasons for your approach. (Reference section: Anorexia Nervosa)

3. Identify home situations that could place a child at risk for child abuse. (Reference section: Child Abuse)

Case Study with Critical Thinking Questions

A 3-month-old infant of a 15-year-old mother is admitted for failure to thrive. The infant was full term and weighed 3.0 kg. The admission weight was 4.4 kg. The mother reports that she is bottle feeding 6 ounces about every 4 to 6 hours and that the infant takes it without difficulty. She also states that the baby has been sleeping through the night since 1 month of age. On physical assessment, it is noted that the infant's anterior fontanel is soft but slightly depressed. The arms and legs are thin with little fatty tissue. When the infant cries, the mother does not respond quickly, especially if she is watching television or talking on the phone. The nurse has to remind the mother that it is time to feed her baby, and the mother says she will do it shortly. The mother and her boyfriend usually leave in the early afternoon, and the mother does not return until late in the evening.

1. What is your impression of this situation?

2. What would be the expectation for a 3-month-old in weight and intake?

3. What topics would be appropriate to discuss with the mother about infant care?

Internet Activities

1. Explore the National Institute on Drug Abuse website (www.nida.nih.gov) for information related to substance abuse. What are the current statistics for marijuana use with preadolescents and adolescents? What are some of the common street names for this drug? From this site, explore other links to related topics.

2. What sites are available to parents and adolescents regarding eating disorders? To start, visit the website for the behavioral health department of the St. Francis Health System (www.laureate.com/behaviorhealth). In addition, visit www.edap.org, the website for Eating Disorder Awareness and Prevention, Inc.

Hematology and Oncology Disorders

Student Name _____   Date _____

Matching Questions

1. ____ Reed-Sternberg cell
2. ____ sickle cell anemia
3. ____ hemarthrosis
4. ____ neutropenic
5. ____ hematology
6. ____ thrombocytes
7. ____ source of iron
8. ____ thrombosis

a. the study of blood and blood-forming tissues
b. dried fruits
c. clot
d. hemorrhage into a joint
e. inherited disease involving the red blood cells
f. decrease in leukocytes
g. double-nucleated cell that is diagnostic for Hodgkin's disease
h. platelets

Multiple Choice

1. A parent needs additional teaching with iron administration if the parent states:
   1. "I will administer the iron with a straw."
   2. "It is okay to give my child Tums while on iron."
   3. "Milk should not be given with iron."
   4. "Orange juice is a good choice to give with iron."

2. The nurse teaches parents that in order to increase the absorption of iron, which vitamin(s) is/are added to the diet?
   1. B complex vitamins
   2. vitamin C
   3. vitamin A
   4. vitamin D

3. The nurse reinforces that a sickle cell crisis can be precipitated by:
   1. exercise
   2. overheating
   3. low altitude
   4. taking antibiotics

4. Nursing care for sickle cell crisis includes:
   1. heating pad application prn
   2. cold packs to the affected area
   3. oxygen at 4 liters per nasal cannula
   4. demerol for pain control

5. Priority preoperative nursing care for a child with a Wilms tumor is to:
   1. avoid abdominal palpation
   2. count wet diapers daily
   3. maintain aseptic technique
   4. reassure parents about prognosis

6. The nurse is caring for a newly admitted child with ALL. Which of the following are often found upon assessment and examination? (**Select all that apply.**)
   1. anemia
   2. elevated hemoglobin
   3. elevated temperature
   4. lymphadenopathy
   5. glucosuria

7. An adolescent who is a model is being treated with chemotherapy for cancer. She is particularly concerned about what the medications will do to her appearance. An important nursing intervention for her would be to:
   1. help her pick out a wig and false eyelashes before treatment begins
   2. reassure her that she will be beautiful even without hair
   3. tell her that the chemotherapy probably will not affect her appearance
   4. advise her that her hair will probably grow back in curly

8. The nurse explains to parents that treatment for Ewing sarcoma can involve the following:
   1. chemotherapy
   2. surgery
   3. radiation
   4. all of the above

9. An important nursing intervention for a child with hemarthrosis is:
   1. apply heat to the injury
   2. active range of motion
   3. compression to the area
   4. administer ibuprofen

10. A 14-year-old child with terminal cancer asks the nurse if he is dying. What is the best response from the nurse?
   1. "Don't you have a minister to talk with?"
   2. "Shouldn't you ask your doctor about this?"
   3. "Why don't you discuss this with your parents?"
   4. "Why do you think you are dying?"

Study Questions

1. Discuss care of the young adolescent facing amputation from osteosarcoma (Reference section: Osteosarcoma)

2. Discuss clinical signs and symptoms of the child with leukemia (Reference section: Leukemia)

3. Create a brochure for a hemophiliac regarding safe sports (Reference section: Hemophilia)

4. Prepare a day's menu for an 11-month-old with anemia (Reference section: Iron Deficiency Anemia)

5. A 7-year-old has a brain tumor. He wishes to go to a summer camp for children with cancer. How would you help the family prepare him for camp? Discuss both the physical and psychological considerations. (Reference section: Brain Tumors)

Case Study with Critical Thinking Questions

A 10-month-old African-American child is admitted to the hospital with a severe infection. The physician suspects that she may also be experiencing a sickle cell crisis. Intravenous fluids are started, and she is medicated for the infection and pain. The child was diagnosed with sickle cell disease at birth by the newborn screen. Her parents have some knowledge about the disease.

1. Develop a care plan for this child that includes her immediate needs for tissue perfusion, fluids, pain, infection, and knowledge deficit related to sickle cell crisis.

2. After being hospitalized for a week, the child's parents are preparing for her discharge in the morning. What information regarding home care is necessary to discuss with them?

Internet Activity

1. Explore the Internet and find sites that provide information regarding sickle cell disease.

2. Explore sites for children with cancer. Include reliable resources/sites for parental use.

End-of-Life Care for Children and Their Families

Student Name _____   Date _____

Matching Questions

1. ____ palliative care
2. ____ anticipatory grief
3. ____ anxiolytics
4. ____ grief
5. ____ pain

a. whatever the person experiencing it says it is and existing whenever he or she says it does
b. a functional category of drugs used in the treatment of anxiety that do not cause excessive sedation
c. occurs before the loss
d. subjective and unique to the individual
e. care and comfort at the end of life

Multiple Choice

1. Which of the following children would realize death is permanent?
   1. a 2-year-old who sees a dead puppy
   2. a 4-year-old whose grandmother dies
   3. a child in kindergarten who hears his friend's grandfather has died
   4. a 10-year-old whose classmate dies of complications from a medical condition

2. Which age group sees death as a person (personification of death)?
   1. toddler
   2. preschooler
   3. school-age child
   4. adolescent

3. In dealing with death, which of the following would be the most positive way for a nurse to cope?
   1. becoming secluded from family and friends
   2. isolating herself from her peers
   3. discussing the event with her supervisor
   4. relating the story to several of her friends

4. The nurse understands that the death of a child will change the dynamics of the family because:
   1. death is final and causes much family conflict
   2. the parents disagree about how the death will affect them
   3. siblings will resent the attention given to the dying child
   4. death is an event during which new mechanisms for coping need to be established

5. The nurse is aware that anticipatory grief begins:
   1. at the time of death
   2. during the dying process
   3. during the funeral
   4. after the loss

6. Shortness of breath and dyspnea can lead to the feeling of "air hunger." Which medication will the nurse administer to help with this discomfort?
   1. Tylenol
   2. morphine
   3. glycerin suppository
   4. Phenergan

7. Nursing care for a 4-year-old who is dying will be based on the knowledge that:
   1. he has no understanding of death
   2. the nurse should provide all the care
   3. his primary fear is separation from his parents
   4. he is too young to sense his parents' anxiety

8. As a dying child's condition deteriorates, the mother angrily shouts at the nurse, "This isn't fair. Why can't you do something?" What is the most appropriate response by the nurse?
   1. "I will not discuss this until you can calm down."
   2. "Please calm down. You are upsetting your daughter."
   3. "You are right. This is not fair. What would you like me to do?"
   4. "Being angry is not going to help anyone. Now what can I help you with?"

9. A dying child's desire is to be at home, and a referral is made to hospice. The nurse understands that hospice will:
   1. provide for the physical needs of the child
   2. teach the family how to care for the child
   3. enhance the quality of life that remains
   4. provide all the care so the family can rest

10. As death is approaching, the child's respirations become labored and noisy. What nursing care would be indicated at this time?
    1. perform deep suctioning
    2. let the family know this is expected
    3. give the child something to drink
    4. call the physician

s knowledge of death,
nts regarding the child's
in? (Reference section: Table

3. What is a cause of the cool hands and feet that the dying child will have? (Reference section: Box 22-3)

Case Study with Critical Thinking Questions

An 8-year-old boy has a diagnosis of advanced lymphoma. A bone marrow transplant has been unsuccessful. There is no longer hope for a cure, and the disease is advancing at a rapid rate. The parents are undecided about what and when to tell their child.

1. How can the nurse help the parents?

2. How can the nurse help the child?

3. What reaction would the nurse expect from the child when he is told that he is dying?

4. When is the most appropriate time to discuss death with the child?

5. When should the recommendation for hospice referral be made?

Internet Activity

1. Explore hospice organizations online such as HospiceNet *(www.hospicenet.org/)* or Hospice International *(www.chionline.org/)*.

2. Explore websites of support groups such as The Compassionate Friends *(www.compassionatefriends. org/home.aspx)*.

3. Search "organ transplant" for criteria for suitable donors.